Cardiology Core Curriculum

A problem-based approach

Cardiology Core Curriculum

A problem-based approach

Edited by

John D Rutherford

Cardiologist, Vice President of Clinical Operations, Professor of Internal Medicine, Gail Griffiths Hill Chair in Cardiology, UT Southwestern Medical Center, Dallas, Texas, USA

First published in 2003
by BMJ Books, BMA House, Tavistock Square,
London WC1H 9JR

www.bmjbooks.com

British Library Cataloguing in Publication Data

A catalog record for this book is available from the British Library

ISBN 0 7279 1690 4

Typeset by SIVA Math Setters, Chennai, India
Printed and bound in Spain by Graphycems, Navarra

Contents

Contributors

Tayo Addo
Cardiology Fellow, UT Southwestern Medical Center, Dallas, Texas, USA

Luis Araujo
Director of Nuclear Cardiology, Associate Professor of Radiology and Medicine, Hospital of the University of Pennsylvania, University of Pennsylvania School of Medicine, USA

John A Bittl
Interventional Cardiologist, Ocala Heart Institute, Ocala, Florida, USA

M Elizabeth Brickner
Cardiologist, Director, Noninvasive Laboratories at Parkland Memorial Hospital, Associate Professor of Medicine, UT Southwestern Medical Center, Dallas, Texas, USA

James A de Lemos
Cardiologist, Medical Director, Coronary Care Unit at Parkland Memorial Hospital, Assistant Professor of Internal Medicine, UT Southwestern Medical Center, Dallas, Texas, USA

Victor A Ferrari
Cardiologist, Associate Director, Noninvasive Imaging Laboratory, Hospital of the University of Pennsylvania, Associate Professor of Medicine, University of Pennsylvania School of Medicine, USA

Daniel B Friedman
Cardiologist, Presbyterian Heart Group, Albuquerque, New Mexico, USA

Samuel Z Goldhaber
Cardiologist, Director of the Anticoagulation Service and the Venous Thromboembolism Research Group, Brigham and Women's Hospital, Associate Professor of Medicine, Harvard Medical School, Boston, Massachusetts, USA

David J Kessler
Cardiologist, Austin Heart, Austin, Texas, USA

Robert C Kowal
Cardiologist, Assistant Professor of Medicine, UT Southwestern Medical Center, Dallas, Texas, USA

Charles Landau
Assistant Professor of Clinical Medicine, Columbia University, College of Physicians and Surgeons, Cardiologist, Cardiac Associates of Southern Connecticut, Bridgeport, Connecticut, USA

Thomas H Lee
Chief Medical Officer, Partners Community Healthcare, Inc., Associate Professor of Medicine, Harvard Medical School, Boston, Massachusetts, USA

Leonard S Lilly
Cardiologist, Chief, Brigham and Women's/Faulkner Cardiology, Associate Professor of Medicine, Harvard Medical School, Boston, Massachusetts, USA

Michael L Main
Consulting Cardiologist, Mid America Heart Institute, Kansas City, Missouri, USA

James D Marsh
Cardiologist, Chief, Division of Cardiology, Professor and Associate Chair for Research, Department of Internal Medicine, Wayne State University, Detroit, Michigan, USA

Rao H Naseem
Cardiology Fellow, UT Southwestern Medical Center, Dallas, Texas, USA

John A Osborne
Cardiologist, Dallas, Texas, USA

Richard L Page
Cardiologist, Head, Division of Cardiology, Robert A Bruce Professor of Medicine, University of Washington School of Medicine, Seattle, Washington, USA

Khether E Raby
Cardiologist, Assistant Professor of Clinical Medicine, Boston University School of Medicine, Massachusetts, USA

Sharon C Reimold
Cardiologist, Medical Director, UT Southwestern Clinical Heart Center, Associate Professor of Internal Medicine, UT Southwestern Medical Center, Dallas, Texas, USA

John D Rutherford
Cardiologist, Vice President of Clinical Operations, Professor of Internal Medicine, Gail Griffiths Hill Chair in Cardiology, UT Southwestern Medical Center, Dallas, Texas, USA

Carlos M Sotolongo
Cardiologist, Diagnostic Cardiology, PA Jacksonville, Florida, USA

Martin G St John Sutton
Cardiologist, Director, Cardiovascular Imaging Program, Hospital of the University of Pennsylvania, John Bryfogle Professor of Cardiovascular Diseases, University of Pennsylvania Health System, Philadelphia, Pennsylvania, USA

Clyde W Yancy Jr
Cardiologist, Medical Director of Heart Failure and Cardiac Transplant Program, Associate Professor of Medicine, Carl H Westcott Distinguished Chair in Medical Research and Dallas Heart Ball Chair in Cardiac Research, UT Southwestern Medical Center, Dallas, Texas, USA

Preface

One could legitimately ask, "Why another book about cardiology and what is its focus?"

The idea for this book arose out of a series of postgraduate extramural educational courses jointly sponsored by UT Southwestern Medical Center and the American College of Cardiology entitled *Clinical Cardiology Management and Diagnostic Dilemmas*, starting in 1996. The format has been a series of 30 minute overview lectures, followed by an interactive discussion of case studies between the attendees (cardiologists, primary care providers, nurses, cardiology trainees, and medical technicians) and an expert panel, led by a UT faculty cardiologist facilitator. This has been a popular educational format, and has provoked intense, thoughtful, and lively discussion. The attachment of core curriculum to the discussion of interesting clinical problems has mirrored the way many physicians trained, building their knowledge by asking questions or reading about cases they encountered. This is what we have tried to capture in this book.

All of the senior chapter authors are experienced clinicians, and educators, who were asked to develop a text composed of essential clinical information amplified by discussion of actual patient cases. Some have been joined in this task by cardiology trainees. Therefore, this book is not encyclopedic, and it is not a book of lists. The text is intended to cover essential information on common cardiovascular diseases, and the case histories will allow the reader to see how mature clinicians approach problems and incorporate differential diagnosis and, when appropriate, practice guidelines and examination findings into patient care.

With the increasing prevalence of cardiovascular diseases, and the aging population, many non-specialist healthcare professionals provide clinical cardiology care. It is hoped that the educational format of this book will appeal to those individuals and to cardiovascular trainees (medical students, house officers, residents, registrars, and fellows), and that it will provide a stimulus for better patient care and further exploration in cardiology.

Acknowledgements

I should like to thank the contributors, many of them longstanding friends, for the lessons they have taught me in patient care, and for their commitment to teaching and scholarship. I thank Mary Banks,

Christina Karaviotis, Lotika Singha and Andy Baker of BMJ Books for their advice, support, and the rapid response to trans-Atlantic emails and attachments. For administrative support I remain indebted to Shirley Crook and Doris Matthews.

John D Rutherford
UT Southwestern Medical Center
Dallas, Texas

1: Cardiac history and examination

TAYO ADDO, JOHN D RUTHERFORD

This introductory chapter provides some basic information about the dominant symptoms of the history and the essentials of the clinical cardiac examination. Too often clinicians rely on non-invasive testing as their primary method of making a clinical diagnosis, or decision, and in our experience auscultatory skills are often deficient in otherwise competent clinicians. Therefore, we give particular emphasis to auscultatory findings in valvular heart disease.

Features of the cardiac history

Angina pectoris ("strangling breast bone or breast") is a discomfort in the chest, or adjacent areas, that is caused by an imbalance between myocardial oxygen demand and oxygen delivery by coronary artery flow. Heberden's initial description of the chest discomfort as conveying "a sense of strangling and anxiety" is still relevant, although other adjectives are frequently used to describe this distress, including "vice-like", "suffocating", "crushing", "heavy", and "squeezing". The patient may not interpret these symptoms as pain. The site of the discomfort is usually retrosternal, but radiation of the pain occurs often and is usually projected to the left shoulder, neck, jaw, and ulnar distribution of the left arm. Radiation to the same areas on the right side and the epigastric area also occurs. Pain referral to the left scapular region of the back occurs but is less common. Typically, angina pectoris begins gradually and reaches a maximum intensity over a period of minutes before dissipating; it is provoked by activity and is relieved within minutes by rest or use of nitroglycerin. Patients with angina prefer to pause, rest, sit, or stop walking during episodes. Angina may be precipitated by activity following a large meal or by cold weather. Severity of angina is assessed by reference to the circumstances associated with its occurrence (Table 1.1).[1]

Characteristics that are not suggestive of angina are fleeting, momentary chest pains described as "needle jabs" or "sharp pains"; discomfort that is aggravated or precipitated by breathing, or a single movement of the trunk or arm; or pain that is localized to a very small area or that is reproduced by pressure on the chest wall. A careful

1

Table 1.1 Severity of angina (Canadian Cardiovascular Society)

Severity of angina	Features
Class I	Angina does not occur with ordinary physical activity; it occurs only with strenuous or prolonged exertion
Class II	Slight limitation of ordinary activity; angina occurs with rapid walking on level ground or up inclines or steps
Class III	Marked limitation or ordinary physical activity; angina occurs when walking
Class IV	Inability to carry out even mild physical activity without angina, which also may occur briefly at rest

Adapted from Campeau [1]

history should uncover risk factors that predispose to coronary artery disease. In general, angina pectoris will tend to occur in males over 40 years of age and females over 50 years of age; a history of cigarette smoking is common, and the presence of diabetes mellitus, hypertension, hypercholestrolemia, or peripheral vascular disease is highly relevant. Similarly, a prior history of myocardial infarction, or a family history of myocardial infarction or sudden death in a male parent or sibling before age 55 years, or a female parent or sibling before age 65 years is important.

Palpitations may be reported by patients as sensations of flipping, stopping, pounding, or fluttering of their heart. Abrupt onset and offset of rapid, sustained palpitations suggests supraventricular or ventricular tachycardia. If the sensation associated with the palpitations is accompanied by dizziness, presyncope, or syncope, then ventricular tachycardia needs to be excluded. If rapid irregular rhythms are reported then atrial fibrillation or flutter or tachycardia with varying block are suggested. Palpitations arising during exercise or in situations of catecholamine excess may be due to ventricular tachycardia arising from the right ventricular outflow tract, and those that arise immediately after exercise may be due to atrial fibrillation and a relative increase in vagal tone. A family history of premature death or arrhythmias is highly relevant. When acquiring the history it can be helpful if the patient can tap out, with their fingers, their perception of normal rhythm and the rhythm associated with their symptoms. (A 12-lead electrocardiogram taken during the abnormal rhythm can be diagnostic. An electrocardiogram taken in normal sinus rhythm can give clues as to the possible primary diagnosis. For example, a short PR interval and δ waves suggest pre-excitation and supraventricular tachycardia; left ventricular hypertrophy, atrial premature beats, or P-wave abnormalities of mitral valve disease may represent substrates for atrial fibrillation; Q waves of prior myocardial infarction may be the substrate for ventricular arrhythmias; and a long QT interval is possibly associated with polymorphic ventricular tachycardia.[2])

Shortness of breath, or dyspnea, is a normal accompaniment of physical exertion and is accentuated by obesity, pregnancy, lack of physical fitness, and advanced age. Normally, shortness of breath limits exercise performance, or physical activity, and individuals have a certain expectation of what is normal for them. The shortness of breath caused by heart disease is similar to that caused by normal exertion, but it is provoked by lower levels of physical activity than has been experienced previously by the individual patient. New symptoms of nocturnal cough or episodic difficulty with breathing when lying supine may also be associated with cardiac dysfunction. Anxious patients may at times experience the sensation that a deeper breath than normal is required to feel comfortable but have normal breathing with physical activity. The clinician must listen carefully to the description provided by the patient and decide whether the symptoms fall into a normal or abnormal category.

Appearance of the patient

The patient may appear to be breathless at rest, which suggests the presence of heart failure or severe pulmonary disease. The appearance of a patient may suggest specific systemic or developmental disorders. For example, in Marfan's syndrome there is a defect in the region of chromosome 15 that encodes the connective tissue protein fibrillin-1; this defect is associated with a well recognized phenotype, including tall stature, joint hypermobility, pectus excavatum, and arachnodactyly. Rarely, arterial pulsations may be immediately obvious after looking at a patient. For example, prominent arterial pulsations might be seen in the neck or the patient's head may be bobbing with each heart beat, possibly indicating the presence of wide pulse pressures as are seen in conditions such as severe aortic regurgitation.

Examination of the skin and mucous membranes is important (Table 1.2). The presence of pale, cool extremities might suggest circulatory insufficiency; the presence of warm extremities with perspiration might suggest increased sympathetic activity (for example, associated with hyperthyroidism) and dry mucous membranes might suggest volume depletion. The patient may exhibit obvious edema,

Table 1.2 Skin and mucous membrane manifestations of cardiac disease

Skin manifestation	Details	Associations
Cyanosis	Bluish discoloration of the skin or mucous membranes might suggest cyanosis, which is usually due to an increased quantity of reduced hemoglobin in the blood	Central cyanosis is associated with a decreased arterial oxygen saturation, either due to right to left shunting of the blood associated with congenital heart disease or to abnormal pulmonary function. Peripheral cyanosis is usually secondary to cutaneous vasoconstriction, low cardiac output, and high oxygen extraction or exposure to cold air or water. Rarely, a patient will have deferential cyanosis confined to the lower half of the body, possibly indicating a right to left shunt through a patent ductus arteriosus in association with an aortic arch abnormality or aortic coarctation
Digital clubbing	Clubbing of the fingers is associated with a wide variety of diseases or may be a congenital abnormality.[3] (The distal part of the finger, including the nail itself, is deformed, and there is swelling and increased sponginess of the tissues overlying the dorsum of the distal phalanx. The shape of the finger is altered so that the widely obtuse angle between the plane of the skin over the nail root and the nail plate itself is filled in)	The commonest cardiac cause is hypoxemia associated with congenital heart disease and right to left shunting. It is seen with chronic infection due to subacute bacterial endocarditis and bronchiectasis. Other important causes include pulmonary malignancy and inflammatory gastrointestinal disorders (Crohn's disease and ulcerative colitis)
Erythema nodosum	Red, raised, tender lesions on shins or forearms	Non-specific allergic reaction to antigens, including rheumatic fever and endocarditis
Facial edema		The presence of facial edema may suggest obstruction of venous return to the heart (superior vena cava obstruction) or constrictive pericarditis

Continued

Table 1.2 Continued

Skin manifestation	Details	Associations
Osler's nodes	Small, red, tender lesions in pulp of fingers and toes and on palms and soles. They fade and become painless over several days	Transient embolic lesions seen with infective endocarditis
Rheumatic nodules	Painless, mobile, subcutaneous lesions about 1 cm around elbows, knees, and knuckles	Rheumatic fever and rheumatoid arthritis
Splinter hemorrhages	Minute, longitudinal hemorrhages that appear like splinters under the nail beds	Embolic phenomena of infective endocarditis or traumatic
Xanthomas	Cholesterol-filled nodules found over tendons or subcutaneously	Eruptive xanthomas are small, yellow, 1–2 mm nodules on an erythematous base found in types I and V hyperlipoproteinemia. Tendinous xanthomas are found in type II hyperlipoproteinemia
Hemochromatosis	Bronze pigmentation of skin and loss of pubic and axillary hair	Associated with cardiomyopathy due to iron deposits in heart
Lentigines	Small brown macular lesions on neck and trunk seen first in childhood	Pulmonary stenosis and hypertrophic cardiomyopathy
Telangiectasias	Multiple capillary hemangiomas of skin, lips, nasal mucosa, and upper respiratory and gastrointestinal tracts	Can cause pulmonary arteriovenous fistulas and be associated with central cyanosis
Arachnodactyly		Marfan's syndrome
Quincke sign	Systolic flushing of nail beds seen by pressing a light against terminal digits	Wide pulse pressure (for example, aortic regurgitation)
Janeway lesions	Non-tender, slightly raised hemorrhagic lesions in palms and soles of feet	Infective endocarditis

especially of the lower extremities, due to hepatic, renal, or cardiac causes, including congestive heart failure and constrictive pericardial disease.

Examination of the optic fundi may provide direct information on a variety of conditions that affect the cardiovascular system. In patients with hypertension the retinal changes are classified according to the Keith–Wagner–Barker method. These changes reflect both atherosclerotic and hypertensive retinopathy. Initially, arterial narrowing is seen (grade 1), and subsequently the arteriolar diameters increase in relation to the venous diameters, manifested as arteriovenous nicking (grade 2 changes). As uncontrolled hypertension progresses, small vessels rupture, and exudates and hemorrhages are seen (grade 3 changes). Eventually, sustained, accelerated, or extreme hypertension is associated with raised intracranial pressure seen as papilledema, usually associated with retinal exudates and hemorrhages (grade 4 changes). Grade 2 changes correlate with other evidence of clinical cardiovascular disease or end-organ damage (left ventricular hypertrophy, renal disease, arterial disease). Overall risk in patients with hypertension correlates with presence, or absence, of conventional cardiovascular risk factors and evidence of uncontrolled hypertension or end-organ damage. In patients with diabetes mellitus (an important cardiovascular risk factor) retinopathy may develop. Increased capillary permeability leads to capillary closure and dilatation, microaneurysms, and dilated veins. Cotton wool spots (microinfarcts), hemorrhages, and hard exudates are seen. New vessel formation and scarring are seen with proliferative retinopathy. Finally, in infective endocarditis evidence of focal retinal hemorrhage (i.e. Roth spots – retinal hemorrhage with a clear center) or embolic phenomena (retinal arterial occlusion) may be found.

Arterial blood pressure and pulses

Blood pressure should initially be measured in both arms. The blood pressure is obtained by sphygmomanometry, and the bladder associated with the cuff should encircle and cover approximately 50% of the length of the upper arm. (If the cuff bladder is too small then inaccurate, abnormally high blood pressure readings may be obtained.) The cuff is inflated rapidly while palpating the pulse until about 20–30 mmHg above the point at which the palpated radial pulse disappears. The cuff is then deflated slowly as the brachial artery is auscultated. The sounds heard are described in five phases (Korotkoff sounds). The initial phase (phase 1) begins with the appearance of clear, tapping sounds and represents systolic blood pressure. Diastolic blood pressure is represented by the disappearance of sounds (phase 5). Just before the sounds disappear they become muffled (phase 4). A discrepancy between blood pressures measured in both arms (of more than 5–10 mmHg) may indicate involvement of the great arteries leaving the heart, in a disease process (arterial occlusive disease, aortic dissection or coarctation).

The major arterial pulses (carotid, brachial, radial, femoral, popliteal, posterior tibial, and dorsalis pedis) should be examined bilaterally. Diminished or absent arterial pulses suggest occlusive disease. The radial and femoral arteries should be palpated simultaneously during the cardiovascular examination. A significant radial–femoral delay (the appearance of the pulses in the lower extremities is delayed as compared with that in the upper extremities) suggests coarctation of the aorta, which needs exclusion. In this instance, an initial step is to measure blood pressures in the lower extremities and compare them with pressures in the upper extremities. Again, if there is a major discrepancy (i.e. the blood pressures measured in the lower extremities are lower) then coarctation of the aorta must be excluded.

When the arterial pulse is palpated (typically in the radial, carotid, and brachial locations initially), rate, rhythm, and quality of the pulse are noted. The rhythm may be regular or irregular. Sinus arrhythmia, a normal finding, may be noted when there is a slight acceleration of the pulse during inspiration and slowing during expiration. This determination can usually be made only when the pulse is relatively slow. An irregularly irregular pulse suggests atrial fibrillation, and occasional dropped or skipped beats may suggest atrial or ventricular premature beats. A rhythm strip, or a 12-lead electrocardiogram, is the only sure way to distinguish these irregularities. The shape of the pulse wave (quality) and the volume of the pulse wave (the amplitude of the pulse is determined by the difference between the systolic and diastolic blood pressures = pulse pressure) each provide important information. Large volume pulses suggest a high cardiac stroke output and may generally be associated with the dilatation of the peripheral blood vessels that is seen normally with exercise, fever, pregnancy, aortic regurgitation, and hyperthyroidism. A small volume pulse might suggest a low cardiac stroke output or obstruction to cardiac outflow, for example significant aortic valve stenosis. During palpation of the arterial pulse or blood pressure measurement an exaggerated decrease in systolic blood pressure with inspiration (pulsus paradoxicus) may suggest cardiac tamponade or may be associated with asthma or, rarely, morbid obesity.

Clinical experience will alert the clinician to any deviation from the shape of the normal arterial pulse wave, which has a smooth, quick rise; a momentary peak; and a smooth, quick fall. In aortic stenosis the upstroke of the pulse may be delayed and associated with a small volume pulse if significant outflow obstruction exists. In patients with significant aortic regurgitation a rapidly rising and falling pulse with a wide pulse pressure may be observed.

Finally, palpation of the pulse (especially the radial and femoral pulses) may provide some indication of "hardening of the arteries", which occurs with advanced atherosclerosis. Certainly in older patients, with loss of elasticity of the arterial walls, the sensation of firmness or hardening of the arteries may be appreciated.

Jugular venous pulse (Figure 1.1)

The level of the jugular venous pulse (JVP) allows estimation of the filling pressure of the right heart (i.e. the central venous filling pressure).[4] It is elevated with heart failure, hypervolemia, conditions that reduce compliance (or increase "stiffness") of the right ventricle, constrictive pericarditis, and obstruction of the superior vena cava. To assess the JVP the right internal jugular vein is usually examined with the patient in a supine position, with back, head, and neck inclined at a 30–45° angle. In the absence of obesity the pulsations of the jugular veins are transmitted to the skin. In contrast to the carotid pulse, which is a fast, localized, single, outward deflection, the JVP is diffuse, usually has two waves, and is a slow rostral deflection. Two phases are evident in the pulsation. An "a" wave occurs just before the first heart sound (S_1) and a "v" wave occurs simultaneously with or just after the second heart sound (S_2; Table 1.3 and Figure 1.1). The "a" wave reflects right atrial contraction and the "v" wave reflects passive atrial filling after systole.

The maximal height of the JVP above the heart, with the patient lying at 45°, closely reflects mean right atrial pressure. A perpendicular plane is extended from the highest point at which the jugular venous pulsation is seen to the sternal angle. The height from the sternal angle is measured. Because the right atrium is approximately 5 cm below the sternal angle, 5 cm is added to the height of the JVP seen above the sternal angle. This approximates JVP in centimeters of water (cmH$_2$O). The upper limit of normal for JVP is 4 cm above the sternal angle or a central venous pressure of 9 cm. With a patient sitting in a 90° upright position, any visible venous waveform is abnormally elevated. Some patients, with severe elevation of right heart filling pressures, will need to sit upright so that the pulses can be visualized and the right atrial pressure estimated.

Table 1.3 Waveforms of jugular venous pressure

Wave	Details	Associations
"a" wave	The rising jugular venous wave due to right atrial contraction; it occurs late in ventricular diastole just before S_1, at a time when the atrium has nearly been filled with blood. A positive venous wave results from blood forced back into the jugular veins from right atrial systole and is normally the highest positive jugular venous wave. The "a" wave follows the P wave of the electrocardiogram	Present with normal sinus rhythm Absent with atrial fibrillation, sinus tachycardia Occurs almost simultaneously with right sided fourth sounds Large "a" waves occur when diastolic filling of the right ventricle is restricted because of hypertrophy or loss of compliance ("stiffness"); for example, pulmonary hypertension, pulmonary stenosis, hypertrophic cardiomyopathy, infiltrative cardiomyopathy, tricuspid obstruction (stenosis, atrial myxoma) "Giant 'a' waves" or "cannon 'a' waves" occur when the atrium contracts and the tricuspid valve is closed; for example, third degree heart block, atrioventricular dissociation (ventricular tachycardia)
X descent	The negative jugular venous wave after right atrial systole has generated the "a" wave is due to more rapid passive filling of the emptied right atrium in late diastole. Normally the end of the X descent is the most negative component of the JVP	The slope of the X descent may be steeper, or enhanced, in constrictive pericarditis or cardiac tamponade when the JVP is elevated to augment right heart filling
"v" wave	A positive pressure wave after the X descent as the passive filling of the right atrium continues and blood backs up in the jugular veins while the tricuspid valve is closed during ventricular systole	In atrial fibrillation the "v" wave is the only positive wave of the JVP A very large "v" wave is seen with tricuspid regurgitation. Tricuspid regurgitation is often accompanied by atrial fibrillation and in this situation the JVP consists of a "v" wave and Y descent A large, sharp peaked "v" wave is seen with atrial septal defect due to increased blood entering the right atrium

Continued

Table 1.3 Continued

Wave	Details	Associations
Y descent	The negative jugular venous wave after the "v" wave, which begins as the tricuspid valve opens and the blood empties into the right ventricle; it is a measure of forward flow across the valve	In tricuspid regurgitation or atrial septal defect, the increased size, and often steeper slope, of the Y descent corresponds to the larger "v" wave Constrictive pericarditis associated with an elevated JVP often has a rapid and deep Y descent followed by a sudden, rapid rebound to a plateau, creating a "square root sign" as the right ventricle has filled to its maximum capacity limited by the abnormal pericardium The Y descent is shallow with tricuspid valve obstruction (atrial myxoma and tricuspid valve stenosis)
"c" wave	A small positive wave sometimes seen on the X descent due to the upward movement of the atrioventricular valve ring during tricuspid closure, creating a retrograde fluid pressure wave	

JVP, jugular venous pressure; S_1, first heart sound

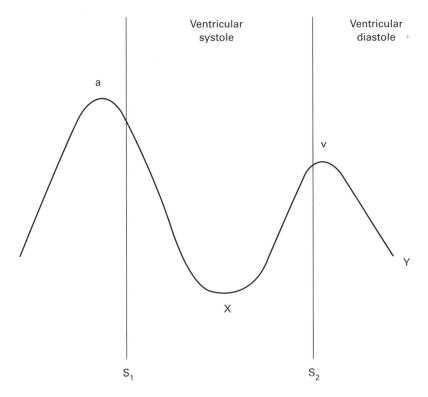

Figure 1.1 The jugular venous pulsation. Two phases are evident in the pulsation. An "a" wave occurs just before the first heart sound (S_1) and a "v wave" occurs simultaneously with, or just after, the second heart sound (S_2). The "a" wave reflects right atrial contraction and precedes ventricular systole and the the "v" wave reflects passive atrial filling after ventricular systole

Cardiac palpation

In most normal adults the apical impulse of the heart (apex beat) lies in the fourth to fifth left intercostal space and is usually within 10 cm from the midline. Its location should be found by palpation of the left anterior chest with the fingers of the right hand. The fingers should extend along the intercostal spaces toward the left axilla. In females the left breast should be lifted out of the way. The apical impulse is then considered the most lateral pulsation of the apex of the heart in the left anterior chest. The apex beat of the heart may not be palpated in patients with major obesity or pulmonary conditions such as emphysema, which distend the lungs more than usual and thus increase the gap between the heart and the chest wall.

Although the value of the position of the apex beat as a physical sign of heart enlargement is limited, some useful information can be obtained by determining its exact position. In normal persons the apex beat pulsation is produced by a small area of left ventricle, most of which lies behind and to the left of the right ventricle. With left ventricular pressure overload the apex beat is forceful and sustained. With left ventricular dilatation and volume overload the apex beat is prolonged, sustained and, when the heart is enlarged, it is displaced leftward and downward. A parasternal lift felt by palpation over the third, fourth, and fifth left intercostal spaces close to the sternum usually indicates right ventricular pressure or volume overload or mitral regurgitation (due to the forceful backflow of blood into the left atrium during left ventricular systole). In patients with abnormal hearts, especially those with valvular heart disease, murmurs may be loud or turbulent enough to be felt as vibrations known as "thrills" (for example, in pulmonic stenosis).

Cardiac auscultation

Successful auscultation of the heart involves recognition of normal heart sounds and detection of abnormal heart sounds associated with cardiovascular disease. In order to concentrate on the appropriate phase of the cardiac cycle, the heart sounds can be timed by assessing their relationship to simultaneous palpation of the carotid pulse in systole. Two heart sounds are heard in all normal people (Figure 1.2).

The first heart sound (S_1) is associated with closure of the atrioventricular valves (mitral and tricuspid) and occurs at the start of ventricular systole. It is usually best heard at the apex of the heart, using the "bell of the stethoscope". S_1 is normally heard as a single sound but actually has two successive components associated with closure of the mitral valve and later closure of the tricuspid valve. In patients with complete right bundle branch block, the delay of the tricuspid component may result in a widely split S_1.

The second heart sound (S_2) is produced by closure of the aortic (A_2) and pulmonary (P_2) valves. S_2 for clinical purposes marks the end of ventricular systole. Normally, the first component (i.e. A_2) and the second component (i.e. P_2) of S_2 separate or "split" during inspiration because P_2 is delayed as a result of the inspiratory increase in capacitance of the pulmonary vascular bed. This splitting is usually best heard in the second left intercostal space (pulmonary area), whereas the louder A_2 can be heard at the base, left sternal edge, and cardiac apex (see Figure 1.2). P_2 is almost never heard at the apex. Fixed splitting of S_2 is heard in most patients with an atrial septal defect, and wide splitting is associated with right bundle branch block and pulmonary valve stenosis. When the patient stands, fixed splitting persists and wide splitting will decrease.

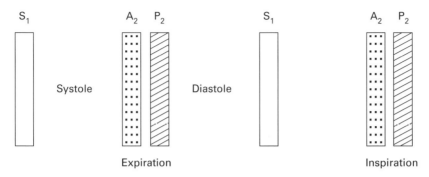

Figure 1.2 Normal heart sounds. S_1, first heart sound; A_2, aortic component of the second heart sound; P_2, pulmonary component of the second heart sound

The "loudness" of the heart sounds can vary in health and disease. The sound associated with S_1 is probably mainly due to mitral valve closure, and its intensity depends on how far into the left ventricular cavity the mitral leaflets are at the onset of the ventricular systole. Therefore, S_1 may be loudest in the presence of a rapid heart rate, a short PR interval, at times in mitral valve prolapse when the mitral valve leaflets are at their maximal point of excursion into the left ventricular cavity at the onset of ventricular systole, and in mitral stenosis with a pliable valve. The intensity of S_1 decreases in situations in which this mobility of the mitral valve leaflets into the ventricular cavity is lost (for example, longstanding mitral valve stenosis with a non-pliable, calcified mitral valve, mitral regurgitation, and a long PR interval). The intensity of S_2 increases with both systemic hypertension (increase in intensity of A_2) and pulmonary hypertension (increase in intensity of P_2).

Added diastolic sounds

Third heart sounds (S_3) are mid-diastolic sounds that are best heard with the stethoscope bell applied lightly and with the patient in the left lateral decubitus position. S_3 occurs during the rapid filling phase of the ventricle, occurring after closure of the aortic and pulmonary valves, and coinciding with the wide ascent of the atrial pressure pulse. In children, young adults, and women during pregnancy, an S_3 may be a normal finding. An abnormal S_3 may be generated if the ventricle is dysfunctional (heart failure) or if there is an increase in flow during the rapid filling phase of the ventricles (mitral and tricuspid regurgitation).

The fourth heart sound (S_4) is probably never a normal finding. An S_4 is a late diastolic (or presystolic) sound and is generated within the ventricle during the atrial filling phase. Active atrial systole is required to generate an S_4 and the sound is not heard in patients with atrial fibrillation when coordinated atrial contraction is absent. An S_4 is typically generated in situations in which the ventricle is "stiff" or "non-compliant", and augmented atrial contraction is needed to fill the ventricle appropriately (for example, left ventricular hypertrophy associated with hypertension or aortic valve stenosis; right ventricular hypertrophy associated with pulmonary hypertension or pulmonary stenosis; and acute myocardial ischemia with a stiff, non-compliant left ventricle). When these sounds originate from the left ventricle they are best heard with the patient in the left lateral decubitus position, applying the bell of the stethoscope lightly to the cardiac apex. When the sounds originate from the right ventricle they may be best heard at the left lower sternal edge with the patient supine and may possibly be accentuated by inspiration.

Cardiac murmurs

In general cardiac murmurs are sounds that result from turbulent blood flow of blood in the heart or great vessels, producing vibrations. When blood vessels or valves are narrowed by disease or when valves leak because of disease the rate of blood flow may result in turbulence and vibrations, and therefore murmurs are heard. It is important to note that turbulence may also occur when blood viscosity is low or when the rate of blood flow through a normal heart or blood vessel is accelerated, as in anemia, fever, or pregnancy.

A grading system for intensity or loudness was proposed by Samuel A Levine on a scale of 1 to 6. A grade 1 murmur is so faint that it is only just heard, a grade 3 murmur is easily heard but not loud, and a grade 5 murmur is very loud. Murmurs may also be described according to their time of onset and termination (for example, mid-systolic, holosystolic [beginning with S_1 and ending with S_2], early systolic, or late systolic) and according to whether they are crescendo, decrescendo, crescendo/decrescendo, or heard as a "plateau".

Murmurs associated with the aortic and pulmonary valves are usually best heard at the base of the heart, those associated with the mitral valve are best heard at the apex, and those associated with the tricuspid valve at the lower left sternal edge. In general, right sided heart murmurs are accentuated by inspiration, aortic diastolic murmurs are best heard with the patient leaning forward in the expiratory phase of respiration, and diastolic mitral murmurs are best heard with the patient lying in the left lateral decubitus position with the bell of the stethoscope lightly applied at the cardiac apex.

Examination of the chest includes the following:

- inspection (shape of the chest – kyphosis, scoliosis; respiratory rate; amplitude and symmetry of chest movement; use of accessory muscles of neck and chest wall with labored respiration)
- listening for noisy breathing (stridor with laryngeal or tracheal obstruction, wheezing with partial bronchial obstruction)
- palpation (position of trachea and upper mediastinum – displaced by masses, collapse or fibrosis of the lung drawing the trachea to the affected side, or tension pneumothorax or a large pleural effusion displacing the trachea to the opposite side)
- measurement of chest expansion (normally 5–10 cm)
- assessment of tactile vocal fremitus.

Vocal tactile vibrations are absent or diminished over a pleural effusion, but are transmitted with greater ease through consolidated lung (for example, in pneumonia) than normally aerated lung. Percussion of the lung yields a resonant note over normally aerated lung, a dull note over fluid, and a tympanitic note or hyperresonant note over collections of gas. Auscultation of normal breath sounds (which are produced in the larynx or throat and conducted down the trachea and bronchial system to the alveoli) reveals bronchial breathing if one listens over the trachea (harsh, low pitched inspiration and longer, high pitched expiration) and normal vesicular breathing over the lungs (lower pitched, less harsh inspiration and faint, short expiration) as normal lung modifies the laryngeal sounds. Normal breath sounds are diminished or absent distal to an occluded bronchus or if fluid or air is between the lung and the chest wall (effusion or pneumothorax). Normal breath sounds change to bronchial sounds if a segment of lung consolidates and allows laryngeal breath sounds to pass with less modification to the chest wall. A variety of abnormal sounds can accompany breath sounds and are known as adventitious sounds. There are two main types of adventitious sounds: crepitations or rales, which are crackling or rustling sounds heard mainly in inspiration when there is fluid in bronchioles and alveoli; and rhonchi, which are louder, coarser sounds associated especially with inflammation or partial obstruction of bronchi (asthma, bronchitis).

The abdomen is examined for evidence of edema, ascites, liver enlargement (heart failure), pulsatile liver (tricuspid regurgitation), enlargement of the abdominal aorta (pulsatile abdominal aortic aneurysm), and bruits (associated with renal artery stenosis or abdominal aortic aneurysm).

Specific cardiac conditions

Certain features of the history, clinical examination, electrocardiogram, and chest x ray film will almost always lead to the correct cardiac diagnosis if carefully and correctly assessed by the clinician. Although many the following conditions[5] are discussed in detail in the relevant chapters of this book, a few are discussed here with particular emphasis on auscultatory findings. It is our opinion that the skilled clinician is very familiar with these findings, actively confirms or excludes their presence during the cardiac examination, and is able to arrive at an informed conclusion regarding the presence and severity of specific cardiac diseases. Furthermore, the physician who has detailed knowledge of the history and clinical examination, electrocardiogram, and chest x ray findings for a patient will be able to interpret accurately the meaning of the non-invasive and invasive cardiac studies and place their findings in perspective. Armed with all of this information, the physician is then in a position to discuss the cardiac diagnosis and options for therapy with the patient. Reliance on the results of non-invasive or invasive testing alone without synthesis of all available clinical information may lead to poor clinical decisions and suboptimal patient care.

Mitral stenosis

In many parts of the world (India, Central America, South Pacific countries) mitral stenosis, caused by rheumatic pancarditis, presents predominantly in young women of child-bearing age, often in association with pregnancy. Elsewhere, the disease presents one or two decades later. The predominant symptom is breathlessness, caused by pulmonary congestion or edema, at times unmasked by the onset of atrial fibrillation.

The clinical examination features of mitral stenosis depend on the following:

- whether the mitral valve apparatus remains "pliable" or mobile, and is fused predominantly along the valve edges, or is "non-pliable" and immobile (a fibrosed, thickened, distorted valve with associated fusion and shortening of the chordae tendinae)
- the presence or absence of pulmonary hypertension
- the presence or absence of atrial fibrillation.

"Pliable" or mobile mitral valve apparatus in sinus rhythm

On physical examination the patient appears normal or is breathless. Pulse is normal or low volume. Blood pressure is normal.

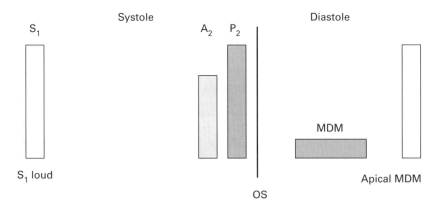

Figure 1.3 Mitral stenosis with pliable valve. S$_1$, first heart sound; A$_2$, aortic component of the second heart sound; P$_2$ is loud and closely followed by the OS. MDM, mid-diastolic murmur; OS, opening snap; P$_2$, pulmonary component of the second heart sound

JVP is normal, or there may be an increased "a" wave if pulmonary hypertension is present. Cardiac impulse is normal or a left parasternal lift is present in pulmonary hypertension.

On auscultation (Figure 1.3), S$_1$ is loud. S$_2$ splits normally on inspiration. P$_2$ is accentuated with pulmonary hypertension. An opening snap (OS) of the mitral valve immediately follows S$_2$ (heard at the apex with the diaphragm), followed by a mid-diastolic, low pitched rumble (with or without presystolic accentuation) that is best heard at the apex with the bell lightly applied and the patient in the left lateral recumbent position. The OS occurs when the opening movement of the mitral apparatus or "doming" into the left ventricle abruptly stops. The loud S$_1$ is the reciprocal sound of the OS and is due to abrupt completion of atrioventricular valve closure. Both sounds arise when the mitral valve apparatus is mobile and pliable, and are lost when it becomes relatively immobile.

On chest examination, crepitations or rales are present with pulmonary congestion. Abdominal examination reveals a normal liver span or pulsatile liver with pulmonary hypertension and secondary tricuspid regurgitation. Peripheral edema may be noted if the patient is pregnant or in the presence of tricuspid regurgitation. The electrocardiogram may indicate left atrial enlargement, which may be manifested as a negative terminal force in the P wave in V$_1$, or as a notched or wide P wave in II. The chest x ray film may show left atrial enlargement with elevation of the left main stem bronchus. Evidence of pulmonary congestion may be seen with prominent upper lobe vessels, and later there may be evidence of interstitial edema and fluid within the interlobular septa (Kerley B lines, which are short, dense, horizontal lines often seen near the lung periphery in the costophrenic angles).

Immobile mitral valve apparatus

The clinical examination features associated with an immobile mitral valve apparatus when the patient has atrial fibrillation, pulmonary hypertension, and secondary tricuspid regurgitation are as follows.

In addition to symptoms of breathlessness and palpitations, the patient may complain of reduced energy and leg swelling. On physical examination the patient may appear normal or be breathless. Pulse is normal or low volume and irregularly irregular (atrial fibrillation). Blood pressure is normal. JVP is elevated to the angle of the jaw with "v" waves. Cardiac impulse is a left parasternal lift due to right ventricular pressure/volume overload.

On auscultation (Figure 1.4), S_1 is soft (and variable). At the base a loud P_2 is heard; S_2 may become single with severe pulmonary hypertension (reduced compliance of the pulmonary vascular bed associated with earlier closure of P_2). A mid-diastolic, low pitched apical rumble is heard at the apex with the patient in the left lateral recumbent position. At the lower left sternal edge a grade 3–4 holosystolic murmur, which increases with inspiration, is heard (tricuspid regurgitation). With right ventricular hypertrophy and dilatation, the murmur of tricuspid regurgitation may be heard at the apex as the enlarging ventricle becomes displaced leftward. In contrast to the patient with the pliable mitral stenotic valve, once the mitral valve becomes fibrosed, distorted, and relatively immobile, S_1 becomes soft and the OS is lost. With the onset of atrial fibrillation the loudness of S_1 becomes variable.

Chest examination reveals crepitations or rales with pulmonary congestion. Abdominal examination indicates increased liver span and a pulsatile liver. Peripheral edema is present. Electrocardiogram findings are atrial fibrillation, evidence of right ventricular hypertrophy with a rightward shift of the mean frontal plane axis greater than 80°, and an R : S ratio greater than 1·0 in V_1. The chest x ray film may show left atrial enlargement, evidence of pulmonary congestion, Kerley B lines, and enlargement of the pulmonary arteries and right ventricle.

Aortic stenosis

Aortic valve stenosis seen in adults is usually secondary to a congenital bicuspid valve or age-related degenerative calcification and

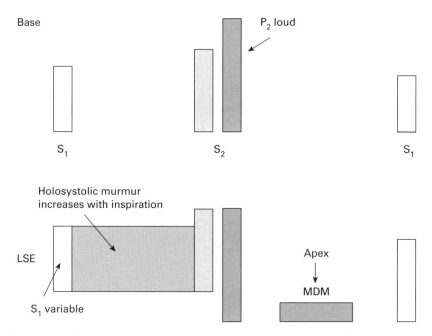

Figure 1.4 Mitral stenosis, pulmonary hypertension, and tricuspid regurgitation. LSE, left sternal edge; MDM, mid-diastolic murmur; S_1, first heart sound; S_2, second heart sound; P_2, pulmonary component of the second heart sound

results in left ventricular pressure overload and concentric hypertrophy. The condition usually presents in patients older than 50 years, with a triad of possible symptoms: angina, increased breathlessness, and exertional syncope (or dizziness).

On physical examination the patient appears normal. Pulse is slow rising, low volume, and sustained. Blood pressure is normal, as is JVP. Cardiac impulse is prominent but usually not displaced (when heart failure ensues late in the natural history, the cardiac impulse becomes displaced inferiorly and laterally).

On auscultation (Figure 1.5), S_1 is normal. S_2 sound is single and/or soft. An ejection systolic murmur is heard at the base of the heart (upper right sternal edge) and is often transmitted to the carotids and cardiac apex. Chest and abdominal examinations are normal. Peripheral arterial pulses are all normal volume and equal. Carotid pulses are slow rising and sustained. A transmitted ejection systolic murmur, from the aortic valve, is often heard over the right carotid. On electrocardiography, left ventricular hypertrophy is found in the majority of patients with severe aortic stenosis. Chest *x* ray film appearances are often normal.

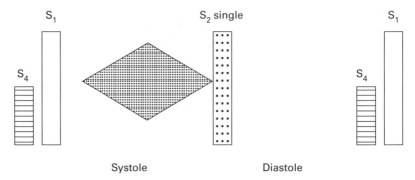

Figure 1.5 Aortic valve stenosis. S_1, first heart sound; S_2, second heart sound; S_4, fourth heart sound. Single S_2 (because A_2 is delayed and merges with P_2); ejection systolic murmur; S_4 often present. A_2, aortic component of the second heart sound; P_2, pulmonary component of the second heart sound

If the pulse is slow rising, low volume, and sustained, S_2 is single, and the typical ejection systolic murmur is long and late peaking, then it is likely that severe, aortic valve stenosis is present. The most useful clinical findings for diagnosing aortic stenosis, in order of importance, are a slow rate of rise of the carotid pulse, a mid to late peaking systolic murmur, and a decreased intensity or absent S_2.

Hypertrophic cardiomyopathy

In this condition, also known as idiopathic hypertrophic subaortic stenosis, there is cardiac hypertrophy, usually involving the interventricular septum, which in a minority of patients can lead to a dynamic left ventricular outflow obstruction. In the patients with obstruction any situation that results in a reduction in left ventricular volume (hypovolemia, Valsalva maneuver) increases the obstruction of the thickened, non-compliant, "restrictive" ventricle. The disease has a genetic basis, at times affecting families, and involves mutations in the coding of β cardiac myosin heavy chains. The majority of patients are asymptomatic but the condition can present, usually in young adults, with syncope, sudden death, or breathlessness. Abnormal cardiac rhythms are poorly tolerated and patients may present with atrial tachyarrhythmias, leading to hypotension, as a result of the loss of the atrial contribution to filling the "restrictive" ventricle.

On physical examination, the pulse is bisferiens or "jerky", with a brisk arterial upstroke. Blood pressure is normal and JVP is usually normal. There is a prominent, forceful, left ventricular impulse.

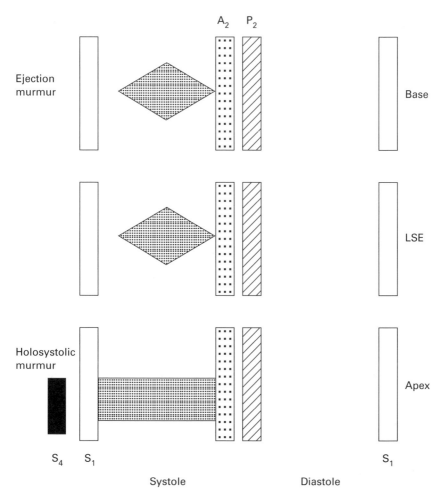

A₂ P₂

Ejection
murmur

Base

LSE

Holosystolic
murmur

Apex

S_4 S_1 S_1

Systole   Diastole

Figure 1.6 Obstructive hypertrophic cardiomyopathy. S_1, first heart sound; P_2, pulmonary component of the second heart sound; A_2, aortic component of the second heart sound; S_4, fourth heart sound; LSE, left sternal edge

On auscultation (Figure 1.6), S_1 is normal and S_2 is split normally on inspiration. There is a prominent S_4. A mid to late systolic ejection murmur is heard at the left sternal edge and apex. The murmur typically increases with Valsalva maneuver. When mitral regurgitation is present, an apical, holosystolic murmur is heard and may be accompanied by an S_3.

The chest and abdominal examinations are normal. There is no peripheral edema. Electrocardiogram findings are left ventricular hypertrophy, ST and T wave abnormalities, and prominent septal Q

Table 1.4 Distinguishing examination features of obstructive hypertrophic cardiomyopathy and aortic valve stenosis

Feature	Obstructive hypertrophic cardiomyopathy	Aortic valve stenosis
Pulse	Bisferiens or "jerky", with a brisk arterial upstroke	Slow rising, low volume, and sustained
Murmur	Ejection systolic; increases with Valsalva (which decreases stroke volume) with or without mitral holosystolic	Ejection systolic; increases with squatting (which increases stroke volume)

waves (narrow and deep) caused by hypertrophy of the septal region (a "pseudo-infarction" appearance). The chest *x* ray film appearance is normal or cardiac enlargement may be present. Certain examination features distinguish obstructive hypertrophic cardiomyopathy (subaortic stenosis) from aortic valve stenosis (Table 1.4).

The clinician needs to be aware that hypertrophic obstructive myopathy can be found in young adults; it may be unmasked by inappropriate hypotension associated with atrial arrhythmias (because of restriction of cardiac filling), and the obstructive variety often has an S_4 and an ejection systolic murmur.

Mitral regurgitation

Acute mitral regurgitation

The commonest causes of significant, acute mitral regurgitation are infective endocarditis, prosthetic valve dysfunction, and acute myocardial infarction associated with papillary muscle dysfunction or chordal rupture (usually posteromedial papillary muscle with inferoposterior infarction). The predominant symptom is acute breathlessness. On physical examination the patient usually has sinus tachycardia and there may be evidence of acute pulmonary congestion/edema. The dominant auscultatory findings are gallop rhythms (S_4 with or without S_3), and the mitral systolic murmur may be relatively unimpressive (soft, short, and barely audible). This is because patients who develop acute, severe mitral regurgitation often have a small "unprepared" left atrium; the pressures in the left sided chambers equilibrate quickly with extremely high left atrial pressures and acute pulmonary edema ensues, with increases in pulmonary vascular resistance and eventually right ventricular hypertrophy.[5]

Chest x ray findings will indicate acute pulmonary congestion/edema. The correct clinical diagnosis is preceded by a high index of suspicion and is confirmed by echocardiography.

Chronic mitral regurgitation

The major causes of chronic mitral regurgitation include cardiomyopathy, ischemic heart disease, infective endocarditis, and rheumatic heart disease. With mitral regurgitation a fraction of stroke volume ejects into the left atrium and initially, because of the reduction in ventricular afterload, there is more complete emptying of the ventricle. Chronic volume overload of the left ventricle eventually results in increased dilatation (which results in further regurgitation) and hypertrophy, so that the heart has a greater volume at any pressure. Left ventricular end-systolic volume or diameter is a more useful indicator of ventricular performance than ejection fraction, which, because of reduced afterload of the ventricle (resulting from the leaking mitral valve), may appear "normal" when ventricular function is depressed. The left atrium can dilate enormously over time and receive the regurgitant blood from the left ventricle without substantial elevations in pressure. Therefore, pulmonary vascular resistance and right ventricular hypertrophy may not result.

Symptoms of breathlessness and fatigue do not occur with chronic mitral regurgitation until ventricular dysfunction develops. On physical examination, the pulse usually has a sharp upstroke and is full volume. The cardiac impulse is hyperdynamic and displaced downward to the left.

On auscultation (Figure 1.7), S_1 is diminished. With regard to S_2, A_2 may be earlier (because of shortened ejection time and the reduced left ventricular outflow resistance), making the S_2 split wider than usual. The murmur of mitral regurgitation is typically holosystolic but may occur early or late in systole. An S_3 is usually present with hemodynamically significant (moderate to severe) mitral regurgitation.

Electrocardiogram findings reveal left atrial enlargement and atrial fibrillation, and chest x ray findings are cardiomegaly with left atrial and ventricular enlargement.

Aortic regurgitation

Diseases of the aortic root (cystic medial necrosis, degeneration with aging, "seronegative" arthritis and inflammation) or the valve (rheumatic fever, infective endocarditis) can present acutely (infective endocarditis) or chronically.

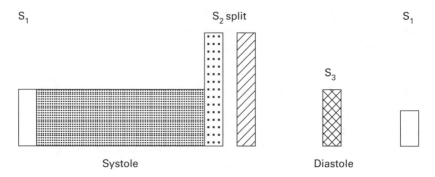

Figure 1.7 Chronic mitral regurgitation. S_1, first heart sound; S_2, second heart sound; S_3, third heart sound; S_1 soft or buried in murmur; holosystolic murmur; S_3 often present

Acute aortic regurgitation

The commonest cause of acute regurgitation is infective endocarditis. In this situation the "unprepared", normal left ventricle suddenly receives a large regurgitant volume from the aorta, in addition to normal inflow from the left atrium, causing a rapid increase in diastolic pressure (above left atrial pressure) and premature closure of the mitral valve (which partially protects the pulmonary venous bed). The ventricle has to eject its entire stroke volume into the high pressure arterial circulation, and a decline in forward stroke volume occurs. Patients present acutely with breathlessness, hypotension, and cardiovascular compromise.

On physical examination the patient appears ill, with breathlessness and peripheral vasoconstriction. Assessment of the pulse reveals tachycardia, and normal or only slightly widened pulse pressure. Blood pressure is normal or hypotensive, with only slightly widened pulse pressure. Cardiac impulse is undisplaced.

On auscultation, S_1 is soft (with premature mitral valve closure). With regard to S_2, P_2 is often accentuated. There is gallop rhythm, with S_3 and S_4. There is a short, soft, early diastolic murmur of aortic regurgitation (patient leaning forward in expiration) and an ejection flow murmur in the aortic area.

Chest examination reveals rales. Abdominal examination is normal. There is no peripheral edema. Peripheral arterial pulses are possibly absent or unequal if aortic dissection is the cause of acute aortic regurgitation. Chest x ray findings reveal evidence of acute pulmonary edema or congestion. Electrocardiogram findings are sinus tachycardia and non-specific ST-T wave changes.

The clinician has to have a high index of suspicion that a compromised patient might have acute aortic regurgitation. This is because the dominant findings relate to the presence of acute left heart failure rather than to full volume pulses or the typical early diastolic murmur associated with chronic aortic regurgitation.

Chronic aortic regurgitation

The left ventricular stroke volume is ejected into the high pressure systemic circulation, and the left ventricular end-diastolic volume (preload) increases. Because wall tension of the ventricle is directly related to the radius of the ventricle and the intraventricular pressure, and inversely related to wall thickness (Laplace's law), dilatation of the ventricle increases the tension required to generate systolic pressure. For many years compensatory hypertrophy occurs (reducing the tension per unit of muscle mass) so that the normal ratio of wall radius to wall thickness is preserved, but eventually the hemodynamic stress overcomes this compensation with a rise in wall stress and a fall in ejection fraction. In concordance with this process, patients remain asymptomatic for many years and only develop breathlessness after myocardial dysfunction has developed.

On physical examination the patient appears normal or breathless. In patients with significant aortic regurgitation, a rapidly rising and falling pulse, with a wide pulse pressure, may be observed. (Several eponyms have been associated with the description of this pulse. Corrigan described the visible pulsation in the arteries of the neck and limbs associated with large volume pulses. The term "water hammer pulse" refers to a sealed tube containing some water in a vacuum. When the tube is inverted, the impact of the falling water imparts a sharp sensation to the hand holding it. Abnormal capillary pulsations can be detected by transmitting a light through the patient's fingertips or pressing a glass slide on the patient's lip [Quincke sign]. Some auscultatory findings also confirm a wide pulse pressure: Traube sign [pistol shot sounds] refers to the loud systolic and diastolic sounds, which may be heard over the femoral artery; and Duroziez sign refers to a systolic murmur heard over the femoral artery when it is compressed proximally, and a diastolic murmur is heard over the femoral artery when it is compressed distally.) Systolic blood pressure is normal or elevated and diastolic blood pressure is low. Cardiac impulse is hyperdynamic, diffuse, and displaced inferiorly and caudally.

On auscultation (Figure 1.8), S_1 is normal. S_2 is normal or accentuated if regurgitation is due to aortic root disease and diminished if it is due to valve disease. An S_3 gallop is a harbinger of ventricular dysfunction. The classic murmur is a high frequency, early

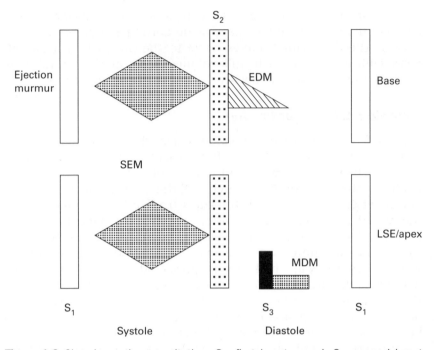

Figure 1.8 Chronic aortic regurgitation. S_1, first heart sound; S_2, second heart sound; S_3, third heart sound; SEM, systolic ejection flow murmur; EDM, early diastolic decrescendo murmur; LSE, left sternal edge; MDM, Austin–Flint mid-diastolic murmur

diastolic, decrescendo murmur[6] beginning with A_2 (best heard using the diaphragm of the stethoscope at the left sternal edge, or base, with the patient leaning forward during expiration). Severe aortic regurgitation can affect the anterior leaflet of the mitral valve in diastole and create a mid-diastolic, rumbling murmur (heard best at the apex with the patient in the left lateral decubitus position), called the Austin–Flint murmur (which is almost always preceded by an S_3). It is common for patients with significant aortic regurgitation to have an aortic ejection systolic flow murmur in the absence of any demonstrable aortic stenosis.

The electrocardiogram reveals left axis deviation and increased voltages, with development of a "strain pattern" of dilatation and hypertrophy. Chest x ray indicates the presence of cardiac and aortic root dilatation. In patients with chronic aortic regurgitation, major indicators of a poor prognosis are progressive symptoms and an abnormal left ventricular end-systolic diameter.

Conclusion

In evaluating a patient with cardiac disease we believe that a careful history and clinical cardiac examination, accompanied by a review of electrocardiogram and chest x ray findings, should precede other non-invasive testing. This approach will usually lead to the correct cardiac diagnosis. Furthermore, correct interpretation of these findings provides an invaluable assessment of the severity of cardiac disease and a basis for the interpretation of subsequent, imperfect cardiac tests. If the clinician who is primarily responsible for the care of the patient carefully follows this approach, then subsequent advice given to the patient regarding options for treatment will have taken into account all the readily available, pertinent background information.

References

1 Campeau L. Grading of angina pectoris. *Circulation* 1976;**54**:522–3.
2 Zimetbaum P, Josephson ME. Evaluation of the patient with palpitations. *N Engl J Med* 1998;**338**:1369–73.
3 Myers KA, Farquhar DRE. Does this patient have clubbing? *JAMA* 2001;**286**:341–7.
4 Cook DJ, Simel DL. Does this patient have abnormal central venous pressure? *JAMA* 1996;**275**:630–4.
5 Carabello BA, Crawford FA. Valvular heart disease. Review article. *N Engl J Med* 1997;**337**:32–41.
6 Choudhry NK, Etchells EE. Does this patient have aortic regurgitation? *JAMA* 1999;**281**:2231–8.

2: Cardiac non-invasive imaging and stress testing

VICTOR A FERRARI, LUIS ARAUJO,
MARTIN G ST JOHN SUTTON

Various non-invasive diagnostic studies are available to investigate patients with diseases of the cardiovascular system, and they can be conveniently categorized as follows.

- Anatomic imaging studies delineate anatomic structures, including cardiac chamber dimensions, shape, and wall thickness; cardiac valves; and coronary arteries.
- Functional imaging studies characterize chamber motion patterns, regional myocardial coronary blood flow and metabolism, and blood flow velocity and direction.
- Physiologic assessments measure cardiac performance, blood flow, and chamber pressure.
- Stress studies test the ability of the circulation to respond to the increased demand of physical exercise and pharmacologic perturbations.

Echocardiography: two-dimensional and Doppler

Echocardiography is the most commonly employed non-invasive imaging modality to evaluate the heart. It provides anatomic, functional, and physiologic information about the heart, and can assess the changes that occur during stress testing. Furthermore, echocardiography can be performed at the bedside.

Two-dimensional echocardiography employs a transducer that transmits ultrasound into the thorax, and reconstructs images of the heart in real time from the ultrasound reflected back to the transducer from the walls of the cardiac chambers, cardiac valves, and great vessels. It is similar in principle to marine sonar used to map the ocean floor or detect schools of fish. Ultrasound energy in the frequency range between 2·0 and 6·2 MHz is directed into the body via a transducer either placed on the chest wall (i.e. transthoracic echo) or less frequently placed in the esophagus or stomach (i.e. transesophageal echo). Transesophageal echo is "minimally invasive" because it involves conscious sedation during passage of the transducer into the esophagus. The echocardiographic images obtained using the transesophageal route are usually of higher quality than those obtained transthoracically because the ultrasound energy is not attenuated by passing through lung tissue. However, echocardiographic images obtained from either route enable measurement of cardiac chamber sizes, geometry, and contractile function.

Doppler echocardiography permits assessment of blood flow velocity and direction within the heart chambers and great vessels. Doppler echocardiography utilizes the principle first described by Christian Doppler, which in cardiac applications involves the interrogation of blood flowing through the heart and great vessels with an ultrasound beam. The velocity of blood flow can be determined by Doppler echocardiography from the shift in frequency between the transmitted and reflected ultrasound, which relates to the direction of flow and the cosine of the angle of incidence between the direction of flow and the ultrasound beam.

Blood flow velocity is defined by the relationship:

$$V = f_d \cdot C / 2 \cdot f_t (\cos \theta)$$

where f_d is the Doppler frequency, f_t is the transmitted frequency, C is the velocity of sound in the body, and θ is the angle between the moving object and the path of the ultrasound beam. Flow toward the transducer results in an increase or upward shift in the frequency of the reflected ultrasonic waves, whereas flow away from the transducer results in a decrease or downward shift in frequency, so that the peak and mean velocities as well as the direction of flow can be determined. The more parallel the ultrasound beam is to the direction of flow in the heart or great vessels (i.e. the smaller the angle of incidence), the more accurate are the measurements of blood flow velocity. Conversely, the greater the angle of incidence between the ultrasound beam and the direction of flow, the greater the underestimation of flow velocity as determined by the cosine function. For example, when the Doppler beam is perpendicular to the direction of flow, the velocity estimate will be zero ($\cos 90° = 0$).

The Doppler principle provides the basis not only for assessment of blood flow velocity and direction, but also for quantitation of volume flow in the heart and great vessels. Blood volume flow (Q) can be assessed as the product of the area under the instantaneous Doppler velocity signal (known as the velocity time integral [VTI]) and the cross-sectional area (CSA) of the flow stream:

$$Q = VTI \times CSA$$

Clinical echocardiography

Echocardiography was first used in the 1950s to detect pericardial effusions and to examine the mitral valve in rheumatic heart disease, and now plays an important role in daily clinical cardiology, cardiac surgery, the interventional catheterization laboratory, and non-invasive stress testing. The heart can be examined by two-dimensional echocardiography in an infinite number of planes, but for practical and comparative purposes the imaging planes have been standardized by the American Society of Echocardiography[1] so that all the cardiac chambers can be evaluated in the same views at sequential examinations, and any changes in size or function with time can be correctly interpreted.

The long axis of the left ventricle is used as a reference plane for obtaining the majority of echocardiographic images. It is represented on the chest wall in the coronal plane by a line connecting the apical impulse of the heart in the fifth left intercostal space in the mid-clavicular line to the junction of the middle and medial thirds of the right clavicle.[2] In the sagittal plane the long axis of the left ventricle is represented by a line connecting the apex of the heart to the body of the second thoracic vertebra.[2] Echocardiographic imaging of the heart through the chest wall is limited to the left parasternal, apical, subxiphoid, and suprasternal regions, where the heart is close to the chest wall. This is because the transmitted and reflected ultrasound signals are attenuated by the air contained in lung tissue. Two-dimensional echocardiographic imaging from the esophagus and stomach is of much higher quality because the esophagus lies directly behind the heart with no intervening lung tissue.

A routine two-dimensional echocardiographic examination consists of obtaining short axis sections at the aortic valve level, the left ventricle and right ventricle at the levels of the mitral valve and papillary muscles, as well as a long axis image of the left ventricle from the left parasternal region. In addition, images from the apex of the heart in the four chamber view are obtained, in which both right and left atria and ventricles are visualized so that their respective sizes can be compared. Images are also recorded of the apical long axis view in which the left ventricular inflow and outflow tracts are side by side, the apical two chamber view in which the left atrium and ventricle are visualized with the mitral valve dividing the two chambers, and from the subcostal region. The ability of two-dimensional echocardiography to image the left ventricle in multiple orthogonal planes allows estimation of cavity volumes and ejection fraction, which are the traditional measurements for assessing ventricular size and efficiency of emptying. Furthermore, these values have corresponded closely to ventricular volumes measured from contrast angiography, which has been the "gold standard" for comparison. The most accurate echocardiographic method used to quantitate left ventricular volumes employs biplane images of the left ventricle in the apical four chamber and the apical long axis views, and the method of discs or modified Simpson's rule. One invaluable, unique feature of echocardiography is the ability to visualize the leaflets of the four cardiac valves in real time, and describe the textural characteristics as well as their opening and closing mechanics.

The combination of Doppler and two-dimensional echocardiographic imaging in valvular heart disease allows assessment of the hemodynamic effects of valve stenosis and regurgitation on right and left ventricular size and function, and estimation of transvalve gradients, valve orifice areas, and regurgitant fractions. Cardiac catheterization is now only necessary for determining the presence and severity of coexistent coronary artery disease, or for diagnostic purposes when the echocardiographic imaging is technically unsatisfactory. Doppler echocardiography is also used to select patients ideally suited for balloon valvuloplasty, to guide valve repair and replacement intraoperatively, to choose the optimal timing for surgical intervention, and to evaluate the efficacy of pharmacologic load perturbations in postponing surgery without compromising left ventricular function. Application of simple principles of fluid mechanics, for example the modified Bernoulli equation (vide infra), has enabled intracardiac hemodynamics to be calculated non-invasively, which correlate closely and consistently with conventional measurements made in the cardiac catheterization laboratory and thus have proved to be of significant clinical value.

Valvular heart disease

Mitral stenosis

The echocardiographic findings in rheumatic mitral stenosis are pathognomonic and demonstrate the mechanism of left ventricular inflow tract obstruction. The leaflets are thickened and motion restricted by fusion of the valve commissures, shortening, and cicatrization of the chordae tendineae, which insert into the tips of the valve leaflets; this gives the narrowed valve orifice a fish mouth-like opening in short axis, and a "hockey stick" deformity in long axis images (Figure 2.1). In the majority of patients with rheumatic mitral stenosis, the valve orifice area can be planimetered under direct vision and the values obtained correlate closely with those calculated from hemodynamic measurements made in the cardiac catheterization laboratory using the Gorlin equation. Doppler blood flow velocities across the stenotic mitral valve are increased, and from these

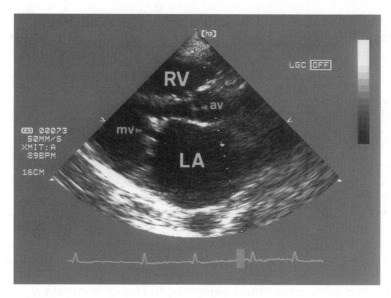

Figure 2.1 Two-dimensional echocardiogram in the parasternal long axis view shows the left atrium (LA), aortic valve (av), and mitral valve (mv). The LA is dilated (>4·0 cm), and the mv exhibits the characteristic features of rheumatic disease: thickened and calcified anterior and posterior leaflets, with restricted mobility. The anterior leaflet (more superior in figure) demonstrates the typical "hockey stick" deformity in diastole, and the narrowed valve orifice may also be seen (arrow). By contrast, the av leaflets are normal (thin) and just perceptible on the image. RV, right ventricle

recordings the peak and mean pressure gradients can be calculated, because velocity and pressure are related by a quadratic function. The relationship between the pressure drop (DP) across a stenotic valve is described by the Bernoulli equation:

$$DP = (p_2 - p_1) = 4 \times V^2$$

where V is the peak velocity recorded distal to the stenosis, p_2 is the pressure distal to the stenosis, and p_1 is the pressure proximal to the stenosis.

The pressure half time ($t_{1/2}$) can be estimated from the rate of velocity decay during diastole, from which the mitral valve orifice area (MVA) can be quantitated using the following equation:

$$MVA = 220/t_{1/2}$$

where 220 is an empiric constant.

The only remaining hemodynamic information to evaluate in the management of patients with mitral stenosis is the presence of concomitant mitral regurgitation or concomitant aortic or tricuspid valve disease, left ventricular function, and pulmonary arterial systolic pressure, all of which can be identified using Doppler echocardiography. The consequences of mitral stenosis are well seen echocardiographically, and consist of an enlarged left atrium and, if the stenosis is severe, pulmonary hypertension develops with enlargement of the right heart chambers and tricuspid regurgitation. To identify patients who are likely to benefit most from balloon valvuloplasty, assessment of the mitral leaflets and subvalve apparatus, and exclusion of significant mitral regurgitation are required. The likelihood of successful balloon mitral valvuloplasty decreases when the valve is heavily calcified, the valve leaflets and chordal structures are thickened and scarred, or when there is significant mitral regurgitation. Similarly, because there is no ideal prosthetic mitral valve replacement, primary valve repair is attempted whenever feasible, and patients are selected on echocardiographic assessment of the mitral valve unit as a whole.

Mitral regurgitation

The cause of mitral regurgitation can usually be ascertained by two-dimensional echocardiography, and is best classified in terms of abnormalities of the valve leaflet texture or motion, the subvalve apparatus, the valve annulus, or the left ventricle. The most striking abnormality of the mitral valve leaflets is caused by rheumatic heart disease or infective endocarditis, in which vegetations are adherent to the valve leaflets, usually from the atrial surface; this results in mitral regurgitation either by perforating or avulsing one or both leaflets, or by interfering with leaflet coaptation (Figure 2.2).

Systolic prolapse of the mitral valve leaflets is a common anomaly that predominates in asthenic women, and is associated with mitral regurgitation and symptoms of atypical chest pain and/or palpitations. Mitral valve prolapse can be unequivocally diagnosed by two-dimensional echocardiographic imaging of the mitral valve apparatus in the parasternal and apical long axis views of the left ventricle (Figure 2.3). The diagnosis is made in these imaging planes if any part of the valve leaflets or the coaptation point cross to the atrial side of the plane of the mitral valve ring by more than 2 mm (see Figure 2.3). When mitral regurgitation is demonstrated by color flow Doppler velocity mapping or thickened valves are seen, antibiotic prophylaxis against endocarditis is recommended for dental treatment.

Mitral regurgitation also frequently results from dilatation of the mitral valve annulus secondary to chronic enlargement of the left

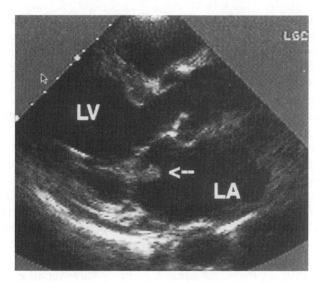

Figure 2.2 Parasternal long axis view demonstrating thickened leaflets and mobile vegetation (arrow) adherent to the mitral valve in a patient with infectious endocarditis. This patient developed endocarditis after a routine dental procedure without antibiotic prophylaxis in the setting of antecedent mitral valve prolapse. The left ventricular cavity (LV) and left atrium (LA) are also identified

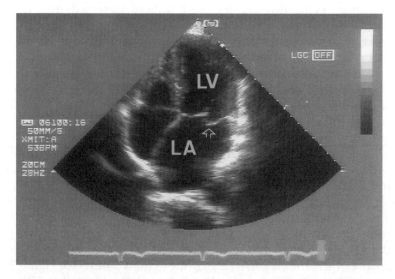

Figure 2.3 Apical four chamber view demonstrating a prolapsing segment of the posterior mitral valve leaflet (open arrow). Note that the leaflet prolapses nearly 1 cm into the left atrium (LA) from the normal plane of the mitral valve (scale to right in 1 cm graduations). The right atrium and right ventricle lie immediately adjacent to the LA and left ventricle (LV), respectively

ventricle, either from primary myocardial dysfunction or coronary artery disease. Dysfunction of the papillary muscles may occur transiently or permanently following inferior myocardial infarction, and this may seriously interfere with the complex mechanism of mitral valve closure, and result in severe mitral regurgitation.

Regardless of the etiology of the mitral regurgitation, the diagnosis is easily established by color flow Doppler mapping, and the effects on left ventricular cavity size and function can be assessed echocardiographically. However, evaluation of the severity of the mitral regurgitation is only semiquantitative (range: 1+ [mild] to 4+ [severe]), and for practical purposes is assessed by color flow Doppler mapping as the size of the regurgitant jet in orthogonal planes expressed as a ratio of left atrial size. The limitations of the Doppler color flow mapping method are that it does not take into account initial jet velocity, the compliance of the left atrium, jet impaction, and the gain settings of the ultrasonoscope. The amount of regurgitant flow can be approximated by calculating the volume of blood entering the left ventricle through the mitral valve and substracting from it the volume of blood ejected through the aortic valve, or by calculating the regurgitant fraction as the regurgitant volume divided by the total volume of blood entering the left ventricle. The volume of blood crossing the mitral or aortic valve during the cardiac cycle is quantitated as the product of the cross-sectional area of the flow stream and the area under the instantaneous velocity signal, known as the velocity time integral (VTI). Regurgitant flow volume and regurgitant fraction estimated by Doppler echocardiography in mitral regurgitation correlate well with those estimated at cardiac catheterization. Proximal to the regurgitant jet at the mitral valve level, there is a hemispherical zone of blood with laminar flow and increased velocity, which can be readily visualized using Doppler color flow mapping, known as the flow convergence zone. The gain settings on the ultrasonoscope can be arranged in such a way that a velocity amplitude can be assigned to the points describing the hemispherical interface at which aliasing occurs. The radius of this hemisphere relates directly to flow (Q), which can be determined from the following equation:

$$Q = (2 \pi r^2) \times V$$

where V is the preassigned aliasing velocity.

The volume of regurgitant flow calculated from Doppler color flow mapping correlates closely with angiographic estimates of the severity of mitral regurgitation. However, both non-invasive and invasive assessments of mitral regurgitation are only approximations, and work is in progress to develop more accurate methods for assessing the severity of regurgitant valvular lesions.

Aortic stenosis

Aortic stenosis may be congenital when it presents at any time from birth to adolescence or early adulthood with symptoms of dyspnea, chest pain, or syncope. It may be rheumatic in origin when there is concomitant mitral valve disease, or it may be due to degenerative or senile calcific stenosis of a tricuspid or bicuspid valve presenting in middle to old age. Aortic valve stenosis results in increased myocardial work, or pressure overload, which induces compensatory hypertrophy in an attempt to normalize left ventricular wall stress and maintain normal contractile function. Left ventricular hypertrophy, cavity volumes, and ejection fraction can readily be estimated echocardiographically, and the pressure gradient across the aortic valve calculated from Doppler velocity recordings obtained proximal and distal to the stenotic valve. The etiology of the aortic stenosis is usually obvious from two-dimensional echocardiography; the number of leaflets (tricuspid or bicuspid), leaflet texture, calcification and mobility, and the presence of coexistent aortic regurgitation are apparent. In aortic stenosis the magnitude of the transvalvular gradient is directly related to left ventricular contractile function. When left ventricular function is preserved, a high transvalvular pressure gradient indicates hemodynamically important aortic stenosis, whereas a low transvalve gradient is associated with mild aortic stenosis. However, when left ventricular function is impaired, a low transaortic valve pressure gradient is difficult to interpret because the left ventricle is unable to generate a high intracavity pressure. In this setting aortic valve orifice area must be calculated because it varies independently of left ventricular function.

Valve orifice area in aortic stenosis can be calculated using the continuity principle, or the law of conservation of momentum. This simply states that in a closed system (such as the cardiovascular system) in which resting cardiac output is relatively constant, the flow proximal to the stenosis is equal to the flow across the stenosis. If blood volume flow is calculated as the product of the flow velocity time integral (VTI) and the cross-sectional area (CSA) of the flow stream proximal to the stenotic aortic valve, and the increased velocity distal to the valve is recorded, then simple substitution in the continuity equation will enable the one unknown[3] (i.e. the aortic valve area CSA [distal]) to be calculated:

$$\text{VTI (proximal)} \times \text{CSA (proximal)} = \text{VTI (distal)} \times \text{CSA (distal)}$$

Non-invasive assessment of aortic valve area in patients with aortic stenosis by Doppler echocardiography correlates closely with hemodynamic measurements obtained invasively across the whole

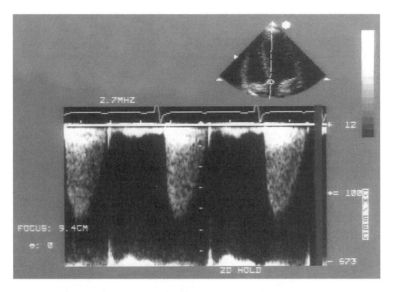

Figure 2.4 A continuous wave Doppler tracing measured across a severely stenotic valve demonstrates the velocity and direction of blood flow relative to the transducer. In this example of the five chamber view (insert at upper right), the continuous wave cursor is directed along a line from the left ventricular apex toward the aortic root. The Doppler velocity signal depicts flow away from the apex (negative values on scale; maximum is 673 cm/s) toward the ascending aorta, as expected. However, the velocity of the flow is significantly higher than normal (100–150 cm/s), at nearly 450 cm/s, which is related to the stenotic aortic valve. This Doppler tracing is used to calculate the velocity time integral for aortic valve area calculations

spectrum of disease severity (Figure 2.4).[4] Valve replacement surgery for aortic stenosis is performed when the patient becomes symptomatic, and the role of the echocardiographer is to demonstrate the presence of severe stenosis by transvalve gradient and a calculated valve orifice area of below 0·75 cm^2 (Figure 2.5).

Aortic regurgitation

The diagnosis of aortic regurgitation can be made with Doppler echocardiography when it is so mild that it is not clinically apparent; this is because the Doppler is very sensitive to high velocity aortic regurgitant flow. Although the presence of aortic regurgitation is easily detected by color flow Doppler, assessment of its severity remains a difficult problem. In addition, nearly one-third of patients with moderate to severe aortic regurgitation remain asymptomatic until late in the course of their disease.

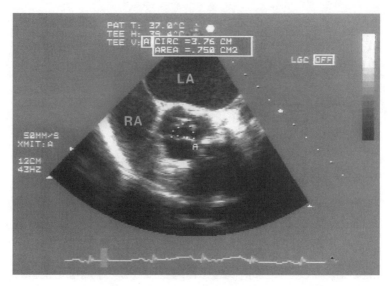

Figure 2.5 In this transesophageal echocardiogram, a short axis view of a stenotic aortic valve is shown. The three leaflets of the aortic valve are seen, which are thickened and calcified with severely decreased mobility. Aortic valve areas can also be estimated by planimetry, as shown. In this patient, the valve area was calculated to be 0·75 cm². The right atrium (RA) and the left atrium (LA) are also identified

Aortic regurgitation results in volume overload of the left ventricle and left ventricular dilatation, which by Laplace's law is associated with increased wall stress. Increased wall stress is a powerful stimulus for ventricular hypertrophy and a major determinant of contractile function, in that wall stress varies inversely with ejection fraction; thus, the higher the wall stress, the lower the ejection fraction. The left ventricular dilatation, hypertrophy and the diastolic regurgitant jet in the left ventricular outflow tract can very easily be detected by two-dimensional Doppler echocardiography, and ejection fraction can be estimated from cavity volume calculations. Importantly, ejection fraction in aortic regurgitation is extremely load dependent and may remain spuriously high and thereby mask the development of underlying irreversible left ventricular dysfunction. Early evidence of insidious left ventricular dysfunction can only be recognized by assessing load independent indices of contractile left ventricular function.

A number of measurements can be made with Doppler echocardiography in patients with aortic regurgitation to assess indirectly the degree of regurgitation. These include regurgitant fraction expressed as the ratio of the velocity time integrals of antegrade systolic (VTIa) and retrograde diastolic (VTIr) flows in the descending thoracic aorta (VTIr/VTIa); the pressure half-time from the Doppler velocity of regurgitant diastolic flow (the shorter the pressure half-time, the more severe the aortic regurgitation); and calculation of the cross-sectional area of the regurgitant aortic jet using the continuity equation during diastole. Initial studies using Doppler color flow velocity mapping of the regurgitant jet indicated that measurement of jet length from the aortic valve correlated with angiographic severity of aortic regurgitation. Subsequently, a better understanding of the factors that influence the length of the jet, such as left ventricular size, compliance, jet velocity, and jet impaction, have demonstrated that these are poor indicators of severity, and the only semiquantitative color Doppler measurement that is reliable is the ratio of the width of the regurgitant jet at the aortic valve and left ventricular outflow diameter. Although these latter assessments have aimed directly at quantitating the degree of aortic regurgitation, assessment of the impact of the aortic regurgitant volume on longitudinal measurements of left ventricular cavity size at end-diastole and end-systole, and ejection fraction have proved more useful prognostically.[5]

Tricuspid and pulmonary valve disease

The pulmonary and tricuspid valves can both be easily visualized in multiple planes from the left parasternal, apical, and subxiphoid regions. However, they are less frequently directly involved with intrinsic valve leaflet pathology than the aortic and mitral valves. Although the pulmonary and tricuspid valves may be involved in rheumatic heart disease and develop leaflet thickening and commissural fusion, this is no longer commonplace. Usually, the right sided cardiac valves are indirectly involved in rheumatic heart disease because of pulmonary hypertension, and secondary right ventricular hypertrophy, dilatation, and alteration in right ventricular chamber architecture associated with tricuspid and pulmonary valve regurgitation. The presence of tricuspid and pulmonary regurgitation are readily appreciated with color flow mapping. The peak velocity of the tricuspid regurgitant jet is used to estimate pulmonary artery systolic pressure, which has prognostic value for conservative and surgical management of patients with valvular and myocardial disease.

Pulmonary artery pressure can be calculated, providing the pulmonary valve is not stenosed, as follows. The Bernoulli equation is used to assess the pressure difference across the tricuspid valve from the peak velocity of the regurgitant jet ($4V^2$). To the result of that calculation is added either a clinical assessment of right atrial pressure from the height of the jugular venous pulse, or by adding 14 mmHg (a value derived from a regression correction of a comparison of simultaneous assessments of invasive and Doppler estimates of pulmonary artery systolic pressures).[6]

The tricuspid valve, and more rarely the pulmonary valve, may be the site of infective or non-infective thrombotic endocarditis either with or without left heart involvement in systemic illness with immune deficiency syndromes or intravenous drug abuse. In addition, the pulmonary valve may be congenitally stenosed either as an isolated anomaly or associated with a ventricular septal defect, part of complex congenital heart disease with narrowing of the right ventricular tract due to malalignment of the outlet septum (tetralogy of Fallot), or discordant connections between the ventricles and great arteries (transposition of the great arteries). Isolated pulmonary valve stenosis is identified by two-dimensional echocardiography because the valve leaflets dome during systole due to failure of the commissures to completely separate or due to dysplasia of the leaflets and valve ring. Furthermore, in children in whom the disease predominates, assessment of the transpulmonary systolic gradient by Doppler enables the severity of the stenosis to be evaluated and decisions made regarding optimal therapy.

Prosthetic valve replacement

Prosthetic cardiac valves can be divided into biological valves (porcine heterograft, homografts) and mechanical valves. The latter consist either of tilting disks (Bjork Shiley and St Jude) or central occluders, of which the ball and cage (Starr-Edwards) is the most common type. The echocardiographic appearance and Doppler hemodynamics of the individual prostheses varies widely. Unlike native cardiac valves, biological and mechanical prosthetic valves present a number of technical problems. This is because many of their components reflect most of the interrogating ultrasound and thereby appear very echogenic, and distort or attenuate ultrasound signals (both imaging and Doppler) returning from adjacent or deeper tissues. Other problems involve interrogation of the prosthetic poppet motion or opening and closing of the tilting disk(s), which are dependent on correct orientation of the ultrasound beam to the plane of blood flow through the prosthesis. In spite of these difficulties, Doppler echocardiography allows accurate assessment of the function of both biologic and mechanical prosthetic valves, quantitation of transvalve gradients and effective orifice areas, and detection of stenoses and perivalvular leaks.

One widely acknowledged problem with transthoracic two-dimensional echocardiography is the unequivocal diagnosis of vegetative infective endocarditis on prosthetic valves. Early recognition of prosthetic endocarditis is of paramount importance because the prognosis is poor. Furthermore, the longer the diagnosis is delayed, the greater the likelihood of adjacent abscess formation, prosthetic obstruction or incompetence, heart failure, and embolization. Therefore, when the clinical diagnosis of prosthetic endocarditis is suspected and the transthoracic two-dimensional echocardiographic diagnosis is equivocal, transesophageal echocardiography, with its superior imaging, is mandatory. Doppler echocardiographic examination of the varying types of prosthetic valves shows that they are all stenotic as compared with their native counterparts. The extent of the prosthetic stenosis can be calculated from the Bernoulli equation in terms of transvalve gradients, which depend on individual valve design, location, and effective orifice area.

Infective endocarditis

Endovascular infection may often be associated with vegetative lesions on the cardiac valve leaflets, which if undiagnosed may progress to leaflet perforation or avulsion, valve ring abscess, or penetrating sinus formation. Two-dimensional echocardiography is currently the most sensitive means of identifying and describing the location and morphology of valvular vegetations in infective endocarditis, and is invaluable in assessing their hemodynamic impact and the presence of complications.

The two-dimensional echocardiographic appearance of valvular vegetations is of shaggy mobile masses varying in size from 2 mm to several centimeters, which are attached to and move with the valve leaflets, interfering with the normal valve leaflet motion pattern (Figure 2.6). The size and mobility of valvular vegetations have recently been demonstrated to correlate with the likelihood of embolization, development of heart failure, and the need for emergent valve replacement. Numerous studies of infective endocarditis have shown that transthoracic two-dimensional echocardiography can detect vegetations in between 50% and 80% of patients, with a greater accuracy for identifying aortic valve vegetations. Detection of vegetations by transesophageal echocardiography is much better than with transthoracic echocardiography, with a sensitivity greater than 90% and a specificity of almost 100%.

Cardiomyopathy

"Cardiomyopathy" is a term that the World Health Organization has recommended be used only to describe primary disorders of the

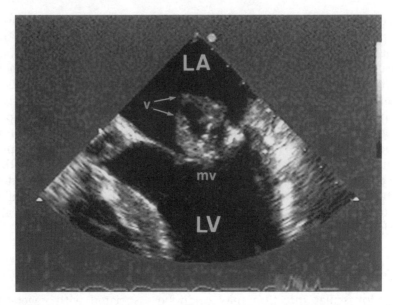

Figure 2.6 A transesophageal echocardiogram demonstrates the mitral valve (mv) and several mobile vegetations (v) attached to both the anterior and posterior leaflets. The left atrium (LA) and left ventricle (LV) are shown for orientation. Transesophageal echocardiography provides excellent views of the mitral valve and left atrium in clinical situations in which endocarditis or potential cardiac sources of embolism (e.g. atrial thrombus) must be evaluated

myocardium in which the etiology is unknown, and which may involve the left ventricle, both ventricles, or rarely the right ventricle alone.[2] However, cardiomyopathy has come to be used commonly to describe myocardial diseases in which the cause is well documented, and include coronary artery disease and cardiac amyloidosis. Traditionally, cardiomyopathy has been divided into three categories – hypertrophic, dilated and restrictive – on the basis of left ventricular architecture, systolic contractile function, and diastolic filling characteristics assessed by contrast angiography and by examination of autopsy specimens.

In dilated cardiomyopathy the left ventricle is markedly enlarged and there is severely impaired global contractile function, often with no recognizable etiology. Two-dimensional echocardiography clearly demonstrates that the increase in left ventricular radius far exceeds the increase in wall thickness, which results in abnormally high wall stress and reduced fractional shortening. The disproportionate increase in cavity size alters left ventricular architecture, and the change in cavity shape impacts on blood flow velocities so that stasis occurs, especially at the apex of the ventricle, which predisposes to thrombus formation (Figure 2.7). Thrombus in the left heart chambers

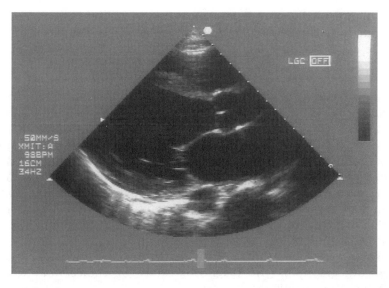

Figure 2.7 Left ventricular long axis image from the parasternal view illustrating a significantly dilated left ventricular cavity, as well as a mildly dilated left atrium. The normal cavity diameter in this plane is up to 5·5 cm, whereas this patient's ventricle measures nearly 7 cm. Cavity dilatation may occur as a result of valvular disease, a myopathic process, or longstanding hypertension

may be associated with systemic embolism (resulting in a stroke, and limb or organ ischemia) and, if present, anticoagulation should be instituted if it is not contraindicated. The left ventricular enlargement changes the geometry of the mitral valve apparatus and normal coaptation of the leaflets, resulting in varying degrees of mitral regurgitation. This in turn leads to further cavity enlargement and contractile dysfunction, as well as left atrial dilatation (see Figure 2.7). When contractile dysfunction involves the right ventricle, which it does in approximately two-thirds of patients with idiopathic dilated cardiomyopathy, the right heart chambers dilate with the concomitant onset of tricuspid valve regurgitation. Right and left sided atrioventricular valve regurgitation are frequently present in dilated cardiomyopathy and can be demonstrated unequivocally with color Doppler velocity flow mapping.

Hypertrophic cardiomyopathy is dominantly inherited and characterized by asymmetric left ventricular hypertrophy (in which the septum is at least 1·3 times thicker than the left ventricular wall), a normal or small left ventricular cavity, and systolic anterior motion of the mitral valve, with dynamic obstruction to left ventricular ejection (Figure 2.8). This type of cardiomyopathy predominantly affects the left ventricle, but may occasionally involve both ventricles.

The asymmetric hypertrophy usually occurs in the basal interventricular septum, but may involve the free ventricular wall or rarely be confined to the apex. The papillary muscles are hypertrophied and displaced anteriorly so that they encroach on the left ventricular outflow tract and predispose to systolic anterior motion of the mitral valve and dynamic systolic obstruction. Systolic contractile function is often supranormal, with ejection fractions in excess of 75% because of almost complete left ventricular obliteration in systole (see Figure 2.8). However, diastolic function may be impaired because of the extensive hypertrophy with reduced transmitral blood flow velocity during passive filling (E wave) and increased velocity during atrial contraction (A wave), with reversal of the normal E/A velocity ratio. In addition, mitral regurgitation occurs in more than half of patients with hypertrophic cardiomyopathy and is accompanied by left atrial dilatation. The left ventricular morphology and ejection dynamics described above are so consistent in hypertrophic cardiomyopathy that two-dimensional echocardiography is the diagnostic study of choice, and cardiac catheterization is only rarely necessary.

Restrictive cardiomyopathy is characterized by abnormal left ventricular diastolic filling, and patients usually present with congestive heart failure even though left ventricular cavity size, wall thickness, and systolic function may be normal. Cardiac amyloidosis is probably the most commonly occurring type of restrictive cardiomyopathy. The left and right ventricular and atrial walls in amyloid appear thickened on two-dimensional echocardiography because of deposition of a non-contractile protein in the intercellular spaces in the myocardium. The abnormal composition of the myocardium alters its acoustic impedance, which is detectable by the brighter appearance of the ventricular walls due to enhanced echo reflectance. This "stiffening" of the walls of the ventricles is associated with elevation in ventricular diastolic pressures, mitral and tricuspid valve regurgitation, and biatrial dilatation. The important impact on left ventricular filling is apparent as a spectrum of abnormalities in transmitral Doppler blood flow velocity patterns, which in their most severe and classic form consist of an increase in E wave velocity with a rapid deceleration slope (<150 ms duration) and a reduced or absent velocity signal during atrial contraction.[7] The early truncation of the passive diastolic phase of left ventricular filling corresponds with the abrupt early increase and subsequently unchanged left ventricular diastolic pressure, the so-called "dip and plateau" or "square root" sign in the diastolic pressure wave form. Two echocardiographic measurements that have proved to be of prognostic value in restrictive cardiomyopathy due to cardiac amyloidosis and of diagnostic value are left ventricular wall thickness and the duration of passive filling.

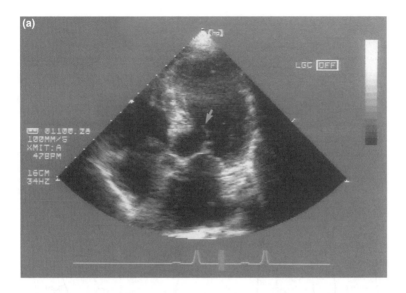

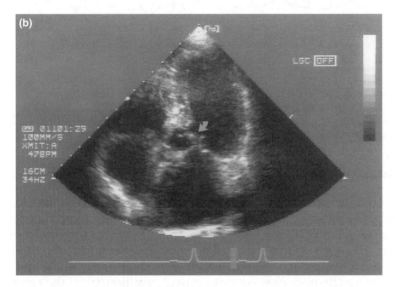

Figure 2.8 Apical five chamber view demonstrating asymmetric septal hypertrophy with systolic anterior motion of the mitral valve in **(a)** early and **(b)** late systole. The mitral apparatus (arrow) is seen to move toward the left ventricular outflow tract (between the left ventricle and aortic valve), and as systole progresses the mitral valve moves further into the outflow tract, resulting in mechanical obstruction to flow

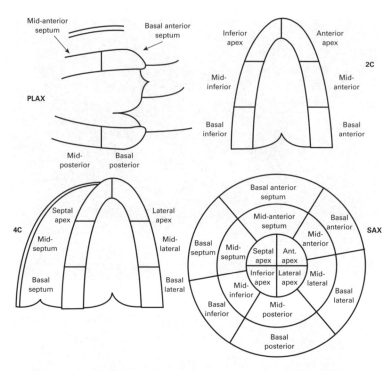

Figure 2.9 Diagrams illustrating segmental approach to nomenclature for wall motion analysis. The left parasternal long (PLAX) and apical four chamber (4C) views (left), as well as the apical two chamber (2C) and composite parasternal short axis (SAX) views (right) comprise the myocardial regions evaluated when assessing segmental function

Ischemic heart disease

Two-dimensional echocardiography is used extensively in exercise and pharmacologic stress testing for risk stratification, early detection of acute infarction, and characterizing left ventricular remodeling in survivors of myocardial infarction. The routine left parasternal views of the left ventricle in short axis and long axis, and the apical four and apical two chamber views serve to provide a silhouette of the coronary artery supply to the left ventricular myocardium (Figure 2.9). When coronary blood flow to a region of myocardium is insufficient for baseline metabolic function, systolic myocardial shortening is either absent or severely attenuated. Sudden and complete interruption of coronary flow in the absence of collateral flow results in myocardial necrosis, which can be recognized early as regional akinesis or dyskinesis (regional left ventricular wall motion abnormality) and at late follow up as a region of thinned and scarred heart wall. The size of the myocardial infarction relates to the extent of the region of contractile dysfunction, and the culprit coronary artery may be determined from the location of the left ventricular wall motion abnormality.

The effects of myocardial infarction on left ventricular size and function can be assessed echocardiographically repeatedly during episodes of hemodynamic instability early or late in the evolution of infarction. Important complications of acute myocardial infarction that necessitate early diagnosis include ventricular septal rupture, acute severe mitral regurgitation, right ventricular infarction, pericardial tamponade, infarct extension with left ventricular aneurysm formation, and heart failure. All of these infarct complications are readily detected with two-dimensional echocardiography. The process of postinfarction left ventricular remodeling has been characterized almost exclusively using echocardiography as a period of expansion of the necrotic infarct zone within the first several days, which is followed by a prolonged period of left ventricular enlargement over months or years that involves myocardium even remote from the infarction zone. Left ventricular size, ejection fraction, and end-systolic dimension have emerged as strong predictors of clinical outcome, and they may demonstrate the efficacy of strategies aimed at restoration of coronary artery patency and reduction in left ventricular loading conditions with vasodilator and angiotensin converting enzyme inhibitor therapies.

The presence of coronary artery disease before infarction can also be demonstrated, and is the fundamental premise upon which stress echocardiography is based. Coronary blood flow limitation and distribution at rest remains normal until a coronary artery stenosis exceeds 90–95% of the vessel diameter. Thus, echocardiographic regional left ventricular wall motion abnormalities may be absent at rest and only develop when there are multiple, similarly severe stenoses in more than one coronary artery, or when myocardial oxygen requirements are increased, as occurs with musculoskeletal exercise. For the purpose of semiquantitating the extent of myocardium at risk, the left ventricle has been divided into 16 wall segments based on the internal anatomy and the distribution of coronary artery blood supply, as recommended by the American Society of Echocardiography.[8] Regional left ventricular contractile function is graded in terms of wall motion as normal, hypokinetic, akinetic, or dyskinetic from 1 through 4 for each myocardial wall segment, and a total score divided by the number of wall segments assessed. These wall motion score indices correlate closely with biochemical assessments of myocardial infarct size. Stress echocardiography employs exercise stress or pharmacologic agents such as adenosine and dobutamine to increase oxygen demand, using conventional protocols that require estimation of wall motion score at rest and repeated either at peak stress or at predefined stages throughout the study protocol.

The appearance of new regional wall motion abnormalities or an increase in the size of the region of wall motion abnormality (involvement of adjacent or remote wall segments) during or after stress denotes the presence of an ischemic territory. There is a high degree of sensitivity and specificity for the correct detection of coronary artery stenoses when compared with perfusion scanning.[9] The limitation of echocardiographic stress testing is that high quality imaging of the entire left ventricle at baseline and during stress is a prerequisite for accurate interpretation.

Pericardial disease

In the normal heart the pericardium is only visible as an increased echo reflection from the surfaces of the visceral and parietal pericardium, which are in contact when there is no effusion. However, echocardiography plays a major role in the diagnosis of pericardial effusions and in assessing their size and impact on hemodynamic function. The pericardium is reflected off the great arteries onto the epicardial surface of the cardiac chambers anteriorly and laterally, around the cardiac apex, and onto the diaphragmatic surface up to the atrioventricular groove at the level of the inferior pulmonary veins. This creates a bare area or pericardial free space behind the left atrium. Use is made of this anatomic information and the spatial relations of the descending thoracic aorta for differentiating pericardial from pleural effusions. Fluid accumulating in the pericardial and pleural spaces appears as an echo-free region anterior and posterior to the heart. The echo-free space formed by a pericardial effusion is anterior to the descending thoracic aorta and is best visualized in the long axis view of the left ventricle from the left parasternal region (Figure 2.10). By contrast, pleural effusions are located lateral and posterior to the descending aorta, which is the most reliable echocardiographic feature for differentiating pleural from pericardial effusions.

Pericardial tamponade is a life-threatening yet correctable condition in which the pressure in the pericardial space is increased due either to rapid accumulation of a small volume of fluid or to chronic accumulation of large volumes of fluid. Thus, diastolic filling of the right and left heart chambers is compromised, with resultant reduction in cardiac output, hypotension, tachycardia, elevated jugular venous pressure, and arterial pulsus paradoxus. There are several echocardiographic findings that can be recorded from the apical four chamber view and, together with the clinical history and physical examination, they can secure the diagnosis of tamponade. The two-dimensional echocardiographic signs of tamponade consist of right atrial and, more importantly, right ventricular collapse with respiration in the presence of a variably sized pericardial effusion, and

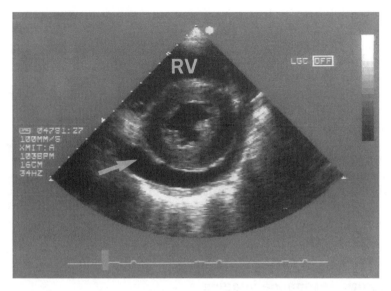

Figure 2.10 A moderate sized hypoechoic (dark) region representing a circumferential pericardial effusion (arrow) is seen in this parasternal short axis view of the left ventricle. The patient also has moderate left ventricular hypertrophy with normal cavity size. The clear space adjacent to the left ventricular septum is the right ventricular cavity (RV)

respiratory variation (>50%) in transmitral and trans-tricuspid Doppler blood flow velocities. When these clinical and confirmatory echocardiographic signs are present, they indicate the urgent need for pericardiocentesis to relieve the tamponade.

Another serious disease of the pericardium that requires definitive diagnosis is constrictive pericarditis, which is often difficult to differentiate from restrictive cardiomyopathy. The pericardium becomes thickened and may also be calcified with fusion of the visceral and parietal layers, either from longstanding tuberculous pericarditis or more commonly from viral pericarditis.

Congenital heart disease

Two commonly occurring congenital lesions that deserve consideration are atrial septal defects and ventricular septal defects, both of which are usually diagnosed in early childhood and are associated with shunting of blood from the higher pressure left heart to the lower pressure right heart chambers. Shunt flow from left to right increases pulmonary blood flow relative to systemic blood flow, which if uncorrected eventually leads to reactive pulmonary hypertension and, in its most severe form, to irreversible pulmonary vascular disease.

Defects in the interatrial septum and interventricular septum can usually be clearly visualized by transthoracic echocardiography using Doppler color flow velocity mapping. When there is difficulty in making the definitive diagnosis clinically, which is more common with atrial septal defects, it may be established unequivocally by transesophageal echocardiography, with which the defects can be visualized directly. The effects of intracardiac shunting at atrial and at ventricular levels can be assessed indirectly in terms of right heart size and function, or pulmonary artery systolic pressure; or directly by quantitating the ratio of pulmonary (Q_p) and aortic (Q_s) blood volume flows (Q_p/Q_s), which are calculated as the respective products of Doppler flow velocity time integrals and cross-sectional areas of the two great arteries.

Magnetic resonance imaging

Magnetic resonance imaging (MRI) provides excellent definition of anatomic structure, assessment of cardiac function, and measurement of blood flow velocity and flow direction.[10] In addition, myocardial metabolism can be evaluated with magnetic resonance spectroscopic techniques at rest and during stress testing, providing information regarding myocardial perfusion. The principle involved in use of nuclear magnetic resonance to construct images of the heart is excitation of the constitutive atoms in a high power magnetic field by radiofrequency energy. The MRI scanner detects the signal produced by the atoms of the heart as they relax or return to their equilibrium energy state. Hydrogen atoms, which are ubiquitous in the body, are most commonly used for magnetic resonance imaging purposes; however, phosphorus or carbon may be used when assessing myocardial metabolism. Differences in tissue composition (muscle, fat, liver, etc.) alter proton relaxation properties and thereby permit differentiation of the tissues from one another. In particular, abnormal myocardial tissue (for example, infarcted or infiltrated by sarcoidosis) can often be detected even before wall thinning or conduction abnormalities occur.

MRI produces images with excellent spatial resolution, and is probably the best technique for complete tomographic imaging of the heart in any planar orientation. The rapid imaging sequence and acquisition with three-dimensional reconstruction algorithms enable detailed assessment of the anatomy of the cardiac chambers, great vessels, and their intrathoracic relations. For this reason MRI is the diagnostic modality of choice for investigating abnormalities of the

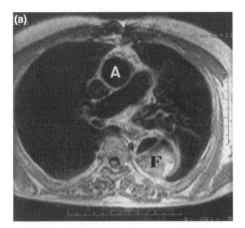 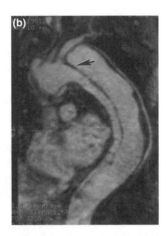

Figure 2.11 (a) Spin echo and **(b)** three-dimensional gadolinium contrast-enhanced magnetic resonance images demonstrating a dissection of the descending aorta. In the transaxial plane **(a)**, the ascending aorta (A) is normal but the descending aorta is dilated and contains a dissection flap that separates the true from the false (F) lumen. Vascular structures containing rapidly moving blood appear dark on spin echo magnetic resonance imaging, whereas slower moving blood has a brighter signal. Thus, the true lumen is dark and the false lumen appears brighter in these images. In the oblique sagittal plane image **(b)**, the dissection flap (arrow) is seen to extend from just distal to the left subclavian artery to the abdominal aorta

pulmonary arterial tree and of the aorta, and in particular for dissecting aortic aneurysms in which precise knowledge of the location of the dissected intimal flap is pivotal in diagnosis, treatment, and surgical repair (Figure 2.11).[11] Echocardiography provides better temporal resolution than MRI, and is therefore better for examining the morphology of rapidly moving structures such as cardiac valves. However, gating the MRI signals to the simultaneously recorded electrocardiographic QRS complex enables dynamic events during the cardiac cycle to be readily appreciated. Assessment of cardiac function including wall motion, wall thickening, and change in chamber size and volume can easily be quantitated.

Stress testing

If the heart or the coronary arteries are diseased, then the heart may not be able to meet the increased metabolic requirements of exercise, and evidence of cardiac disease may only be unveiled when the heart is stressed.

Cardiac stress tests are designed to quantitate the cardiovascular responses to controlled incremental increases in metabolic demands using conventional protocols. Stress tests fall into two categories: physical exercise and pharmacologic. Irrespective of the type of stress test protocol used, the measurements routinely obtained include heart rate and blood pressure, electrocardiograms at each incremental increase in workload, and a continuous account of symptoms. Stress testing is frequently performed in combination with imaging techniques, or various nuclear cardiac imaging techniques, which allow additional measurements to be made during stress testing, including ventricular contractile performance (i.e. ejection fraction, regional left ventricular wall motion, and myocardial perfusion and metabolism).

Exercise stress tests

Exercise stress tests are conducted either on a treadmill or a bicycle ergometer. Exercise is begun at a low workload that the patient can easily sustain. The workload is then increased in increments at regular intervals predefined by the exercise protocol until the patient:

- achieves the maximum exercise workload of the protocol
- achieves 85% of their predicted heart rate for age and sex
- achieves his or her anaerobic threshold
- develops typical symptoms with electrocardiographic evidence of ischemia
- becomes hypotensive, or
- develops ventricular dysrhythmias.

All of these are reasons to terminate any and every stress test, whether exercise or pharmacologic.

Pharmacologic stress tests

Pharmacologic stress tests are used in patients who cannot engage in physical exercise for various reasons. They are conducted by administering a drug that either increases myocardial workload (dobutamine) or vasodilates the coronary microvasculature (dipyridamole or adenosine).

Abnormal findings

Abnormal findings during stress that reflect impaired performance of the coronary circulation and the myocardium are as follows.

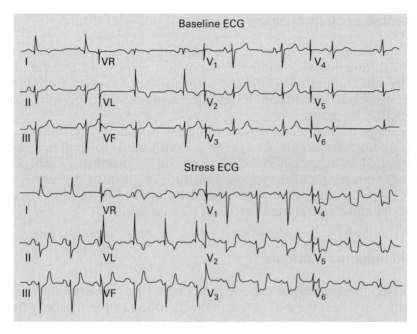

Figure 2.12 A pre-exercise (upper) and post-exercise (lower) 12-lead electrocardiogram (ECG) demonstrating normal ST segments at rest, which become significantly depressed (below baseline) diffusely in both anterolateral (leads V$_2$–V$_6$) and inferior (leads II, III, and aVF) distribution. The diffuse changes and ST elevation in lead aVR suggest severe left mainstem or proximal left anterior descending coronary artery stenosis as the anatomic lesion responsible for the electrocardiographic abnormalities

- Characteristic electrocardiographic changes occur during exercise when the increased myocardial metabolic activity provokes myocardial ischemia, that is ≥2 mm of planar depression of the ST segments in the electrocardiographic leads that represent the distribution of the stenotic coronary artery (Figure 2.12).
- Myocardial ischemia is frequently accompanied by a decline in left ventricular contractile performance heralded by hypotension, which denotes proximal severe triple coronary artery stenoses, stenosis of the left main coronary artery, or ventricular dysfunction. Decline in left ventricular contractile function can be detected by imaging studies conducted during or immediately following stress.
- The increased cardiac workload associated with stress may provoke abnormalities and non-uniformities of myocardial coronary perfusion, which may be detected by imaging studies conducted immediately following stress. Alternatively, they may result in electrical irritability and ventricular arrhythmias that are evident electrocardiographically.

Cardiac nuclear imaging

Cardiac nuclear imaging provides important information on cardiac function by employing radiotracer techniques and external detection equipment. The most frequently used nuclear techniques are myocardial perfusion imaging, radionuclide angiography, and metabolic imaging.

Cardiac nuclear imaging is based on the detection of γ rays emitted by radiopharmaceutical agents administered to patients and measured by large detectors (i.e. γ cameras) outside the body. The images created represent various functions of the heart depending on the type of radiopharmaceutical employed. We briefly discuss radiopharmaceuticals and detection systems below.

Radiopharmaceuticals

Radiopharmaceuticals are compounds that have two distinct elements. One is the radioactive material, called a radionuclide, which is attached to a molecule that distributes in the body according to a given physiologic function. Radionuclides are unstable elements that decay to a more stable state by emitting particles or photons from their nuclei that can be detected. This process is called radioactive decay. In general, radioactive decay may occur in one of three forms: α, β, and γ. Both α and β decay involve the emission of particles, whereas γ decay is characterized by the emission of γ rays (electromagnetic radiation). Clinical nuclear imaging is based entirely on γ emitting radionuclides because γ rays pose the least harmful effect to tissues while having sufficient penetrating power to traverse the body tissues and be detected externally.

The most widely used radionuclide for clinical testing is technetium-99m (Tc-99m). This radionuclide is produced by a generator made of molybdenum-99, which decays to Tc-99m and emits γ rays of 140 KeV (kiloelectron volts) energy. Tc-99m decays with a half-life of 6 hours. Another type of radionuclide used in cardiac imaging is the positron emitting radioisotope. This element decays by emitting a "positron" from the nuclei, which is a particle of the same energy (511 KeV) as an electron but is positively charged. This particle immediately interacts with an electron in the surrounding matter in a process known as annihilation. Two γ rays of the same energy and opposite direction are emitted from that process. An example of a positron emitting radionuclide is fluorine-18, which has a half-life of 110 min.

The radionuclides above can be attached to other molecules that have a known distribution in the body and thus form a radiopharmaceutical agent. An example of a radiopharmaceutical is Tc-99m sestamibi, which is a myocardial blood flow (MBF) tracer made of two components: the radionuclide (i.e. Tc-99m) and the pharmaceutical (i.e. sestamibi). Sestamibi distributes in the myocardium in proportion to MBF, and its distribution pattern can be detected because of the presence of technetium in the molecule. In patients who have suffered heart attacks, abnormal distribution of tracer helps to define the area of infarction.[12]

Detection systems

The overall principle of the detection system is based on the theory that certain types of crystal emit light when struck by γ rays. One example of this type of crystal is sodium iodide, which is used in most clinical scanners. The light output of the crystal is amplified many times by photomultiplier tubes and by complex electronic circuitry. This light output can be localized to represent a three-dimensional map of radionuclide distribution within the myocardium. With the aid of computers, this information is digitized and images produced and displayed on computer screens or x ray film.

Large detectors, called γ cameras, are used to image large parts of the body. The cameras may produce a single image in a given projection (planar technique) with respect to the organ of interest (for example, heart or liver), or multiple projections that can be reconstructed into images known as tomograms. The advantage of the tomographic method is that the three-dimensional distribution of the radiopharmaceutical may be determined in detail while avoiding the overlap of structures that occurs with planar images. This technique is called single photon emission computed tomography (SPECT) and is designed to image radionuclides that emit single photons. The other major technique available is known as positron emission tomography (PET), which is an imaging method used to detect positron emitting radionuclides. This is a more complex, but more accurate method and is based on a principle called coincidence counting. Positron emitting isotopes decay by giving off two γ rays in exactly opposite directions, each with the same energy. Using sophisticated electronics, the origin of the γ rays may be localized within the body more precisely, resulting in a three-dimensional map of perfusion or metabolism, depending on the tracer used (see below).

Myocardial perfusion imaging

Myocardial perfusion tracers are used to estimate non-invasively the relative amounts of blood flow to various regions of the heart.

Table 2.1 Summary of tracers used in myocardial perfusion imaging

Type of tracer		Examples
Retained in myocardium	Mechanical retention (based on microsphere size)	Technetium-99,[*] carbon-11[†] or gallium-68[†] labeled albumin microspheres
	Metabolic retention	Thallium,[*] rubidium-82,[†] potassium analogs (Na/K energy requiring pump), nitrogen-13 ammonia[†] (retained as glutamine)
	Retained in proportion to electrical membrane gradients	Technetium-99 sestamibi
Diffusible	Hydrophilic	Oxygen-15 water[†]
	Lipophilic	Carbon-11 or oxygen-14 butanol[†]
Partially diffusible		Technetium-99 teboroxime[*]

These tracers may be used in [*]single photon emission computed tomography (SPECT) and [†]positron emission tomography (PET).

This test is the most commonly used technique in cardiac nuclear imaging. In this section we briefly discuss the various radiotracers available for the assessment of regional myocardial perfusion. We review a number of tracers based on the mechanism by which these radiopharmaceuticals measure MBF.

Broadly speaking, there are two major categories of myocardial perfusion tracers (Table 2.1): those that are retained in the myocardium and those that are diffusible.

Mechanically retained, or labeled albumin microspheres are not used clinically because they are large particles (15 μm in diameter), which if injected intravenously become trapped in the lung capillaries rather than in the myocardium. In order to be used as myocardial perfusion tracers, these microspheres must be injected into the left sided circulation via a catheter placed into the left atrium or ventricle, which involves a more invasive procedure.

Tracers retained in the myocardium via non-mechanical means are the most commonly used perfusion agents in clinical practice. These tracers are retained in the myocardium in proportion to MBF, and include thallium-201 and Tc-99m sestamibi for SPECT imaging, and nitrogen-13-ammonia and rubidium-82 for PET imaging.

The retention process takes place during the first few minutes after tracer injection, and the distribution of activity represents the blood flow at the time of the injection. This characteristic allows us to image patients beginning several minutes after the injection, and permits longer scan times, which improves image resolution. Further improvements in resolution are possible using a new acquisition method synchronized to the cardiac cycle, which also provides information on left ventricular wall thickening – a measure of regional function. The ability of tracers to remain in the myocardium for minutes to hours after administration allows us to perform interventions such as exercise or pharmacologic stress testing in patients and then image MBF during flexible time intervals afterward. The most typical example is the perfusion study performed with exercise. Exercise is performed in the exercise laboratory, adjacent to the imaging room, with patients using a treadmill or bicycle ergometer. The perfusion tracer is administered at peak exercise, and the patient is allowed to recover for a few minutes to an hour (depending on the radioisotope), followed by perfusion imaging. Typically, with thallium agents, a resting scan is performed approximately 3 hours after the stress imaging, to allow for comparison with the stress state (Figure 2.13). A smaller dose of thallium is usually given just before the rest image in order to detect better ischemic but viable myocardium. Patients with severely ischemic myocardium may be imaged at 24 hours to allow for further redistribution of the isotope. Using a tracer with a longer half-life and higher energy such as technetium sestamibi has an important practical advantage in that higher quality images are obtained. Thus, the stress intervention can be performed before the resting examination and, should the stress perfusion images be normal, this will eliminate the need for a resting examination.

None of the diffusible tracers are used clinically because of the complicated scanning techniques required. However, these techniques are very accurate for quantifying MBF and are used mainly for clinical research. An example of this group of agents is oxygen-15 water, which is employed with PET scanning.

Imaging protocols Myocardial perfusion imaging is usually performed with some form of stress test when used for the diagnosis of coronary artery disease (CAD) or for evaluation of treatment in patients with known CAD (for example, angioplasty, bypass surgery, or medications). Stress testing is necessary to detect regional differences in myocardial perfusion due to occlusive CAD, because MBF at rest is not decreased even in the presence of coronary stenoses with up to 80% reduction in normal vessel diameter. By increasing MBF with exercise or coronary vasodilators such as dipyridamole or adenosine, myocardial regions supplied by significantly diseased coronary vessels may be detected because of their inability to increase MBF to a degree similar to that in regions supplied by normal vessels.

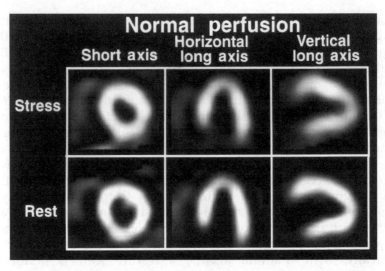

Figure 2.13 A normal thallium perfusion scan is shown that illustrates the three views used for planar clinical cardiac imaging. In the short axis view the right ventricle is faintly seen to the left of the image, adjacent to the interventricular septum. The left ventricular (LV) lateral wall is seen to the right of the image. In the horizontal long axis image, the LV apex is at the top of the image, and the lateral wall is to the right. In the vertical long axis view, the anteroseptum is seen at the top of the image, and the LV apex is to the right. Note the homogeneous intensity pattern in all LV myocardial regions

Given that the radiopharmaceuticals are carried in the blood and extracted by the myocardium, significantly less tracer is distributed to areas supplied by diseased vessels, and therefore the total amount of radiotracer delivered to these regions is less than to normal areas. This result produces a low intensity segment, or defect, on the scan in regions subserved by diseased vessels, and permits not only the detection of the presence of CAD but also assists with localizing the disease to specific coronary arteries (Figure 2.14).

The most frequently used stress test in clinical practice is the exercise test. With exercise, there is an increment in heart rate, blood pressure, and contractility that increases with myocardial metabolism, and in turn increases MBF in order to increase oxygen delivery to meet the increased myocardial oxygen demand. An appropriate increment in MBF in response to the oxygen demand can be reached in those segments of the myocardium that are supplied by non-stenotic arteries. This increment in MBF with maximal exercise or maximal vasodilatation is called the coronary flow reserve, and is approximately three to four times the normal resting MBF.

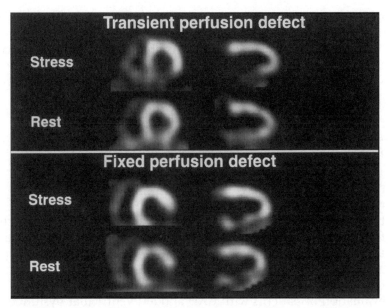

Figure 2.14 Perfusion defects. A transient perfusion defect is seen in the upper panel that is consistent with exercise-induced ischemia. During stress, the inferior walls in both the short axis and vertical long axis views exhibit decreased signal intensity, and therefore decreased perfusion, relative to the remaining walls. The signal intensity normalizes or reverses in the resting image, demonstrating a reversible defect. In the lower panel, a fixed defect in a similar location is shown. A defect noted on the stress images show no reversibility upon rest, which is consistent with infarction or non-viable tissue. Reinjection of a small amount of thallium at the time of rest images improves detection of severely ischemic but viable myocardium

However, in segments perfused by a stenotic artery there is an additional resistance in the vessel that prevents an appropriate increment in MBF. Therefore, patients with CAD will not match their increased myocardial oxygen demand, resulting in an imbalance between oxygen demand and supply and producing myocardial ischemia. This supply/demand mismatch and ischemia may result in a typical syndrome of retrosternal chest pain associated with sweating, shortness of breath, and radiation of the pain along the left arm to the elbow or fingers (angina). In other patients, there may be few or no symptoms at all, despite electrocardiographic changes demonstrating myocardial ischemia (silent ischemia). Under these conditions normally perfused myocardium will demonstrate high MBF and the region supplied by the stenotic vessel will have lower MBF. If we inject a myocardial perfusion tracer at this point, the resulting image will show a regional perfusion imbalance or defect that is not present in a resting image, when MBF would be more comparable.

There are pharmacologic stress tests that can be used to provoke these same transient perfusion defects, which involve the use of potent coronary vasodilators or β-agonists that increase myocardial oxygen consumption in a similar manner to exercise.

Clinical applications The major clinical applications of myocardial perfusion imaging are:

- diagnosis of CAD
- risk stratification in patients with known chronic CAD
- treatment evaluation in patients with known CAD, in particular following revascularization techniques such as percutaneous transluminal coronary angioplasty or coronary artery bypass grafting
- risk stratification after acute myocardial infarction
- evaluation of patients with CAD and left ventricular dysfunction
- evaluation of patients with "silent ischemia".

Radionuclide angiography

Ventricular function is most commonly assessed with a technique called multigated image acquisition scanning, which uses a "blood pool" method approach. Blood labeled with technetium-99 remains in the intravascular space, or blood pool, and provides a means to measure the end-diastolic and end-systolic volumes (EDV and ESV, respectively) of the heart non-invasively. The ejection fraction, or (EDV − ESV)/EDV, is a common measure of global ventricular performance. If a stress test is performed after baseline imaging, then the cardiac "reserve" can be estimated, with a fall in exercise ejection fraction indicating abnormal reserve.

Metabolic imaging

PET scanning is a technique that can assess myocardial perfusion and metabolism somewhat more rigorously than thallium scanning.[13] Nitrogen-13-ammonia is a common perfusion isotope, while [18]fluorine deoxyglucose is used as the metabolic tracer that evaluates the ability of myocytes to use glucose (Figure 2.15). One potential advantage to PET scanning is that the study may be performed at rest; however, the use of the above isotopes requires a cyclotron for production.

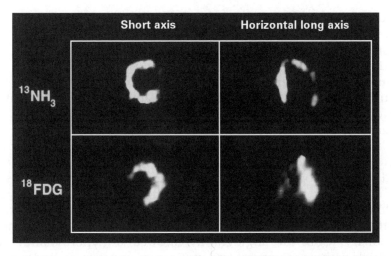

Figure 2.15 In this positron emission tomography (PET) image, the perfusion agent nitrogen-13 ammonia ($^{13}NH_3$; upper panels) demonstrates decreased resting blood flow to the lateral wall, as seen in both the short axis and horizontal long axis views. The metabolic tracer 2-deoxy-2-[^{18}F]fluoro-D-glucose (^{18}FDG) depicts regions in which the conversion from free fatty acid substrate use (normal metabolism) to glycolytic metabolism (ischemic zones) has occurred. High signal intensities in the ^{18}FDG images (bottom panels) are seen in segments corresponding to the hypoperfused regions, which is indicative of ischemia-related changes in metabolism

Case studies

Case 2.1

A 32-year-old male tax accountant presented with a 2 year history of progressive shortness of breath on exertion such that he could only walk two blocks on flat ground or climb five stairs. He had never complained of chest pain or palpitations, and was a non-smoker and non-drinker.

When aged 15 years, at a school sports medical examination, a cardiac murmur was detected. In his remote past he had sustained two unexplained syncopal episodes that were unrelated to exertion or posture. His father, who had always enjoyed good health as an active athlete and non-smoker, died suddenly from a "heart attack" at age 37 years. His father's death prompted an office visit to a cardiologist who, in addition to eliciting an ejection systolic murmur at the left sternal edge, recorded a 12-lead electrocardiogram, which revealed left ventricular hypertrophy and repolarization abnormalities. A clinical working diagnosis of congenital aortic valve stenosis was made, and an outpatient two-dimensional echocardiogram was scheduled, which excluded aortic valve stenosis, but showed left ventricular hypertrophy with normal systolic function, and no further recommendations were made. At age 30 years he noticed reduction in his exercise tolerance and was found to have moderate mitral regurgitation, and because of the family history of premature heart disease he underwent cardiac catheterization and coronary arteriography.

Catheterization demonstrated a cardiac index of 4·1 l/min per m²; ejection fraction 73%; end-diastolic volume index 55 ml/m²; end-systolic volume index 15 ml/m²; left ventricular pressure 135/23 mmHg; aortic pressure 102/65 mmHg; a "v" wave in the pulmonary capillary wedge pressure of 41 mmHg; pulmonary artery systolic pressure 46 mmHg; and right atrial pressure 9/7 mmHg (mean 6 mmHg). Contrast angiography showed a hyperdynamic left ventricle with no segmental wall motion abnormality, grade 3+ mitral regurgitation, an enlarged left atrium, and normal coronary arteries. In view of the progressive reduction in exercise capacity, the moderate pulmonary hypertension, and moderately severe mitral regurgitation, he was referred for mitral valve repair/replacement.

Examination. Physical examination: the patient was comfortable lying flat. Pulse: 78 beats/min, brisk upstroke, full volume. Blood pressure: 105/60 mmHg in the right arm. Jugular venous pulse: normal. Cardiac impulse: forceful, double impulse, regular rhythm. First heart sound: normal. Second heart sound: reversed splitting. Fourth heart sound was present. Apical grade 3/6 holosystolic murmur radiating to axilla, grade 2/6 ejection systolic murmur at mid-left sternal edge, which increased with Valsalva. Chest examination: normal air entry, no rales or rhonchi. Abdominal examination: soft abdomen, no tenderness, and no masses. Normal liver span. No peripheral edema. Femoral, popliteal, posterior tibial, and dorsalis pedis pulses: all normal volume and equal. Carotid pulses: full volume, rapid upstroke, no bruits. Optic fundi: normal.

Investigations. Laboratory findings: normal. Electrocardiogram: sinus rhythm at 78 beats/min, normal intervals and frontal QRS axis, severe left ventricular hypertrophy with small Q waves, and 2 mm ST segment depression and T-wave inversion in leads V_4 through V_6 consistent with strain or lateral ischemia. Chest *x* ray: mild cardiomegaly with left atrial enlargement and normal lung fields. 24-Hour ambulatory electrocardiographic monitoring: predominant cardiac rhythm was sinus, occasional isolated premature ventricular depolarizations, and three episodes of non-sustained ventricular tachycardia, with the longest being an 11-beat run at a maximum rate of 178 beats/min.

Transthoracic   two-dimensional   echocardiogram.   Asymmetric hypertrophy of the interventricular septum; a small hyperdynamic left ventricle; systolic anterior motion of the mitral valve; a 30 mmHg left ventricular outflow tract gradient in systole at rest, which increased to 64 mmHg with Valsalva in late systole; enlarged left atrium; and moderately severe mitral regurgitation by color flow Doppler velocity mapping.

Clinical course. The patient underwent mitral valve surgery, from which he made an excellent recovery and was discharged from hospital on postoperative day 7 on β-adrenergic blocking agents. At 3 month follow up his exercise tolerance had increased to 12 blocks on flat ground.

Questions

1. What are the differential diagnoses of a systolic murmur and electrocardiographic left ventricular hypertrophy?
2. What is the diagnosis in this patient, and on what clinical and echocardiographic criteria is the correct diagnosis based?
3. The patient married 6 months after discharge from hospital and wished to start a family. What is the pattern of genetic inheritance of his disease and how would you counsel the patient in this regard?
4. Explain the mechanism of the increase in left ventricular outflow tract gradient with Valsalva.
5. Why was the patient placed on β-adrenergic receptor blocking agents?
6. What is the prognostic significance of non-sustained ventricular tachycardia in this disease?

Answers

Answer to question 1   The differential diagnosis of an ejection systolic murmur and left ventricular hypertrophy by electrocardiography includes discrete anatomic lesions causing obstruction to left ventricular ejection and increased pressure work on the left ventricle; discrete subaortic stenosis; aortic valve stenosis; supravalvular stenosis; bicuspid aortic valve with associated coarctation of the aorta; hypertrophic obstructive cardiomyopathy; and systemic hypertension with an unrelated innocent systolic murmur.

Answer to question 2   The diagnosis in this patient was hypertrophic obstructive cardiomyopathy. This diagnosis was based clinically on the auscultatory findings of an ejection systolic murmur with a forceful double apical impulse, brisk pulses with rapid upstroke to the carotid pulses, and augmentation of the cardiac murmur with Valsalva. The confirmatory two-dimensional echocardiographic findings comprised asymmetric septal hypertrophy, systolic obliteration of the left ventricular cavity with supranormal ejection fraction, systolic anterior motion of the mitral valve, with the left ventricular outflow tract gradient at rest increasing with Valsalva in late systole.

Answer to question 3 The genetic pattern of inheritance of hypertrophic cardiomyopathy is dominant, and the patient should be counseled so that he is cognizant of the likelihood of his progeny having the same disease. The sudden and unexpected death of his father, who was otherwise healthy, suggests that he had died from the same disease.

Answer to question 4 Valsalva increases intra-thoracic pressure and reduces venous return to the heart so that left ventricular end-diastolic volume is reduced and systolic anterior motion of the mitral valve more easily obstructs the left ventricular outflow tract and thereby augments the systolic gradient.

Answer to question 5 The patient was placed on β-adrenergic receptor blocking agents to reduce augmentation of the systolic outflow tract gradients in order to prevent or attenuate the increase in left ventricular outflow tract gradient with exercise, which is at least partly mediated by increased catecholamines. Another reason is to slow the heart rate, which allows longer diastolic filling and greater left ventricular end-diastolic volume. Furthermore, β-adrenergic blocking agents may be efficacious in the treatment of non-sustained ventricular tachycardia.

Answer to question 6 Non-sustained ventricular tachycardia correlates with sudden death, which accounts for the yearly attrition rate of approximately 5–8% of patients with familial hypertrophic cardiomyopathy.

Case 2.2

A 47-year-old female Asian immigrant was brought to the emergency room with a dominant sided dense hemiplegia and severe expressive dysphasia. The history obtained from a relative was limited but included long-term shortness of breath on minimal exercise and at night, requiring three pillows to sleep, and weight loss over the previous 6 months.

In early childhood she spent 1 year away from school convalescing following an acute illness, which consisted of a painful migratory arthralgia with swelling of both knees and ankles but with no other stigmata. She was discouraged from playing games and took penicillin tablets once daily until adulthood. She remained well and next saw a physician during the last trimester of her second pregnancy, when she developed an episode of palpitations and became light-headed. When she was seen by a cardiologist she was in regular rhythm and in no distress. However, a murmur was detected, which was thought to be due to increased blood flow velocity associated with the volume overload state of pregnancy, and no follow up was arranged.

Five years later she noted progressive shortness of breath, intermittent palpitations provoked by exertion, and was finally admitted for investigation following hemoptysis. She declined cardiac catheterization but agreed to have an echocardiogram and was discharged home on digoxin 0·25 mg/day, furosemide 40 mg/day, potassium supplements, and warfarin at a dose to maintain an International Normalized Ratio of 2·5–3·0.

Examination. Physical examination: the patient had a right-sided neurologic deficit. She was only comfortable at 45°. Pulse: 152 beats/min, irregularly irregular. Blood pressure: 95/70 mmHg. Jugular venous pulse: 12 cm at 45°. Cardiac impulse: parasternal lift, palpable P_2. First heart sound: loud. Second heart sound: split with loud P_2. At apex was opening snap close to P_2. Mid-diastolic murmur at apex. Chest examination: normal air entry, basal crepitations. Abdominal examination: enlarged, tender liver. No peripheral edema. Carotid pulses: normal, no bruits.

Investigations. Laboratory findings: normal hemoglobin, hematocrit, white blood cell count, platelets, electrolytes, and creatinine. Aspartate aminotransferase 198 U/l (3·3 μkat/l); alanine aminotransferase 33 U/l (5·6 μkat/l); International Normalized Ratio 1·3. Electrocardiogram: atrial fibrillation at 167 beats/min, right axis deviation, right ventricular hypertrophy, and T-wave and ST-segment depression throughout the limb and chest leads. Chest *x* ray: cardiomegaly, enlargement of the left and right atria and main pulmonary artery, prominence of the left atrial appendage, and elevation in the left main bronchus at the carina. Calcification of the mitral annulus, small left pleural effusion, septal (Kerley B) lines, and cephalization of the upper lobes of the lung were also noted.

Echocardiogram. Echocardiography demonstrated a heavily calcified, severely stenotic mitral valve with shortened chordae, and calcification extending from the valve leaflets to the tips of the papillary muscles, but with no mitral regurgitation. Left ventricular size, wall thickness, and function were normal. The left atrium was dilated with laminated mural thrombus on the left atrial wall behind the posterior aortic root. The aortic valve was trileaflet and normal, the right atrium and right ventricle were both dilated with moderate tricuspid regurgitation through a normal tricuspid valve. A small hemodynamically unimportant pericardial effusion was present. Doppler assessment revealed a peak gradient across the mitral valve of 28 mmHg (mean 14 mmHg) and a valve orifice area of 0·7 cm^2 calculated from the pressure half-time, and a pulmonary artery systolic pressure of 68 mmHg calculated from the tricuspid regurgitant jet.

Hospital course. The patient was not considered a candidate for mitral balloon valvuloplasty because of the extensive calcification of the valve leaflets and subvalve apparatus, and the presence of left atrial thrombus. She underwent mitral valve replacement with a mechanical prosthesis 3 months later when the risk of exacerbating her neurologic deficit by cardiopulmonary bypass was considered to be less likely, and she was discharged on warfarin with an International Normalized Ratio of 2·9.

Questions

1. What are the clinical diagnoses? What was her childhood illness and the likely rhythm disturbance during pregnancy?
2. What factors contributed to the neurologic event?
3. Explain the auscultatory findings of a loud first heart sound, loud P$_2$, and the clinical significance of the closeness of the opening snap to P$_2$.
4. Why was the liver enlarged and the liver function tests deranged?
5. Explain the abnormalities on the electrocardiogram.
6. Describe the chest *x* ray findings that support the clinical diagnosis.
7. What additional hemodynamic information would be obtainable at cardiac catheterization?
8. Why was a mechanical rather than a biologic mitral prosthesis selected for mitral valve replacement in so young a woman?

Answers

Answer to question 1 The clinical diagnoses are mitral stenosis and cerebral thromboembolism. The disease in childhood was rheumatic fever, which caused her polyarthralgia even though during the acute phase there was no rheumatic carditis or cardiac murmur detected. The rhythm disturbance with light-headedness during the last trimester of pregnancy was probably paroxysmal rapid atrial fibrillation, which spontaneously reverted to normal sinus rhythm.

Answer to question 2 The factors that contributed to her neurologic event include mitral valve stenosis with resultant slow flow in the left atrium, left atrial enlargement, atrial fibrillation, and poor anticoagulant status with an International Normalized Ratio of 1·3.

Answer to question 3 The loud first heart sound is due to the closure of rheumatically thickened mitral valve leaflets; the loud P_2 is due to the presence of pulmonary hypertension. The closeness of the opening snap to P_2 relates to the amplitude of left atrial pressure and the severity of the mitral stenosis, so that the closer the opening snap is to P_2, the more severe the mitral stenosis.

Answer to question 4 The liver is enlarged because of systemic venous hypertension from tricuspid regurgitation, and the deranged liver function tests indicate acute distension of the liver from congestive heart failure or from chronic elevation of systemic venous pressure and "cardiac cirrhosis".

Answer to question 5 Atrial fibrillation occurs from atrial dilatation and is part of the natural history of chronic rheumatic heart disease. The right axis deviation and right ventricular hypertrophy are due to pulmonary hypertension, and the T and ST abnormalities are digitalis effects.

Answer to question 6 Left atrial enlargement, prominence of the left atrial appendage and main pulmonary artery, elevated left main bronchus, intracardiac calcification of the mitral valve apparatus, and cephalization of the upper lobes of the lungs.

Answer to question 7 None.

Answer to question 8 The patient is postmenopausal and so problems with subsequent pregnancy are not an issue. She is in established atrial fibrillation with a dilated left atrium, and will therefore require anticoagulation. Importantly, the primary failure rate of bioprostheses at 10 years is approximately 20%, so she would need to undergo at least two additional valve replacements. Therefore, the use of a durable prosthesis over the long term is desirable, and thus a mechanical prosthesis is the treatment of choice.

Case 2.3

A 59-year-old male business executive was brought to the emergency room complaining of sudden onset of severe central chest pain (which he graded 10/10) radiating through to his back, associated with diaphoresis and nausea. He had never had chest pain previously and played golf once weekly without any exercise intolerance or shortness of breath. His past medical history included an arthroscopy for meniscectomy at age 37 years, and hypertension treated for 11 years initially with β-adrenergic blocking agents but for the past 4 years with once daily angiotensin-converting enzyme inhibitor therapy. Risk factors for coronary artery disease included a family history (his father had sustained a myocardial infarction at age 61 years and underwent coronary artery bypass vein grafting; his mother and younger brother had hypertension), he was not diabetic or a smoker, and had a cholesterol of 230 mg% (5·9 mmol/l).

Examination. Physical examination: the patient was in acute distress, and was cold, clammy, and complaining of pain in his mid-back. Pulse: 110 beats/min, normal character. Blood pressure: 160/100 mmHg in right arm. Jugular venous pulse: 8 cm. Cardiac impulse: prominent, displaced to anterior axillary line. First heart sound: normal. Second heart sound: split normally on inspiration. No added sounds. Decrescendo murmur at upper left sternal border. Chest examination: normal air entry, no rales or rhonchi. Abdominal examination: soft abdomen, no tenderness, and no masses. Normal liver span. No peripheral edema. Pulses absent below femoral on the right, and his right foot was colder than his left. Carotid pulses: normal, no bruits. Optic fundi: normal.

Investigations. Laboratory findings: normal electrolytes and creatinine. Two sets of cardiac enzymes normal. Electrocardiogram: sinus tachycardia, left axis deviation (−32°), minor QRS widening, left ventricular hypertrophy with non-specific T wave abnormalities throughout. Chest *x* ray (anteroposterior): widening of the mediastinum and an "unfolded aorta", with cardiomegaly but clear lung fields. Two-dimensional echocardiogram: mildly dilated left ventricle with concentric hypertrophy; normal systolic function; no segmental wall motion abnormalities; mild aortic regurgitation by color flow Doppler; a dilated aortic root with an intimal flap in the ascending aorta, which could be identified as extending to the abdominal aorta from the subxiphoid images; and no pericardial effusion. Magnetic resonance imaging confirmed the diagnosis and delineated the extent of the disease and the complications.

Clinical course. Following his echocardiogram, the patient complained of a further episode of severe interscapular pain only partly relieved by intravenous morphine, after which his blood pressure dropped to a systolic pressure of 70 mmHg. Examination demonstrated that he could no longer move his legs, his right leg remained cold and pulseless, he had a sensory level at his mid-thorax (T9), and had not passed urine since admission, although he was still mentating normally. Heart sounds and aortic regurgitant murmur were unchanged. On his way to the operating room he became profoundly hypotensive and developed sinus bradycardia, which was followed quickly by a cardiac arrest from which he could not be resuscitated. A postmortem was conducted.

Questions

1. What was the differential diagnosis of the patient's chest pain?
2. What in the clinical history and physical examination made you select your working diagnosis?
3. Explain the possible mechanisms for aortic regurgitation. Did any of these potential etiologies elucidate the seriousness or emergent nature of the patient's management? Does any classification of the disease in question spring to mind?
4. What was the significance of the cold right leg?
5. Why was the patient unable to move his legs, and what was the significance of the sensory level at T9?
6. The presence of the intimal flap seen by echocardiography and magnetic resonance imaging was indicative of what?
7. What additional information was provided by magnetic resonance imaging that was unavailable by transthoracic two-dimensional echocardiography?
8. What findings would you anticipate at postmortem examination?

Answers

Answer to question 1   Acute myocardial infarction and acute aortic dissection.

Answer to question 2   A history of hypertension associated with chest pain radiating to the back does not distinguish between myocardial infarction and aortic dissection, and the presence of aortic regurgitation is a common feature of type A aortic dissection, but aortic regurgitation may also occur in patients with hypertension. However, the diagnosis of aortic dissection is strongly suggested by the loss of pulses in the right leg.

Answer to question 3   The probable mechanisms for the aortic regurgitation include acute dissection of the ascending aorta, involving the aortic root with prolapse of the valve leaflets, and dilatation of the aortic root due to longstanding systemic hypertension. Aortic dissections are classified as type A if they involve the ascending aorta or aortic arch, and as type B if they are limited to the descending thoracic aorta, usually beginning at the origin of the left subclavian artery. The treatment of acute type A dissection is urgent surgical repair, whereas type B dissections without rupture or compromise of an organ or limb have a similar outcome with medical or surgical repair. The presence of aortic regurgitation and the two-dimensional echocardiographic confirmation of type A dissection necessitated emergent surgical repair (transesophageal echocardiography would have been a better choice than transthoracic echocardiography).

Answer to question 4 The cold pulseless right leg was caused by dissection and subsequent occlusion of the right common iliac artery, resulting in an ischemic right leg.

Answer to question 5 The type A dissection had occluded the arteria magna, which has a mid-thoracic origin and supplies the anterior spinal arteries to the mid-thoracic cord. The anterior spinal artery supplies the corticospinal (motor), and anterior and lateral spinothalamic tracts (sensory), interruption of which resulted in motor paralysis of the legs and the sensory level at T9.

Answer to question 6 The intimal flap is the dissection between the intimal and medial layers of the aortic wall. The free intimal flap is identified by both two-dimensional echocardiography and magnetic resonance imaging.

Answer to question 7 The magnetic resonance imaging scan demonstrated the extent of the aortic dissection, the sites of the entrance and exit of the dissection, as well as the occlusion of the right common iliac artery, which were unavailable by echocardiography. Because the transesophageal echocardiography probe cannot be passed beyond the stomach, the proximal abdominal aorta is the limit of echocardiographic evaluation.

Answer to question 8 Postmortem examination demonstrated similar anatomic findings in terms of the dissection, but in addition exsanguination caused by rupture of the descending thoracic aorta into the left pleural cavity.

Case 2.4

A 48-year-old male physician saw his local physician complaining of a sensation of heaviness in the chest associated with weakness and light-headedness that had progressed over the prior 3 weeks. The pain did not radiate, but was provoked by anxiety and by decreasing amounts of exertion over the 3 weeks following its onset and was relieved quickly by rest. He had brought forward his medical appointment because of an episode the day before in which his chest discomfort occurred while at rest reading the newspaper. His past medical history was unremarkable, with no previous illness or admissions to hospital. His risk factors included a remote smoking history (he had quit 15 years previously), no hypertension or diabetes, unknown cholesterol, and a positive family history for early coronary disease (his father had had two myocardial infarctions at ages 50 and 57 years, one brother had coronary artery bypass graft surgery at age 53 years, and his eldest brother had a myocardial infarction at age 56 years but is now symptom free on medical therapy).

Examination. Physical examination: the patient appeared normal. Pulse: 78 beats/min, normal character. Blood pressure: 135/80 mmHg. Jugular venous pulse: normal. Cardiac impulse: normal. First heart sound: normal. Second heart sound: split normally on inspiration. No added sounds or murmurs. Chest examination: normal air entry, no rales or rhonchi. Abdominal examination: soft abdomen, no tenderness, and no masses. Normal liver span. No peripheral edema. Femoral, popliteal, posterior tibial, and dorsalis pedis pulses: all normal volume and equal. Carotid pulses: normal, no bruits. Optic fundi: normal.

Investigations. Laboratory findings: normal levels of sodium, potassium, blood urea nitrogen, creatinine, creatine phosphokinase, and creatine kinase-MB. Total cholesterol: 285 mg/dl (7·4 mmol/l). Electrocardiogram: sinus rhythm, normal QRS axis and intervals, T-wave flattening in leads V_1–V_3. Chest *x* ray: normal heart size and clear lung fields. Stress thallium was performed using a standard (Bruce) protocol. The patient developed his typical chest heaviness, became hypotensive and presyncopal after 3 min exercise, and had 3 mm planar depression of the ST segments in leads V_1 through V_4 with multiple ventricular extrasystoles. Thallium scan revealed a large reversible defect involving the whole of the anterior left ventricular wall and anterior septum. Emergent cardiac catheterization: left ventricular end-diastolic pressure 19 mmHg; no left ventricular angiogram was performed, and during intubation of the left coronary artery arterial systolic pressure dropped to 70 mmHg, so that only limited views of the left coronary artery were obtained; the right coronary artery was normal. The patient was referred for urgent cardiac surgery.

Clinical course. The patient underwent surgery without any complications and was discharged home on postoperative day 6.

Questions

1. What was the underlying reason for the hypotension and presyncope at such a low workload, the electrocardiographic changes and electrical instability?
2. What were the likely diagnoses?

3. Explain the significance of the "reversible" defect on the thallium scan and the urgency for the cardiac catheterization.
4. Why did hypotension supervene during left coronary angiography and not during injection of the right coronary artery?
5. What were the likely findings of the cardiac catheterization?
6. Why was the patient referred for surgery rather than undergoing angioplasty?
7. What medical therapy, if any, would you institute following hospital discharge?

Answers

Answer to question 1 Hypotension during stress testing indicates that the myocardium cannot meet the increased demands of exercise and fails to generate a normal blood pressure response. This is usually due to severe proximal triple vessel disease (left anterior descending, left circumflex, and right coronary artery) or left mainstem coronary artery stenosis, or severe ventricular dysfunction. The impressive anterior electrocardiographic ST-segment depression demonstrates extensive anterior ischemia at a low workload in the territory of the left anterior descending coronary artery. The electrical instability and ventricular ectopy are probably induced by myocardial ischemia.

Answer to question 2 Left mainstem coronary artery stenosis or severe proximal triple coronary artery disease.

Answer to question 3 The reversible defect on the thallium scan indicates a large region of left ventricular myocardium that has severely reduced perfusion, even during mild exertion, which is completely viable and is normally perfused at rest. This suggests that if occlusion of the vessel occurred, then the area at risk for infarction would be large. The reason for the urgent cardiac catheterization was the probable diagnosis of left main coronary stenosis.

Answer to question 4 Hypotension supervened during left coronary artery injection because when the catheter engaged the severely diseased left coronary artery it completely obstructed flow, resulting in myocardial ischemia. The right coronary artery was normal and the catheter did not occlude antegrade flow.

Answer to question 5 Coronary arteriography demonstrated a 95% stenosis of the left main coronary artery and an 80% tubular stenosis in the mid left anterior descending artery, with normal left circumflex and right coronary arteries.

Answer to question 6 The treatment of left main coronary stenosis is left internal mammary artery graft to the left anterior descending artery and saphenous venous graft to the left circumflex artery. Angioplasty is contraindicated for left main disease because of risk for severe acute global ischemia and for acute dissection and closure should complications occur.

Answer to question 7 Long-term cholesterol lowering therapy should be instituted because this reduces the incidence of late cardiovascular events in patients with coronary artery disease.

References

1 Henry WL, DeMaria A, Gramiak R, *et al*. Report of the American Society of Echocardiography Committee on Nomenclature and Standards in Two-dimensional Echocardiography. *Circulation* 1980;**62**:212–7.
2 St John Sutton M, Kotler M, Oldershaw P, eds. *Textbook of adult and pediatric echocardiography and Doppler*. London: Blackwell Science, 1996.
3 Skjaerpe T, Hegrenaes L, Hatle L. Noninvasive estimation of valve area in patients with aortic stenosis by Doppler ultrasound and two-dimensional echocardiography. *Circulation* 1985;**72**:810–8.
4 Currie P, Seward J, Reeder G, *et al*. Continuous wave Doppler echocardiographic assessment of the severity of calcific aortic stenosis: a simultaneous Doppler-catheter correlative study in 100 adult patients. *Circulation* 1985;**71**:1162–9.
5 Bonow R, Lakatos E, Maron B, Epstein S. Serial long-term assessment of the natural history of asymptomatic patients with chronic aortic regurgitation and normal left ventricular systolic function. *Circulation* 1991;**84**:1625–35.
6 Chan K, Currie P, Seward J, Hagler D, Mair D, Tajik A. Comparison of three Doppler ultrasound methods in the prediction of pulmonary artery pressure. *J Am Coll Cardiol* 1987;**9**:549–54.
7 Klein A, Cohn G. Clinical applications of doppler echocardiography in the assessment of diastolic function. In: St John Sutton M, Kotler M, Oldershaw P, eds. *Textbook of adult and pediatric echocardiography and Doppler*. London: Blackwell Science, 1996:83–96.
8 Schiller N, Shah P, Crawford M, *et al*. Recommendations for quantitation of the left ventricle by two-dimensional echocardiography. *J Am Soc Echocardgr* 1989;**2**: 358–67.
9 Marvick T, Nemec J, Stewart W, Salcedo E. Diagnosis of coronary artery disease using exercise echocardiograph and positron emission tomography: comparison and analysis of discrepant results. *J Am Soc Echocardgr* 1992;**5**:231–9.
10 Marcus M, Schelbert H, Skorton D, Wolf G, eds. *Cardiac imaging: a companion to Braunwald's heart disease*. Philadelphia: WB Saunders Co, 1991.
11 Nienaber C, von Kodolitsch Y, Nicholas V, *et al*. The diagnosis of thoracic aortic dissection by noninvasive imaging procedures. *N Engl J Med* 1993;**328**:1–9.
12 Zaret B, Beller G, eds. *Nuclear cardiology: state of the art and future directions*. St Louis: Mosby, 1993.
13 Marshall R, Tillisch H, Phelps M, *et al*. Identification and differentiation of resting myocardial ischemia and infarction in man with positron emission tomography, ^{18}F-labeled fluorodeoxyglucose and N-13 ammonia. *Circulation* 1983;**67**:766.

3: Cardiac catheterization

CHARLES LANDAU

The advent of improved equipment and techniques plus an increasing number of non-surgical options for the treatment of cardiovascular disorders has increased the role of the cardiac catheterization laboratory in the management of patients with a variety of diseases that affect the vascular and valvular structures of the heart.

Diagnostic cardiac catheterization

Definitions and overview

The term "cardiac catheterization" refers to the placement of hollow plastic tubes (catheters) into the chambers of the heart or into the epicardial coronary arteries with fluoroscopic guidance for the purpose of acquiring pressure measurements, collecting blood samples, and injecting radiographic contrast material in order to opacify coronary arterial and ventricular anatomy. The latter procedures are frequently referred to as arteriography or angiography. A catheterization procedure usually consists, at a minimum, of acquiring arterial pressures and coronary arteriography.

Right heart catheterization involves the passage of a catheter from the venous access site via the vena cava to the right atrium, right ventricle, and pulmonary artery. Pulmonary capillary wedge pressure (PCWP), a reflection of left atrial pressure as transmitted retrograde through the pulmonary vasculature, is determined by advancing the catheter to a terminal segment of the pulmonary arterial tree. Pressures are measured in each of the chambers, and blood samples are drawn for the determination of oxygen saturations when clinically indicated. Determinations of cardiac output are also a routine aspect of this protocol in most catheterization laboratories. When clinically indicated, an endomyocardial biopsy can be taken from the right ventricle using a flexible biopsy forceps after hemodynamic measurements have been acquired.

Left heart catheterization denotes the passage of a catheter from the arterial access site retrograde to the left ventricle through the aortic valve. In order to avoid the consequences of systemic emboli, patients undergoing a left heart catheterization are usually systemically anticoagulated with heparin. Pressure is recorded sequentially in the left ventricle and then, after pull-back of the catheter, in the ascending aorta. This series of measurements is performed to exclude a pressure gradient across the aortic valve, a finding indicative of aortic stenosis. Following these measurements a ventriculogram is performed with a contrast injection into the left ventricle. The images of the opacified left ventricle are used to assess regional wall motion, determine ventricular volumes, calculate global left ventricular function as an ejection fraction, and assess the presence and severity of mitral regurgitation, which manifests as the appearance of contrast in the left atrium during ventricular systole as a result of an incompetent mitral valve. Selective coronary angiography is routinely performed after ventriculography, during which the left main and right coronary arteries are selectively cannulated, followed by contrast injections to define coronary anatomy, including stenoses and vascular distribution.

Right and left heart catheterization combines the components described above. In addition to the protocols outlined, simultaneous measurements of the PCWP and left ventricular pressures are made in order to evaluate the presence of a pressure gradient across the mitral valve. This is a pathologic finding that is usually indicative of mitral stenosis.

Indications

In clinical practice the majority of diagnostic cardiac catheterizations are undertaken primarily for three reasons (Table 3.1).

- To obtain anatomic information regarding the coronary arteries and left ventricular function.
- To quantify hemodynamic abnormalities, including valvular lesions.
- To determine the site and magnitude of an intracardiac shunt.

Cardiac catheterization should not be undertaken in any patient who is unable or unwilling to provide informed consent. In addition, the procedure is contraindicated in those circumstances that increase the risks associated with the procedure, such as bleeding diatheses, decompensated congestive heart failure, worsening renal function, systemic infections and untreated hyperthyroidism, and in those unwilling to provide informed consent. Because catheterization involves radiation exposure, pregnancy should be excluded in women of childbearing age.

Table 3.1 Indications for cardiac catheterization

Indication		Reasons
Definition of cardiac anatomy	To facilitate the diagnosis of coronary artery disease	Equivocal non-invasive evaluation
		Persistent chest pain despite negative non-invasive tests
		Dilated cardiomyopathy
		Sudden cardiac death
	Patients refractory to medical therapy for ischemia	Intolerant of medications
		Limiting angina despite adequate drug therapy
		Unstable angina
		Postmyocardial infarction angina
		Positive predischarge exercise test following myocardial infarction
	Patients with suspected high-risk anatomy (i.e. left main or severe three-vessel disease)	Markedly positive exercise test
		Diffuse ECG changes (ST depression) during spontaneous episodes of ischemia
		Rapid onset pulmonary edema, presumably due to ischemia
Hemodynamic assessment	To determine the severity of valvular abnormalities	Aortic stenosis
		Aortic regurgitation
		Mitral stenosis
		Mitral regurgitation
		Pulmonic stenosis
	To assess the severity of hemodynamic derangements in myocardial or pericardial disease	Dilated cardiomyopathy*
		Hypertrophic obstructive cardiomyopathy*
		Restrictive cardiomyopathy
		Constrictive pericarditis
		Left ventricular diastolic dysfunction
Intracardiac shunt assessment		Atrial septal defect
		Ventricular septal defect
		Aorto-pulmonary window
		Patent ductus arteriosus

*Can also be utilized to assess the efficacy of treatment.

Procedural techniques

Cardiac catheterization begins with vascular access. Because this portion of the procedure involves some patient discomfort, it is important that it be accomplished in its entirety at the beginning of catheterization so that the patient may return to a steady-state condition for the hemodynamic measurements that follow. It is routine for patients to be premedicated with a combination of diazepam and diphenhydramine hydrochloride, or similar medications, to lessen anxiety and to reduce the severity of an allergic reaction to contrast should one occur. In order to detect vagal episodes, which manifest as a rapid decrement in blood pressure and/or heart rate with the associated symptoms of diaphoresis, nausea, pallor, hyperventilation, yawning, and/or mydriasis, it is essential that vital signs be continuously monitored during this portion of the procedure. The vascular access site is first infused with lidocaine (lignocaine) to achieve local anesthesia.

Vascular access is achieved through either brachial, femoral, or radial sites. Femoral access is used most frequently because the larger size of the femoral artery decreases the potential for vascular complications. The Seldinger technique is utilized to place a sheath in the femoral artery (for left heart access via the aorta) and/or the femoral vein (for right heart access via the inferior vena cava). A small skin incision is made and the vascular structure is located using a hollow 18-gauge needle. Next, a non-traumatic guidewire is introduced through the needle into the vessel, the needle is removed while leaving the wire in place, and then a plastic sheath is advanced over the wire into the vascular lumen before removing the wire. The sheath, which is a hollow tube 2·0–3·0 mm in diameter and approximately 10 mm in length, with a proximal one-way valve resting outside the patient to prevent back bleeding, is then used as a conduit through which the longer catheters are advanced into the heart or its vessels.

A similar technique can be used at the brachial site for arterial access only because the course of venous structures in the antecubital fossa is highly variable. Alternatively, a cutdown can be performed to visualize directly the brachial artery with access achieved through an arteriotomy in the superior surface of the artery, which is repaired at the conclusion of the procedure. The advantage of this method over the Seldinger technique is that a brachial vein can be located and used for right heart access. The brachial approach is most commonly used in patients with severe iliofemoral vascular disease in whom arterial access may be troublesome or marked by an increased potential for vascular complications. Other clinical circumstances that favor the brachial approach because of difficulties in attaining hemostasis include marked obesity, poorly controlled hypertension, or a wide pulse pressure (i.e. aortic regurgitation). Additionally, the radial artery can be accessed percutaneously.

Following vascular access, catheters are placed in the cardiac chambers of interest and hemodynamic measurements are made before the injection of any contrast material. This strategy is followed because intravascular contrast injections alter cardiac physiology and conduction such that measurements made following the administration of these agents do not reflect the baseline hemodynamics of the patient.

Angiography is the final phase of the procedure and involves rapid infusion of radiopaque contrast material into the ventricle and then the coronary arteries. Contrast temporarily replaces the blood volume, resulting in opacification of the ventricular chamber and coronary arterial lumen, respectively. This technique only provides information about the portions of these organs in contact with the blood pool; no direct data regarding the structure of the ventricular or vascular wall is obtained.

When the catheterization procedure has been completed, protamine is given to reverse the effects of heparin. The vascular sheaths are removed and hemostasis is achieved with direct pressure applied either manually or with a mechanical device for 15–30 min, depending on sheath size. Following hemostasis, the utilized limb is immobilized for 6–8 hours to permit the clot that has formed at the vascular puncture site to stabilize. Alternatively, a vascular closure device may be utilized. These devices employ either bovine collagen (which is thrombogenic and focally positioned at the puncture site) or resorbable suture (which is introduced percutaneously through the arteriotomy site created by the sheath) to achieve rapid hemostasis with minimal compression. If successfully deployed, patients can ambulate in 2 hours, which facilitates discharge when catheterization is performed in the outpatient setting.

Risks associated with cardiac catheterization

Complications arising from cardiac catheterization are due to vascular access, catheter manipulations, or administration of drugs and contrast material. The most serious complications of death, stroke, and myocardial infarction occur in approximately 0·1%, 0·07%, and 0·06% of cases, respectively. Other complications include allergic reactions, arrhythmias, cardiac perforation, and vascular complications, which occur in 0·5–4% of cases. Examples of vascular complications include hematoma formation, bleeding, thrombosis, embolism, pseudoaneurysm, and arteriovenous fistula.

An additional consideration in patients who will undergo angiography during their procedure is the risk for developing renal insufficiency from exposure to iodinated contrast material. Patients with pre-existing renal insufficiency, diabetes mellitus, recent (within the past 48 hours) contrast exposure, and female gender or advanced age are at increased risk for this complication. In patients with multiple myeloma, contrast exposure is associated with an especially high incidence of irreversible renal dysfunction.

Hemodynamic measurements

Usually reliable pressure measurements are obtained using a fluid-filled system in which the catheter is connected to a pressure transducer with a short length of tubing. The transducer converts the kinetic energy of the pressure signal to an electrical impulse, which is then recorded on paper or digitized for archiving using optical or magnetic storage media. Pressures are reported in millimeters of mercury.

The accuracy of the pressures measured is dependent on the system components. The ideal catheter (i.e. one that provides the truest reflection of intracardiac pressures) is rigid and possesses a large lumen because these characteristics are consistent with the best frequency response. These properties must be balanced with those involving patient safety because maximizing these characteristics would result in a catheter with increased risk for cardiac perforation. The saline-filled connection between catheter and transducer must be devoid of blood or air, either of which can cause dampening of the pressure signal. Reliable pressure references are also required, and this is achieved by calibrating the system to zero pressure at the level of the heart and against a fixed standard, usually a mercury sphygmomanometer.

Right heart pressures

Evaluation of right heart pressures begins in the right atrium, where care is taken to direct the catheter tip toward the lateral wall of the chamber, away from the tricuspid annulus where a regurgitant jet could result in a measuring artifact. The normal pressure tracing consists of an "a" wave and a "v" wave, which are analogous to those observed in jugular venous pulsations (Figure 3.1). The "a" wave represents the pressure increase resulting from atrial contraction at the conclusion of diastole, and is followed by the X descent. The "v" wave represents the pressure increase resulting from upward movement of the tricuspid annulus during ventricular systole (which decreases the effective size of the atrium) and the continued inflow of blood into an atrium that is unable to drain in the presence of a closed tricuspid valve. The rapid decrement in pressure that results from opening of the valve is termed the Y descent (Table 3.2). Examples of conditions that result in an elevated right atrial pressure include constrictive pericarditis, restrictive cardiomyopathy, right ventricular infarction, and right sided congestive heart failure.

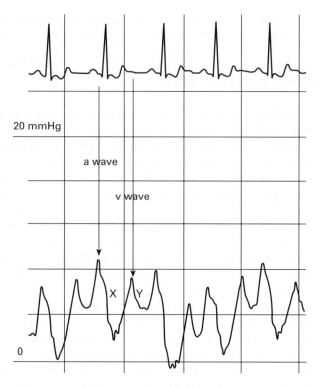

20 mmHg

a wave

v wave

X Y

0

Figure 3.1 Simultaneous recording of electrocardiogram and right atrial pressure. The "a" wave, a reflection of atrial systole, follows the "p" wave. The "v" wave peak occurs just before tricuspid valve opening during diastole. X and Y descents are also shown

Right ventricular pressure is measured next, after the catheter is passed through the tricuspid valve. Ventricular ectopy may be encountered with this maneuver because of catheter contact with the endocardial surface, and so care must be taken to find a location in the mid-portion of the chamber so that an accurate pressure recording can be taken. The operator should carefully observe the morphology of the waveform because the "dip and plateau" of the diastolic pressure may be the first indication that the patient has constrictive/restrictive physiology. Because of the proximity of the right bundle to the ventricular septum, a transient right bundle branch block can be induced in up to 5% of patients during catheter manipulations in the right ventricle. This complication is well tolerated except in those with a pre-existing left bundle branch block, in which case all three conducting fascicles are jeopardized, resulting in complete heart block. The hemodynamic compromise that occurs in this circumstance can be lessened by placing a temporary pacing catheter in the right

Table 3.2 Normal values for cardiac catheterization

Parameter (unit)	Value
O_2 consumption index (ml/min per m²)	110–150
Cardiac index (l/min per m²)	2·7–4·2
Pressures	
Right atrium (mean; mmHg)	0–8
Right ventricle (mmHg)	15–30/0–8
Pulmonary artery (mmHg)	15–30/4–12
Pulmonary capillary wedge (mean; mmHg)	1–10
Aorta (mmHg)	100–140/60–90
Left ventricle (mmHg)	100–140/3–12
Resistances	
Pulmonary vascular (dyne·s/cm⁵)	20–120 (0·25–1·5 Woods units)
Systemic vascular (dyne·s/cm⁵)	770–1500 (9·6–18·7 Woods units)
Angiographic volumes	
Left ventricular end-diastolic volume index (ml/m²)	50–90
Left ventricular end-systolic volume index (ml/m²)	15–30
Left ventricular stroke volume index (ml/m²)	35–75
Left ventricular ejection fraction (%)	50–80

ventricle before right heart catheterization in patients with a left bundle branch block. Alternatively, use of a balloon-tipped catheter instead of a rigid one may reduce, but does not eliminate, the risk of catheter-induced right bundle branch block.

Pulmonary artery pressure is next determined after the catheter is passed through the pulmonic valve into the proximal pulmonary arterial tree. Because the right ventricular outflow tract is especially thin, great care must be taken during this portion of the catheterization procedure to prevent puncture of the right ventricle. If the pulmonary arterial systolic pressure is lower than the right ventricular systolic pressure, then a gradient is present between the two chambers. This is consistent with a stenotic lesion, which may be valvular, subvalvular, or supravalvular. This finding should be confirmed with a continuous pressure recording as the catheter is pulled back from the pulmonary artery to the right ventricle.

The right heart pressure measurements are concluded with a measurement of PCWP, which is obtained by advancing the catheter until it comes to rest in the distal pulmonary vasculature. This can be facilitated by having the patient inspire while the catheter is pushed distally, and then having the patient cough. Adequate catheter position should be confirmed by drawing an oxygen saturation that is 95% or greater. This establishes that the waveform recorded is not contaminated by pulmonary arterial pressure, because inclusion of pulmonary artery blood in the sample would decrease the measured saturation to a value below 95%. The PCWP is an accurate reflection of left atrial pressure, as reflected retrograde through the pulmonary venous system.

There are several differences in the morphology of pulmonary arterial pressure and PCWP tracings. First, the pulmonary arterial pressure (PA) has a single peak for each QRS complex of the electrocardiogram, whereas the PCWP, like the right atrial pressure tracing, inscribes an "a" and "v" wave for each QRS. On those occasions where a large "v" wave is present, or when the patient has no "a" wave (i.e. atrial fibrillation), the pulmonary arterial and PCWP pressures may appear similar, but because of the delay in pressure transmission through the pulmonary bed the "v" wave peak occurs later in the cardiac cycle (usually in the region of the T wave of the electrocardiogram) than the peak of the pulmonary arterial tracing (usually near the end of the QRS complex). In addition, unlike the PA tracing, "v" waves do not possess a dicrotic notch on the downslope of the pressure waveform. Finally, the mean of the PCWP is always less than the mean pulmonary arterial pressure.

Left heart pressures

In those cases in which an accurate PCWP is not obtainable, left atrial pressure can be measured directly by passing a catheter from the right atrium, through the interatrial septum, and into the left atrium. This technique, known as transseptal catheterization, requires the use of a long metal Brockenbrough needle, which is introduced from the right femoral vein. Once the needle has punctured the septum, a catheter is usually passed over the needle into the left atrium. This method increases the risk for chamber rupture because a sharp object is deliberately positioned within the cardiac chambers, and so it is not routinely utilized for pressure measurements. Circumstances in which the transseptal approach is used include the following: inability to obtain a satisfactory PCWP tracing when this information is vital; mitral valvuloplasty, where balloon dilating equipment must be placed antegrade across the mitral valve; and procedures in which left ventricular pressure measurements or angiography are critical and the left ventricle cannot be entered retrograde through the aortic valve, such as severe aortic stenosis or the presence of a tilting disk valve prosthesis in the aortic position. Passing a catheter through these types of mechanical valves can result in catheter entrapment. In such cases, the left ventricle is entered by a passing a catheter from the right atrium through the left atrium to the left ventricle.

In most situations, left ventricular pressure can be sampled by passing a catheter across the aortic valve and maneuvering it to a position where ventricular ectopy is not encountered. Because of differences in magnitude between left ventricular systolic and diastolic pressures, waveforms are usually recorded on two different scales. Left ventricular end-diastolic pressure (LVEDP) is measured at the time corresponding to the peak of the QRS complex, and is similar in magnitude to the a wave peak of the PCWP tracing, which also occurs temporally at the conclusion of diastole. The LVEDP is dependent on factors other than the volume state of the left ventricle, and does not reflect left ventricular pressure during the earlier portions of diastole. Consequently, the PCWP is a more accurate reflection of the pressure experienced by the pulmonary vasculature. When left ventricular pressure sampling is completed, pressure is measured continuously as the catheter is withdrawn into the ascending aorta in order to determine whether a gradient is present between the left ventricle and aorta, a condition consistent with left ventricular outflow obstruction below the valve (as in hypertrophic obstructive cardiomyopathy) or at the level of the aortic valve (aortic stenosis).

Cardiac output

The determination of cardiac output is an important component of hemodynamic measurements. It is the amount of blood ejected by the heart in liters/min, and its value is used in the calculation of vascular resistances, valve areas, and intracardiac shunt magnitudes. Because of the relationship between metabolic demands and body size, it is also reported as the quotient of cardiac output/body surface area, termed the cardiac index. Normal values are listed in Table 3.2. The two most popular methods for measuring cardiac output are the Fick and indicator dilution methods.

The Fick principle states that the consumption or release of a substance by an organ is equal to the product of the blood flow through the organ and the concentration difference of the substance entering and exiting the organ. For the purposes of determination of cardiac output, the organ of interest is the lung and the consumed substance is oxygen. Transposing the terms of the Fick equation results in the following relationship.

$$\text{Cardiac output} = O_2 \text{ consumption}/(\text{pulmonary venous } O_2 \text{ concentration} - \text{pulmonary arterial } O_2 \text{ concentration})$$

The oxygen concentration is calculated as the product of the oxygen saturation (ml O_2/dl), the hemoglobin (g/dl), and the oxygen carrying capacity of hemoglobin (1·39 ml O_2/g). The result, in milliliters/deciliter, is multiplied by 10 to convert the concentration to milliliters/liter. Oxygen consumption (in ml/min) is measured using a timed collection of expired air that depends on a comparison of expired to room air oxygen content, or a metabolic rate measuring device that samples expired air directly and reports an oxygen consumption. The quotient of oxygen consumption and the oxygen concentration difference across the lungs returns a value in liters/min. In the absence of an intracardiac shunt, pulmonary and systemic blood flows are equal, and so the cardiac output determined using the Fick equation also represents the blood flow through the systemic circuit.

Errors in cardiac output determinations using this technique are most frequently due to incomplete or inadequate determinations of oxygen consumption. It is also less accurate in patients with a high cardiac output in whom the oxygen difference across the lungs is narrow, which tends to magnify the obligate error in the measurement of oxygen saturation.

The indicator dilution technique is based on the principle that a bolus injection of an indicator dissipates at a rate that is inversely proportional to the cardiac output. Most frequently, the indicator utilized is an injection of cooled saline and temperature is sampled distal to the infusion site, a task readily accomplished using a Swan–Ganz catheter with its distal tip positioned in the pulmonary artery. A temperature sensing thermistor permits creation of a temperature versus time plot following the saline injection, and a computer derives a value for the cardiac output by dividing a constant (which is dependent on the catheter properties, amount and temperature of saline injected, and blood temperature) by the area under the temperature–time curve. This is known as the thermodilution technique. This method is prone to errors in patients with tricuspid regurgitation, which yields a falsely low value for cardiac output. It is least accurate in patients with a low cardiac output, in whom the temperature–time curve is distorted, leading to artifacts in the calculation of cardiac output.

Once pressures and the cardiac output are known, vascular resistances are calculated using the following formula (which is essentially Ohm's law):

$$\text{Resistance} = \text{pressure/flow}$$

Pulmonary vascular resistance (PVR) and systemic vascular resistance (SVR) are both calculated in this way using mean pressures:

$$PVR = [(PA - PCWP)/CO] \times 80$$

$$SVR = [(Ao - RA)/CO] \times 80$$

where PA is the pulmonary arterial pressure, CO is the cardiac output, Ao is the aortic pressure, and RA is the right arterial pressure.

The result is reported in dynes·s/cm^5. These values are also commonly reported in Woods units, which are obtained by eliminating the 80 multiplicand in the above equations.

Oxygen saturations and shunt calculations

Oxygen saturations in a given cardiac chamber can be determined by drawing approximately 2 ml blood for analysis in a reflectance oximeter or similar device. These measurements are utilized to determine the presence of an intracardiac communication, which results in shunting of oxygenated blood from the left heart to the less saturated right heart. The hallmark of such a defect is an increase in oxygen saturation between the chamber proximal to the shunt and the chamber where shunting occurs; this is referred to as a step-up in oxygen saturation. Because of individual variations and incomplete blood mixing, measured saturations are not identical in all right heart chambers (Table 3.3). A pathologic step-up can be expressed in terms of an increase in either oxygen saturation or oxygen content expressed as volume percentage (ml O_2/100 ml blood). Screening oxygen saturations are usually drawn from the superior vena cava, right atrium, and pulmonary artery during initial right heart catheterization. If an abnormal step-up is detected, then a full oximetry run with multiple samples from each chamber is undertaken, and the criteria presented in Table 3.3 are again applied to the oxygen contents to determine the precise location of the intracardiac shunt.

The detection of a shunt is followed by a calculation of the shunt ratio, defined as the quotient of the pulmonary blood flow (PBF) and the systemic blood flow (SBF), using formulae based on the Fick principle:

$$PBF = O_2 \text{ consumption}/[Hb \times 1·39 \times 10 \times (Ao\ SO_2 - PA\ SO_2)]$$

$$SBF = O_2 \text{ consumption}/[Hb \times 1·39 \times 10 \times (Ao\ SO_2 - \text{mixed venous } SO_2)]$$

where SO_2 is the oxygen saturation, Hb is the hemoglobin concentration, Ao is the aorta, and PA is the pulmonary artery. The mixed venous saturation is the mean value in the chamber proximal to the site of the shunt. If the shunt occurs at the atrial level, that is the patient has an atrial septal defect, then a weighted average of the vena caval saturations [(3 × superior vena cava SO_2) + inferior vena cava SO_2]/4 is most commonly utilized. The above equations are valid if no right to left shunt is present because the equation for PBF assumes that the oxygen saturation in the pulmonary vein is equal to that in aorta. The determination of shunt ratio is important because

Table 3.3 Differences in blood oxygen concentrations consistent with an intracardiac left to right shunt

Oxygen parameter	Value
Oxygen content difference (using only the highest value in each chamber)	
Superior vena cava to right atrium	>1·9 ml O_2/100 ml
Right atrium to right ventricle	>0·9 ml O_2/100 ml
Right ventricle to pulmonary artery	≥0·5 ml O_2/100 ml
Oxygen saturation difference (single sample from each chamber)*	
Superior vena cava to right atrium	>9%
Right atrium to pulmonary artery	>6%
Superior vena cava to pulmonary artery	>9%
Oxygen saturation difference (mean of samples from each chamber)	
Superior vena cava to right atrium	>8%
Right atrium to right ventricle	>4%
Right ventricle to pulmonary artery	>3%

*These criteria are used to analyze the screening saturations for the presence of an intracardiac left to right shunt.

corrective surgery is usually recommended for PBF/SBF values of 1·5 or greater.

Transvalvular gradients and the calculation of valve area

The presence of valvular stenosis leads to a drop in pressure across the affected valve. The pressure difference between the chambers proximal and distal to the valve is referred to as the transvalvular gradient. Although gradients for the pulmonic and aortic valves can be measured by sequentially recording waveforms during a catheter pull-back, gradients are more accurately determined with simultaneous recordings of the pressure on either side of the valve. For the mitral valve, PCWP and left ventricular pressure are recorded, whereas for the aortic valve, left ventricular and aortic pressures are sampled. From the recorded pressures, a mean gradient during the period of blood flow through the valve (diastole for the mitral valve, systole for the aortic valve) is derived.

Because the gradient is proportional to the amount of blood passing through the valve, decisions regarding the severity of valvular stenosis are based on the calculated flow-independent valve area (in cm^2), which is obtained using the Gorlin equation.

$$\text{Valve area} = [CO/(HR \times FP)]/[k \times (\text{mean gradient})^{1/2}]$$

where CO is the cardiac output (ml/min) and HR is the heart rate. For the aortic valve, FP is the systolic filling period (in seconds) and k equals 44·3. For the mitral valve, FP is the diastolic filling period and k equals 37·7. Valve replacement is appropriate in patients who are symptomatic and have a valve area of 1·0 cm^2 or less.

Angiography

Angiography is an integral part of the catheterization procedure and involves the injection of radiopaque contrast material while simultaneously recording the radiographic image on cine film, usually at a rate of 30 frames/second. This technique is utilized so that images can be obtained throughout the cardiac cycle, thus increasing the information content of the study. Cine films are screened on an appropriate projector system that permits the operator to view the images both forward and backward at an adjustable speed, thus allowing attention to be focused on regions of interest. Alternatively, images can be acquired and stored digitally, with viewing on a high-resolution video screen.

Coronary angiography

Coronary angiography provides a detailed picture of the epicardial coronary arterial tree, with resolutions of approximately 0·1 mm. To achieve this goal, it is essential that each coronary artery be imaged in multiple views such that the artery of interest is adequately opacified, is freed of overlap by other coronary arteries, and is viewed in a plane parallel to its course along the epicardial surface such that features of the artery are not foreshortened. The left and right coronary arteries are selectively engaged with preshaped catheters, and cine film is recorded as 2–10 cm^3 of contrast is hand injected for each view. The imaging system moves about the patient in order to provide the various angulations required, and the table on which the patient lies supine is moved during the cine run to capture the dye as it flows distally within the coronary tree. The left coronary is usually imaged with five to seven injections, and the right coronary artery with two to three injections. In patients who have undergone previous coronary artery bypass surgery, each of the vein graft and internal mammary artery conduits are also selectively engaged and imaged in appropriate views, with special emphasis on visualizing the anastomoses of the grafts to the aorta and to the native coronary arteries (Figure 3.2).

Dominance of the coronary tree refers to the coronary artery that gives rise to the posterior descending artery (PDA), which supplies the posterior interventricular septum. The left main coronary artery is a short segment that gives rise to the left anterior descending artery

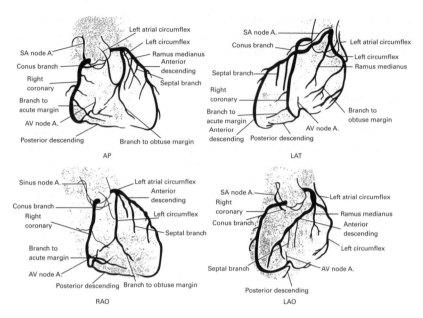

Figure 3.2 Normal coronary anatomy, as seen from the anteroposterior (AP), lateral (LAT), right anterior oblique (RAO), and left anterior oblique (LAO) projections. Reprinted with permission of the *New England Journal of Medicine*, from Abrams HL, Adams DF. The coronary arteriogram. *N Engl J Med* 1969; **281**:1277, Massachusetts Medical Society

(LAD) and the left circumflex (LCx) coronary arteries. The LAD usually supplies the largest portion of the myocardium, including the anterior and portions of the lateral wall, as well as the interventricular septum. Branches supplying the anterior interventricular septum are called septals, and those that fan out over the anterior and lateral walls are called diagonals. The proximal LAD is that portion between the left main coronary artery bifurcation and either the first septal or first diagonal branch. The mid and distal LAD represent the proximal and distal portions of the remaining vessel. The LCx supplies blood to the left atrium and the lateral and posterolateral portions of the left ventricular wall as it courses along the posterior atrioventricular groove. The right coronary artery (RCA), which arises from an ostium separate from the left, courses through the anterior atrioventricular groove and gives rise to right atrial branches, acute marginals, which supply the right ventricle, and the conus branch, which supplies the right ventricular outflow tract. In the majority of cases, it terminates in a bifurcation of the PDA, which supplies the inferior interventricular septum, and the posterior left ventricular branch, which supplies the posterolateral portion of the left ventricular wall.

There is a great deal of individual variation with respect to the size and territory of myocardium supplied by each of the three main coronaries, namely the LAD, LCx, and RCA. In approximately 90% of patients, the PDA arises from the distal RCA as described above, a situation referred to as right dominance. Occasionally, the distal RCA gives rise to a large posterior left ventricular system in conjunction with a diminutive distal LCx, which is called a super-dominant RCA. In approximately 7% of patients, the distal LCx terminates in the PDA, which is known as a left dominant system. The remaining patients are codominant, and there is a dual PDA system arising from both the distal LCx and RCA. The atrioventricular node is supplied by the artery of the same name, which is a terminal branch of the dominant artery. The sinoatrial node is supplied by an atrial branch of the RCA in 60% of patients and from the LCx in the other 40%. On occasion, the left main coronary artery can trifurcate with the middle vessel, designated the ramus medianus or ramus intermedius.

Stenoses in the coronary tree represent regions of luminal narrowing when compared with segments that appear smooth and larger in contour. Lesions are reported as a percentage stenosis, which is represented by the following equation.

$$\% \text{ Stenosis} = 100 \times [(\text{luminal diameter}_{normal} - \text{luminal diameter}_{diseased})/\text{luminal diameter}_{normal}]$$

When a vessel abruptly halts the lesion is referred to as an occlusion, which represents a 100% stenosis. The vessel distal to an occlusion is often filled retrograde by collateral vessels, which may arise from the same coronary artery, or from either or both of the other coronaries.

Descriptors are also attached to coronary lesions. An eccentric stenosis is one in which the lumen is not centered with respect to the adjacent segment. A long lesion is one that is greater than two luminal diameters in length. Calcified lesions possess radiodense linear densities in the vessel wall. Certain angiographic appearances are characteristic of intraluminal thrombus, including a hazy lumen morphology, jagged lesion borders, filling defects within the diseased lumen, and lesion borders that overhang the stenosis.

Ventriculography

The purpose of ventriculography is to opacify the entire left ventricular chamber, which permits observation of wall motion, determination of ventricular volumes, and assessment of overall systolic function through calculation of the left ventricular ejection fraction. To achieve this goal, a catheter is placed retrograde across the aortic valve into the left ventricle and positioned such that no

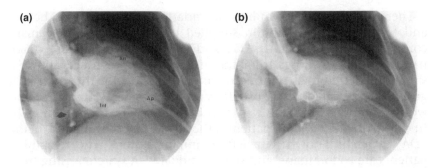

Figure 3.3 Frames from **(a)** diastole and **(b)** systole of a normal ventricle in the right anterior oblique view. If mitral regurgitation were present, then contrast would be seen filling the left atrium, marked with an arrow. An, anterior wall; Ap, apical region; Inf, inferior wall

ventricular ectopy occurs. The catheter is connected to a power injector – a device that rapidly infuses contrast material into the left ventricular chamber. The volume of contrast required to opacify the left ventricle is 40–50 cm^3 injected over a period of 3–4 seconds, a rate that is not feasible with manual injection. As dye is injected, the image is recorded on cine film. The camera is positioned in the right anterior oblique projection, which places the left ventricle in profile such that the anterior, apical, and inferior walls may be visualized. Segmental wall motion of the septal, posterior, and lateral walls can be assessed by repeating the ventriculogram in the left anterior oblique view. Alternatively, some catheterization laboratories can obtain both views with a single contrast injection if they are equipped with a biplane cine system that acquires images simultaneously from two different orientations. In order to correct for magnification differences in the final image, which are dependent on body habitus and the location of the left ventricle in the thorax, it is common practice to film also an object of known dimensions placed adjacent to the patient at the level of the heart (Figure 3.3).

Ventriculography also provides an estimate of the severity of mitral regurgitation by grading the intensity of contrast that refluxes into the left atrium during ventricular systole. The degree of regurgitation is graded semiquantitatively on a scale from 1 to 4 (Table 3.4). Complications that can occur with ventriculography include ventricular arrhythmias as a result of catheter motion during rapid contrast injection; myocardial staining due to subendocardial infusion of contrast under pressure, which can result in persistent ventricular ectopy; and embolic events caused either by dislodgement of a pre-existing ventricular thrombus by catheter contact, or by inadvertent injection of thrombus or air through the catheter.

Table 3.4 Semiquantitative system for angiographic grading of valvular regurgitation

Grade	Description*
0	No regurgitation
1+	Regurgitation into the atrium, which clears with each subsequent cardiac cycle
2+	Regurgitation with persistence of contrast in the atrium, which does not appear as dense as the ventricle
3+	Regurgitation with persistence of contrast in the atrium, which appears as dense as the ventricle
4+	Regurgitation with persistence of contrast in the atrium, which appears denser than the ventricle, or filling of the atrium in a single beat

*Criteria for mitral regurgitation supplied. For aortic regurgitation, substitute "ventricle" for "atrium", and "aorta" for "ventricle".

Aortography

Contrast injection in the ascending aorta is not a routine procedure during cardiac catheterization. It is reserved for patients with aortic regurgitation, in whom retrograde filling of the left ventricle during the aortogram is used as an estimate of the severity of the valvular lesion using a grading scale similar to that utilized for mitral regurgitation. Other circumstances in which aortography is helpful include patients with the following: saphenous vein bypass grafts (to identify the location of the proximal graft anastomoses); anomalous coronary artery origins (to locate the ostium of the congenitally abnormal vessel); aortic dissections; thoracic aortic aneurysms; aortic coarctation; and arteriovenous connections, such as aortopulmonary window, patent ductus arteriosus, or fistulas between the aorta and either the right atrium or right ventricle. Typically a power injector is utilized to infuse 50–60 cm^3 contrast over 2–3 seconds in the ascending aorta. The use of aortography solely to provide a measurement of the aortic root as an aid to aortic valve surgery has been largely supplanted by non-invasive imaging techniques such as echocardiography, computed tomography, and magnetic resonance imaging.

Case studies

Case 3.1

A 67-year-old male with a history of smoking, hypertension, and insulin-dependent diabetes mellitus complained of substernal chest discomfort, which was exertional and had occurred for the past

6 months. He noted severe dyspnea accompanying these episodes. Since decreasing his activity level, the frequency of his symptoms had diminished. Past medical history: diabetes, on insulin therapy for the past 15 years; hypertension, treated for the past 10 years; claudication; and history of transient ischemic attacks, quiescent since being placed on aspirin therapy. Medications: aspirin 325 mg/day, enalapril 10 mg/day, and NPH insulin (human insulin of recombinant DNA origin) 40 U/day in the morning.

Examination. Physical examination: the patient appeared overweight; no abnormalities of skin, nail beds, or oral mucosa. Temperature: normal. Pulse: 84 beats/min, normal character. Blood pressure: 140/84 mmHg in right arm. Jugular venous pulse: normal. Cardiac impulse: normal. First heart sound: normal. Second heart sound: split normally on inspiration. Fourth heart sound: present. No murmurs. Chest examination: normal air entry, bibasilar rales. Abdominal examination: soft abdomen, no tenderness, and no masses. Normal liver span: no peripheral edema. Femoral, popliteal, posterior tibial, and dorsalis pedis pulses: all normal volume and equal. Carotid pulses: normal, left carotid bruit. Optic fundi: normal.

Investigations. Normal hematology and biochemistry profile. Creatinine: 1·4 mg/dl (88·4 µmol/l). Electrocardiogram: normal sinus rhythm, normal intervals, left ventricular hypertrophy with strain. Chest x ray: hyperexpanded lung fields. Exercise tolerance test: the patient exercised for 3 min and halted because of chest pain and shortness of breath. During exercise his heart rate increased from 88 to 124 beats/min, with a fall in his blood pressure from 150/88 to 110/70 mmHg. He achieved a workload of 4·7 METs (Metabolic Equivalents for exercise = a unit of resting oxygen uptake = 3·5 ml/kg/min). At peak exercise, the electrocardiogram changes were diagnostic of ischemia and his electrocardiographic abnormalities and symptoms persisted for 10 minutes after exercise was terminated, resolving after two nitroglycerin tablets were administered sublingually.

Cardiac catheterization (see Table 3.2). Aortic pressure: 160/80 mmHg. Left ventricular pressure: 160/26 mmHg. The left ventricle exhibited normal wall motion, no mitral regurgitation, and an ejection fraction of 63%. Left ventricular dimensions were within normal limits. The left main had a 75% distal stenosis. The left anterior descending artery was free of significant disease, the first obtuse marginal had a 60% stenosis, and the right coronary artery had a 90% stenosis distally.

Questions

1. What role did the exercise test play in this patient's management?
2. What is the significance of the elevated left ventricular diastolic pressure? How does it help to explain the patient's symptom complex?

3. Should the recent improvement in his symptoms influence his management?
4. What therapeutic options should be offered to the patient?
5. Are there any other clinical problems that require evaluation?

Answers

Answer to question 1   Exercise testing is performed to diagnose the presence of significant coronary artery disease (CAD); to determine the efficacy of therapy for coronary disease, either with medication or mechanical revascularization with angioplasty or bypass surgery; or to assess the exercise capacity of a patient with known heart disease due to valvular, myocardial, or coronary artery disease. This patient's history and risk factor profile make the diagnosis of coronary disease a likely one, so use of the exercise test to confirm the presence of CAD is optional. An alternative strategy in this patient would be to institute appropriate medical therapy for CAD, and then to perform an exercise test to assess the adequacy of drug treatment. In a patient with unstable angina (i.e. with symptoms of increasing duration, frequency, and severity, or angina at rest), exercise testing is generally contraindicated and prompt catheterization should be considered. The exercise test in this case demonstrated ischemic changes at a low level of activity and a drop in blood pressure during the test, both of which are suggestive of severe, possibly multivessel, coronary disease. When such an early positive result is found, catheterization is recommended to assess lesion severity specifically.

Answer to question 2   An elevated left ventricular end-diastolic pressure results from either an elevated diastolic volume or a decrease in the compliance of the left ventricle. In this patient with normal ventricular volumes found at catheterization, the latter is the case. A decrease in compliance, which results in a stiffer ventricle, is due to the combination of hypertension and coronary artery disease in this patient. In the presence of ischemia, there is a further reduction in left ventricular compliance, leading to levels of diastolic pressure even higher than those measured at the time of catheterization. Consequently, left atrial and pulmonary venous pressures rise when the patient experiences angina, leading to an increase in pulmonary capillary pressure, which is manifested as dyspnea accompanying his ischemia-induced chest discomfort. This pathophysiology can also lead to shortness of breath in patients who are ischemic but who have normal left ventricular diastolic pressures at rest.

Answer to question 3   Although the patient's symptoms are stable, the anatomic information obtained at catheterization should dictate his management. Because unstable angina carries a worse prognosis than does stable angina, more aggressive management of the patient's coronary disease is generally recommended. In this particular case it is likely that the improvement in his symptoms is due to a lower activity level with a resultant decrease in myocardial oxygen demand, rather than any meaningful improvement in his underlying condition.

Answer to question 4 Coronary artery disease (CAD) is managed with medical therapy, percutaneous revascularization using balloon angioplasty (PTCA) and allied techniques, or coronary artery bypass grafting (CABG). The decision regarding which is most appropriate is based on several factors, including the severity of coronary disease, left ventricular function, degree of symptoms, and current medical management. The presence of a stenosis of 50% or greater in the left main coronary artery is usually a firm indication for bypass surgery, regardless of left ventricular function, because CABG reduces the high mortality in these patients to a greater extent than does medical therapy. PTCA is hazardous and carries a low success rate in the left main coronary artery, and is therefore not an option for this patient. Other common indications for bypass surgery include the following: three vessel CAD in the presence of impaired left ventricular systolic function (ejection fraction <50%); two vessel CAD, in which one of the stenoses involves the proximal segment of the left anterior descending coronary artery with impaired left ventricular function; and refractory anginal symptoms in which PTCA is not a viable option because of anatomic lesion factors or patient preference.

Answer to question 5 The finding of a carotid bruit and a history of transient ischemic attacks suggests that significant carotid atherosclerosis may be present. The presence of such disease increases the risk for stroke at the time of coronary artery bypass grafting (CABG) because mean blood pressure while the patient is on cardiopulmonary support (with the heart–lung machine) is below physiologic levels, and results in cerebral hypoperfusion in the presence of a flow-limiting carotid stenosis. Non-invasive carotid imaging and potentially a carotid angiogram should be considered preoperatively, with plans for a simultaneous carotid endarterectomy and CABG if a severe stenosis is identified.

Case 3.2

A 44-year-old woman presented to hospital with new onset shortness of breath. She had been in good health with the exception of a prolonged febrile illness in childhood. She had no regular medical follow up, but was told of a murmur by her gynecologist at the time of her examination. She had one child after an uneventful pregnancy 12 years earlier. She claimed to have no prior symptoms of dyspnea, but her husband commented that she always walked at an extremely slow pace. She presented with 24 hours of palpitations and orthopnea. In the emergency department, she was found to be in atrial fibrillation at a rate of 160 beats/min, with examination findings consistent with pulmonary edema. She was treated with digoxin to slow her heart rate, diuresed with furosemide, and spontaneously converted to sinus rhythm 1 day later.

Examination (at presentation). Physical examination: the patient appeared thin and was breathless. Pulse: 110 beats/min, irregularly irregular. Blood pressure: 110/70 mmHg. Jugular venous pulse: 10 cm. Cardiac impulse: normal. First heart sound: loud. Second heart sound: split normally on inspiration with a loud P_2. No added sounds. Grade 3/6 mid-diastolic murmur heard at apex (with bell lightly applied). Chest examination: normal air entry, rales one-third up the lung fields. Abdominal examination: soft abdomen, no tenderness, and no masses. Normal liver span. No peripheral edema. Femoral, popliteal, posterior tibial, and dorsalis pedis pulses: all normal volume and equal. Carotid pulses: normal, no bruits. Optic fundi: normal.

Investigations. Chemistry and hematologic parameters within normal limits. Electrocardiogram: atrial fibrillation at 110 beats/min, normal intervals, right axis deviation, non-specific ST-segment and T-wave changes consistent with digoxin effect. Chest x ray: left atrial enlargement, pulmonary congestion with Kerley B lines.

Cardiac catheterization (Figure 3.4). Heart rate: 60 beats/min. Pressures (in mmHg): right atrium 12; right ventricle 75/9; pulmonary artery 75/23 (mean 42); pulmonary capillary wedge pressure 23 (mean); left ventricle 108/7; aorta 108/66. Mitral valve gradient: 16 mmHg. Diastolic filling period: 0·65 s. Cardiac output: 3·4 l/min.

Questions

1. What is the likely duration of her atrial fibrillation? How does the presence of this arrhythmia influence her symptom complex?
2. What is the patient's mitral valve area?
3. What is her pulmonary vascular resistance? What is the natural history of an abnormal pulmonary vascular resistance following repair/replacement of a stenotic mitral valve?
4. What would the left atrial pressure be if the cardiac output in this patient were to increase by 25%?
5. The patient undergoes a percutaneous valvuloplasty in which a balloon is placed across the stenotic valve and inflated.

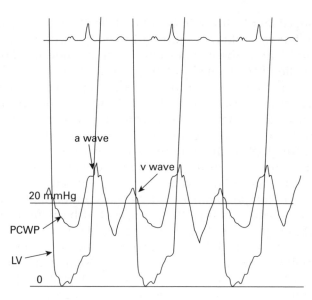

Figure 3.4 Simultaneous pulmonary capillary wedge (PCWP) and left ventricular (LV) pressures in a patient with mitral stenosis. Normally these two pressures would be superimposed during diastole, but the presence of a pressure difference is consistent with the diagnosis. (See text for full discussion)

Hemodynamic data was again obtained following balloon inflation. Heart rate: 60 beats/min. Pressures (in mmHg): right atrium 8; right ventricle 45/9; pulmonary artery 45/8 (mean 20); pulmonary capillary wedge pressure 10 (mean); left ventricle 115/7; aorta 115/66. Mitral valve gradient: 4 mmHg. Diastolic filling period: 0·65 s. Cardiac output: 4·3 l/min. What are the postprocedural mitral valve area and pulmonary vascular resistance?

Answers

Answer to question 1 Patients with mitral stenosis will frequently present when they first develop atrial fibrillation. The increase in heart rate compared with sinus rhythm results in a decrease in the diastolic filling period as the majority of the decrement in the R–R interval (beat to beat time period) with rising heart rates is derived from diastole because of the obligate time period required for the mechanical events that occur during systole. Referring to the transposed formula for the mitral valve area (MVA):

$$\text{Mean gradient}_{\text{mitral valve}} = [CO/(HR \times DFP)/(33\cdot7 \times MVA)]^2$$

where CO is the cardiac output (ml/min), HR is heart rate, and DFP is the diastolic filling period. A fall in the DFP results in an increase in the mean gradient across the mitral valve, which leads to increased left atrial pressures. Patients in this situation will acutely develop symptoms of pulmonary congestion. It is therefore likely that this patient had 1 day of atrial fibrillation, which she experienced as palpitations, and that her orthopnea is a result of an increase in her left atrial and consequently pulmonary venous pressures.

Answer to question 2 Using the formula for mitral valve area (MVA):

$$MVA = [3400/(70 \times 0.65)]/[37.7 \times (16)^{1/2}] = 0.5 \text{ cm}^2$$

Answer to question 3 Using the formula for pulmonary vascular resistance (PVR):

$$PVR = [(42 - 23)/3.4] \times 80 = 447 \text{ dyne·s/cm}^5$$

This is substantially greater than the normal value of 50–150 dyne·s/cm^5. An elevated PVR results in a second level of abnormal impedance to flow in addition to the anatomic barrier posed by the stenotic mitral valve (Figure 3.5). The resultant pressure load on the right ventricle leads to right ventricular hypertrophy and eventual right ventricular failure if the stenotic valve area is not augmented by either mitral valve surgery (valve commissurotomy or mitral valve replacement) or balloon mitral valvuloplasty. The latter procedure is performed by placing a guidewire across the stenotic valve using the transseptal technique to gain access to the left atrium via the right femoral vein. An appropriately sized balloon catheter is advanced over the guidewire, positioned in the annulus of the mitral valve, and rapidly inflated and deflated (Figure 3.6). PVR declines immediately following successful enlargement of the mitral valve area, and continues to decrease over the ensuing weeks, indicating a component of reversible pulmonary vasoconstriction.

Answer to question 4 The left atrial pressure can be calculated using the sum of the left ventricular end-diastolic pressure and the mean mitral valve gradient, although this usually results in an overestimation of left atrial pressure. Using the formula in answer 1 above and a cardiac output of 4250 ml/min with our calculated mitral valve area of 0.5 cm^2, the computed mean gradient is 42 mmHg. The resultant left atrial pressure would be approximately 49 mmHg, which is substantially greater than the value of 17 mmHg at rest.

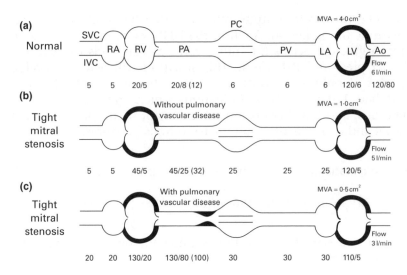

Figure 3.5 Schematic diagrams representing three hypothetical patients with **(a)** a normal mitral valve, **(b)** mitral stenosis without pulmonary vascular disease, and **(c)** mitral stenosis with pulmonary vascular disease. In the absence of pulmonary vascular disease, elevations of pulmonary arterial pressures are due primarily to passive pressure increases resulting from the mitral pressure gradient. With concomitant pulmonary vascular disease, pulmonary arterial pressures are substantially higher in order to overcome the additional stenosis in the pulmonary vascular tree. IVC, inferior vena cava; LA, left atrium; LV, left ventricle; MVA, mitral valve area; PA, pulmonary artery; PC, pulmonary capillary; PV, pulmonary vein. Reprinted with permission of Williams and Wilkins from Grossman W. Profiles in valvular heart disease. In: Grossman W, Baim DS, eds. *Cardiac catheterization, angiography and intervention, 4th ed.* Philadelphia: Lea & Febiger, 1991:559

Because the gradient is a function of the square of the cardiac output, relatively modest changes in this parameter lead to large and clinically significant alterations in pulmonary venous pressures.

Answer to question 5 The new mitral valve area (MVA) is 1.6 cm^2 and the pulmonary vascular resistance (PVR) has fallen to 186 dyne·s/cm^5. This represents a typical result following balloon valvuloplasty with a fall in mitral valve gradient, an increase in MVA, an augmentation in cardiac output, and an immediate decrease in PVR. This represents a palliative procedure that does not restore the normal MVA of 4.0–6.0 cm^2, but nonetheless replaces severe with mild mitral stenosis. The result is a return to near normal hemodynamics at rest and improvement in the patient's symptomatic status.

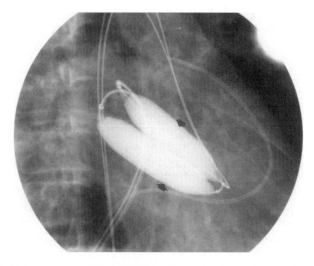

Figure 3.6 Right anterior oblique (RAO) radiograph of a patient undergoing mitral balloon valvuloplasty using the double balloon technique. Each inflated balloon is marked by an arrow, and is positioned across the mitral valve annulus

Case 3.3

A 73-year-old male with a past history remarkable only for hypertension presented to the emergency room with a complaint of the recent onset of exertional chest pressure. He last saw a physician 4 years previously, at which time a systolic murmur was detected. On further questioning, the patient also related an episode of syncope 6 months earlier that occurred after climbing several flights of stairs. Medications: enalapril 5 mg/day.

Examination. Physical examination: the patient appeared normal; no abnormalities of skin, nail beds, or oral mucosa. Pulse: 60 beats/min, slow upstroke. Blood pressure: 160/100 mmHg in right arm. Jugular venous pulse: normal. Cardiac impulse: sustained, non-displaced. First heart sound: normal. Second heart: single. Fourth heart sound: loud. Late peaking 2/6 ejection systolic murmur at left upper sternal border radiating to carotids. No diastolic murmur. Chest examination: normal air entry, no rales or rhonchi. Abdominal examination: soft abdomen, no tenderness, and no masses. Normal liver span. No peripheral edema. Carotid pulses: reduced bilaterally with slowed upstrokes. Optic fundi: normal.

Investigations. Electrocardiogram: normal sinus rhythm, left atrial enlargement, and voltage criteria for left ventricular hypertrophy.

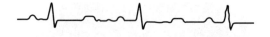

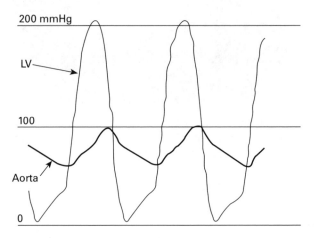

Figure 3.7 Simultaneous tracing of left ventricular (LV) and aortic pressures in a patient with aortic stenosis. Note the slowed systolic upstroke of the aortic pressure wave as compared with the LV upstroke, which is consistent with valvular stenosis. (See text for full discussion)

Chest *x* ray: normal cardiac silhouette, calcification in the region of the aortic valve.

Cardiac catheterization (Figure 3.7). Heart rate: 76 beats/min. Pressures (in mmHg): right atrium 6; right ventricle 25/6; pulmonary artery 35/15 (mean 22); pulmonary capillary wedge pressure 15 (mean); left ventricle 208/20; aorta 102/62. Aortic valve gradient: 74 mmHg. Systolic ejection period: 0·34 s. Cardiac output: 5·9 l/min. Coronary angiography: normal coronaries, left dominant system.

Questions

1. Does the presence of hypertension exclude the presence of significant aortic stenosis?
2. What is the aortic valve area? Is valve replacement surgery warranted?

3. Is it unusual that the patient has symptoms consistent with angina in the absence of coronary artery disease?
4. Why is the syncope related to aortic stenosis exertional or postexertional?

Answers

Answer to question 1 In aortic stenosis, the peak left ventricular systolic pressure is equal to the sum of the systemic systolic pressure and the gradient across the aortic valve. Even in the presence of severe aortic stenosis it is possible for a patient to manifest systemic hypertension because it is feasible for the left ventricle to generate systolic pressures of up to 250 mmHg. If such a patient had a peak gradient across the aortic valve of 90 mmHg, then the measured systolic pressure would be 160 mmHg.

Answer to question 2 Using the Gorlin formula with the aortic valve constant of 44·3 and the cardiac catheterization data provided above:

$$\text{Aortic valve area} = [5900/(76 \times 0{\cdot}34)]/[44{\cdot}3 \times (74)^{\frac{1}{2}}] = 0{\cdot}6 \text{ cm}^2$$

Surgery is generally recommended in the presence of symptoms, manifest as syncope, angina, or congestive heart failure, if the calculated valve area is less than 1·1 cm². Because of the morbidity and mortality of valve surgery and the knowledge that the event rate in asymptomatic patients is low, the presence of aortic stenosis alone is not an indication for surgery.

Answer to question 3 Angina pectoris is caused by an imbalance of oxygen supply and demand. Aortic stenosis leads to marked increases in left ventricular mass caused by the presence of chronic pressure overload. In addition, wall stress, a major determinant of myocardial oxygen demand, is elevated because of the high intracavitary pressures. These circumstances can lead to a resting level of myocardial oxygen demand such that minor increases as a result of exertion can produce ischemia due to the "supranormal" needs of the hypertrophied myocardium, which cannot be met by even a "normal" coronary tree.

In addition, there are physiologic constraints on myocardial blood flow in the patient with aortic stenosis. As with all patients, because of increased intramyocardial pressures during systole, the majority of coronary blood flow occurs during diastole. The gradient for blood flow during this period is the difference between the pressure at the origin of the coronary artery (aortic diastolic pressure) and at the endocardial surface (left ventricular end-diastolic pressure [LVEDP]). Because of increased ventricular stiffness resulting from left ventricular hypertrophy, the LVEDP is frequently elevated in patients with aortic stenosis, leading to a decrease in the pressure difference driving coronary blood flow.

Because aortic stenosis results in both increased myocardial oxygen demand and a relative decrease in supply, it is not unusual that angina is experienced by such patients, even in the absence of coronary artery disease.

Answer to question 4 During exercise the increased metabolic demands of the skeletal muscle lead to vasodilatation and a decrease in systemic vascular resistance. The ventricle normally responds to this decreased impedance to ejection by increasing stroke volume. Coupled with the increased heart rate that is typically seen with exertion, the cardiac output (which is the product of heart rate and stroke volume) increases. In the patient with significant aortic stenosis, the major source of afterload is the stenotic valve rather than the impedance of the resistance vessels. Consequently, the exercise-induced fall in peripheral resistance may not be matched by an appropriate increase in cardiac output, leading to a fall in blood pressure (which is the product of cardiac output and peripheral vascular resistance). This decrease in perfusion pressure can reduce myocardial blood flow, resulting in myocardial ischemia and further decrements in blood pressure caused by ischemia-induced left ventricular dysfunction. Once blood pressure falls to the point that central nervous system perfusion is affected, syncope may ensue.

An additional insult occurs during the postexertional state due to the rapid fall in skeletal muscle augmented venous return that accompanies the halting of exercise. Because the ventricle in patients with aortic stenosis is stiff as a result of the ventricular hypertrophy that accompanies this condition, maintaining cardiac output is highly dependent on the presence of adequate ventricular filling during diastole. This dependence on preload results in marked decreases in cardiac output and consequently blood pressure when ventricular filling is reduced, as is the case immediately following exercise. For the same reason, aggressive use of diuretic therapy in patients with aortic stenosis can be hazardous.

Case 3.4

A 28-year-old woman presented with a 1 year history of gradually increasing dyspnea on exertion and easy fatigability. She had an uneventful prior medical history, with two uncomplicated pregnancies 3 and 8 years previously. She had no risk factors for coronary artery disease.

Examination. Physical examination: the patient appeared normal. No cyanosis or clubbing. Pulse: 60 beats/min, normal character. Blood pressure: 108/70 mmHg in right arm. Jugular venous pulse: 5 cm. Cardiac impulse: fifth intercostal space 2 cm lateral to mid-clavicular line. Parasternal lift present. First heart sound: normal. Second heart sound: fixed splitting with no increase in intensity of P_2. No added sounds. Grade 3/6 systolic ejection murmur heard best in pulmonic area. Chest examination: normal air entry, no rales or rhonchi. Abdominal examination: soft abdomen, no tenderness, and no masses. Normal liver span. No peripheral edema. Femoral, popliteal, posterior tibial, and dorsalis pedis pulses: all normal volume and equal. Carotid pulses: normal, no bruits. Optic fundi: normal.

Investigations. Electrocardiogram: normal sinus rhythm, axis 120°, incomplete right bundle branch block, no ST or T wave abnormalities. Chest x ray: enlarged cardiac silhouette with right atrial and right ventricular prominence, enlargement of both pulmonary arteries.

Cardiac catheterization. Pressures (in mmHg): right atrium 4 (mean); right ventricle 26/4; pulmonary artery 26/9 (mean 16); pulmonary capillary wedge pressure 9 (mean); aorta 122/75 (mean 98). Oxygen saturations (in %; mean of all saturations drawn in each chamber): inferior vena cava (IVC) 70; superior vena cava (SVC) 58; vena cava 61; right atrium 83; right ventricle 83; pulmonary artery 83; aorta 95. Oxygen content (ml/100 ml): IVC 12·9; SVC 10·7; vena cava 11·3; right atrium 15·3; right ventricle 15·3; pulmonary artery 15·3; aorta 17·6. Oxygen consumption: 213 ml/min. Hemoglobin: 13·3 g/dl. Oxygen contents were calculated using the following formula (for explanation, see the section on Oxygen saturations and shunt calculations, above):

$$O_2 \text{ content (ml/100 ml)} = O_2 \text{ saturation (\%)}$$
$$\times \text{ hemoglobin (g/100 ml)} \times 1·39 \text{ (ml } O_2/\text{g hemoglobin)}$$

Questions

1. What findings on physical examination, electrocardiogram, and chest x ray film are consistent with an atrial septal defect?
2. Based on the oxygen saturation data, where is the site of the shunt? What is the shunt ratio (Q_p/Q_s)?
3. What are the peripheral and systemic resistances?
4. What arguments can be used for counseling surgical closure of the atrial septal defect?

Answers

Answer to question 1 Patients with an atrial septal defect (ASD) usually have shunting of blood from the left to right sided cardiac chambers at the level of the atrium. In fact, the size of the defect essentially converts the two atria into a common chamber. As a result, the augmented filling of the right atrium with inspiration, which normally causes the A_2–P_2 interval of the second heart sound to increase, is negated. Consequently, physiologic splitting of the second heart sound is replaced by fixed splitting. Electrocardiogram findings in patients with an ASD typically include incomplete right bundle branch block with right axis deviation in secundum defects and left axis deviation in primum defects. The chest x ray findings reflect the increased right heart flows, which result from the left to right shunting of blood. Right atrial and ventricular enlargement are common, and increased flow to the pulmonary bed is manifested as enlargement of the pulmonary arteries and pulmonary plethora, a generalized increase in the caliber of smaller order pulmonary arteries. Because of normal left heart hemodynamics, evidence of pulmonary venous hypertension is not observed.

Answer to question 2 Inspection of the saturation data is necessary to determine the shunt site. Using the values presented in Table 3.3, the oxygen saturation differences between vena cava and right atrium, right atrium and right ventricle, and right ventricle and pulmonary artery are therefore 12%, 0%, and 0%, respectively. Only the value of 12% crosses the threshold for a pathologic step-up using mean saturations from each chamber, and therefore the sole site of the left to right shunt is the atrium.

The left to right shunt results in an increase in flow in the pulmonary circulation (Q_p) as compared with the systemic circulation (Q_s), whereas these two values are equal in individuals without an intracardiac shunt. The Fick principle is utilized to calculate these values. The modified equations (see the section on Oxygen saturations and shunt calculations, above) use the oxygen contents entering and leaving each of the two blood flow circuits. The value for the mixed venous saturation is taken from the chamber proximal to the shunt, which in the case of an atrial septal defect is the vena cava. Because of differential contributions from the superior vena cava (SVC) and inferior vena cava (IVC), the weighted average $[(3 \times SVC\ SO_2) + IVC\ SO_2]/4$ is most frequently used.

$$\text{Pulmonary blood flow} = Q_p = 213/[13{\cdot}3 \times 1{\cdot}39 \times 10 \times (0{\cdot}95{-}0{\cdot}83) = 9{\cdot}6 \text{ l/min}$$

$$\text{Systemic blood flow} = Q_s = 213/[13{\cdot}3 \times 1{\cdot}39 \times 10 \times (0{\cdot}95{-}0{\cdot}61) = 3{\cdot}4 \text{ l/min}$$

The shunt ratio $Q_p/Q_s = 9{\cdot}6/3{\cdot}4 = 2{\cdot}8{:}1$.

Answer to question 3 The pulmonary vascular resistance (PVR) and systemic vascular resistance (SVR) are calculated using a modification to the formulae (see the formulae under Cardiac output, above) with the appropriate blood flow substituted in the denominator.

$$PVR = [(PA-PCWP)/Q_p] \times 80 = [(16-9)/9{\cdot}6] \times 80 = 58 \text{ dyne}{\cdot}\text{s/cm}^5$$

$$SVR = [(Ao-RA)/Q_s] \times 80 = [(98-4)/3{\cdot}4] \times 80 = 2212 \text{ dyne}{\cdot}\text{s/cm}^5$$

These values are both within normal limits and are typical of patients with atrial septal defect, who infrequently develop pulmonary vascular abnormalities as a result of the increased flow that accompanies the left to right shunt. Such alterations, which can lead to pulmonary hypertension as a result of a permanent increases in PVR, are more common with more distal shunts, for example a ventricular septal defect or patent ductus arteriosus. When the abnormality is so severe that the ratio of PVR to SVR is 1 or more, patients are said to exhibit Eisenmenger's physiology.

Answer to question 4 Surgical closure of atrial septal defect is generally recommended in patients with a shunt ratio (Q_p/Q_s) of 1·5 or greater. Elimination of the increased right heart blood flow will alleviate the long-term complications of right heart failure and atrial arrhythmias that accompany this disorder. In addition, ASD closure theoretically eliminates the risk of paradoxic emboli resulting from transit of small thrombi or air through the interatrial septum into the systemic circulation. There is also strong evidence that ASD repair prolongs life, as long as the operation can be performed with acceptable levels of surgical mortality. If the PVR/SVR ratio is 0·25 or less, then a mortality of below 1% should be expected. Higher ratios, reflecting pulmonary vascular disease, increase surgical mortality and a value of 0·75 or more is generally a contraindication to closure because of unacceptable surgical risk. Percutaneous ASD closure using an implanted "clamshell" device is performed in some cardiovascular centers.

Case 3.5

A 53-year-old male presented with 3 months of increasing lower extremity edema and exertional fatigue. He was in excellent health with the exception of previous pulmonary tuberculosis, for which he was treated with appropriate drug therapy 5 years ago. He first noted the inability to complete the task of mowing his lawn without frequent rests because of marked fatigue. He noticed swelling of his feet and legs shortly thereafter, which had gradually increased in severity. He currently takes no medications.

Examination. Physical examination: the patient appeared thin. Respiratory rate: 18/min. No abnormalities of skin, nail beds, or oral mucosa. Pulse: 110 beats/min, normal character. Blood pressure: 108/60 mmHg in right arm. Jugular venous pulse: pulsations observed near the angle of jaw with further elevations during inspiration (Kussmaul's sign). Cardiac impulse: normal. First heart sound: distant. Second heart sound: split normally on inspiration. No added sounds or murmurs. Chest examination: normal air entry, bibasilar rales. Abdominal examination: soft abdomen, liver span 17 cm, non-pulsatile. Peripheral edema to mid-thighs. Femoral, popliteal, posterior tibial and dorsalis pedis pulses: all normal volume and equal. Carotid pulses: normal, no bruits. Optic fundi: normal.

Investigations. Hematology and chemistry profile within normal limits. Electrocardiogram: sinus tachycardia PR interval 0–16 s; QRS duration 0·08 s, frontal axis 60°. Low QRS voltage with diffuse T-wave flattening. Chest *x* ray: normal heart size with pericardial calcification, mild pulmonary venous congestion, apical scarring unchanged from chest *x* ray film 5 years earlier. Calcified hilar nodes.

Cardiac catheterization. Heart rate: 110 beats/min. Pressures (in mmHg): right atrium 20 (prominent X and Y descents); right ventricle 43/20; pulmonary artery 43/23; pulmonary capillary wedge pressure PCWP 20; left ventricle 110/24; aorta 110/76. Body surface area: 1·60 m². Left ventriculography: normal wall motion, ejection fraction 67%. End-systolic volume index: 20 ml/m². End-diastolic volume index: 45 ml/m².

Questions

1. What physical examination findings are helpful in the diagnosis?
2. What cardiac catheterization findings are consistent with the diagnosis?
3. Why did the patient present primarily with findings of right sided heart failure?
4. Why did the patient develop exertional fatigue?

Answers

Answer to question 1 The physical examination and hemodynamic manifestations of constrictive pericarditis are caused by the impaired ventricular filling caused by the ensheathment of the heart within a rigid structure. As a result, there is an elevation and equalization in all chamber pressures during diastole. This circumstance also results in a small stroke volume due to the inability of the ventricles to fill normally. On physical examination, right atrial pressure is most readily assessable by observation of the level of the jugular venous pressure wave, and is invariably elevated in constrictive pericarditis. Other signs of right sided failure develop with time, and included hepatomegaly and peripheral edema in this patient.

Kussmaul's sign is a paradoxic rise in the jugular venous pressure with inspiration, which reflects the increase in right atrial pressure that accompanies this maneuver. Normally, the augmented venous return that accompanies inspiration is countered by the reduction in intrathoracic pressure transmitted to the heart, resulting in a decrease in right atrial pressure. In constrictive pericarditis, venous return still increases with inspiration because the vena cavae are exposed to intrathoracic pressure excursions, but the rigid pericardium does not transmit the fall in intrathoracic pressure to the heart. As a result, this transient volume load leads to an elevation in right atrial pressure.

The presence of rales also indicates elevation in left atrial pressure. The severity of pulmonary congestion is dependent on the level to which the equalized diastolic pressures rise.

Answer to question 2 Because of impaired diastolic filling, the majority of ventricular inflow occurs in the early part of diastole followed by early onset of diastasis. This leads to the "dip and plateau" appearance of the diastolic portion of the right ventricular pressure tracing (Figure 3.8). The "dip" coincides with the rapid and prominent Y descent of the right atrial pressure tracing. The prominent X descent follows a peaked "a" wave as the atrium attempts to eject into a right ventricle that can accept no additional volume.

Diastolic equalization of pressures at an elevated level is another hallmark finding, and is most frequently demonstrated with simultaneous right ventricular and left ventricular pressure tracings, with diastolic values within 5 mm of each other (see Figure 3.8). Typically, left ventricular ejection fraction is normal, with small systolic and diastolic volumes resulting from the increased resistance to ventricular filling that accompanies this condition.

Answer to question 3 The right atrial and left atrial pressures (as reflected by the pulmonary capillary wedge pressure) are both elevated to similar levels in this case. The pulmonary vascular system has great capacity to compensate for gradually increasing left atrial pressure by increasing the ability of the lymphatic system to remove the obligate increase in interstitial fluid accompanying the shift in hydrostatic forces that occurs with elevations in left atrial pressures. As a result, there is a limited degree of interstitial fluid accumulation in the alveoli, which results in less pulmonary congestion than would have occurred if the rise in left atrial pressures occurred abruptly. The

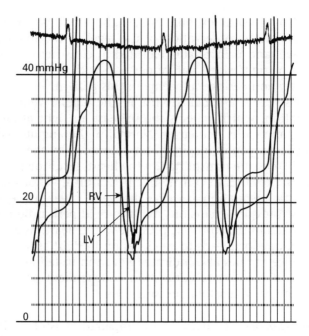

Figure 3.8 Simultaneous left ventricular (LV) and right ventricular (RV) pressures in a patient with constrictive pericarditis. Note the dip and plateau configurations of both pressures in diastole. (See text for full discussion)

systemic venous system has a far more limited ability to compensate for the increases in right atrial pressure, and findings of systemic venous congestion become clinically manifest.

Answer to question 4 Because of small and fixed ventricular volumes, the patient with constrictive pericarditis maintains cardiac output with an increase in resting heart rate (cardiac output = heart rate × stroke volume). In this case:

Stroke volume = EDV–ESV = body surface area × (ESVI–EDVI) = 40 ml

Cardiac output = 110 × 40 = 4400 ml/min

where EDVI is end-diastolic volume index and ESVI is end-systolic volume index. During exercise, the patient is unable to increase stroke volume significantly, and therefore increases in cardiac output are dependent solely on increased heart rate. Assuming an exercise rate of 160 beats/min and the same stroke volume, cardiac output = 160 × 40 = 6400 ml/min. This augmentation in cardiac output is far less than expected for an exercising patient, and is unable to meet the increased metabolic demands of the exercising skeletal muscle. As a result, the patient experiences fatigue and suffers from diminished exercise tolerance.

Percutaneous transluminal coronary angioplasty

The term percutaneous transluminal coronary angioplasty (PTCA) refers to the dilatation of a coronary artery lesion using a balloon catheter placed within the lumen of the affected vessel. Since its inception in 1977, PTCA has been utilized in many patients with stable angina, unstable angina, and acute myocardial infarction. Its use was initially limited to discrete stenoses in proximal segments of a coronary artery, but improvements in equipment and techniques have led to its use in more complex stenoses, in distal coronary arterial segments, and in relatively high risk patients.

The mechanisms by which PTCA increases the size of the arterial lumen include cracking, splitting, and disruption of the atherosclerotic plaque; dehiscence of the intima and plaque from the underlying media; and stretching or tearing of the media and adventitia, with resultant aneurysmal dilatation. These morphologic alterations result in new pathways for blood flow, leading to an augmentation in the effective luminal size. At the same time, balloon inflation may be deleterious, causing plaque hemorrhage, extensive dissection (resulting in luminal compromise), platelet deposition, and thrombus formation. Periprocedural antiplatelet and antithrombotic therapy (aspirin and heparin, respectively) is administered to reduce the incidence of the latter two events. In the weeks after successful PTCA, favorable remodeling of the disrupted plaque and endothelialization at sites of intimal injury result in increased luminal size. The major limitation to PTCA is the recurrence of the stenosis (restenosis) in the months following a successful procedure.

Indications

Stable, exertional angina

PTCA provides effective relief of stable angina in most patients with single-vessel coronary artery disease. In those with multivessel disease it is less likely to achieve complete long-term alleviation of angina because the incidence of lesion recurrence is increased when multiple stenoses are dilated, and because incomplete revascularization results when only "culprit" stenoses – those deemed most likely to be responsible for symptoms – are dilated.

The relatively short-term results of several randomized trials comparing PTCA and bypass surgery in patients with stable angina and single or multivessel coronary artery disease have been reported. The studies are in agreement that the end-points of death and non-fatal myocardial infarction are equivalent with either revascularization strategy. However, patients treated with PTCA have more additional procedures (because of restenosis), take more antianginal medication, and have less optimal anginal relief in the first years following the index procedure than are their surgical counterparts. On the other hand, the procedure is less traumatic and has low morbidity and mortality.

Unstable angina

When treated medically, patients with unstable angina have an in-hospital mortality rate of 1–5%, and up to 10% sustain a myocardial infarction before hospital discharge. A few patients with unstable angina can be managed successfully with aggressive medical therapy; however, most patients are also investigated with coronary angiography and revascularization when appropriate. Initial success with PTCA is slightly lower in patients with unstable angina than in those with stable angina, and the incidence of vessel closure and restenosis is somewhat higher. Nevertheless, with the use of coronary stents and new antiplatelet medications, excellent results are obtained acutely.

Acute myocardial infarction

Recent randomized trials comparing primary PTCA with intravenous thrombolytic therapy in patients with evolving infarction have demonstrated that antegrade flow in the infarct-related artery can be restored in about 95% of those undergoing PTCA, which is greater than that achieved (75–90%) with thrombolytic therapy. Those having primary PTCA had fewer in-hospital adverse events (non-fatal reinfarction or death) and were less likely to have recurrent ischemia or to require coronary revascularization during follow up. As compared with thrombolytic therapy, PTCA is particularly advantageous in "high risk" patients (those older than 65 years, those with anterior infarction, or those with persistent tachycardia). Many major medical centers with equipment and resources available perform primary angioplasty, provided they have the ability to open occluded vessels within 60–90 min of the patient's arrival in hospital; however, the majority of patients who are not treated in these settings receive thrombolytic therapy.

In patients with myocardial infarction complicated by cardiogenic shock, the in-hospital mortality with medical therapy is approximately

80%. Consideration of emergent PTCA in this group of patients is supported by several retrospective studies that suggested that some patients with cardiogenic shock have a markedly improved outcome if patency of the infarct-related artery is restored. The randomized SHOCK trial confirmed the benefit of early revascularization with PTCA or coronary artery bypass grafting (for those patients with left main or severe coronary artery disease in whom PTCA is not feasible) in this patient population, especially for those younger than 75 years.

Following thrombolytic therapy

Although thrombolytic therapy restores antegrade perfusion of the infarct-related artery in most patients, some are left with a severe residual stenosis of the infarct artery, which may lead to recurrent thrombotic occlusion. In these patients, PTCA after thrombolysis could theoretically reduce the severity of the residual stenosis and the likelihood of recurrent occlusion, thereby improving morbidity and mortality. This hypothesis has been tested by performing PTCA in lytic treated patients acutely, days, and up to 1 week following the infarct. It has been convincingly demonstrated that routine PTCA of the infarct-related artery following thrombolytic therapy confers no benefit, and patients managed in this manner are at increased risk for adverse events if the intervention is performed acutely. Following thrombolytic therapy, therefore, PTCA should be reserved for the patient with symptomatic or objective evidence of ischemia.

Summary of techniques

Medications

Aspirin is routinely given periprocedurally to reduce the incidence of abrupt closure of the artery being dilated. Clopidogrel (an inhibitor of platelet aggregation that inhibits binding of adenosine diphosphate to its platelet receptor, and thus interferes with activation of the glycoprotein IIb/IIIa complex) is routinely administered for up to 1 month following PTCA and stent placement. Intravenous glycoprotein IIb/IIIa inhibitors (abciximab, tirofiban, eptifibatide) are frequently administered in selected cases because of their ability to reduce periprocedural myocardial infarction, although they do not reduce restenosis or mortality. Heparin is administered intravenously during the procedure to decrease the incidence of coronary arterial thrombosis. In patients with a history of heparin-induced thrombocytopenia, direct thrombin inhibitors (lepirudin, argatroban, bivalirudin) are alternatives. Nitroglycerin (sublingual and/or

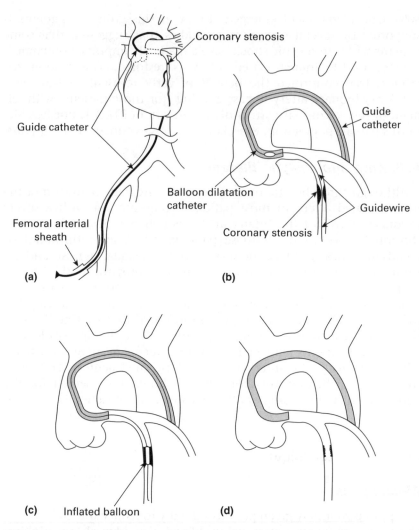

Figure 3.9 Sequence in percutaneous transluminal coronary angioplasty. **(a)** Advancement of guide catheter. **(b)** Passage of flexible guidewire through catheter to the distal arterial segment and subsequent placement of balloon dilatation catheter. **(c)** Inflation of the balloon. **(d)** Withdrawal of balloon dilatation catheter and guidewire. (See text for full discussion.) Reprinted by permission of the *New England Journal of Medicine*, from Landau C, Lange RA, Hillis LD. Percutaneous transluminal coronary angioplasty. *N Engl J Med* 1994;**330**:983, Massachusetts Medical Society

intracoronary) and, at times, a calcium antagonist are given to prevent coronary vasospasm and to diminish ischemia during balloon inflation (by reducing myocardial oxygen demand while coronary flow is interrupted).

Procedure

PTCA equipment consists of a large lumen "guide" catheter, a flexible guidewire, and a balloon dilatation catheter. Vascular access is usually attained using techniques similar to those for diagnostic catheterization. A guide catheter is advanced through the arterial sheath to the ostium of the coronary artery to be dilated (Figure 3.9a). The guide catheter is stiffer than the catheters used for diagnostic angiography, and it has a larger internal diameter to permit delivery of radiographic contrast material and visualization of the artery when the guidewire and balloon dilatation catheter are within the guide catheter.

With the guide catheter positioned in the coronary ostium, angiography of the diseased artery is performed to visualize the stenosis and the artery proximal and distal to it. The flexible guidewire is advanced through the guide catheter, navigated or "steered" across the stenosis, and positioned in the distal arterial segment (Figure 3.9b). With the guidewire across the stenosis, the deflated balloon dilatation catheter is advanced over the guidewire and positioned at the stenosis. The position of the guidewire and balloon dilatation catheter are confirmed periodically by visualizing the artery as contrast material is injected through the guide catheter. Once positioned, the balloon is usually inflated for 1–2 min at 2–8 atmospheres of pressure with a mixture of saline and contrast material, so that balloon inflations can be visualized fluoroscopically (Figure 3.9c). The patient often has angina and/or electrocardiographic evidence of ischemia during balloon inflation, because the coronary artery is temporarily occluded. If an adequate result is achieved, then the guidewire and balloon dilatation catheter are removed. If the stenosis is not adequately dilated, then the guidewire remains across the stenosis, and the initial balloon dilatation catheter may be replaced with a larger one. Once balloon inflations are completed, a final angiogram is obtained to confirm that the result is satisfactory and that other segments of the artery, including branches, have not been compromised (Figure 3.9d).

Postprocedural management

Over the 4–8 hours after PTCA, the patient is observed as the anticoagulant effect of heparin subsides. The femoral arterial sheath is then removed, and hemostasis is achieved. If there is angiographic evidence of extensive coronary arterial dissection or thrombosis, some operators continue heparin overnight. If the procedure is uncomplicated, then the patient is discharged within 24 hours. Discharge medications are determined by the patient's underlying cardiac condition; no post-PTCA regimens are recommended routinely.

Procedural success and risks

Success rates

With modern equipment, PTCA of a non-occluded coronary artery is successful in approximately 90–95% of patients, with success defined as a luminal diameter narrowing of 50% or less (by visual estimation) on the post-PTCA angiogram. In the remaining 10%, PTCA is unsuccessful because the stenosis cannot be crossed with the guidewire; the stenosis is crossed with the wire but cannot be crossed with the balloon dilatation catheter; the stenosis does not dilate adequately despite the use of an appropriately sized balloon; or the vessel abruptly occludes (so-called "abrupt closure"). PTCA of stenoses that are chronically occluded, long, eccentric, angulated, calcified, ostial, located at the site of a branch point, associated with intraluminal thrombus, or located within a saphenous vein bypass graft have a lower success rate. Clinical variables associated with a lower success rate include unstable angina, advanced age, and possibly female sex.

Short-term complications

Although PTCA is generally safe, complications occasionally occur, including myocardial infarction in 2–4%, the need for emergency bypass surgery in 2–5%, and death in 0–2%. These events are usually caused by extensive coronary arterial dissection, intracoronary thrombosis, or both, with resultant vessel occlusion.

Acute or abrupt closure occurs in 1–6% of patients undergoing PTCA and accounts for most of the short-term morbidity and mortality associated with the procedure. In the majority of patients with abrupt closure, it manifests within minutes of PTCA, at a time when they are still in the catheterization laboratory; in the others, it usually occurs within 24 hours of the procedure. Several clinical, anatomic, and procedural variables are associated with an increased incidence of abrupt closure with PTCA, including the following: female sex; unstable angina; intracoronary thrombus; lesions that are long, eccentric, in a diffusely diseased artery, calcified or located on a bend; and extensive dissection as a result of PTCA. The likelihood of abrupt closure escalates with increasing numbers of these factors being present.

The consequences of abrupt closure are variable and depend on collateral supply and the size of the territory supplied by the acutely occluded vessel. Most commonly, abrupt closure is accompanied by chest discomfort and electrocardiographic evidence of ischemia, and requires urgent revascularization of the occluded vessel to prevent or limit myocardial injury.

When abrupt closure occurs, redilatation with a standard balloon dilatation catheter is usually attempted and is successful in about half of the patients. When this strategy fails, a perfusion balloon catheter may be introduced if the coronary anatomy is suitable. The catheter design maintains perfusion of the distal artery during prolonged (10–30 min) inflations. If these strategies are unsuccessful in restoring and stabilizing antegrade flow, then placement of an intracoronary stent may be considered. Although this device initially restores flow in over 90% of patients with abrupt closure, procedure-related infarction of some magnitude may occur, and subacute closure in the ensuing days to weeks occurs in up to 10–15% of patients so treated.

If percutaneous methods fail to restore antegrade flow in the abruptly occluded artery, then the patient is usually referred for emergency bypass grafting. Although the early mortality associated with emergency bypass surgery is higher than for an elective procedure, survivors of emergency surgery appear to have a good long-term prognosis. Despite successful surgery, 25–50% of patients with abrupt closure evolve a Q-wave myocardial infarction.

Long-term complications

In patients who have undergone successful PTCA, the major limitation to long-term, event-free survival is recurrence of the stenosis, a process termed restenosis. Restenosis is most commonly defined as a greater than 50% stenosis at the site of a previously successful PTCA. Restenosis occurs in about 30–50% of patients in whom a narrowed artery is successfully dilated and in about 60% of those in whom a chronically occluded artery is dilated. Restenosis most often occurs 1–3 months after PTCA, and 95% of those who develop it do so within 6 months.

Patients with restenosis after successful PTCA usually experience recurrent angina, but up to half of those in whom angiographic restenosis occurs are asymptomatic. Because these patients have a good prognosis, repeat PTCA should be reserved for those with recurrent symptoms. Restenosis is often treated successfully with a second PTCA. In comparison to the initial PTCA, the second procedure is more likely to be successful and less likely to be associated with an acute complication. The incidence of restenosis after a second PTCA is thought to be similar to that after the initial dilatation. Thus, sustained clinical success is likely to be achieved in 80–90% of patients following one or two angioplasties.

Numerous pharmacologic approaches and new devices have been evaluated in an attempt to prevent restenosis. To date, only intracoronary stent placement (see below) has convincingly demonstrated an ability to reduce the incidence of restenosis.

Intracoronary stents

There is a wide variety of intracoronary stents available for deployment in the coronary arteries after PTCA. These will reduce the rate of restenosis, as compared with PTCA alone, when introduced into vessels of sufficiently large caliber. Two randomized trials compared Palmaz-Schatz stent placement following PTCA versus PTCA alone for elective procedures in large vessels ($\geq 3 \cdot 0$ mm) and convincingly demonstrated that angiographic restenosis and need for repeat interventions were lower in stented patients. This benefit was derived at the cost of longer hospital stays and a greater incidence of vascular complications in the stented group because of the need for aggressive anticoagulation following stent placement. The incidence of stent thrombosis, for which a patient is at risk for approximately 30 days following the procedure, was less than 4% in those studies. Because stent deployment strategies now include only aspirin and clopidogrel for 1 month instead of a combination of aspirin and coumadin, there are currently no disadvantages to using stents, other than cost.

Although the incidence of lesion recurrence is decreased with stenting, in-stent restenosis is a difficult situation to treat because of a high incidence (up to 70%) of a second restenosis, especially if the renarrowing involves the majority of the stent length. Intravascular radiation (brachytherapy) using either β or γ emitters have been demonstrated to reduce conclusively the incidence of recurrent in-stent restenosis, although at a greater risk for stent thrombosis. Consequently, patients receiving coronary brachytherapy are treated with aspirin and clopridogel for 6–9 months rather than the usual 30 days. A promising alternative is the use of coated stents, which locally release antiproliferative pharmaceuticals continuously over several weeks. Initial results using paclitaxel and sirolimus eluting stents have shown a marked reduction in in-stent restenosis, although further studies are needed.

Coronary atherectomy

Atherectomy refers to a procedure that employs a class of percutaneously introduced devices to actually remove or pulverize plaque within the coronary arteries. Like balloon angioplasty, a guide catheter and guidewire are used with all of these devices.

Directional coronary atherectomy involves the use of a device with a windowed cylindrical housing that is compressed against the stenosis as the attached balloon is inflated against the opposite wall of the artery. Once positioned, a rotating metal cutting blade inside the housing is advanced, shaving plaque from the vessel wall and depositing the shaved debris in the catheter's nose cone. An increased luminal area is achieved by the dilating effect of the device itself, angioplasty effect from balloon inflation, and the removal of atherosclerotic material. When used for non-calcified stenoses, the incidence of initial success, abrupt closure, and restenosis with atherectomy is similar to that with PTCA. At present, atherectomy offers no obvious benefit as compared with PTCA.

Transluminal extraction atherectomy is a different device that employs a rotating conical blade that is attached to a hollow shaft through which suction is applied. The contents of the vessel cut by the blade are liquefied and removed by the vacuum, which is transmitted to the tip of the device. It has been less well studied than directional atherectomy, and appears to have a role primarily in lesions with intracoronary thrombus or in old, degenerated saphenous vein grafts, which are usually lined with friable atheromatous material.

Rotational atherectomy utilizes a high speed burr that pulverizes plaque as it is passed through the diseased vessel over the guidewire. Its utility is greatest in heavily calcified lesions, diffusely diseased vessels, and ostial stenoses. As with transluminal atherectomy, most lesions treated with the device are subjected to adjunctive balloon angioplasty or stenting to achieve an optimal result. Rotational atherectomy is utilized primarily in circumstances in which primary PTCA is an unattractive option because of high-risk lesion characteristics.

Case studies

Case 3.6

A 58-year-old diabetic hypertensive man with a several-year history of exertional angina presented to the hospital with a prolonged episode of pain at rest. He was admitted and was rendered pain-free with the addition of intravenous nitroglycerin and heparin to his regimen. A myocardial infarction was excluded with serial cardiac enzymes and electrocardiograms. He had several recurrent episodes of angina on hospital day 2 and, because of his refractory ischemia, he was sent to the cardiac catheterization laboratory. Medications: aspirin 325 mg/day, nitroglycerin 150 micrograms/min intravenously, heparin 1200 U/hour intravenously, metoprolol 100 mg twice per day, diltiazem 60 mg four times per day, and glyburide 5 mg/day.

Examination. Physical examination: the patient appeared normal. Pulse: 54 beats/min, normal character. Blood pressure: 100/60 mmHg in right arm. Jugular venous pulse: 6 cm. Cardiac impulse: normal. First heart sound: normal. Second heart sound: split normally on inspiration. No added sounds or murmurs. Chest examination: normal air entry, no rales or rhonchi. Abdominal examination: soft abdomen, no tenderness, and no masses. Normal liver span. No peripheral edema. Femoral, popliteal, posterior tibial, and dorsalis pedis pulses: all normal volume and equal. Carotid pulses: normal, no bruits. Optic fundi: normal.

Investigations. Hematology and biochemistry: normal. Electrocardiogram: sinus bradycardia; PR interval 0·24 s; QRS duration 0·09 s. Flattened T waves in leads I and aVL. During anginal episodes, 1·5 mm of horizontal ST depression in these same leads. Chest *x* ray: normal cardiac silhouette, no pulmonary venous congestion.

Cardiac catheterization. Aortic pressure: 98/60 mmHg. Left ventricular pressure: 98/20 mmHg. Normal left ventricular wall motion, ejection fraction 55%, no mitral regurgitation. Left ventricular systolic and diastolic volumes were within normal limits. The left main had a normal contour without stenoses. The left anterior descending artery had a 30% lesion in its mid-portion, there was a 90% lesion of the proximal left circumflex artery that measured 2·5 mm, and the right coronary artery had a 50% lesion in its distal segment.

Questions

1. Is it reasonable to continue medical therapy alone?
2. What revascularization options can be offered to the patient?
3. Should stenting be considered as a primary modality for this patient?

Answers

Answer to question 1 Although many patients with unstable angina can successfully be treated with medications, this patient is experiencing ongoing ischemia despite an aggressive regimen. One of the objectives of medical therapy is to reduce myocardial oxygen demand by decreasing heart rate and blood pressure. This patient already exhibits excellent control of both parameters, and in addition has first-degree atrioventricular block on the electrocardiogram that may be drug induced. Increased doses of his calcium antagonist or β-blocker may result in bradyarrhythmias and/or hypotension. The

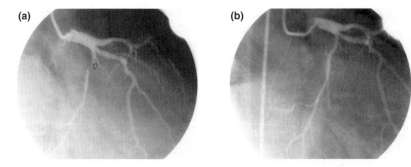

Figure 3.10 Cineangiographic frames revealing **(a)** a 90% stenosis in the proximal left circumflex coronary artery (arrow), which was **(b)** successfully dilated to a 10% residual stenosis. The left anterior descending artery is seen in the upper portion of this right anterior oblique view

presence of electrocardiogram changes with pain also places this patient in a high-risk subgroup for adverse events, and so an aggressive approach in this case is most appropriate.

Answer to question 2 Using the normal threshold of a lesion of 70% or greater as denoting a significant stenosis, this patient is classified as having single vessel coronary disease of the left circumflex artery. Because of his medically refractory symptoms, mechanical revascularization is indicated. Although bypass surgery is likely to offer symptomatic relief, in the case of single vessel disease the lower morbidity and mortality of PTCA make it the preferred approach in these circumstances. In the absence of the adverse lesion characteristics mentioned above, a success rate in excess of 90% can be expected with an approximately 30% risk of recurrent symptoms caused by restenosis over the ensuing 6 months (Figure 3.10).

Answer to question 3 The use of intracoronary stents appears to diminish restenosis when used in *de novo* (i.e. not previously dilated) lesions. Because of the 2·5 mm caliber vessel in this case, stenting may not be the best option for this patient. Other lesion characteristics that may dissuade the use of stents (and that were excluded from the studies comparing stent with PTCA) include excessive length, marked vessel tortuosity, intracoronary thrombus, or lesion location at a branch point or in a diffusely diseased vessel. On the other hand there is growing evidence that in diabetic patients PTCA and stenting is preferred to PTCA alone because of the high rate of restenosis after PTCA.

Further reading

Bittl JA. Advances in coronary angioplasty. *N Eng J Med* 1996;**335**:1290–302.

Boehrer JD, Lange RA Willard JE, Grayburn PA, Hillis LD. Advantages and limitations of methods to detect, localize, and quantitate intracardiac left-to-right shunting. *Am Heart J* 1992;**124**:448–55.

Ellis SG, da Silva ER, Heyndrickx G, *et al*. Randomised comparison of rescue angioplasty with conservative management of patients with early failure of thrombolysis for acute anterior myocardial infarction. *Circulation* 1994;**90**:2280–4.

Grines RJ, Browne KF, Marco J, *et al*. A comparison of primary angioplasty with thrombolytic therapy for acute myocardial infarction. *N Engl J Med* 1994;**331**:673–9.

Grossman WG, Baim DS, eds. *Cardiac catheterization, angiography, and intervention, 4th ed*. Philadelphia: Lea and Febiger, 1991.

King SB, Lembo NJ, Weintraub WS, *et al*. A randomised trial comparing coronary angioplasty with coronary bypass surgery. *N Engl J Med* 1994;**331**:1044–50.

Nobuyoshi M, Hamasaki N, Kimura T, *et al*. Indications, complications, and short term clinical outcome of percutaneous transvenous mitral commissurotomy. *Circulation* 1989;**80**:782–92.

Serruys PW, Jaegere P, Kiemeneij F, *et al*. A comparision of balloon expandable stent implantation with balloon angioplasty in patients with coronary artery disease. *N Engl J Med* 1994;**331**:489–95.

Shabetai R, Fowler NO, Guntheroth WG. The hemodynamics of cardiac tamponade and constrictive pericarditis. *Am J Cardiol* 1980;**46**:570–5.

Topol EJ, Leya F, Pinkerton CA, *et al*. A comparison of directional atherectomy with coronary angioplasty in patients with coronary artery disease. *N Engl J Med* 1993; **329**:221–7.

4: Hypertension

SHARON C REIMOLD

Hypertension is a major common cardiovascular disease, affecting up to 75% of the population by the eighth decade of life. Although hypertension is defined as a blood pressure exceeding 140/90 mmHg, the cardiovascular risk associated with elevated blood pressure forms a continuum. The primary reason for treating hypertension is to reduce the risk for vascular complications, including hemorrhagic and atherothrombotic stroke, congestive heart failure, coronary artery disease, aortic dissection, sudden death, nephrosclerosis, and peripheral vascular disease. The risks for these complications rise with increasing severity of hypertension.

Definitions

The Joint National Committee on the Detection and Treatment of Hypertension Guidelines[1] form the basis for diagnosis, classification (Table 4.1),[2] and treatment of hypertension. Although hypertension is defined as a blood pressure greater than 140/90 mmHg, the guidelines draw attention to the population of patients with systolic blood pressure ranging from 130 to 139 mmHg and diastolic blood pressure from 85 to 89 mmHg as a "high normal group". This group is important because blood pressures in this range may be associated with increased risk for adverse outcomes.

The most typical form of hypertension involves elevation in both the systolic and diastolic blood pressures. Systolic hypertension, or isolated elevation in systolic blood pressure to a level greater than 140 mmHg with normal diastolic pressure, is common in the elderly. It is now recognized that patients with increased pulse pressure (systolic blood pressure − diastolic blood pressure) are at higher risk for cardiovascular complications than are those with lower pulse pressure.[3] For example, a patient with a blood pressure of 180/90 mmHg has greater cardiovascular risk than does a patient with a blood pressure of 150/95 mmHg.

Blood pressure is determined as the product of cardiac output and total peripheral resistance. Early in the course of the hypertensive disease process, cardiac output is elevated and total peripheral resistance is essentially normal. As the disease progresses, cardiac output normalizes but total peripheral resistance becomes elevated.

Table 4.1 Classification of adult blood pressure

Category	Systolic pressure (mmHg)	Diastolic pressure (mmHg)
Optimal	<120	<80
Normal	<130	<85
High normal	130–139	85–89
Hypertension		
Stage I	140–159	90–99
Stage II	160–179	100–109
Stage III	≥180	≥110

From the Sixth Report of the Joint National Committee on Prevention, Detection, Evaluation, and Treatment of High Blood Pressure[2]

Table 4.2 Voltage criteria for left ventricular hypertrophy

Lead	Criteria
Limb lead	R amplitude in aVL >11 mm
	R wave in aVF >14 mm
	R wave in lead I plus S wave in lead III >25 mm
Precordial lead	R wave in V_5–V_6 plus S wave in V_1 >35 mm
	R wave in V_5 or V_6 >26 mm

Blood pressure therapies can work by decreasing cardiac output or peripheral resistance, or both.

In response to the elevated systolic arterial blood pressure, the myocardium hypertrophies. Several electrocardiographic criteria exist for the detection of hypertrophy. Voltage criteria are the most helpful (Table 4.2). Left ventricular hypertrophy may be detected on echocardiography as increased wall thickness and increased myocardial mass. Echocardiography is more sensitive for the detection of hypertrophy than is electrocardiography. Detection of left ventricular hypertrophy is a marker for end-organ damage from hypertension. This increased wall thickness may lead to systolic and/or diastolic dysfunction of the myocardium. Individuals who develop systolic dysfunction may have had an inadequate hypertrophic response of the ventricle and develop decreased myocardial contractile function in response to increased afterload. Systolic dysfunction in hypertension may be identified as a reduction in ejection fraction accompanied by a small increase in chamber volumes. Advanced cases of systolic dysfunction may present with a low cardiac output state.

It is more common for patients with hypertension and left ventricular hypertrophy to develop diastolic dysfunction (Figure 4.1).[4] In these patients, the relaxation or compliance of the left ventricle is

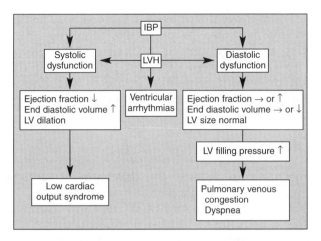

Figure 4.1 Impact of elevated blood pressure on systolic and diastolic function of the left ventricle. IBP, arterial blood pressure; LVH, left ventricular hypertrophy. From Shepherd et al.[4]

abnormal. The ejection fraction may be normal or increased with normal chamber volumes. For these normal volumes, however, left ventricular filling pressures are elevated, leading to pulmonary venous congestion and symptoms of decreased exercise tolerance or dyspnea. Patients with systolic dysfunction also have underlying diastolic dysfunction of the ventricle. The hypertrophy produced by hypertension predisposes patients to the development of ventricular arrhythmias and sudden death.

Approximately 95% of all patients with high blood pressure have essential hypertension. Essential hypertension may also be referred to as primary or idiopathic. Although no underlying etiology is identified for patients with essential hypertension, it is likely that multiple factors play a role in the development of hypertension. Up to 5% of patients have secondary hypertension. Secondary hypertension implies that a specific etiology for the elevated blood pressure has been identified. Treatment of secondary hypertension is based on the specific underlying etiology (see Secondary hypertension, below).

The frequency of hypertension increases with age and varies by race. African-American and Hispanic patients are more likely to have hypertension before age 40 years than are Caucasian patients. Genetic abnormalities may be responsible for the development of hypertension in many of these patients. Only a few single gene mutations capable of producing hypertension have been identified. Abnormalities in the gene encoding aldosterone synthase/ 11β-hydroxylase and 11β-hydroxysteroid dehydrogenase deficiency are examples of monogenic forms of hypertension. The development of hypertension may also be polygenic, requiring several genetic abnormalities to be present at one time. Multiple genes may contribute to the regulation of blood pressure, and the ultimate development of hypertension may relate to the interaction of a genetic substrate with environmental and dietary factors.

Pathophysiology

Several mechanisms underlie the development of hypertension. These mechanisms include sympathetic nervous system overactivity, renin–angiotensin excess, abnormal nephron number, genetic abnormalities, obesity, and endothelial abnormalities.

The renin–angiotensin system is important in the development of hypertension (Figure 4.2).[5] The juxtaglomerular cells of the kidneys secrete renin. Renin works together with renin substrate to produce angiotensin I. Angiotensin-converting enzyme converts angiotensin I to angiotensin II. The biologic effect of angiotensin II is to directly produce vasoconstriction and to upregulate aldosterone synthesis. Aldosterone facilitates sodium retention. The combined effects of angiotensin II and aldosterone production lead to elevated blood pressure. Elevated blood pressure results in negative feedback on renin production by the juxtaglomerular cells. On the basis of this negative feedback loop, it would be expected that patients with essential hypertension would have low renin states. However, many of these patients may actually have elevated renin states. Several explanations for elevated renin have been suggested, including catecholamine mediated release of renin from the kidney.

Patients with single or multiple genetic mutations may have abnormal enzymes or proteins, which alter either sodium and volume regulation in the kidney, sympathetic nervous system activity, or the vasculature. Reduced nephron number may be present in patients with low birth weight and prematurity. The reduced renal sodium excretion and decreased filtration surface of the kidney may predispose these patients to hypertension.

Extrinsic and intrinsic stressors lead to sympathetic nervous overactivity. Activation of the sympathetic nervous system produces increased contractility of the ventricle and may lead to arterial and venous constriction. Elevated circulating catecholamine levels also lead to increased renin release.

The association between hypertension and hyperinsulinemia is most pronounced in patients with truncal obesity. Patients who are obese or hypertensive may demonstrate augmented sympathetic

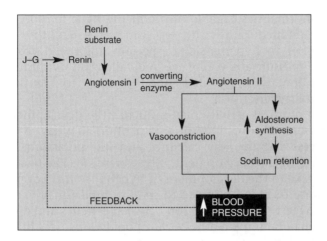

Figure 4.2 Renin–angiotensin system and its role in hypertension. J–G, renal juxtaglomerular cell. From Kaplan[5]

pressor activity and/or decreased vasodilatory response to insulin. These abnormalities may result in elevation of blood pressure in this patient population. Non-obese hypertensive persons may have abnormal vascular responses to circulating insulin. Increasing age is associated with the development of hypertension. This may be related to increased vascular stiffness that occurs with advancing age.

Other growth factors and endothelial cell dysfunction may play a role in the control of blood pressure. Patients with high blood pressure may fail to synthesize sufficient nitric oxide, a substance that is important to the maintenance of vascular tone and smooth muscle cell relaxation. In addition, patients with hypertension have abnormal nitric oxide mediated vasodilatation. The absence of appropriate nitric oxide mediated vasodilatation may lead to abnormal vascular remodeling and promote vascular damage, predisposing the patient to atherosclerosis. Nitric oxide mediated forearm vasodilatation may be normalized by treatment with antihypertensive therapy. Endothelin and related factors produce vasoconstriction but have not been shown to have a role in human hypertension.

Risk factors for the development of hypertension

Genetic predisposition to hypertension is an extremely important risk factor for the development of hypertension. Although very few genetic abnormalities capable of producing hypertension have been found, a detailed family history can often identify a familial predisposition to hypertension, especially for the development of high blood pressure at a young age. A detailed history should be taken from a patient with elevated blood pressure to identify familial clustering of hypertension.

Diet and physical activity may influence the development of high blood pressure. Chronic ingestion of alcohol (30 g/day) has a pressor effect. Excess sodium, low calcium, and low potassium intake are associated with the development of hypertension. The relationship of sodium intake to the development of hypertension is not predictable. The response of blood pressure to sodium intake may vary between families, suggesting an interaction between genetics and diet. Sodium retention may be impaired in certain populations (low birth weight) because of a deficit in nephron development.

Obesity, physical inactivity, and psychologic stress predispose patients to the development of hypertension. Individuals with truncal (high waist/hip ratios) obesity have a greater likelihood of developing hypertension than do those with other distributions of obesity. Truncal obesity is associated with insulin resistance and hyperlipidemia in the "metabolic syndrome". Such patients are at high risk for the subsequent development of coronary artery disease. There is an inverse relationship between physical activity and hypertension risk; individuals with decreased physical activity have a higher risk for the development of hypertension. Obesity is also associated with decreased physical activity, and may explain a portion of the hypertensive risk in this population.

Hypertension is more common in smokers because of enhanced sympathetic nervous system activity provoked by nicotine. Abnormal peripheral vascular compliance can be seen in smokers, and this may contribute to the development of hypertension. Sleep apnea, which is often related to obesity, is associated with hypertension. The mechanism of hypertension in patients with sleep apnea is related to enhanced catecholamine and possibly endothelin release in the setting of hypoxia.

Laboratory evaluation of the patient with hypertension

Performing diagnostic testing in the patient with hypertension is aimed at assessing overall cardiovascular risk, identifying end-organ damage related to hypertension, and highlighting potential secondary etiologies of hypertension. The laboratory evaluation of a patient with hypertension should include a variety of serologic tests and an electrocardiogram (Box 4.1). Identification of end-organ damage, such as renal dysfunction or left ventricular hypertrophy, should lead to a decision to institute pharmacologic therapy. The identification of glucose intolerance or dyslipidemia should prompt patient education, dietary interventions, and/or drug therapy, depending on the severity and type of underlying disorder. Baseline renal dysfunction may also be the etiology rather than the result of hypertension. Detection of renal dysfunction should lead to further imaging or diagnostic studies to determine the etiology of the problem. These studies can include a variety of tests, including 24-hour urine collection for protein and creatinine, renal ultrasound, and magnetic resonance angiography.

Box 4.1 Basic laboratory evaluation of the patient with new onset hypertension

Electrolytes
Blood urea nitrogen, creatinine
Calcium
Phosphate
Liver function tests
Glucose
Uric acid
Lipoproteins
Urinalysis
Electrocardiogram

Secondary hypertension

A small proportion of patients with hypertension (approximately 5%) has a secondary, or definable, cause for the hypertension. The decision to pursue the evaluation of a secondary cause of hypertension may be based on several clinical features (Box 4.2).[2] The onset of hypertension at a young or old age is suggestive of a secondary etiology. Severe hypertension and end-organ damage may signal a secondary cause of hypertension. Of those patients with secondary hypertension (Table 4.3),[2] chronic renal disease and renovascular hypertension account for the vast majority of underlying causes. Endocrine etiologies such as pheochromocytoma and Cushing's syndrome each account for 0·1–0·3% of hypertensive cases.

Box 4.2 Clinical features of "unusual hypertension"

Diagnosis before age 20 years or after age 50 years

Blood pressure greater than 180/110 mmHg

Organ damage: creatinine ≥1·5 mg/dl, cardiomegaly, grade 2 or higher fundoscopic findings

Features suggestive of secondary causes: unprovoked hypokalemia; abdominal bruit; syndrome of variable pressure with tachycardia, sweating, tremor; family history of renal disease; unequal upper/lower extremity pressures

Poor response to therapy that is usually effective

Table 4.3 Secondary causes of hypertension

Secondary cause	Examples
Renal disorders	Renal parenchymal disease (diabetic nephropathy, hydronephrosis, polycystic disease, nephritis, acute glomerulonephritis), renin producing tumors
	Renovascular (renal vascular stenosis, renal vasculitis)
	Primary sodium retention (Liddle syndrome, Gordon syndrome)
Cardiac	Coarctation of the aorta[6]
Neurologic disorders	Increased intracranial pressure (brain tumor, encephalitis)
	Sleep apnea
	Quadriplegia
	Miscellaneous (acute porphyria, familial dysautonomia, lead poisoning, Guillain–Barré syndrome)
Pregnancy-induced hypertension	
Endocrine disorders	Thyroid disorders (hypothyroidism, hyperthyroidism)
	Acromegaly, hyperparathyroidism, carcinoid
	Adrenal disorders: Cushing syndrome, primary aldosteronism,[7] congenital adrenal hyperplasia, pheochromocytoma, apparent mineralocorticoid excess (licorice intake)
	Exogenous hormones
Acute stress	Surgery, burns, postresuscitation, sickle cell crisis
Alcohol and drug use	

From the Sixth Report of the Joint National Committee on Prevention, Detection, Evaluation, and Treatment of High Blood Pressure[2]

Establishing the diagnosis of hypertension

The physical examination of the patient with suspected hypertension should focus on appropriate recording of blood pressure. The patient should be seated in a quiet place for 5 min without exogenous adrenergic stimulants. Caffeine and smoking should be avoided for up to 1 hour before measuring the blood pressure. The blood pressure cuff should cover two-thirds of the length of the arm. Using a smaller cuff results in inappropriately high readings. At least two recordings should be made at each visit. At the initial visit, blood pressure should be taken in both arms. The highest arm blood pressure should be used. A minimum of three recordings should be made at least a week apart to establish the diagnosis of hypertension. To record the blood pressure, the cuff should be inflated to a pressure 20 mmHg above the systolic pressure. The cuff should be deflated at a rate of 3 mmHg/second. The disappearance of the beat (Korotkoff phase V) should be recorded in adults.

A discrepancy between the blood pressures measured in both arms (of more than 5–10 mmHg) may indicate involvement of the great arteries leaving the heart in a disease process (arterial occlusive disease, aortic dissection, or coarctation).

The radial and femoral arteries should be palpated simultaneously during the cardiovascular examination. A significant radial–femoral delay (the appearance of the pulses in the lower extremities is delayed as compared with their appearance in the upper extremities) suggests coarctation of the aorta and must be excluded. In this instance, an initial step is to measure blood pressures in the lower extremities and compare them with the pressures in the upper extremities. Again, if there is a major discrepancy (i.e. if the blood pressures measured in the lower extremities are lower than those in the upper extremities), then coarctation of the aorta must be excluded.

Some patients have a phenomenon known as "white coat hypertension"; in the presence of healthcare personnel, their blood pressure is elevated. Measuring home or ambulatory blood pressures or use of a 24-hour blood pressure monitor may provide a more accurate assessment of blood pressure levels in these patients. Recommendations for follow up of blood pressure have been established (Table 4.4).[2] Patients with normal blood pressure should have it rechecked approximately every 2 years. Because high normal blood pressure (130–139/85–89 mmHg) is associated with an increased risk for adverse events, lifestyle modifications should be introduced and the blood pressure followed more closely. Patients with significant elevation in blood pressure should be evaluated as outlined in Box 4.1. As expected, those patients with more dramatic elevation in blood pressure should be seen and evaluated more

Table 4.4 Follow up of blood pressure based on initial blood pressure recordings

Systolic blood pressure (mmHg)	Diastolic blood pressure (mmHg)	Follow up
<130	<85	Recheck in 2 years
130–139	85–89	Recheck in 1 year; lifestyle modifications
140–159	90–99	Confirm within 2 months; lifestyle modifications
160–179	100–109	Evaluate or refer to source of care within 1 month
≥180	≥110	Evaluate or refer for care immediately or within 1 week, depending on clinical presentation

From the Sixth Report of the Joint National Committee on Prevention, Detection, Evaluation, and Treatment of High Blood Pressure[2]

promptly. Hypertensive patients with evidence of acute end-organ involvement, including pulmonary edema, intracranial bleeding, encephalopathy, and acute renal dysfunction, should be seen and treated emergently.

Although the blood pressure criteria involve resting measurements, some patients may develop a pronounced hypertensive response to exercise. These patients have an increased likelihood of developing hypertension subsequently and should be evaluated carefully.

Physical examination of the patient with hypertension

In addition to recording the degree of blood pressure elevation and heart rate, eye examination with an ophthalmoscope to evaluate blood vessels is an important aspect of the physical examination in patients with hypertension. The most common cardiac finding in patients with hypertension is an S_4 (fourth heart sound) gallop, caused by the atria contracting against a stiff ventricle. Evidence of clinical heart failure such as elevated central venous pressure, rales, cardiac enlargement, peripheral edema, and the presence of a third heart sound should be sought. A careful vascular examination should be performed, looking for abdominal/renal bruits or delayed or reduced lower extremity pulses suggestive of renal vascular disease or aortic coarctation, respectively. Blood pressure should be recorded from both arms and legs when assessing for a coarctation.

In patients' with hypertension the retinal changes are classified according to the Keith–Wagner–Barker method. These changes reflect both atherosclerotic and hypertensive retinopathy. Initially arterial narrowing is seen (grade 1) and subsequently the arteriolar diameters increase in relationship to the venous diameters, manifested as arteriovenous nicking (grade 2 changes). As uncontrolled hypertension progresses small vessels rupture, and exudates and hemorrhages are seen (grade 3 changes). Eventually, sustained, accelerated, or extreme hypertension is associated with raised intracranial pressure seen as papilledema, usually associated with retinal exudates and hemorrhages (grade 4 changes). Grade 2 changes correlate with other evidence of clinical cardiovascular disease or end-organ damage (left ventricular hypertrophy, renal disease, arterial disease). The overall risk in patients with hypertension correlates with presence, or absence, of conventional cardiovascular risk factors and evidence of uncontrolled hypertension or end-organ damage.

Non-pharmacologic treatment of hypertension

Dietary and environmental factors contribute to risk for developing hypertension. By modifying these factors it is possible to decrease blood pressure. In addition, these lifestyle modifications may be important adjuncts to pharmacologic therapy, decreasing overall medication requirements. Although no trials have been performed to assess the impact of lifestyle modifications on cardiovascular end-points or mortality, they are believed to be an important part of antihypertensive therapy (Table 4.5).[2] Patients in the high normal blood pressure group are likely to develop hypertension and are at risk for complications. Lifestyle modifications should be initiated in all patients. Drug therapy should be initiated in this population if there is evidence for target organ damage, cardiovascular disease, or diabetes. Patients with stage 1 hypertension should undergo a trial of lifestyle modifications depending on risk profile. If lifestyle modifications are not successful in decreasing blood pressure, then pharmacologic therapy should be initiated. All patients with stage 2 and 3 hypertension should receive pharmacologic therapy.

Lifestyle modification includes a variety of changes to dietary and physical activity (Box 4.3). Moderate sodium restriction is associated with a reduction in blood pressure. It is recommended that sodium intake be decreased to about 100 mmol/day. This reduction in sodium intake is associated with a 5·4 mmHg decrease in systolic pressure and a 6·5 mmHg decrease in diastolic pressure.[3] Individual responses to

Table 4.5 Strategy for lifestyle modifications and pharmacologic therapy of hypertension

Blood pressure stage	Risk group A[*]	Risk group B[†]	Risk group C[‡]
High normal	Lifestyle modifications	Lifestyle modifications	Drug therapy
Hypertension stage I	Lifestyle modifications (up to 12 months), then drug therapy	Lifestyle modifications (up to 6 months), then drug therapy	Drug therapy
Hypertension stages II and III	Drug therapy	Drug therapy	Drug therapy

For definition of blood pressure stages, see Table 4.1. *No cardiovascular risk factors or disease; no target organ disease. [†]At least one risk factor, not including diabetes; no target organ disease or clinical cardiovascular disease. [‡]Target organ damage; clinical cardiovascular disease; diabetes with or without other risk factors. From the Sixth Report of the Joint National Committee on Prevention, Detection, Evaluation, and Treatment of High Blood Pressure[2]

decreased sodium intake are variable. Weight reduction is associated with a reduction in blood pressure. Systolic blood pressure drops by 1·6 mmHg and diastolic blood pressure by 1·3 mmHg for each 1 kg drop in body weight.[3] The diet of patients on weight loss programs often includes decreased sodium content. This reduction in sodium content may account for some of the blood pressure reduction in this population. Reduction in alcohol intake is associated with a reduction in blood pressure.

Regular moderate exercise is associated with a reduction in blood pressure. Walking, jogging, running, swimming, and cycling are examples of isotonic activities that may be effective in decreasing blood pressure. Regular exercise also promotes weight loss and increases levels of high-density lipoproteins, thereby further reducing cardiovascular risk. Combining these modifications has been shown to have a moderate impact on blood pressure reduction (approximately 9 mmHg fall in systolic and diastolic blood pressures).

Box 4.3 Lifestyle modifications for the treatment of hypertension

Regular moderate exercise
Weight loss
Smoking cessation
Decreased sodium content in diet
Reduced alcohol intake
Increased calcium intake

Pharmacologic treatment of hypertension

Pharmacologic therapy for hypertension is indicated for patients in whom lifestyle modification is inadequate and for those patients with target organ damage or other cardiovascular risk factors (see Table 4.5). The goal of pharmacologic therapy is not only to reduce blood pressure, but also to reduce adverse outcomes, including stroke, coronary artery disease, congestive heart failure, and mortality. In a meta-analysis of randomized, placebo controlled trials in hypertension using diuretics or β-blockers,[8] both agents were effective in reducing the risks for stroke and heart failure (Figure 4.3). The influence of those agents on coronary artery disease was less apparent. There was a trend for a 10% reduction in mortality due to those agents. As new agents are evaluated for the treatment of hypertension, the impact of therapy on stroke, heart failure, and death is extremely important.

The target blood pressure for therapy has been debated. Cruickshank called attention to the "J curve" associated with hypertension.[9] This curve reflects the concept that small to moderate blood pressure lowering is associated with a reduction in adverse events but further blood pressure lowering is associated with an increase in adverse outcomes. To investigate this hypothesis, the Hypertension Optimal Treatment trial was conducted, which included nearly 19 000 patients.[10] Patients were randomized to groups with three different target diastolic blood pressures: 90, 85, or 80 mmHg. Felodipine, a long-acting dihydropyridine, was the primary therapy initiated. Other agents were given as needed. A small difference in diastolic pressure was achieved in the three treatment groups. No detrimental effect of lowering diastolic blood pressure to 80 mmHg was noted. Diabetic patients who achieved a diastolic blood pressure below 80 mmHg had a markedly reduced risk for major cardiovascular events. The data from that study support lowering of blood pressure to less than 140/90 mmHg in all persons, and to less than 130/85 mmHg in high risk patients such as those with diabetes.

The major classes of pharmacologic agents for hypertension are reviewed below (Table 4.6).[11,12]

Diuretics

Several classes of diuretics exist. These agents may be classified according to their site of action in the kidney. Carbonic anhydrase inhibitors exert their action on the proximal tubule. Loop diuretics such as furosemide are most effective for patients with renal insufficiency or resistant hypertension. Thiazides and potassium-sparing agents

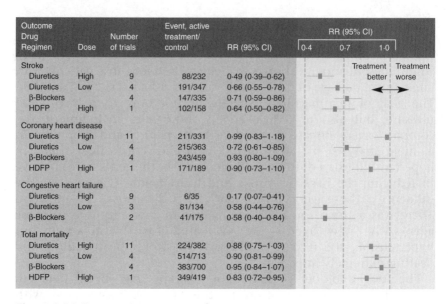

Outcome Drug Regimen	Dose	Number of trials	Event, active treatment/ control	RR (95% CI)	RR (95% CI)
Stroke					
Diuretics	High	9	88/232	0·49 (0·39–0·62)	
Diuretics	Low	4	191/347	0·66 (0·55–0·78)	
β-Blockers		4	147/335	0·71 (0·59–0·86)	
HDFP	High	1	102/158	0·64 (0·50–0·82)	
Coronary heart disease					
Diuretics	High	11	211/331	0·99 (0·83–1·18)	
Diuretics	Low	4	215/363	0·72 (0·61–0·85)	
β-Blockers		4	243/459	0·93 (0·80–1·09)	
HDFP	High	1	171/189	0·90 (0·73–1·10)	
Congestive heart failure					
Diuretics	High	9	6/35	0·17 (0·07–0·41)	
Diuretics	Low	3	81/134	0·58 (0·44–0·76)	
β-Blockers		2	41/175	0·58 (0·40–0·84)	
Total mortality					
Diuretics	High	11	224/382	0·88 (0·75–1·03)	
Diuretics	Low	4	514/713	0·90 (0·81–0·99)	
β-Blockers		4	383/700	0·95 (0·84–1·07)	
HDFP	High	1	349/419	0·83 (0·72–0·95)	

Figure 4.3 Influence of diuretics and β-blockers on stroke, coronary heart disease, congestive heart failure, and total mortality in patients with hypertension. From Psaty *et al*.[8]

work more distally and have a major role in the treatment of hypertension.

The initial effect of diuretics is to increase sodium excretion and decrease plasma and extracellular fluid volume. After 6–8 weeks of therapy, volume returns to normal but blood pressure remains lowered because of a reduction in peripheral resistance. As blood pressure falls and blood volume is reduced, renin and aldosterone are secreted, blocking further excretion of sodium and reduction of blood volume.

The net effect of diuretic administration is to lower blood pressure by approximately 10 mmHg. The actual reduction in blood pressure is variable and may be influenced by underlying renal function, the response of the renin–aldosterone system to therapy, severity of blood pressure elevation, and sodium intake. Excess sodium intake (>8 g/day) can overwhelm the effects of these agents. The most frequently used diuretic is hydrochlorothiazide, a thiazide diuretic. Doses as low as 12·5 mg/day may be effective in patients with creatinine levels of 2·0 mg/dl (177 mmol/l) or less. Patients with renal dysfunction may benefit from one or two daily doses of a loop diuretic such as furosemide or torsemide, or an intermittent dose of metolazone. Diuretics may be effective single agent therapy for patients with hypertension and are important adjuncts to other agents, increasing the efficacy of those agents by diminishing intravascular volume.

Table 4.6 Drugs used in the treatment of hypertension

Drug	Trade name	Usual dose range, total mg/day (frequency/day)	Selected side effects and comments
Diuretics (partial list)			
			Short-term: increase cholesterol and glucose levels; biochemical abnormalities; decrease potassium, sodium, and magnesium levels; increase uric and calcium levels. Rare: blood dyscrasias, photosensitivity, pancreatitis, hyponatremia
Chlorthalidone	Hygroton	12·5–50 (1)	
Hydrochlorothiazide (G)	Hydrodiuril, Microzide, Esidrix	12·5–50 (1)	
Indapamide	Lozol	1·25–5 (1)	(Less or no hypercholesterolemia)
Metolazone	Zaroxolyn	2·5–10 (1)	
Loop diuretics			
Bumetanide (G)	Bumex	0·5–4 (2–3)	(Short duration of action, no hypercalcemia)
Ethacrynic acid	Edecrin	25–100 (2–3)	(Only non-sulfonamide diuretic, ototoxicity)
Furosemide (G)	Lasix	40–240 (2–3)	(Short duration of action, no hypercalcemia)
Torsemide	Demadex	5–100 (1–2)	
Potassium-sparing agents			
Amiloride hydrochloride (G)	Midamor	5–10 (1)	
Spironolactone (G)	Aldactone	25–100 (1)	(Gynecomastia)
Triamterene (G)	Dyrenium	25–100 (1)	
Adrenergic inhibitors			
Peripheral agents			
Guanadrel	Hylorel	10–75 (2)	(Postural hypotension, diarrhea)
Guanethidine monosulfate	Ismelin	10–150 (1)	(Postural hypotension, diarrhea)
Reserpine (G)	Serpasil	0·05–0·25 (1)	(Nasal congestion, sedation, depression, activation of peptic ulcer)

Continued

Table 4.6 Continued

Drug	Trade name	Usual dose range, total mg/day (frequency/day)	Selected side effects and comments
Central α-agonists			Sedation, dry mouth, bradycardia, withdrawal hypertension
Clonidine hydrochloride (G)	Catapres	0·2–1·2 (2–3)	(More withdrawal)
Guanabenz acetate (G)	Wytensin	8–32 (2)	
Guanfacine hydrochloride (G)	Tenex	1–3 (1)	(Less withdrawal)
Methyldopa (G)	Aldomet	500–3000 (2)	(Hepatic and "autoimmune" disorders)
α-Blockers			Postural hypotension
Doxazosin mesylate	Cardura	1–16 (1)	
Prazosin hydrochloride (G)	Minipress	2–30 (2–3)	
Terazosin hydrochloride	Hytrin	1–20 (1)	
β-Blockers			Bronchospasm, bradycardia, heart failure; may mask insulin-induced hypoglycemia. Less serious: impaired peripheral circulation, insomnia, fatigue, decreased exercise tolerance, hypertriglyceridemia (except agents with intrinsic sympathomimetic activity)
Acebutolol	Sectral	200–800 (1)	
Atenolol (G)	Tenormin	25–100 (1–2)	
Betaxolol	Kerlone	5–20 (1)	
Bisoprolol fumarate	Zebeta	2·5–10 (1)	
Carteolol hydrochloride	Cartrol	2·5–10 (1)	
Metoprolol tartrate (G)	Lopressor	50–300 (2)	
Metoprolol succinate	Toprol-XL	50–300 (1)	
Nadolol (G)	Corgard	40–320 (1)	
Penbutolol sulfate	Levatol	10–20 (1)	

Continued

Table 4.6 Continued

Drug	Trade name	Usual dose range, total mg/day (frequency/day)	Selected side effects and comments
Pindolol (G)	Visken	10–60 (2)	
Propranolol (G)	Inderal	40–480 (2)	
	Inderal LA	40–480 (1)	
Timolol maleate (G)	Biocadren	20–60 (2)	Postural hypotension, bronchospasm
Combined α- and β-blockers			
Carvedilol	Coreg	12·5–50 (2)	
Labetalol hydrochloride (G)	Normodyne, Trandate	200–1200 (2)	Headaches, fluid retention, tachycardia
Direct vasodilators			
Hydralazine hydrochloride (G)	Apresoline	50–300 (2)	(Lupus syndrome)
Minoxidil (G)	Loniten	5–100 (1)	(Hirsutism)
Calcium channel blockers			
Non-dihydropyridine			Conduction defects, worsening in systolic dysfunction, gingival hyperplasia
Diltiazem hydrochloride	Cardizem SR	120–360 (2)	(Nausea, headache)
	Cardizem CD	120–360 (1)	
	Dilacor XR, Tiazac		
Mibefradil dihydrochloride (T-channel calcium channel blocker)	Posicor	50–100 (1)	(No worsening of systolic dysfunction; contraindicated with terfenadine [Seldane], astemizole [Hismanal], and cisapride [Propulsid]. Removed from the market in the USA)
Verapamil hydrochloride	Isoptin SR, Calan SR	90–480 (2)	(Constipation)
	Verelan, Covera HS	120–480 (1)	
Dihydropyridine			Edema of the ankle, flushing, headache, gingival hypertrophy
Amlodipine besylate	Norvasc	2·5–10 (1)	
Felodipine	Plendil	2·5–20 (1)	

Continued

Table 4.6 Continued

Drug	Trade name	Usual dose range, total mg/day (frequency/day)	Selected side effects and comments
Isradipine	DynaCirc	5–20 (2)	
	DynaCirc CR	5–20 (1)	
Nicardipine	Cardene SR	60–90 (2)	
Nifedipine	Procardia XL, Adalat CC	30–120 (1)	
Nisoldipine	Sular	20–60 (1)	
Angiotensin-converting enzyme inhibitors			Common: cough. Rare: angioedema, hyperkalemia, rash, loss of taste, leukopenia
Benazepril hydrochloride	Lotensin	5–40 (1–2)	
Captopril (G)	Capoten	25–150 (2–3)	
Enalapril maleate	Vasotec	5–40 (1–2)	
Fosinopril sodium	Monopril	10–40 (1–2)	
Lisinopril	Prinivil, Zestril	5–40 (1)	
Moexipril	Univasc	7.5–15 (1–2)	
Quinapril hydrochloride	Accupril	5–80 (1–2)	
Ramipril	Altace	1.25–20 (1–2)	
Trandolapril	Mavik	1–4 (1)	
Angiotensin II receptor blockers			Angioedema (very rare), hyperkalemia
Losartan potassium	Cozaar	25–100 (1–2)	
Valsartan	Diovan	80–320 (1)	
Irbesartan	Avapro	150–300 (1)	

These dosages may vary from those listed in the *Physicians' desk reference 51st ed.*[11] which may be consulted for additional information. The listing of side effects is not all-inclusive, and side effects are for the class of drugs except where noted for individual drugs (in parentheses); clinicians are urged to refer to the package insert for a more detailed listing. (G) indicates generic available.

Adverse metabolic effects of diuretics include elevated glucose, cholesterol, and uric acid levels. In those individuals who develop gout as a result of diuretic-induced hyperuricemia, long-term therapy with a uricosuric agent may be beneficial.

Hypokalemia may be seen with loop diuretics or thiazides due to kaliuresis. The degree of hypokalemia is generally related to the dose of the agent. Low doses of hydrochlorothiazide (12·5 mg/day) may not be accompanied by significant potassium losses. Because hypokalemia may blunt the blood pressure lowering effect of these agents as well as lead to ventricular ectopy, muscle weakness, and leg cramps, prevention and treatment of hypokalemia is important. Some of these patients may develop hypomagnesemia. Repletion of magnesium may be necessary if hypomagnesemia develops. Strategies for preventing potassium depletion include using a low dose of diuretic, restricting sodium intake (100 mmol/day), increasing dietary potassium intake, or use of additional agents such as a potassium-sparing diuretic, angiotensin-converting enzyme inhibitor, or angiotensin II receptor blocker. Potassium-sparing therapy should be used with caution in patients with underlying renal dysfunction or in those on other therapies associated with elevated potassium levels such as angiotensin-converting enzyme inhibitors, angiotensin receptor blocking agents, or non-steroidal anti-inflammatory drugs. Potassium-sparing diuretics include spironolactone (an aldosterone antagonist), and triamterene and amiloride (direct inhibitors of potassium secretion).

Adrenergic inhibitors

Several classes of agents that inhibit the adrenergic nervous system are available to treat hypertension. Reserpine and guanethidine are peripheral neuronal inhibitors. Reserpine inhibits the uptake of norepinephrine (noradrenaline) into storage vesicles within the ganglion. Guanethidine inhibits the release of norepinephrine from the adrenergic neurons but is not commonly used because of its association with orthostatic hypotension.

Central α-agonists work by stimulating central adrenergic receptors, reducing sympathetic outflow from the central nervous system. This action results in a decrease in peripheral vascular resistance, thereby reducing systemic blood pressure. Drugs in this class include methyldopa, clonidine, and guanabenz. Methyldopa is used infrequently because of the incidence of abnormal liver function tests; however, it remains an important and relatively safe form of antihypertensive therapy during pregnancy.

The mechanism of action of α-adrenergic receptor antagonists is the blockade of presynaptic or postsynaptic receptors. Phenoxybenzamine and phentolamine block presynaptic and postsynaptic α-receptors. Blockage of presynaptic receptors leads to stimulation of norephinephrine release from the neuron. This increased norepinephrine release may overwhelm the postsynaptic receptors, blunting the effect of the agents. Phenoxybenzamine and phentolamine are used infrequently because of side effects and limited efficacy. Phentolamine may be used in hypertensive crises.

Examples of selective postsynaptic α-receptor blockers include prazosin, terazosin, and doxazosin. The postsynaptic α-receptor mediates vasoconstriction. By blocking these receptors, a decrease in peripheral resistance is seen because of arterial and venous dilatation. Norepinephrine release from the neuron is inhibited by the intact α_2-receptor on the neuron. This inhibition of norepinephrine release may be responsible for the first-dose hypotensive responses observed with prazosin. Terazosin and doxazosin have a slower onset of effect and longer duration of action. These agents are less likely to produce orthostasis. These agents are effective in lowering blood pressure in patients on multiple agents and in those with renal dysfunction. They also reduce smooth muscle tone in the bladder and prostate, and have been used extensively in patients with benign prostatic hypertrophy. The most common side effects are weakness, fatigue, headaches, and dizziness. The ongoing Antihypertensive and Lipid-Lowering Treatment to Prevent Heart Attack Trial is a double-blind, randomized trial of antihypertensive therapy in patients older than 55 years.[13] Compared with cholorthalidone which was superior to other agents in lowering systolic blood pressures, and was cheaper, doxazosin had 25% more cardiovascular events and caused more heart failure and was not recommended as a first choice agent to lower blood pressure.

β-Adrenergic blocking agents are a popular class of antihypertensive agent. These agents are associated with a reduction in mortality if taken at the time of or after a myocardial infarction, and have now been shown to decrease mortality in patients with congestive heart failure. In large clinical trials of hypertension, however, diuretics are better at reducing the likelihood of a primary cardiac event than are β-blockers.[8] β-Blockers work by reducing cardiac output. These agents reduce renin levels up to 60% by blocking the sympathetic release of renin by the juxtaglomerular cells. These agents may also block central nervous system sympathetic release.

β-Blockers differ in their lipid solubility, intrinsic sympathomimetic activity, and cardioselectivity. The antihypertensive effect of the various agents does not depend on lipid solubility. Nadolol and atenolol have reduced lipid solubility and cross the blood–brain barrier to a lesser extent than do other agents, thereby reducing central nervous system side effects. β-Blocking agents with intrinsic sympathomimetic action such as pindolol or acebutolol block the agonist effects of endogenous catecholamines. These agents lower blood pressure but lead to a smaller decrease in heart rate and cardiac output as compared with other agents.

β-Receptors exist as β_1-receptors in the heart and β_2-receptors in the bronchi and peripheral blood vessels. Non-selective agents such as nadolol, propranolol, and timolol may lead to a greater propensity to develop bronchoconstriction as an adverse side effect. Although selective agents may be less likely to influence β-receptors in the lung, doses of these agents used to treat hypertension are sufficient to block bronchial receptors.

Some β-blocking agents possess α-blocking activity. Labetalol, bucindolol, and carvedilol are examples of agents in this class. Blood pressure is reduced by these agents primarily by reducing peripheral resistance. Intravenous labetalol can be used to treat hypertensive emergencies. Carvedilol can be used to treat hypertension as well as heart failure. The advantage of carvedilol for the treatment of heart failure is that it provides both β-blocking effects and vasodilating action.

Vasodilators

Direct vasodilating agents are effective antihypertensive agents because they reduce peripheral resistance. Hydralazine was used extensively in the 1970s and is still used in selected patients. Use of hydralazine alone can result in tachycardia, flushing, and angina. Combining hydralazine therapy with a β-blocker and a diuretic may blunt the tachycardia and angina, as well as decrease fluid retention related to the agent. Its use has decreased because of the incidence of side effects and frequent dosing (4 times/day). Minoxidil acts as a direct vasodilator and is extremely effective in achieving blood pressure control. Concomitant use of an adrenergic receptor blocker and diuretic is needed to avoid the increase in cardiac output and fluid retention associated with this agent. Facial hirsutism prevents the widespread use of this agent.

Calcium channel blockers

Calcium channel blockers are a popular class of antihypertensive agents. Myocardial contractility is reduced by verapamil more than by diltiazem or the dihydropyridines (nifedipine, amlodipine, felodipine). A decrease in heart rate and altered atrioventricular nodal conduction can be seen with diltiazem and verapamil. Vasodilatation is more prominent with the dihydropyridines than with diltiazem and verapamil. In trials comparing short-acting calcium channel blockers with other therapy, there was a suggestion of a hazard associated with these agents. Those data, as well as the demonstration of adverse events following use of liquid nifedipine, has led to withdrawal or decreased use of the short-term agents. Several trials investigating long-acting dihydropyridines have demonstrated safety and efficacy of these agents.[14]

Angiotensin-converting enzyme inhibitors and angiotensin receptor blockade agents

The renin–angiotensin system is activated in hypertension. β-Blocking agents block renin release. Angiotensin-converting enzyme (ACE) converts the inactive angiotensin I to the active angiotensin II. This action may be blocked by ACE inhibitors, agents that bind to the converting enzyme and prevent the formation of angiotensin II. This results in decreased vasoconstriction and decreased aldosterone synthesis, decreasing sodium retention. ACE inhibitors block the degradation of bradykinin. This effect may lead to vasodilatation from the kinin and may be responsible for producing the cough associated with these agents. Angiotensin receptor blockers (ARBs) work further downstream in the pathway, blocking the effects of angiotensin II on vascular tone and aldosterone synthesis.

Captopril was the first agent developed in the ACE inhibitor class. This short-acting agent is an effective hypertensive agent but must be taken two to three times per day. Most other agents in this class may be administered one to two times per day, increasing the likelihood of drug compliance. ACE inhibitors may be least effective in the African-American population, who tend to have lower renin levels. In treating hypertension, captopril is as efficacious as diuretics and β-blockers in preventing adverse cardiovascular events.[15] ACE inhibitors are associated with improved survival of patients with congestive heart failure and those with acute myocardial infarction. Patients at high risk for cardiovascular events, including those with diabetes mellitus, benefit from treatment with ramipril.[16]

In comparison with other agents, ACE inhibitors have little effect on metabolic parameters such as glucose or lipids. Development of a dry cough is one of the most common side effects of an ACE inhibitor. Other potential side effects include a rash, leukopenia, angioedema, and loss of taste. Patients with renal dysfunction may be prone to develop worsening of renal function and hyperkalemia. Caution must be exercised when administering ACE inhibitors with other potassium-sparing agents (diuretics or non-steroidal anti-inflammatory drugs).

The use of ARBs is generally reserved for patients who are intolerant of ACE inhibitors, largely because of the lack of outcome data from large trials. The effects of ARBs on the kidney are similar to those of ACE inhibitors, but cough does not tend to occur because of the intact degradation of bradykinin by ACE. As more data concerning outcome for patients treated with ARBs become available, indications for their use may broaden.

Algorithm for the treatment of hypertension

The goals of therapy should be communicated to the patient. Lifestyle modifications should be instituted in all patients. For those patients with other risk factors and those in whom adequate antihypertensive control is not achieved, pharmacologic therapy is appropriate. Initial pharmacologic therapy should begin with initiating a single agent at small doses, and titrating the agent and/or additional agents upward as needed to achieve the treatment goal. Long-acting once daily agents may provide better antihypertensive effect and are associated with better patient compliance (Figure 4.4). Low dose combinations of some agents may allow for increased therapeutic effect with decreased risk for toxicity. The choice of the initial agent depends on whether the hypertension is uncomplicated or associated with other disorders such as heart failure, diabetes mellitus, and myocardial infarction. Initial therapy can be titrated to achieve the desired pharmacologic response. Additional agents may be needed if this response is inadequate or if side effects occur (Table 4.7).

Efficacy of therapy is influenced by many variables. White coat hypertension is said to be present when blood pressure is more elevated when the patient presents for evaluation at the doctor's office. Home blood pressure measurement systems may be used to monitor the efficacy of therapy and may offer a realistic assessment of ambient blood pressure. Twenty-four-hour monitoring of blood pressure may provide a more complete view of blood pressure control. Non-compliance with a medical regimen may occur because of side effects, inconvenient dosing regimen, cost of drugs, and inadequate patient education. Adverse lifestyle patterns such as increasing weight, alcohol intake, and anxiety may reduce the effectiveness of a given regimen. Patients with secondary causes of hypertension and those with volume overload may be resistant to antihypertensive therapy.

Lack of drug efficacy may be related to use of inadequate drug doses or inappropriate combinations. Coexisting use of non-steroidal anti-inflammatory agents, steroids, caffeine, cocaine, and various over

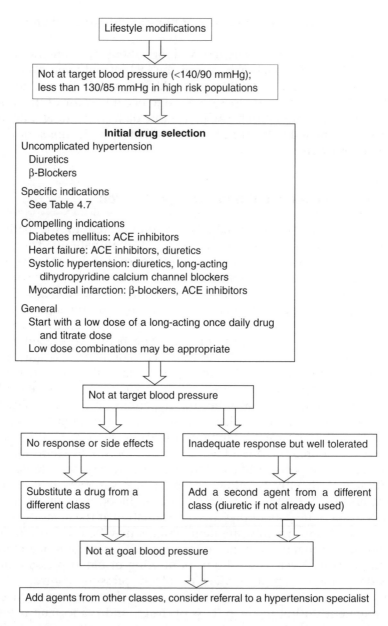

Figure 4.4 Algorithm for treating hypertension. ACE, angiotensin-converting enzyme. From the Joint National Committee on Prevention, Detection, Evaluation, and Treatment of High Blood Pressure[2]

Table 4.7 Considerations for individualizing antihypertensive drug therapy*

Indication	Drug therapy
Compelling indications unless contraindicated	
Diabetes mellitus (type 1) with proteinuria	ACE inhibitor
Heart failure	ACE inhibitor, diuretics
Isolated systolic hypertension (older patients)	Diuretics (preferred), CCB (long-acting DHP)
Myocardial infarction	β-Blockers (non-ISA), ACE inhibitor (with systolic dysfunction)
May have favorable effects on comorbid conditions	
Angina	β-Blockers, CCB
Atrial tachycardia and fibrillation	β-Blockers, CCB (non-DHP)
Cyclosporin-induced hypertension (caution with the dose of cyclosporin)	CCB
Diabetes mellitus (types 1 and 2) with proteinuria	ACE inhibitor (preferred), CCB
Diabetes mellitus (type 2)	Low dose diuretics
Dyslipidemia	α-Blockers
Essential tremor	β-Blockers (non-CS)
Heart failure	Carvedilol, losartan potassium
Hyperthyroidism	β-Blockers
Migraine	β-Blockers (non-CS), CCB (non-DHP)
Myocardial infarction	Diltiazem hydrochloride, verapamil hydrochloride
Osteoporosis	Thiazides
Preoperative hypertension	β-Blockers
Prostatism (BPH)	α-Blockers
Renal insufficiency (caution in renovascular hypertension and creatinine ≥3 mg/dl [265·2 mol/l])	ACE inhibitor
May have unfavorable effects on comorbid conditions	
Bronchospastic disease	β-Blockers
Depression	β-Blockers, central α-agonists, reserpine
Diabetes mellitus (types 1 and 2)	β-Blockers, high dose diuretics
Dyslipidemia	β-Blockers (non-ISA), diuretics (high dose)

Continued

Table 4.7 Continued

Indication	Drug therapy
Gout	Diuretics
Second or third degree heart block	β-Blockers, CCB (non-DHP)
Heart failure	β-Blockers (except carvedilol), CCB (except amlodipine besylate, felodipine)
Liver disease	Labetalol hydrochloride, methyldopa
Peripheral vascular disease	β-Blockers
Pregnancy	ACE inhibitor, angiotensin II receptor blockers
Renal insufficiency	Potassium-sparing agents
Renovascular disease	ACE inhibitor, angiotensin II receptor blockers

Conditions and drugs are listed in alphabetical order. For initial drug therapy recommendations, see Figure 4.4. For references, see Chapter 4 of the *Physicians' desk reference 51st ed.*[11] and Kaplan and Gifford.[12] ACE, angiotensin-converting enzyme; BPH, benign prostatic hyperplasia; CCB, calcium channel blocker; DHP, dihydropyridine; ISA, intrinsic sympathomimetic activity; MI, myocardial infarction; non-CS, non-cardioselective the counter decongestants or appetite suppressants may blunt or ameliorate the effect of the pharmacologic regimen. Patients who have undergone organ transplantation often develop cyclosporin-mediated hypertension.

Treatment of hypertensive emergencies

Marked increases in blood pressure may result in encephalopathy, pulmonary edema, aortic dissection, intracranial hemorrhage, and renal dysfunction. The critical blood pressure for the development of these symptoms is variable, although a diastolic blood pressure greater than 130 mmHg is associated with acute vascular damage. Patients with hypertensive crisis may exhibit hemorrhage, exudates, and papilledema on fundoscopic examination. The neurologic examination may be variable but headache, coma, confusion, stupor, focal neurologic deficits, and seizures may occur. Evidence for heart enlargement and/or failure may be present. Decreased urine output, hematuria, proteinuria, and elevated creatinine are renal manifestations of hypertensive crisis.

Those patients who are in immediate danger from elevated blood pressure should be treated with parenteral agents. An infusion of nitroprusside is associated with rapid blood pressure reduction and may be titrated to the desired level. Nitroglycerin and hydralazine are alternative parenteral agents. Nitroglycerin may be particularly useful in those patients with coexisting myocardial ischemia. Intravenous labetalol (α- and β-blocker) is effective as an acute blood pressure lowering agent, and has the advantage of providing additional cardiac protection for patients with ischemia. Intra-arterial monitoring of therapy is advisable in the patient population who may have rapid and dramatic changes in blood pressure. Many oral agents have been used to treat hypertensive urgencies (moderate blood pressure elevation with normal mental status and no cardiovascular distress). β-Blockers, α-blockers, and vasodilators have also been used in this context.

Hypertension after 60 years

After age 60 years approximately 60–70% of the population have hypertension; it is often systolic hypertension, and symptoms of an orthostatic fall in blood pressure while taking pharmacotherapy are common. A number of important trials address treatment in this age group, for example the Systolic Hypertension in the Elderly Program (SHEP).[17] In this trial 4736 patients, aged 60 years or older, with

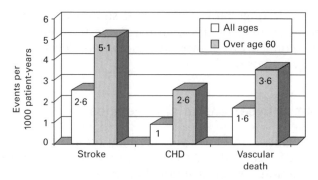

Figure 4.5 Absolute reduction in incidence of events with antihypertensive therapy. Data are taken from 17 randomized trials. Reductions in systolic and diastolic blood pressures were 10–14 mmHg and 5–6 mmHg, respectively. CHD, coronary heart disease. From MacMahon and Rodgers.[18]

systolic blood pressures from 160 mmHg to 219 mmHg and diastolic blood pressures less than 90 mmHg were randomly assigned to chlorthalidone (12·5–25 mg/day) or placebo. After a follow up of 4·5 years the average blood pressures (and pulse pressures) for placebo and diuretic treated patients were 155/72 mmHg (83 mmHg) and 143/68 mmHg (75 mmHg), respectively. Treatment with a diuretic was associated with a reduction in fatal and non-fatal stroke (relative risk 0·64) – the primary end-point. In addition, as compared with placebo, diuretic therapy had a favorable impact on secondary end-points including coronary artery disease death and myocardial infarction (relative risk 0·73) and all causes of death (relative risk 0·87).

Analyses of the influence of antihypertensive therapy in 17 randomized trials (which achieved reductions in systolic pressure of 10–14 mmHg and in diastolic pressure of 5–6 mmHg) showed that therapy was more likely to reduce cardiovascular events in patients over the age of 60 years than among all patients treated (Figure 4.5).[18] In a study that evaluated monotherapy for hypertension in this age group, diuretics were better than β-blockers at controlling blood pressure (66% were well controlled on diuretic monotherapy versus less than 33% on β-blocker monotherapy) and at preventing cerebrovascular events, fatal stroke, and both cardiovascular and all-cause mortality.[19]

Joint National Committee VI recommendations advocate starting therapy with weight loss and modest salt reduction, and then initiating low-dose thiazide diuretics.[1] An important European trial, the Systolic Hypertension in Europe (Syst-Eur) trial, with a design similar to that of SHEP, compared placebo with a dihydropyridine calcium channel blocker (nitrendipine 10–40 mg/day) as treatment for systolic hypertension.[20] Placebo and nitrendipine respectively lowered systolic (13 and 23 mmHg) and diastolic (2 and 7 mmHg) blood pressures during 2 years of follow up. It was found that treatment with nitrendipine reduced the total rate of strokes (from 13·7 to 7·9 per 1000 patient-years) and all cardiac end-points, including sudden death.[14] The rate of dementia also appeared to be slowed.[20] Joint National Committee VI recommendations include long-acting dihydropyridines as the next therapeutic option after thiazide diuretics.[1] Because of the similar designs of SHEP and Syst-Eur, the relative efficacy of diuretics and nitrendipine were compared in diabetic and non-diabetic patients,[21] and it was found that nitrendipine appeared to be associated with greater reductions in mortality, cardiovascular events, and strokes.

Hypertension during pregnancy

Hypertension during pregnancy is a common problem and is associated with increases in maternal and perinatal mortality.[22] Gestational hypertension is the development of high blood pressure for the first time after 20 weeks of gestation, in the absence of features of pre-eclampsia, and generally the outcome of pregnancy is satisfactory without drug treatment. Some of the patients develop pre-eclampsia and others develop chronic hypertension.

Pre-eclampsia is the occurrence of hypertension plus hyperuricemia or proteinuria after 20 weeks of gestation in a previously normotensive woman. It is categorized as mild or severe, depending on the degree of elevation in blood pressure and proteinuria. In this condition there is a defect in placentation (failure of the second wave of trophoblastic invasion into the spiral arteries of the uterus) and secondarily of normal cardiovascular adaptations (increased plasma volume and reduced systemic vascular resistance). Thus, both cardiac output and plasma volume are reduced and systemic vascular resistance is increased. Maternal risks include convulsions and cerebral hemorrhage, coagulopathy, renal failure and liver hemorrhage, abruptio placentae, and death. Fetal risks include growth retardation, hypoxia, acidosis, prematurity, and death. The ultimate treatment of the condition is delivery of the child; however, the aim of antihypertensive treatment is to keep the mean arterial blood pressure below 126 mmHg and the diastolic pressure below 105 mmHg. Agents often used include methyldopa, labetalol, and nifedipine.

Coarctation of the aorta

Surgical repair of coarctation of the aorta results in normalization of blood pressure in most patients for 5–10 years after operation. During longer follow up the prevalence of hypertension is much greater than in a normal population.[6] Late hypertension is more common in individuals undergoing surgical repair after the age of 20 years.

Case studies

Case 4.1

A 27-year-old woman presented 2 months after delivering her first child with palpitations, headache, and fatigue lasting 1 hour. She feels nauseated at the time of the episodes but has never had syncope. She has had seven episodes of palpitations, described as a sudden onset rapid regular heart beat, since the time of delivery. These episodes resolved spontaneously. During the third trimester of pregnancy the patient had a blood pressure of 160/90 mmHg that improved with bed rest and treatment with labetalol 200 mg orally twice a day. The patient has no other cardiovascular history.

Her past medical history is notable for childhood asthma. She has not had any prior operations. There are no known drug allergies. Her current medications include multivitamins. She reports no tobacco or illicit drug use, and rare (<1 can of beer/week) alcohol intake. Her family history is notable for hypertension and diabetes mellitus in her mother at age 50 years, and diabetes in a maternal aunt.

Examination. Physical examination: the patient appeared normal. Temperature: normal. Pulse: 80 beats/min, normal character. Blood pressure: 145/90 mmHg in right arm. Jugular venous pulse: normal. Cardiac impulse: normal. First heart sound: normal. Second heart sound: split normally on inspiration. No added sounds or murmurs. Chest examination: normal air entry, no rales or rhonchi. Abdominal examination: soft abdomen, no tenderness, and no masses. Normal liver span. No peripheral edema. Femoral, popliteal, posterior tibial, and dorsalis pedis pulses: all normal volume and equal. Carotid pulses: normal, no bruits. Optic fundi: normal.

Investigations. Laboratory tests: sodium 141 mg/dl (mmol/l), potassium 3·2 mEq/l (mmol/l), chloride 108, bicarbonate 25, blood urea nitrogen 14 (5·0 mmol/l), and creatinine 0·8 mg/dl (70 μmol/l). The hematocrit was 36, with a normal white blood cell and platelet count. The electrocardiogram demonstrated normal sinus rhythm at a rate of 90 with a PR interval of 0·16, QRS of 0·08, and QT interval of 0·44 ms.

Questions

1. The differential diagnosis includes (A) essential hypertension, (B) pheochromocytoma, (C) primary hyperaldosteronism, or (D) all of these?

Answers

Answer to question 1 The correct answer is D – all of these. Some patients with essential hypertension will have labile blood pressure recordings. Onset of hypertension during pregnancy may be due to pre-eclampsia or to chronic hypertension.[22] Thyroid disorders may develop during and shortly after pregnancy, and may be associated with palpitations and hypertension.

Hyperaldosteronism is associated with potassium loss, sodium retention, and renin suppression because of increased levels of aldosterone.[7] Increased levels of aldosterone may be due to an aldosterone producing adrenal adenoma or, less commonly, to an aldosterone secreting carcinoma. Hyperaldosteronism can also result from adrenal hyperplasia. Hypertension associated with spontaneous hypokalemia should raise the suspicion of this disorder. If dietary sodium intake is low, then serum potassium may be normal. The diagnosis may be made by demonstrating elevated plasma aldosterone levels (or increased urinary aldosterone secretion), along with suppressed plasma renin activity. Imaging techniques such as magnetic resonance imaging or computed tomography may be used to identify tumors. In some instances, these imaging techniques may be inadequate to detect small tumors. Radionuclide imaging with radioionated cholesterol may be used in this situation to identify the abnormal tissue.

The diagnosis of pheochromocytoma should be suspected when the constellation of clinical symptoms is present to support the diagnosis. The findings of hypertension, sweating, headaches, and palpitations (tachycardia) are suggestive of this diagnosis. A family history pheochromocytoma should also be ascertained. The first step in establishing this diagnosis is to identify excess release of catecholamines. Pheochromocytomas differ in the composition of free catecholamines and their metabolites. A 24-hour urinary collection is ideal to assess for increased norepinephrine, epinephrine (adrenline), vanillylmandelic acid, and metanephrine levels. Multiple collections may be necessary to confirm the diagnosis. Elevated plasma catecholamine levels may be suggestive of the diagnosis if they are obtained during an episode. Normal levels do not exclude the diagnosis of pheochromocytoma because some tumors may secrete catecholamines episodically.

In patients with borderline elevations of catecholamine levels, clonidine suppression testing may be used to confirm the diagnosis. Clonidine decreases central nervous system sympathetic activity and inhibits norepinephrine release in the periphery. In normal individuals, therefore, administration of clonidine leads to a suppression in norepinephrine levels. In a patient with pheochromocytoma, levels of norepinephrine will not be suppressed because it is autonomously produced from the tumor. After the diagnosis is made, anatomic localization of the tumor can usually be made by computed tomography or magnetic resonance imaging. Scintigraphy with radioiodinated metaiodobenzylguanidine may be used to localize pheochromocytomas and has been particularly useful in identifying extra-adrenal tumors.

In this case, markedly elevated urinary catecholamine levels supported the diagnosis of pheochromocytoma. A computed tomography scan localized the tumor to the right adrenal. The tumor was resected with resolution of her hypertension.

Case 4.2

A 70-year-old Asian man is referred to you for evaluation of new onset hypertension. Other than a history of gastroesophageal reflux disease and a history of tobacco smoking (1 pack per day for 40 years), he has been healthy. He is on no medications at the time of his visit and has not had any operations. He does not drink alcohol.

Examination. Physical examination: the patient appeared thin and undistressed. Pulse: 80 beats/min, normal character. Blood pressure: 175/105 mmHg in right arm. Jugular venous pulse: normal. Cardiac impulse: normal. First heart sound: normal. Second heart sound: split normally on inspiration. No murmurs. Fourth heart sound: present. Chest examination: normal air entry, no rales or rhonchi. Abdominal examination: soft abdomen, No tenderness and no masses. Paraumbilical bruit. Normal liver span. No peripheral edema. The aorta is not palpated and no masses are appreciated. A soft right femoral bruit is heard. Pulses in the feet are present bilaterally.

Investigations. Laboratory tests: normal electrolytes and glucose, blood urea nitrogen 37 mg/dl (13·2 mmol/l), creatinine 2·1 mg/dl (186 mmol/l). Resting electrocardiogram reveals normal sinus rhythm at a rate of 80 beats/min with left ventricular hypertrophy. No ST-segment changes were noted.

Questions

1. Additional diagnostic evaluation should include which of the following: (A) 24-hour urine collection for catecholamines, (B) urinalysis, (C) thyroid function tests, (D) renal ultrasound, and (E) aldosterone level?

Answers

Answer to question 1 The correct answers are B and D. This patient presents with new onset hypertension and evidence of renal disease.

Although it is not clear whether the renal dysfunction is the cause or the result of the hypertension, the presence of an abdominal bruit raises the suspicion of renal vascular disease. The initial evaluation of such a patient should include a urinalysis to assess for proteinuria and active urine sediment. Proteinuria and hematuria would be suggestive of a renal parenchymal process. The renal ultrasound can be used to assess kidney size and asymmetry, as well as evidence of obstruction. In many centers Doppler flow studies may be performed in conjunction with ultrasound to assess for renal artery stenosis.

In addition to ultrasound, several strategies for non-invasive detection of renal artery stenosis have been developed. Resting plasma renin activity is not useful in distinguishing essential hypertension from renovascular hypertension. Administration of captopril 25 mg orally followed by measurement of plasma renin level 90 min later may help to identify the patient with renovascular disease. In the patient who is off antihypertensive medications, administration of captopril results in inhibition of conversion of angiotensin I to angiotensin II.

Renal scintigraphy with captopril is capable of detecting patients who are most likely to benefit from renal revascularization. The administration of captopril is followed by dilatation of the efferent arteriole, decrease in glomerular filtration, and decreased excretion by the involved kidney. Severe lesions may result in decreased uptake or excretion of the radiotracer, or both.

Magnetic resonance angiography may be useful to identify the anatomy of the renal vasculature and identify possible sites of stenosis. This non-invasive imaging technique provides excellent definition of the renal vessels but does not establish the diagnosis as precisely as does renal angiography and collection of blood from the renal veins for measurement of renin. Angiography may be performed to confirm the diagnosis of renovascular disease. Selected patients with renovascular disease may be treated with percutaneous stenting of the renal arteries to improve renal blood flow.

References

1 Anonymous. The Sixth Report of the Joint National Committee on Prevention, Detection, Evaluation, and Treatment of High Blood Pressure. *Arch Intern Med* 1997;157:2413–46.
2 Anonymous. *Sixth Report of the Joint National Committee on Prevention, Detection, Evaluation, and Treatment of High Blood Pressure*. NIH Publication No. 98–4080. Bethesda, MD: National Institutes of Health, National High Blood Pressure Educational Program, 1997.
3 Franklin SS, Khan SA, Wong ND, Larson MG, Levy D. Is pulse pressure useful in predicting risk for coronary heart disease. The Framingham Study. *Circulation* 1999;100:354–60.
4 Shepherd RF, Zachariah PK, Shub C. Hypertension and left ventricular diastolic function. *Mayo Clin Proc* 1989;64:1521–32.

5 Kaplan NM. Systemic hypertension: mechanisms and diagnosis. In: Braunwald E, Zipes D, Libby P, eds. *Heart disease*, 6th ed. W.B. Saunders Co, 2001:941–94.

6 Clarkson PM, Nicholson MR, Barratt-Boyes BG, Neutze JM, Whitlock RM. Results after repair of coarctation of the aorta beyond infancy: a 10–28 year follow-up with particular reference to late systolic hypertension. *Am J Cardiol* 1983;**51**:1481–8.

7 Ganguly A. Current concepts: primary aldosteronism. *N Engl J Med* 1998;**339**: 1828–34.

8 Psaty BM, Smith NL, Siscovick DS, *et al.* Health outcomes associated with antihypertensive therapies used as first-line agents. *JAMA* 1997;**277**:739–45.

9 Cruickshank JM. Coronary flow reserve and the J curve relation between diastolic blood pressure and myocardial infarction. *BMJ* 1988;**297**:1227–30.

10 Hansson L, Zanchetti A, Carruthers SG, *et al.* Effects of intensive blood-pressure lowering and low-dose aspirin in patients with hypertension: principal results of the Hypertension Optimal Treatment (HOT) randomised trial. *Lancet* 1998;**351**: 1755–62.

11 *Physician's desk reference 51st ed* (www.PDR.net). Montvale, New Jersey: Medical Economics Co, 2002.

12 Kaplan NM, Gifford RW. Choice of initial therapy for hypertension. *JAMA* 1996;**275**:1577–80.

13 The ALLHAT Trial. Major outcomes in high-risk hypertensive patients randomized to angiotensin-converting enzyme inhibitor or calcium channel blocker vs diuretic. *JAMA* 2002;**288**:2981–97.

14 Staesson JA, Fagard R, Thijis L, *et al.* Randomised double-blind comparison of placebo and active treatment for older patients with isolated systolic hypertension. *Lancet* 1997;**350**:757–64.

15 Hansson L, Lindholm LH, Niskanen L, *et al.* Effect of angiotensin-converting enzyme inhibition compared with conventional therapy on cardiovascular morbidity and mortality in hypertension: the Captopril Prevention Project (CAPP) randomized trial. *Lancet* 1999;**353**:611–6.

16 HOPE, the Heart Outcomes Prevention Evaluation Study Investigators. Effects of an angiotensin-converting-enzyme inhibitor, ramipril, on cardiovascular events in high-risk patients. *N Engl J Med* 2000;**342**:145–53.

17 SHEP Cooperative Research Group. Prevention of stroke by antihypertensive drug treatment in older persons with isolated systolic hypertension. *JAMA* 1991;**265**:3255–64.

18 MacMahon S, Rodgers A. The effects of blood pressure reduction in older patients: an overview of five randomized controlled trials in elderly hypertensives. *Clin Exp Hypertens* 1993;**15**:967–78.

19 Messerli FH, Grossman E, Goldbourt U. Are β-blockers efficacious as first-line therapy for hypertension in the elderly? *JAMA* 1998;**279**:1903–7.

20 Forette F, Seux M, Staessen JA, *et al.* Prevention of dementia in randomised double-blind placebo-controlled Systolic Hypertension in Europe (Syst-Eur) trial. *Lancet* 1998;**352**:1347–51.

21 Tuomilehto J, Rastenyte D, Birkenhager WH, *et al.* Effects of calcium-channel blockade in older patients with diabetes and systolic hypertension. *N Engl J Med* 1999;**340**:677–84.

22 Sibai BM. Treatment of hypertension in pregnant women. *N Engl J Med* 1996;**335**:257–65.

5: Lipid disorders

DANIEL B FRIEDMAN

Coronary heart disease (CHD) is the leading cause of death in Western civilizations, and it has become apparent that reductions in morbid and fatal events resulting from CHD can result from modifying specific risk factors. Certainly, modification in high blood cholesterol is important for both primary and secondary prevention[1,2] but other risk factors (Table 5.1) are important and act synergistically to increase risk. For example, obesity, hyperinsulinemia, hypertriglyceridemia, low high-density lipoprotein (HDL), and hypertension have been shown to interact in a way that markedly increases risk for CHD.[1-3] The genetic relationships that exist are also becoming clearer; hypertension is related both to diabetes mellitus and to obesity.

Cigarette smoking is the leading cause of premature death in the developed world in individuals aged 35–69 years and is associated with a substantially increased risk for cardiovascular mortality in men and women.

In the Western world the prevalence of hypertension is high and increases with age. Prospective studies have repeatedly identified an increased risk for myocardial infarction, as well as stroke, congestive heart failure, and renal insufficiency, with progressively high levels of systolic and diastolic blood pressures. Although the link between treatment of this disease and reduction in CHD mortality is not firmly established,[3] most physicians consistently recommend therapy.

Obesity, defined as a body/mass index (weight in kg/height in m^2) greater than 27 kg/m^2, is associated with an increased risk for CHD in both men and women. The influence of obesity is indirect and mostly related to its association with diabetes mellitus, hypertension, and lipid abnormalities (especially low HDL).[4]

Both insulin and non-insulin-dependent diabetes mellitus increase the risk for CHD. Even glucose intolerance in association with insulin resistance can play a major role in the development of CHD. Metabolic "syndrome X", defined as a genetic disorder, is characterized by abdominal obesity, insulin resistance, hyperinsulinemia, hypertension, decreased HDL, elevated triglycerides, and small dense apolipoprotein-B-rich low-density lipoprotein (LDL) particles.[5] Some component of this interaction is probably important to many patients with CHD.

Physical inactivity is possibly an independent risk factor for CHD, and exercise can improve other risk factors for CHD, including hypertension, diabetes mellitus, and obesity.

Table 5.1 Risk factors for coronary heart disease

Modifiable risk factors	Non-modifiable risk factors
LDL-cholesterol >159 mg/dl (>4·1 mmol/l)	Male >44 years
HDL-cholesterol <40 mg/dl (<1·0 mmol/l)	Female >54 years
Cigarette smoking	Family history of myocardial infarction or sudden death: male – parent or sibling before age 55 years; female – parent or sibling before age 65 years
Hypertension	
Diabetes	
Physical inactivity	
Obesity	
Subtract one risk factor if HDL >60 mg/dl (>1·6 mmol/l)	

HDL, high-density lipoprotein; LDL, low-density lipoprotein

Older persons have a higher incidence of CHD than do younger ones. For example, a 65-year-old man has a 500-fold greater likelihood of dying from heart disease during the next 12 months than does a 22-year-old man, and lowering cholesterol possibly influences the prognosis of older individuals to a greater extent in the short term, in addition to the beneficial effects on endothelial function.

Sex is an important determinant of risk for CHD. During their 40s men are four times as likely as women to suffer the consequences of CHD, and this decreases to twice as likely in the eighth decade of life.[6] In fact, CHD is relatively rare before the menopause; this may be mediated in part through the loss of estrogen, resulting in a rise in LDL.[7] This difference between men and women has important therapeutic implications, because men aged over 45 years and women over 55 years are considered to have an additional risk factor for CHD. It also helps to define the role of estrogen replacement.

A family history of clinically significant CHD before age 55 years in a man and 65 years in a woman is a risk factor for first-degree relatives. This is true even when other risk factors are controlled for. Although less critical, a history of early CHD in second-degree relatives (aunts, uncles, and grandparents) is also important. A significant family history alerts the physician to an even greater necessity for altering modifiable factors such as smoking, hypertension, lipid abnormalities, obesity, and a sedentary lifestyle.

Race may also play a role in risk of CHD. For example, CHD death rates are higher among African-American persons than among whites. This may relate to hypertension, diabetes, and higher serum levels of lipoprotein(a). Hispanic persons have a high incidence of diabetes and obesity. Persons from India now living in the West have a particularly high incidence of CHD. This is only partly related to differences between Eastern and current diets. Although the algorithm for cholesterol treatment does not take race into account, physicians should be aware of certain high risk groups.

Over the past 15 years the relationship between lipid abnormalities and CHD has been refined. This resulted in the first National Cholesterol Education Program (NCEP) presented in 1985, which was updated in 1993 and 2001.

Rationale for cholesterol lowering

There is strong evidence from animal and human investigations that elevated cholesterol is causally related to atherosclerosis. In animal studies, in many species, both diet-induced and spontaneous hypercholesterolemia result in atherosclerosis, which can be reversed by drug- or diet-induced cholesterol lowering. Genetic disorders involving the metabolism of lipoproteins have been recognized, and the most dramatic entity is homozygous familial hypercholesterolemia, in which an individual essentially lacks any functional receptors for LDL. This very rare condition causes an LDL-cholesterol level approaching 1000 mg/dl (26 mmol/l), and affected individuals may develop atherosclerosis in the first decade of life. Patients with heterozygous familial hypercholesterolemia have approximately half the normal number of LDL receptors, resulting in cholesterol levels in the 300–400 mg/dl (7·7–10·3 mmol/l) range. They develop atherosclerosis during their 40s and 50s.

Epidemiologic data in humans show a consistent relationship between elevated total cholesterol and LDL levels with an increased risk of coronary heart disease,[6,8] and an inverse relationship between HDL-cholesterol levels and risk for CHD. Clinical studies have demonstrated that a 1% lowering in cholesterol results in an approximately 2% reduction in the incidence of CHD in men. There is overwhelming evidence from randomized, controlled trials that effective LDL lowering therapy for primary and secondary prevention can reduce the risk for CHD and all-cause mortality.[9]

Angiographic studies have demonstrated that cholesterol lowering slows progression and may in fact cause regression of atherosclerosis. Brown et al.[10] followed 120 men with high apolipoprotein B levels and a family history of CHD. Angiographic evaluation was conducted at baseline and after 2·5 years of therapy. Aggressively treated patients experienced a greater degree of coronary artery disease regression than did control individuals. However, the angiographic differences were not as impressive as clinical outcomes. Coronary-related events occurred in 19% of control patients and only 5% of those receiving combination lipid lowering therapy. This led to the theory that cholesterol lowering may stabilize the atherosclerotic plaque such that rupture with subsequent thrombus formation and myocardial infarction is prevented or attenuated.

The greatest initial benefit of LDL lowering, and risk factor modification, is likely to occur in patients with the most severe disease who have the highest likelihood of an event in the near future. In fact, high risk patients may achieve as much as a 3% reduction in the incidence of cardiac end-points for every 1% reduction in cholesterol. This justifies recommendations in guidelines for especially intense treatment of hyperlipidemia in secondary prevention. Because as many as one-third of patients will die during their first myocardial infarction, identifying patients at risk is also critical and forms the basis for the primary prevention treatment guidelines. As in the first National Cholesterol Education Program report, LDL continues to be the main target of the Third Expert Panel.[1] This is based on the known atherogenesis associated with this molecule and the relative ease by which it can be estimated:

$$\text{LDL-cholesterol} = \text{total cholesterol} - \text{HDL-cholesterol} - (\text{triglycerides}/5)$$

If the triglyceride level is greater than 400 mg/dl (4·5 mmol/l), then this relation breaks down, and LDL should be measured by ultracentrifugation in a capable laboratory. Both total cholesterol and HDL-cholesterol can be measured at any time of the day, regardless of whether the patient has been fasting. In contrast, measurement of triglyceride levels requires fasting, and so therefore does estimation of LDL-cholesterol. Of note, patients who are pregnant, acutely ill, or have had a recent myocardial infarction or recent trauma may demonstrate a falsely depressed cholesterol. It may take 12 weeks after a myocardial infarction for the cholesterol to rise to its baseline level.

Therapeutic goals center on LDL, but HDL and triglyceride levels have implications for CHD risk and treatment.[11] Low HDL-cholesterol levels may be associated with cigarette smoking and insulin resistance (overweight, physical inactivity, type 2 diabetes, elevated triglycerides). In all persons with low HDL the primary goal is initially to achieve optimal LDL levels (<100 mg/dl [<2·6 mmol/l]) and then shift to weight reduction and increased physical activity. Low HDL as a risk factor is defined as a level below 40 mg/dl (1·0 mmol/l). Elevated triglycerides are an independent risk factor for CHD and are most often found in patients with metabolic syndrome.[1] The most atherogenic triglycerides are probably "remnant proteins", or partially degraded very-low-density lipoprotein (VLDL). Thus, the sum of VLDL-cholesterol and LDL-cholesterol (equivalent to non-HDL-cholesterol, or total cholesterol minus HDL-cholesterol) becomes a secondary target of therapy in persons with high triglycerides (>200 mg/dl [>5·2 mmol/l]).

Cholesterol testing

The total cholesterol and HDL-cholesterol should be measured at least every 5 years in persons older than 20 years. The prime rationale for measuring HDL-cholesterol is to establish the risk for CHD. This screening can take place in any laboratory that can achieve accurate determinations. However, linking this screening to a physician visit allows one to discuss other important risk factors such as smoking, hypertension, diabetes mellitus, obesity, and need for regular physical activity. Patients with LDL-cholesterol and HDL-cholesterol within the desirable range can be given information on a healthy lifestyle and lipid screening repeated in 5 years (Table 5.2). Patients with borderline values and fewer than two risk factors should be counseled regarding an American Heart Association diet (Table 5.3). For secondary prevention of CHD, currently an LDL-cholesterol below 100 mg/dl (<2·6 mmol/l) is optimal, an HDL-cholesterol below 40 mg/dl (<1·0 mmol/l) is low, and triglyceride concentrations of 150–199 mg/dl (1·7–2·2 mmol/l) are considered borderline high.[1]

Patients with diabetes, but no known CHD, are thought to have equivalent risk to those with CHD and are treated more aggressively.

If LDL-cholesterol is elevated then causes of secondary dyslipidemia should be excluded (i.e. diabetes, hypothyroidism, renal failure, obstructive liver disease, or drugs that raise LDL and lower HDL [steroids and progestins]).

Treatment of hypercholesterolemia

Dietary therapy

Although dietary intervention does not reduce LDL levels as quickly or as much as pharmacologic therapy, diet plays an important role in treating patients with dyslipidemia. Diets high in saturated fat have been shown to be atherogenic whereas substances in fruits, vegetables, whole grains, and fish may be protective, in addition to the antioxidant vitamin effects. Weight loss in obese patients will reduce VLDL and raise HDL. The current recommendations for dietary

Table 5.2 Goals for LDL cholesterol

Risk category LDL goal (mg/dl)
CHD, PVD, or DM <100
Multiple (2+) risk factors <130
0–1 risk factor <160

CHD, coronary heart disease; DM, diabetes mellitus; PVD, peripheral or symptomatic cerebral vascular disease

Table 5.3 Recommended nutrient proportions in diets

Nutrient	AHA dietary guidelines
Total fat	30% or less of total calories
Saturated fat	<7% of total calories
Polyunsaturated fat	Up to 10% of total calories
Monounsaturated fat	Up to 15% of total calories
Carbohydrates	55% or more of total calories
Protein	15% of total calories
Cholesterol	<200 mg/day

All Americans should be encouraged to maintain the AHA diet. Calories from alcohol are not included.

therapy are shown in Table 5.3. If the goals are not reached after 3 months, or the patient has established CHD or other atherosclerosis, then the AHA diet is recommended. It is important for patients to recognize that these alterations represent a way of life and not a temporary fix. If diet does not result in the goals outlined above, then pharmacologic intervention is considered.

Physical activity

Exercise probably reduces the likelihood of CHD, and physical activity has a favorable effect on HDL-cholesterol in persons who exercise consistently over several years.[12,13] Wood et al.[13] demonstrated that the value of exercise is synergistic with that of weight loss in lowering the LDL/HDL ratio in moderately obese men. Also, both a single bout of exercise and chronic vigorous activity lowers triglycerides.[12,13] As little as 30 min brisk walking three or four times weekly (or its equivalent) probably provides nearly the maximal cardiovascular benefit. Exercise reduces other CHD risk factors, including hypertension and diabetes.

Drug treatment

Antioxidants

There is currently little evidence that antioxidants may reduce the atherogenicity of the LDL molecule. Vitamin C, vitamin E, and β-carotene are antioxidants that may be clinically useful. We currently recommend that appropriate patients take 500 mg of vitamin C twice and 400 IU of vitamin E every day. There are supplements that contain these and other potentially useful antioxidants.

Estrogen

Some studies have suggested that estrogen may result in a reduction in coronary heart disease in postmenopausal women.[7,14] A major component of this protective effect results from the effect of estrogen on lipid levels. Orally administered conjugated estrogen at a dose of 0·625 mg/day will reduce the LDL and raise the HDL by about 15%, although triglycerides may rise. Recently, the Heart and Estrogen/ Progestin Replacement Study reported 6·8 years of follow up and showed that hormone replacement therapy did not reduce the risk for cardiovascular events in women with coronary heart disease.[15] Furthermore, the Women's Health Initiative showed that a combination of estrogen plus progestin used as primary prevention in healthy postmenopausal women was associated with an increased risk for coronary heart disease events, stroke, pulmonary embolism, and invasive breast cancer.[16] The results of trials of therapy of estrogen alone, compared with placebo, are awaited.

For many high risk patients specific drug treatment will be necessary to achieve the LDL-cholesterol goals noted above.[17] The major drugs include bile acid sequestrants (cholestyramine, colestipol, nicotinic acid) and 3-hydroxy-3-methylglutaryl coenzyme A reductase inhibitors (i.e. "statins": lovastatin, pravastatin, simvastatin, fluvastatin); other drugs include fibric acid derivatives (gemfibrozil, clofibrate) and probucol (Box 5.1).

Box 5.1 Cholesterol lowering drugs

Major classes of drugs are:
  Bile acid sequestrants
  Nicotinic acid
  3-Hydroxy-3-methylglutaryl coenzyme A reductase inhibitors (statins)
Other classes of drugs are:
  Fibric acid derivatives
  Probucol

Bile acid sequestrants

Bile acid sequestrants will lower LDL by 15–30% and raise HDL by 3–5%, but may increase triglycerides. Thus, they are relatively contraindicated with a triglyceride level greater than 200 mg/dl (>2–3 mmol/l) and absolutely contraindicated when levels are greater than 500 mg/dl (>5–6 mmol/l). They are not absorbed and thus tend to be very safe. However, they do interfere with absorption of digoxin, warfarin, thiazides, thyroxine, β-blockers, and perhaps other drugs. Thus, for patients taking these agents, it is recommended that the resin be taken at night if the other medicines are taken in the morning. In fact, resins probably should be avoided in patients taking agents that require very exact dosing. Very high doses can reduce the absorption of essential fat soluble vitamins.

Resin binders are especially useful in treating patients with an isolated LDL elevation. They are generally the first drugs employed in males younger than 45 years and females younger than 55 years with an LDL in the range 160–220 mg/dl (4·1–5·7 mmol/l). The usual daily doses of cholestyramine and colestipol are 4–16 g and 5–20 g, respectively, with an additional 50% making the dose maximal. They often cause gastrointestinal symptoms such as constipation, bloating, fullness, and flatulence. Because they are safe, patients should receive these agents to the dose that they tolerate; even small doses may result in a lower required dose of other agents such as statins. Of note, this combination is known to be effective in patients with very high LDL levels.

Nicotinic acid

Niacin, or nicotinic acid, is a B vitamin that lowers the LDL-cholesterol by 10–25% and triglycerides by 20–50% while raising HDL-cholesterol by 15–35%. It has been shown to reduce mortality in patients with CHD. If tolerated, it is an ideal therapeutic agent. Patients frequently experience flushing and headache. Aspirin reduces the symptoms. Also, the slow release niacin preparations are associated with fewer side effects, although there may be a slight increase in the risk for hepatic toxicity. Doses of 1500–3000 mg/day are required. Often, beginning at a very low dose such as 125–250 mg twice daily and advancing the dose on a weekly basis will improve tolerance. It should not be used in patients with active liver disease or diabetes mellitus because the latter will be harder to control. It is effective in combination with other major lipid lowering agents, particularly if raising HDL is an important therapeutic goal.

Statins

These agents are used for primary and secondary prevention in order to reduce CHD events and mortality.[2] These agents (i.e.

lovastatin, pravastatin, simvastatin, and fluvastatin) reduce hepatic synthesis of cholesterol, increasing the number of LDL receptors. These receptors then help to remove LDL and VLDL from the circulation. These drugs reduce LDL-cholesterol by 20–40% and triglycerides by 10–20%, and raise HDL-cholesterol by 5–10%.

Studies beyond 5 years have shown these agents to be quite safe. They may be hepatotoxic, particularly in combination with niacin, although the risk is low. They may also cause an important myositis. This is particularly true in combination with fibric acids such as gemfibrozil. Although the combination is used rarely, it can be effective in some patients, who must be followed carefully. Generally, the myopathy is resolved with cessation of the drug, but cases of rhabdomyolysis have been reported. Diarrhea may also occur, but this generally is self-limiting.

Most of the agents are started at 20 mg/day and simvastatin at 10 mg/day. The dose can be increased by about fourfold with continued benefit. Beyond that there may be some additional benefit, but it is small and probably not worth the risk. Because lowering LDL-cholesterol is the central feature of current therapy and the relative easy utility and safety of the statins, they play a central role in lipid treatment.

Fibric acids

Fibric acids include gemfibrozil, clofibrate, and fenofibrate. The former is the most often used, at a dose of 600 mg twice daily. It has been shown to reduce the risk for myocardial infarction. However, total mortality may be as high or even higher on these drugs. They are very effective in lowering triglycerides by 20–50% and are somewhat effective in raising HDL-cholesterol (10–15%). They are generally well tolerated. Because they have little impact on LDL-cholesterol, they are not classified as major drugs and are generally used only in cases of very high triglycerides, particularly in the setting of a low HDL-cholesterol concentration.

Case studies

Case 5.1

A 53-year-old man with no history of heart disease, diabetes, hypertension, or tobacco use is asymptomatic. His father and two paternal uncles had clinically significant CHD by age 55 years. He walks 30–40 min 5 days per week, and eats a diet similar to that of the American Heart Association guidelines. He has no significant past history.

Examination. Physical examination: the patient appeared normal. Height: 70 inches (177·8 cm). Weight: 167 lb (75·7 kg). No abnormalities of skin, nail beds, or oral mucosa. Pulse: 62 beats/min, normal character. Blood pressure: 120/75 mmHg in right arm. Jugular venous pulse: 4 cm. Cardiac impulse: normal. First heart sound: normal. Second heart sound: split normally on inspiration. No added sounds or murmurs. Chest examination: normal air entry, no rales or rhonchi. Abdominal examination: soft abdomen, no tenderness, and no masses. Normal liver span. No peripheral edema. Femoral, popliteal, posterior tibial, and dorsalis pedis pulses: all normal volume and equal. Carotid pulses: normal, no bruits. Optic fundi: normal.

Investigations. Total cholesterol 190 mg/dl (4·9 mmol/l); HDL-cholesterol 38 mg/dl (1·0 mmol/l); triglycerides 105 mg/dl (1·2 mmol/l); LDL-cholesterol 142 mg/dl (3·7 mmol/l); blood glucose 97 mg/dl (5·4 mmol/l). Urinalysis and thyroid function test: normal.

Questions

1. What is the goal for his LDL-cholesterol?
2. What other factors might be relevant in his family history?
3. How should he be treated?

Answers

Answer to question 1 Based on the National Cholesterol Education Program guidelines,[1] in this patient with two risk factors (family history of premature CHD, and being a male over 45 years old) the goal is an LDL-cholesterol of 130 mg/dl (3·6 mmol/l).

Answer to question 2 The family history is very important in CHD. He had several relatives with CHD, including his father. Nevertheless, it would be important to know whether these individuals had other risk factors for CHD. For example, if they were obese, inactive, and smoked, then the family history itself is less concerning. In contrast, if otherwise their risk was similar to that of our patient, then one must be worried that he has a high probability of developing CHD. Thus, when taking a family history, knowing the risk factor profile of individuals affected with CHD is important.

Answer to question 3 One might consider performing a treadmill test to exclude highly significant CHD. If the test was negative, then one would recommend a diet (see Table 5.3). One would also encourage him to continue his walking and keep his weight down.

Vitamin E and C, and perhaps even a baby aspirin would be considered. Cholesterol lowering drugs would not be employed unless his family history was very worrisome.

Case 5.2

A 47-year-old woman with diabetes has no known CHD, peripheral vascular disease, or family history of CHD. She is approximately 20 pounds (9 kg) overweight. She experienced menopause 18 months ago. Her diet includes about 40% of calories from fat, and she is essentially sedentary. She has mild exertional dyspnea but no chest pain. She is on an oral hypoglycemic agent but no other medications.

Examination. Physical examination: the patient appeared normal. Height: 62 inches (157·5 cm). Weight: 136 lb (61·6 kg). No abnormalities of skin, nail beds, or oral mucosa. Pulse: 81 beats/min, normal character. Blood pressure: 145/90 mmHg in right arm. Jugular venous pulse: 5 cm. Cardiac impulse: normal. First heart sound: normal. Second heart sound: split normally on inspiration. Soft fourth heart sound. No murmurs. Chest examination: normal air entry, no rales or rhonchi. Abdominal examination: soft abdomen, no tenderness and no masses. Normal liver span. No peripheral edema. Femoral, popliteal, posterior tibial, and dorsalis pedis pulses: all normal volume and equal. Carotid pulses: normal, no bruits. Optic fundi: normal.

Investigations. Total cholesterol 269 mg/dl (6·9 mmol/l); HDL-cholesterol 42 mg/dl (1·1 mmol/l); triglycerides 863 mg/dl (9·7 mmol/l); LDL-cholesterol not calculated; blood glucose 235 mg/dl (13 mmol/l). Urinalysis: 2+ glucose without protein. Thyroid function tests: normal. Electrocardiogram: normal.

Questions

1. What is her LDL?
2. What is the goal for her LDL-cholesterol?
3. How should she be treated?

Answers

Answer to question 1   Unfortunately, with her triglyceride level well above 400 mg/dl (>4·5 mmol/l), her LDL cannot be calculated. Traditionally, direct measurement of LDL has been difficult. If her diabetes becomes better controlled, her triglycerides are likely to drop significantly.

Answer to question 2 In patients with diabetes mellitus, the LDL goal is 100 mg/dl (2·6 mmol/l) regardless of other risk factors.

Answer to question 3 This is a type of patient who will benefit greatly from an increase in physical activity and weight loss. She might also benefit from some form of structured preventive oriented exercise program with other individuals like herself. This kind of support can make significant differences in compliance. This will improve her diabetes mellitus control, blood pressure, and lipid profile. She would also benefit greatly from nutritional counseling. With continued strong encouragement, her laboratory results should be repeated in approximately 3 months. If despite weight loss and a normal glucose her triglycerides remain elevated, then she should have a direct measurement of her LDL-cholesterol.

Case 5.3

A 64-year-old man is referred to you because of an abnormal electrocardiogram. He has had no symptoms, quit smoking 3 years ago, and is on no special diet. He is quite vigorous, exercising at least 30 min 5 days per week. His father had a myocardial infarction at age 55 years, and he has no history of hypertension.

Examination. Physical examination: the patient appeared normal. Height: 72 inches (182·9 cm). Weight: 156 lb (70·7 kg). No abnormalities of skin, nail beds, or oral mucosa. Pulse: 52 beats/min, normal character. Blood pressure: 120/60 mmHg in right arm. Jugular venous pressure: 5 cm. Cardiac impulse: normal. First heart sound: normal. Second heart sound: split normally on inspiration. No added sounds or murmurs. Chest examination: normal air entry, no rales or rhonchi. Abdominal examination: soft abdomen, no tenderness, and no masses. Normal liver span. No peripheral edema. Femoral, popliteal, posterior tibial, and dorsalis pedis pulses: all normal volume and equal. Carotid pulses: normal, no bruits. Optic fundi: normal.

Investigations. Total cholesterol 210 mg/dl (5·4 mmol/l); HDL-cholesterol 42 mg/dl (1·1 mmol/l); triglycerides 163 mg/dl (1·8 mmol/l); LDL-cholesterol (calculated) 135 mg/dl (3·5 mmol/l). Electrocardiogram: normal sinus rhythm with Q waves in leads II, III, and aVF. No previous tracing available.

Questions

1. Does he have CHD despite the fact that he has no symptoms?
2. Should he undergo further cardiac evaluation?

3. How likely is his LDL-cholesterol to respond to dietary therapy?
4. How should he be treated?

Answers

Answer to question 1 Certainly people can have false Q waves on an electrocardiogram, but it is more likely that he has at some point suffered a silent myocardial infarction. As many as 25% of myocardial infarctions may be associated with no symptoms.

Answer to question 2 One simple way to confirm whether he has had a previous myocardial infarction would be to do an echocardiogram looking for an inferior wall motion abnormality. He should also undergo stress testing. This could be combined with echocardiography to improve sensitivity. In addition to the diagnostic utility, a fair amount of prognostic information comes from exercise testing.

Answer to question 3 Although LDL-cholesterol has been shown to decrease by only about 5% with diet, this cannot be predicted on an individual basis. We have all seen persons who experience a marked lipid improvement with dietary therapy. Thus a 2–3 month trial of diet is generally indicated.

Answer to question 4 If we confirm that he has CHD, then his LDL goal will be 100 mg/dl (2·6 mmol/l). Generally drug therapy would be reserved for individuals who cannot get their LDL to below 130 mg/dl (3·3 mmol/l) despite a good diet. Thus, after a 2–3 month period on an American Heart Association diet his lipids should be remeasured. If his LDL remains near or above 130 mg/dl (3·3 mmol/l), then one would likely initiate drug therapy, probably with a statin drug. A resin binder or niacin could certainly be considered.

Case 5.4

A 54-year-old woman is admitted with an acute myocardial infarction. The following morning lipids are checked along with other laboratory results. She is now pain free and stable having received thrombolytic therapy. She has hypertension, which has been treated, and a late family history of CHD. She does not smoke or have diabetes mellitus, and she does not recall having her lipids determined previously. She walks 2 miles three times weekly, but is on no specific diet.

Examination. Physical examination: the patient appeared mildly obese. Height: 68 inches (172·7 cm). Weight: 158 lb (71·6 kg). No abnormalities of skin, nail beds, or oral mucosa. Pulse: 74 beats/min, normal character. Blood pressure: 140/60 mmHg in right arm. Jugular venous pulse: 5 cm. Cardiac impulse: normal. First heart sound: normal. Second heart sound: split normally on inspiration. No added sounds or murmurs. Chest examination: normal air entry, no rales or rhonchi. Abdominal examination: soft abdomen, no tenderness, and no masses. Normal liver span. No peripheral edema. Femoral, popliteal, posterior tibial, and dorsalis pedis pulses: all normal volume and equal. Carotid pulses: normal, no bruits. Optic fundi: normal.

Investigations. Total cholesterol 262 mg/dl (6·8 mmol/l); HDL-cholesterol 47 mg/dl (1·2 mmol/l); triglycerides 192 mg/dl (2·2 mmol/l); LDL-cholesterol (calculated) 176 mg/dl (4·5 mmol/l). Electrocardiogram: normal sinus rhythm with ST elevation and Q waves in leads II, III, and aVF suggestive of an evolving inferior myocardial infarction.

Questions

1. How valid are her lipid values?
2. How likely is she to respond to diet?
3. In terms of her lipids, how should she be treated?

Answers

Answer to question 1   It is often said that at the time of a myocardial infarction the lipids decrease. Although this is true, usually within the first 24–48 hours, the values are valid. They then may fall below the baseline for as many as 3 months. Irrespectively, if a patient has an elevated cholesterol, one should assume that it is at least that high, and therapy should be outlined accordingly.

Answer to question 2   Diet is unlikely to get her LDL to the goal of 100 mg/dl (2·6 mmol/l). Still, it is not unreasonable to start with diet. Diet can be very effective in some patients, and without measuring specific apolipoproteins it is hard to predict which patients will respond. Furthermore, it is important to educate patients and their families about the appropriate diet.

Answer to question 3   If after a trial of diet the LDL-cholesterol remains above 130 mg/dl (>3·3 mmol/l), then drug therapy would be initiated to attempt to get the value to 100 mg/dl (2·6 mmol/l). Any of the primary drugs that lower LDL could be considered. This would include niacin, a statin, or a resin binder. The statins are probably the most convenient, and are supported by the most data. A combination is also a reasonable choice, such as a low dose of a resin, which may lower the statin requirement. Once a statin or niacin is initiated, liver function tests should be done in 6 weeks and again at 12 weeks, along with a repeat lipid profile.

Case 5.5

A 32-year-old man recently underwent coronary artery bypass surgery. He now feels quite well. He is running 4–6 miles five times per week. He eats a vegetarian diet with 20–30 g fat/day. He has a family history of coronary artery disease, with both grandfathers suffering myocardial infarctions in their early to mid 50s. Both parents are now in their 50s and are healthy. The patient does not know their lipid status. His only medications include aspirin 81 mg/day and fluvastatin 80 mg each night. He drinks one alcoholic beverage weekly.

Examination. Physical examination: The patient appeared thin. Height: 70 inches (177·8 cm). Weight: 149 lb (67·5 kg). No abnormalities of skin, nail beds, or oral mucosa. Pulse: 54 beats/min, normal character. Blood pressure: 110/55 mmHg in right arm. Jugular venous pulse: normal. Cardiac impulse: normal. First heart sound: normal. Second heart sound: split normally on inspiration. No added sounds or murmurs. Chest examination: normal air entry, no rales or rhonchi. Abdominal examination: soft abdomen, no tenderness and no masses. Normal liver span. No peripheral edema. Femoral, popliteal, posterior tibial, and dorsalis pedis pulses: all normal volume and equal. Carotid pulses: normal, no bruits. Optic fundi: normal.

Investigations. Total cholesterol 262 mg/dl (6·8 mmol/l); HDL-cholesterol 28 mg/dl (0·7 mmol/l); triglycerides 114 mg/dl (1·3 mmol/l); LDL-cholesterol (calculated) 211 mg/dl (5·4 mmol/l). Electrocardiogram: Normal.

Questions

1. What should you tell him about his diet?
2. Might he benefit from vitamins or antioxidants?
3. Should he increase his alcohol intake?
4. How might one change his lipid lowering therapy?

Answers

Answer to question 1   His low fat diet is to be commended. At the same time, it is possible that his reduction in monounsaturated fatty acids has actually worked to lower his HDL-cholesterol. He probably should be referred to a dietician and consider a slightly increased intake of monosaturated fatty acids.

Answer to question 2   Controlled clinical studies are lacking, and so it is not possible to assure this patient that antioxidant therapy will have a positive impact on his outcome. Nevertheless, there is growing evidence that he might benefit from such therapy. In appropriate doses, however, the risk is low, and the benefit should be considered. He should consider beginning vitamin C (500–1000 mg/day), vitamin E (400–800 IU/day), and β-carotene (15 mg/day).

Answer to question 3   It is still not absolutely clear which component of alcohol results in an improved outcome from CHD. If wine is superior to other beverages, then is it possible that grape juice and other fruits may provide some protective effect? Still, there may be some specific protective effect from alcohol, and some of this may be mediated through its positive impact on HDL-cholesterol. In a culture in which alcohol-related deaths are considerable, it is hard for some physicians to recommend that people increase their consumption. At the same time one would not discourage a daily alcoholic beverage.

Answer to question 4   There are a number of medication changes that one might make that are likely to result in an improved lipid status and outcome. In this patient, one would want to be very aggressive, trying to get his LDL-cholesterol close to 100 mg/dl (2·6 mmol/l). First of all, not all statins are equally effective. One should probably consider a different drug. Possibilities include pravastatin, lovastatin, simvastatin, or atorvastatin at a maximal dose of 80 mg.

It is still almost certain that a second and/or even a third drug will have to be added to achieve our goal. Although the risk for complications may rise, it is certain that if he does not experience a significant reduction in LDL-cholesterol then he will succumb to serious sequelae of CHD at an early age. Adding niacin might be most helpful. In addition to lowering LDL-cholesterol, one might achieve a significant improvement in HDL-cholesterol. He should begin at a low dose such as 50–100 mg orally three times daily and gradually increase the dose to 500 mg orally three times daily. Liver function tests should be checked at 6 weeks and again at 12 weeks, along with a lipid profile. The slow release niacin preparations cause fewer side effects but may increase the risk for drug-induced hepatitis. Liver function tests should be followed carefully in all patients on a combination of a statin and niacin, and in particular when the slow release preparation is employed.

Some bile acid sequestrant could be added with the hope of some additional LDL lowering. Finally, if the LDL-cholesterol remains high despite this triple therapy combination, then LDL apheresis should be considered. This system washes the plasma of LDL-cholesterol. However, it requires connection to a dialysis-like machine on a regular basis, and at the present time it is available only in limited centers.

Case 5.6

A 52-year-old man presents with diffuse myalgias, which have gradually worsened over the past 2–3 months. He experiences pain in all of his large skeletal muscles, particularly after physical activity. He has known CHD, having suffered a myocardial infarction 2 years previously, at which time he was started on lovastatin. He denies chest pain or shortness of breath. Up until the time of the myalgias he was walking three miles on six days each week. He eats a fairly good diet with occasional increases in his fat intake. Medications include aspirin 81 mg/day, metoprolol 50 mg twice daily, and lovastatin 40 mg each evening.

Examination. Physical examination: the patient appeared normal. No abnormalities of skin, nail beds, or oral mucosa. Pulse: 67 beats/min, normal character. Blood pressure: 130/85 mmHg in right arm. Jugular venous pulse: 4 cm. Cardiac impulse: normal. First heart sound: normal. Second heart sound: split normally on inspiration. No added sounds or murmurs. Chest examination: normal air entry, no rales or rhonchi. Abdominal examination: soft abdomen, no tenderness, and no masses. Normal liver span. No peripheral edema. Femoral, popliteal, posterior tibial, and dorsalis pedis pulses: all normal volume and equal. Carotid pulses: normal, no bruits. Optic fundi: normal.

Investigations. Total cholesterol 182 mg/dl (4·7 mmol/l); HDL-cholesterol 39 mg/dl (1·0 mmol/l); triglycerides 127 mg/dl (1·4 mmol/l); LDL-cholesterol (calculated) 118 mg/dl (3·0 mmol/l). Creatinine 1·0 mg/dl (88·4 μmol/l); creatinine phosphokinase (normal range) 1054 (50–350) mg/dl (17·5 [0·8–5·8] μkat/l). Electrocardiogram: normal sinus rhythm, with inferior Q waves

Questions

1. What is the most likely cause of his muscle pain?
2. What should be done in regard to his muscle pain?
3. What should be done with his lipid therapy?

Answers

Answer to question 1 In addition to liver function test abnormalities, mild elevations in creatinine kinase are common with statin drugs, and usually do not require any change in therapy. However, if myopathy develops to the point of development of symptoms, then the drug should be stopped and the patient followed clinically. Although there may be a slight difference in the incidence of myopathy with different statins, it can occur with any of them. It is also more common in combination with cyclosporin or gemfibrozil.

Answer to question 2   Lovastatin should be stopped and the patient seen back in 4–6 weeks. If he remains well then pravastatin or fluvastatin could be tried, which may have a slightly lower incidence of myopathy. Nevertheless, there is a good chance that the symptoms and enzyme elevation will recur.

Answer to question 3   One should probably consider the use of a different type of lipid lowering agent. Niacin might be considered and started as suggested in Case 5.5. A bile acid sequestrant would be another alternative to attempt to keep his LDL-cholesterol down.

References

1 Anonymous. Executive Summary of The Third Report of The National Cholesterol Education Program (NCEP) Expert Panel on Detection, Evaluation, and Treatment of High Blood Cholesterol in Adults (Adult Treatment Panel III). *JAMA* 2001;**285**:2486–97.
2 Grundy SM. Statin trials and goals of cholesterol-lowering therapy. *Circulation* 1998;**97**:1436–9.
3 Carretero OA, Oparil O. Essential hypertension treatment: part II. *Circulation* 2000;**101**:446–53.
4 Garrison RJ, Wilson PW, Castelli WP, Feinleib M, Kannel WB, McNamara PM. Obesity and lipoprotein cholesterol in the Framingham offspring study. *Metabolism* 1980;**29**:1053–60.
5 Evans DJ, Murray R, Kissebah AH. Relationship between skeletal muscle insulin resistance, insulin-mediated glucose disposal, and insulin binding: effects of obesity and body fat topography. *J Clin Invest* 1984;**74**:1515–25.
6 Castelli WP, Garrison RJ, Wilson PW, Abbot RD, Kalousdian S, Kannel WB. Incidence of coronary heart diseases and lipoprotein cholesterol levels. *JAMA* 1986;**256**:2835–8.
7 Wenger NK. Coronary disease in women. *Annu Rev Med* 1985;**36**:285–94.
8 MRFIT research group, personal communication, 1989, as reported in National Cholesterol Education Program. Report of the Expert Panel on Population Strategies for Blood Cholesterol Reduction. *Circulation* 1991;**83**:2154–232.
9 La Rosa JC, He J, Vupputuri S. Effect of statins on risk of coronary disease. A meta-analysis of randomized controlled trials. *JAMA* 1999;**282**:2340–6.
10 Brown BG, Albers JJ, Fisher LD, *et al.* Regression of coronary artery disease as a result of intensive lipid-lowering therapy in men with high levels of apolipoprotein B. *N Engl J Med* 1990;**323**:1289–98.
11 Anonymous. NIH Consensus Conference. Triglyceride, high-density lipoprotein, and coronary heart disease. NIH Consensus Development Panel on Triglyceride, High-Density Lipoprotein, and Coronary Heart Disease. *JAMA* 1993;**269**:505–10.
12 Leon AS, Haskell WL. The influence of exercise on the concentrations of triglyceride and cholesterol in human plasma. *Exerc Sport Sci Rev* 1984;**12**:205–44.

13   Wood PD, Stefanick ML, Williams PT, Haskell WL. The effects on plasma lipoproteins of a prudent weight-reducing diet, with or without exercise, in overweight men and women. *N Engl J Med* 1991;**325**:461–6.

14   Barret-Connor E, Bush TL. Estrogen and coronary heart disease in women. *JAMA* 1991;**265**:1861–7.

15   Grady D, Herrington D, Bittner V, *et al.* Cardiovascular disease outcomes during 6·8 years of hormone therapy: Heart and Estrogen/progestin Replacement Study follow-up (HERS II). *JAMA* 2002;**288**:49–57.

16   Writing Group for the Women's Health Initiative Investigators. Risks and benefits of estrogen plus progestin in healthy postmenopausal women: principal results from the Women's Health Initiative randomized controlled trial. *JAMA* 2002;**288**: 321–33.

17   Knopp RH. Drug treatment of lipid disorders. *N Engl J Med* 1999;**341**:498–511.

6: Acute coronary syndromes

JAMES A DE LEMOS

Ischemic heart disease can be viewed on a spectrum ranging from stable angina to acute myocardial infarction (MI) and sudden cardiac death. The term "acute coronary syndrome" (ACS) describes the spontaneous presentation of acute ischemic heart disease, and encompasses the diagnoses of unstable angina, non-ST-segment elevation MI (non-Q-wave MI) and ST-segment elevation MI (Q-wave MI). The pathophysiology of the different ACSs can be viewed as points on a single continuum of plaque rupture and thrombus formation (Figure 6.1).[1]

Because patients with coronary atherosclerosis typically have numerous atherosclerotic plaques of varying size and configuration throughout their coronary arteries, intense research has focused on identifying which characteristics make an individual plaque vulnerable to rupture and initiation of an ACS. Of interest is that lesions that subsequently cause an acute MI typically are not associated with critical stenosis before rupture. More important is the content of the plaque; those that have a large lipid core and a thin fibrous cap appear particularly vulnerable, especially if there is an accumulation of inflammatory cells at the critical "shoulder" region of the plaque. These inflammatory cells secrete matrix degrading enzymes that can destabilize the fibrous cap and promote plaque rupture, initiating the cascade of events that lead to ACS (Figure 6.2).[2,3]

Electrocardiographic characterization
of acute coronary syndrome

Patients with ST-segment elevation MI experience a substantial benefit from fibrinolytic therapy, whereas those with non-ST-segment elevation (ST-segment depression or T-wave inversion) ACS do not. The explanation for this difference is that patients with ST-segment elevation exhibit 100% occlusion of the infarct-related artery, whereas patients without ST-segment elevation exhibit a severely stenotic but nevertheless patent coronary artery (Figure 6.3).[4] As opposed to the distinction of ST-segment elevation versus non-ST-segment elevation MI, the determination of Q-wave versus non-Q-wave MI can only be made retrospectively, and is a less useful classification in the early hours of patient management. Untreated, most patients with ST-segment

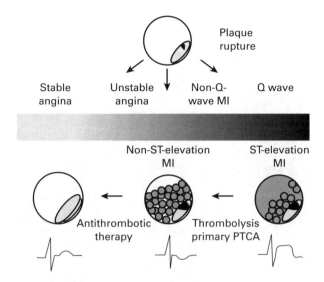

Figure 6.1 The spectrum of coronary artery disease, ranging from patients with stable angina to those with ST-segment elevation myocardial infarction (MI). In patients with acute coronary syndromes, rupture of an atherosclerotic plaque leads to coronary artery thrombosis; in acute ST-segment elevation MI, complete thrombotic occlusion of the infarct artery is present. In those with unstable angina or non-Q-wave MI, the thrombus partially occludes the vessel and limits blood flow at rest. Thrombus is rarely present in patients with stable angina. PTCA, percutaneous transluminal coronary angioplasty. Adapted from Cannon[1]

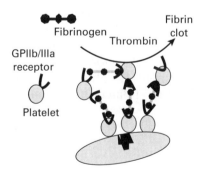

Figure 6.2 The pathophysiologic events that lead to the development of an acute coronary syndrome. The process begins when an atherosclerotic plaque ruptures. Platelets then adhere and become activated, undergoing a conformational change and expressing a greater number of glycoprotein (GP)IIb/IIIa receptors, which makes them receptive to fibrinogen binding. Fibrinogen aggregates platelets by binding to the GPIIb/IIIa receptors on adjacent platelets. On the platelet surface, thrombin is activated, leading to conversion of fibrinogen to fibrin, forming the occlusive thrombus that is responsible for the acute coronary syndrome. From de Lemos *et al.*[3]

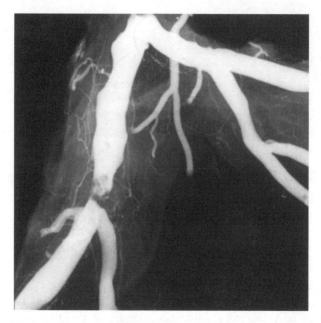

Figure 6.3 Atherosclerotic plaque rupture with subtotal coronary artery occlusion, leading to non-ST-segment elevation acute coronary syndrome. Shown is a coronary angiogram with a ruptured plaque in the proximal left anterior descending coronary artery. Because flow is still present past the lesion, ST elevation does not typically develop. The irregular echolucent area represents thrombus. From Davies[4]

elevation MI evolve a transmural infarction, and develop Q waves on the surface electrocardiogram. With successful reperfusion therapy, however, many patients with ST-segment elevation MI have necrosis limited to the subendocardial regions, and do not develop Q waves. Patients without ST-segment elevation at baseline generally do not develop Q waves because infarction is limited to subendocardial regions.

Diagnosis

History

Distinguishing ischemic heart disease from other non-cardiac diseases is especially challenging for physicians, because only about 15% of patients with the symptom of chest pain at rest will have an ACS. Classically, the chest pain of ACS occurs at rest, and is described as a severe, pressure-type discomfort in the mid-sternum, often radiating to the left arm, neck, or jaw. The pain may be accompanied by dyspnea, diaphoresis, nausea, vomiting, and weakness. Characterization of the quality of pain may help to distinguish it from other conditions that also cause chest discomfort at rest, such as aortic dissection and pericarditis (Table 6.1). Many patients, particularly the elderly and those with diabetes mellitus, present with atypical symptoms, which include dyspnea, indigestion, unusual locations of pain, agitation, altered mental status, profound weakness, and syncope. Furthermore, MI may be "silent" in more than 25% of cases.[5]

Physical examination

The majority of patients with ACS have a normal cardiovascular examination. Thus, the initial examination should focus on narrowing the differential diagnosis and assessing the stability of the patient. A focused examination can help to eliminate diagnoses such as pericarditis, pneumothorax, pulmonary embolus, and aortic dissection, which may mimic acute MI (see Table 6.1). A careful examination can also exclude aortic stenosis, which may complicate patient management. In addition, hemodynamic and mechanical complications of acute MI can often be detected by close attention to physical findings.

Patients with acute MI often appear pale, cool, and clammy; in many cases they are in obvious distress. Elderly patients in particular may be agitated and incoherent, whereas those with cardiogenic shock are often confused and listless. Blood pressure and pulses should be checked in both arms because a diminished pulse or decreased blood pressure in the left arm suggests the possibility of aortic dissection. A pericardial friction rub, although often difficult to hear, suggests that pericarditis may be the cause of a patient's chest discomfort.

A brief survey for signs of congestive heart failure should be performed. Cool extremities or altered mental status suggests decreased tissue perfusion, whereas elevated jugular venous pressure and wet rales on chest examination suggest elevated cardiac filling pressures. Examination of the peripheral circulation may reveal peripheral or cerebral vascular disease, which increase the probability of coronary artery disease.[5]

Electrocardiographic findings

The 12-lead electrocardiogram remains the foundation of initial diagnosis and triage for patients with suspected ACS. If ST-segment

Table 6.1 Distinguishing acute coronary syndrome from other conditions that cause chest pain

Condition	Characterization of pain	Physical findings	ECG findings	Helpful diagnostic tests
Acute coronary syndrome	Pressure type pain at rest, often radiating to neck or left arm	Examination often normal; check for signs of cardiogenic shock or congestive heart failure	ST elevation, ST depression, T-wave abnormalities	Measurement of cardiac enzymes
Aortic dissection	"Tearing" pain radiating to back	Diminished pulse or blood pressure in left arm	Usually normal or with non-specific changes, LVH; ST elevation if dissection involves coronary ostia (5% of patients)	Chest x ray, CT scan, or MRI; transesophageal echocardiography; contrast aortography
Pulmonary embolism	Pleuritic chest pain with dyspnea and cough	Tachypnea; tachycardia; pleural rub; right parasternal lift	Tachycardia with non-specific ST- and T-wave changes; $S_1Q_3T_3$ pattern classic but rarely seen	Ventilation–perfusion lung scan; high resolution chest CT; pulmonary angiogram
Pericarditis	Pain worse lying flat, better sitting forward; may radiate to trapezius ridge	Pericardial friction rub	Diffuse, concave ST elevation with PR-segment depression	Echocardiogram

CT, computed tomography; LVH, left ventricular hypertrophy; MRI, magnetic resonance imaging elevation is seen and the patient is hemodynamically stable, then sublingual nitroglycerin should be given while patient assessment continues. If chest pain and ST-segment elevation resolve completely with sublingual nitroglycerin, then the diagnosis may be coronary vasospasm (Prinzmetal's variant angina), or possibly spontaneous reperfusion of a thrombotic coronary occlusion. Persistent ST-segment elevation is virtually diagnostic of occlusive thrombus, and immediate reperfusion therapy should be given (see Initial therapy for acute coronary syndrome, below). ST-segment elevation from acute MI must be distinguished from that seen in acute pericarditis and the normal early repolarization variant. In pericarditis, ST-segment elevation is typically diffuse and associated with depression of the PR segment (Figure 6.4). In both pericarditis and the early repolarization variant, the contour of the elevated ST segment is concave rather than convex. Patients with prior MI and aneurysm formation may have persistent ST-segment elevation, but this generally occurs in presence of Q waves.

The presence of new, or presumed new, left bundle branch block is suggestive of a large anterior MI, and these patients should receive reperfusion therapy as well. In patients with a pre-existing left bundle branch block, alternative methods are needed to diagnose acute MI because electrocardiographic findings are not sufficiently reliable to guide therapy.

ST-segment depression, or T-wave inversions, as opposed to ST-segment elevation, are suggestive of subendocardial ischemia. Downsloping ST depression is a more specific finding for ischemia than is upsloping depression or T-wave inversion. Unfortunately, many other conditions cause ST and T wave changes that can mimic those of ischemia, including left ventricular hypertrophy, electrolyte and metabolic disorders, and drug effects. Comparison with a patient's prior electrocardiograms is frequently helpful for determining whether the ST and T wave changes seen represent new ischemic changes. In general, dynamic ST changes (those that get worse with chest pain and improve when pain is resolved) are highly suggestive of ACS.

Serum cardiac markers

Although creatinine kinase (CK) is a sensitive marker of myocardial necrosis, this enzyme is present in adult skeletal muscle and thus can rise with skeletal muscle injury as well. The myocardial isoform of CK (i.e. CK-MB) is more specific for cardiac tissue, although it is also present to some degree in other organs and skeletal muscle. CK and CK-MB are detectable 3–6 hours after the onset of chest pain, peak at

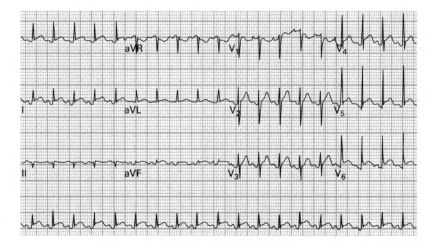

Figure 6.4 Electrocardiographic changes characteristic of pericarditis. Concave (upsloping) ST elevation is seen diffusely, together with PR-segment depression. Importantly, T waves are essentially normal, which is another distinguishing feature from ST-segment elevation myocardial infarction

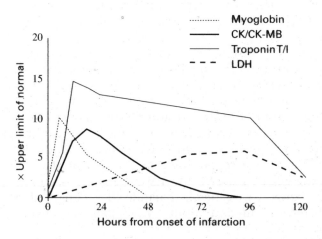

Figure 6.5 Time course of serum marker release in acute myocardial infarction. (See text for details.) CK, creatinine kinase; LDH, lactate dehydrogenase. Adapted with permission from Antman[6]

approximately 18 hours, and return to normal in approximately 3 days (Figure 6.5).[6]

Cardiac troponins T (cTnT) and I (cTnI) are contractile proteins that are released in response to myocardial necrosis. Like CK and CK-MB, these enzymes are detectable 3–6 hours after the onset of chest pain and peak at approximately 14–20 hours (see Figure 6.5). They differ, however, in that they remain elevated for up to 14 days after infarction. This prolonged detection window facilitates the diagnosis of remote infarction (i.e. an infarct that occurred in the days or weeks before presentation) but makes the diagnosis of early recurrent infarction difficult. Because cTnT and cTnI are not found in adult skeletal muscle, they are highly specific for myocardial injury and thus are excellent markers for confirming the diagnosis of MI. The normal reference range for the cardiac troponins is set at a very low level; as a result, troponins are very sensitive for the detection of small amounts of myocardial necrosis. Indeed, it has recently been shown that patients with minor myocardial necrosis, as evidenced by low level troponin elevation in the absence of CK and CK-MB elevation, are at increased risk for the development of adverse clinical outcomes.[7] This finding has led to a revised, more liberal definition of myocardial infarction that now includes patients with low level troponin elevation, even if CK and CK-MB are normal.

Myoglobin is a small cytosolic molecule that is rapidly released from ischemic muscle and promptly cleared by the kidney. Serum levels of myoglobin rise earlier than other available markers, and elevated levels can be detected as early as 2 hours after the onset of chest pain. Myoglobin peaks at approximately 6 hours and returns to normal levels within 18–24 hours (see Figure 6.5). Widespread use of serum myoglobin for the detection of MI has been limited by concerns about poor cardiac specificity. Skeletal muscle trauma and renal failure can raise serum myoglobin levels in a non-specific manner. Nevertheless, myoglobin remains a very useful early marker because of its rapid release and renal clearance, and it is more sensitive than CK-MB for detecting MI within the first few hours after presentation. An elevated myoglobin should be confirmed with a more specific marker at a later time point, such as CK-MB, cTnT, or cTnI.[8]

Radionuclide imaging

New high-resolution agents, such as ^{99m}Tc-sestamibi and ^{99m}Tc-tetrofosmin, are now available for myocardial perfusion imaging. These radionuclides, unlike thallium-201, do not redistribute after their initial deposition. This property allows these agents to be given by intravenous injection during an episode of suspected ischemic pain, with imaging performed following stabilization and/or therapy. The images obtained provide a "snapshot" of myocardial perfusion at the time the tracer was injected. This strategy may be a particularly useful means of excluding ischemia as a cause of prolonged chest pain in patients with a non-diagnostic electrocardiogram.

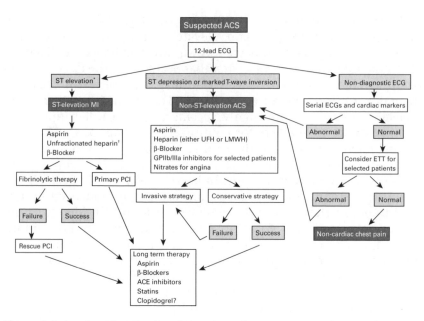

Figure 6.6 An algorithm for the diagnosis and management of suspected acute coronary syndromes (ACS). Dark boxes indicate diagnostic categories; white boxes indicate diagnostic or therapeutic procedures; and gray boxes indicate interpretation of tests or procedures. *New, or presumed new left bundle branch block should be considered together with ST elevation. †Intravenous unfractionated heparin is not indicated as adjunctive therapy with streptokinase. ACE, angiotensin-converting enzyme; ECG, electrocardiogram; ETT, exercise tolerance test; GP, glycoprotein; LMWH, low molecular weight heparin; MI, myocardial infarction; PCI, percutaneous coronary intervention; UFH, unfractionated heparin

Initial therapy for acute coronary syndromes

All patients should be given oxygen and an aspirin tablet to chew. Morphine is an extremely effective agent to relieve the pain of acute myocardial ischemia and MI; in addition, because morphine dilates venous capacitance vessels, it also relieves symptoms of pulmonary congestion or edema. Beyond this, the initial management of patients with suspected ACS depends on the presenting electrocardiogram (Figure 6.6). Patients with ST-segment elevation are directed to immediate reperfusion therapy, whereas those without ST-segment elevation are treated initially with antiplatelet and antithrombotic therapy, and aggressive antianginal medical therapy to minimize ischemia.

Reperfusion therapy for ST-segment elevation myocardial infarction

Options for reperfusion therapy include fibrinolytic therapy and primary percutaneous coronary intervention (PCI), either with percutaneous transluminal coronary angioplasty or intracoronary stenting. Primary PCI is the preferred method in centers with sufficient resources and expertise to perform successful PCI within 90 min of presentation to the hospital; however, if the "door to balloon" time is greater than 90 min, then fibrinolytic therapy is preferred. Clinical studies suggest that mortality is slightly lower with primary PCI than with pharmacologic reperfusion therapy when PCI is performed in expert institutions. In addition, recurrent MI and intracranial hemorrhage are observed less frequently with primary PCI than with fibrinolytic therapy.

Because of resource limitations, fibrinolytic therapy is much more widely available than PCI, and is the reperfusion method of choice in the majority of hospitals. The speed at which reperfusion therapy is administered is much more important than the choice between PCI and fibrinolytic therapy, or the choice between individual fibrinolytic agents. For each hour earlier that reperfusion therapy is administered, there is an absolute 1% decrease in mortality.[9] All of the fibrinolytic agents currently available are plasminogen activators. Reteplase (recombinant plasminogen activator [rPA]) and tenecteplase have a prolonged half-life and can be given as a bolus injection, as compared with the prolonged infusion required with alteplase (recombinant tissue plasminogen activator [tPA]) and streptokinase. Because tPA, rPA, and tenecteplase are more potent than streptokinase, they are associated with slightly lower mortality at a cost of slightly increased bleeding. The cost/benefit ratio favors these agents over streptokinase in patients presenting early after symptom onset with a large area of injury (for example acute anterior MI) and a low risk for intracranial hemorrhage. In groups with smaller potential for survival benefit and a greater risk for intracranial hemorrhage, streptokinase may be the agent of choice, particularly in view of the cost. Additional considerations include avoiding readministration of streptokinase or anistreplase to patients for at least 4 years (preferably indefinitely) because of a high prevalence of potentially neutralizing antibodies, and because there is a risk of anaphylaxis upon re-exposure to these drugs.

There are contraindications to fibrinolytic therapy (Table 6.2). In addition, fibrinolytic therapy is not indicated for patients with non-ST-segment elevation ACS because it increases bleeding complications without a measurable clinical benefit.[10]

Table 6.2 Contraindications to thrombolytic therapy

Absolute contraindications	Relative contraindications
Active internal bleeding	Blood pressure consistently
Prior intracranial hemorrhage	>180/110 mmHg
Stroke within past year	Stroke or TIA at any time in past
Recent head trauma or brain neoplasm	Known bleeding diathesis
Suspected aortic dissection	Proliferative diabetic retinopathy
Major surgery or trauma within 2 weeks	Prolonged CPR
	Pregnancy

CPR, cardiopulmonary resuscitation; TIA, transient ischemic attack

Antiplatelet and antithrombotic therapy

For patients with both ST-segment elevation and non-ST-segment elevation ACS, aspirin reduces mortality, recurrent ischemia, and MI, and therefore should be given to all patients.[11] If a true aspirin allergy is present, then clopidogrel may serve as an effective alternative.

For patients with ST-segment elevation MI, intravenous unfractionated heparin (UFH) should be administered as an adjunct to reperfusion therapy with tPA, rPA, and tenecteplase. With streptokinase, on the other hand, there is no clear benefit of adjunctive heparin, and it should not be given routinely. In non-ST-segment elevation ACS, the addition of intravenous UFH to aspirin reduces the rate of death and recurrent infarction,[12] and therefore should be given unless there is a bleeding contraindication or the patient has a history of heparin associated thrombocytopenia. Heparin should be administered as a weight adjusted bolus and infusion, and titrated to a partial thromboplastin time of approximately 2 × control.

Recently, several novel antiplatelet and antithrombotic therapies have been introduced that appear to be beneficial in patients with non-ST-segment elevation ACS. Ticlopidine and clopidogrel are thienopyridine agents that block adenosine diphosphate mediated platelet aggregation, and appear to provide protection similar to that with aspirin in patients with established vascular disease.[13] Clopidogrel causes fewer hematologic side effects than does ticlopidine, and thus is the agent of choice in this drug class. The combination of clopidogrel and aspirin has recently been shown to be even more beneficial than either agent alone, and prolonged therapy with these two agents following ACS will probably become commonplace in the near future.

Glycoprotein IIb/IIIa inhibitors are intravenous compounds that block the final common pathway of platelet aggregation, namely fibrinogen mediated cross-linking at the glycoprotein IIb/IIIa receptor. These agents provide platelet inhibition that is several times greater than that with aspirin or clopidogrel. Two of the glycoprotein IIb/IIIa inhibitors, namely tirofiban and eptifibatide, have been shown to reduce the probability of recurrent ischemic events among patients with non-ST-segment elevation ACS. The benefit of these agents is greatest in high risk patients (those with dynamic ST changes or elevated cardiac enzymes) who are managed with an early aggressive strategy, including routine angiography and percutaneous revascularization.[14,15]

Low molecular weight heparins (LMWHs) are created by depolymerization of standard UFH and selection of those fragments with lower molecular weight. LMWH is active early in the clotting cascade, inhibiting factor Xa to a greater extent than does UFH, thereby inhibiting both thrombin activity and its generation. The high bioavailability and reproducible anticoagulant response of LMWH allows for subcutaneous administration without monitoring of the anticoagulant effect. In high-risk patients with non-ST-segment elevation ACS, the LMWH heparin compound enoxaparin is associated with modestly lower risk for death and MI versus UFH.[16] Other LMWH compounds appear to be roughly equivalent to UFH. Predominantly because of its ease of use, it is likely that LMWH will replace UFH for most patients with non-ST-segment elevation ACS in the near future.

β-Blockers

β-Blockers exert their beneficial effect in ACS by decreasing myocardial contractility and especially heart rate, thereby improving the balance between oxygen supply and demand. As such, they may reduce infarction size and lower short-term mortality rates. In addition, β-blockers prevent atrial and ventricular arrhythmias in patients following MI, and may prevent ventricular rupture following transmural MI. Long-term therapy is indicated with β-blockers following ACS to prevent recurrent infarction.

Angiotensin-converting enzyme inhibitors

Angiotensin-converting enzyme (ACE) inhibitors have become a mainstay in the treatment of patients with all types of ACS. Following ST-segment elevation MI, ACE inhibitors are administered because they prevent deleterious left ventricular chamber remodeling and subsequent heart failure.[17] In addition, long-term therapy with ACE inhibitors prevents ischemic events in patients with established coronary artery disease.[18] ACE inhibitors should be initiated early (but not emergently) after the presentation of ACS and continued indefinitely.

Nitrates

Nitrates favorably effect both myocardial oxygen supply and demand, and thus are of particular value early in ACS. Nitrates dilate both normal and atherosclerotic resistance coronary arteries, and redistribute blood flow from epicardial to ischemic endocardial regions. Central venodilatation and modest peripheral arterial dilatation reduce myocardial oxygen demand. Nitrates are effective in relieving symptoms of ischemia in patients with ACS, and may be particularly useful in patients with concomitant congestive heart failure (CHF) because of the venodilating properties of this class of drugs. In unstable patients intravenous nitroglycerin should be given because it is easily titratable and rapidly reversible. In more stable patients topical or oral nitrates are usually adequate. It is reasonable to use nitroglycerin for the first 24–48 hours in patients with ACS and recurrent ischemia, CHF, or hypertension. Long-term nitrate therapy should only be used in patients with ongoing symptoms of ischemia because there is no evidence that chronic nitrate therapy prevents MI or death.

Calcium channel blockers

Calcium channel blockers have a limited role in the contemporary management of ACS. Unlike β-blockers and ACE inhibitors, the calcium channel blockers have not been shown to reduce mortality. Thus, they should only be used for patients with contraindications or intolerance to β-blockers and ACE inhibitors, or if refractory hypertension or tachycardia is present. In patients with non-ST-segment elevation ACS diltiazem and verapamil may reduce recurrent ischemia and infarction, but these agents are harmful for patients with left ventricular dysfunction or clinical heart failure. Dihydropyridine calcium channel blockers such as nifedipine should not be used in patients with ACS unless a β-blocker is used in combination to prevent reflex tachycardia. Because of safety concerns, short-acting preparations of nifedipine should not be used.

In-hospital management

Risk stratification

Risk stratification in ACS begins at the moment a patient arrives in the emergency room and should continue through hospital discharge and beyond. When the patient is first seen, history, physical examination, electrocardiogram, and serum marker information are rapidly integrated, both to arrive at a diagnosis and to estimate a patient's risk for adverse outcome. Older age, presence of diabetes, three or more risk factors, and a history of prior MI or CHF are all associated with increased risk. In addition, tachycardia or bradycardia, hypotension, and evidence for CHF are markers of increased risk that are easily obtained from a focused examination. The electrocardiogram provides incremental prognostic value. An anterior location of infarction (or an inferior infarction with right ventricular extension or anterior ST depression), and a greater amount of ST deviation are associated with larger MI and increased risk. Finally, elevated serum cardiac markers at presentation and ACS despite aspirin use during the past week are associated with an increased risk for morbidity and mortality.

Patients are initially triaged based on the presence or absence of ST-segment elevation on the presenting electrocardiogram (see Figure 6.6). Subsequent risk stratification steps should focus on identifying patients at risk for electrical, mechanical, and ischemic complications (see Figure 6.6), and on selecting those patients who will benefit most from particular therapies, such as revascularization. It should be remembered that with many therapies absolute risk reduction is highest in those patients at greatest risk; therefore, the higher the risk in an individual patient, the more aggressive the care should be.

Left ventricular function

Left ventricular function is the single most important determinant of long-term survival in patients with coronary artery disease. Because of the importance of left ventricular function to risk assessment, most patients should have an ejection fraction measurement following an acute MI. Because reversible left ventricular dysfunction may follow an ischemic insult (myocardial "stunning"), initial measurements may significantly underestimate true left ventricular function. Therefore, unless clinically indicated because of CHF, suspected valvular heart disease, or pericardial effusion, measurement of ejection fraction can be deferred until approximately 5–7 days after the MI. Although echocardiography, contrast ventriculography, and radionuclide angiography are all reliable methods for assessing left ventricular ejection fraction, echocardiography has the advantage of providing structural information as well.

Coronary angiography and revascularization

Routine adjunctive percutaneous coronary intervention following fibrinolysis has not been shown to improve clinical outcomes.

However, selected patients with ST-segment elevation MI should be managed with an early invasive strategy, including routine catheterization and revascularization if the coronary anatomy is suitable. Urgent catheterization is indicated for patients with cardiogenic shock and those with evidence of failed fibrinolysis (i.e. those without resolution of ST elevation 90–180 min after fibrinolytic therapy). Elective catheterization should be considered for patients at high risk, including those with significant left ventricular dysfunction and those with spontaneous ischemia or ischemia that is inducible on a predischarge exercise test.

Patients with non-ST-segment elevation ACS have lower initial mortality rates than do patients with ST-segment elevation MI, but have higher rates of recurrent ischemia and reinfarction, so that at the end of 1 year outcomes are similar. There has been considerable controversy as to whether an early invasive or early conservative management strategy is preferred for patients with non-ST-segment elevation ACS. Recent studies suggest that in the modern interventional era, with the use of coronary stents, glycoprotein IIb/IIIa inhibitors, low molecular weight heparins, and careful attention to groin hemostasis, an early invasive approach is associated with modestly lower rates of recurrent ischemic events (MI and recurrent ischemia) but not mortality. In addition to preventing morbidity, an early invasive approach may shorten the hospital stay and is not associated with excess overall costs. The advantages of an early invasive approach appear to be limited to patients at intermediate or high risk for ischemic complications, such as those with dynamic electrocardiographic changes and those with elevation in cardiac enzymes.

A more conservative approach utilizing vigorous medical therapy may be appropriate in low risk patients, especially those who have never previously received antianginal medication. After a "cool-off" period with antiplatelet and antithrombotic therapy, treadmill exercise testing with or without adjunctive imaging may help to define patient management further. If the pattern of angina remains unstable or if electrocardiographic changes suggest ongoing ischemia, then coronary angiography is warranted. In addition, significant ischemia on the predischarge exercise test is considered an indication for coronary angiography and revascularization.

Risk factor modification

Because hospitalization for an ACS is such a significant event in the life of a patient, the hospital stay presents a unique opportunity to address lifestyle factors that contribute to the development and

Table 6.3 Risk factor modification following admission for acute coronary syndromes

Risk factor	Goal of therapy	Treatment options
Smoking	Permanent smoking cessation	Behavioral therapy; pharmacotherapy; hypnosis
Obesity	BMI <25 kg/m^2	Diet; exercise; anorexigen drug therapy as last resort
Diabetes	Hemoglobin A$_{1c}$ <7·0%	Insulin; oral sulfonylureas; metformin; insulin sensitizing agents; diet
Hypertension	Blood pressure <130/85 mmHg	Drug therapy; diet; exercise
Hyperlipidemia	LDL <100 mg/dl (<2·6 mmol/l)	Drug therapy with statins or fibrates; low fat, low cholesterol, or Mediterranean diet

BMI, body mass index; LDL, low-density lipoprotein

progression of coronary atherosclerosis (Table 6.3). Smoking cessation and weight loss should be emphasized, and patients can begin cardiac rehabilitation before leaving the hospital. Treatment of diabetes and hypertension should be optimized. Most importantly, lipid lowering therapy should be initiated for virtually all patients with ACS, regardless of low-density lipoprotein level. Although diet (either a low fat, low cholesterol diet, or a Mediterranean diet) should be instituted, the benefit of statin therapy has been unequivocally demonstrated in patients with established coronary artery disease; therefore, statins are the agents of choice for treating hyperlipidemia following ACS (Table 6.4).

Complications of acute myocardial infarction

The mechanical and electrical complications of acute MI are summarized in Tables 6.5 and 6.6, respectively.

Infarct expansion and remodeling

Following a large MI, the infarct area may expand and cause thinning of the necrotic myocardium. Over weeks to months, the left ventricular cavity may enlarge and assume a more globular shape. This process is termed left ventricular remodeling, and frequently leads to clinical congestive heart failure. Angiotensin-converting

Table 6.4 Summary of treatments for patients with acute coronary syndromes

Treatment	ST-segment elevation MI	Non-ST-segment elevation ACS	Comments
Oxygen	+++	+++	
Morphine	++	++	For pain or CHF symptoms
Antiplatelet therapy			
Aspirin	++++	++++	
Clopidogrel	?	+++	Combine with aspirin
Glycoprotein IIb/IIIa inhibitors	++	+++	Most effective in patients undergoing PCI
Antithrombotic therapy			
Unfractionated heparin	+++	+++	Not indicated with SK
Low molecular weight heparins	?	+++	Enoxaparin superior to UFH in high risk patients
Reperfusion therapy			
Fibrinolytic therapy	++++	NO	
Primary PCI	++++	+	
β-Blockers	++++	+++	Avoid with severe asthma or bradycardia
ACE inhibitors	++++	+++	Avoid in severe renal failure
Nitrates	++	++	For ongoing angina or CHF
Calcium channel blockers	+	+	Avoid with CHF or bradycardia
Statins	++++	++++	Indicated for all patients except those with a very low LDL (<125 mg/dl)

Therapies with a greater number of "+" signs are of greater value. CHF, congestive heart failure; LDL, low-density lipoprotein; PCI, percutaneous coronary intervention; SK, streptokinase; UFH, unfractionated heparin

enzyme inhibitors have been shown to prevent adverse ventricular remodeling after MI.

Recurrent ischemia and infarction

Even when fibrinolytic therapy has been successful, reocclusion of the infarct artery may occur in up to 10–15% of patients by hospital

Table 6.5 Mechanical complications of acute myocardial infarction

Complication	Clinical presentation	Risk of death from complication	Therapy
Remodeling	Late CHF	Moderate	ACE inhibitors
Recurrent MI	Chest pain	Moderate	Emergent PCI; repeat fibrinolytic therapy
Cardiogenic shock	CHF; hypotension; confusion; oliguria	Very high	Emergent PCI; IABP; inotropic therapy
Right ventricular MI	Hypotension with clear lungs, elevated JVD; ST elevation in V_4R	Moderate	Early reperfusion; intravenous fluids; inotropic support
Free wall rupture	Tamponade; sudden death	>90%	Emergent surgery
Septal rupture	Acute CHF; new holosystolic murmur	High	Stabilize with inotropic agents/IABP; surgery
Acute mitral regurgitation	Acute CHF; new holosystolic murmur	High	Stabilize with inotropic agents/IABP; surgery
Aneurysm	Arrhythmias; embolic events; CHF	Moderate	Anticoagulation; surgery in rare instances
Pseudoaneurysm	Late rupture	High	Surgery
Pericarditis	Pleuritic/positional pain	Low	Aspirin

CHF, congestive heart failure; JVD, jugular venous distension; PCI, percutaneous coronary intervention; IABP, intra-aortic balloon pump

Table 6.6 Electrical complications of acute myocardial infarction

Complication	Prognosis	Treatment
Ventricular tachycardia/fibrillation		
Within first 24–48 hours	Good	Immediate cardioversion; lidocaine; β-blockers
After 48 hours	Poor	Immediate cardioversion; electrophysiology study/ implantable defibrillator; amiodarone
Sinus bradycardia	Excellent	Atropine for hypotension or symptoms
Second-degree heart block		
Mobitz type I (Wenkebach)	Excellent	Atropine for hypotension or symptoms
Mobitz type II	Guarded	Temporary pacemaker
Complete heart block		
Inferior myocardial infarction	Good	Temporary pacemaker
Anterior myocardial infarction	Poor	Temporary pacemaker followed by permanent pacemaker

discharge and 30% of patients by 3 months; this complication is associated with recurrent infarction in approximately 50% of cases and a twofold to threefold increase in mortality. Reocclusion rates after primary percutaneous transluminal coronary angioplasty are also high, but this complication may be reduced by the use of adjunctive stenting and glycoprotein IIb/IIIa inhibition. Recurrent ischemia, without infarction, is also a frequent complication following MI. Because patients with postinfarction angina are at high risk for recurrent MI, cardiac catheterization should be considered.

Cardiogenic shock

Infarction of 40% or more of the left ventricle is associated with the development of cardiogenic shock. Other, less common causes of cardiogenic shock include septal rupture, free wall rupture, acute mitral regurgitation, and right ventricular infarction. Cardiogenic shock is characterized by tissue hypoperfusion, hypotension, low cardiac output, and elevated intracardiac filling pressures. Even in the modern era the prognosis of cardiogenic shock is dismal, with mortality rates in excess of 70%. Given the poor prognosis of cardiogenic shock, early aggressive care is indicated. Invasive hemodynamic monitoring with a Swan–Ganz catheter can help to confirm the etiology of shock in difficult cases, and to tailor appropriate inotropic and vasodilator therapy. The intra-aortic balloon pump has been used with success in patients with cardiogenic shock following MI; this device is of particular value in patients with mechanical complications such as acute mitral regurgitation or septal rupture. The intra-aortic balloon pump augments cardiac output by creating a low resistance zone for left ventricular outflow, and enhances coronary blood flow by inflating during diastole and increasing coronary perfusion pressure.

Dobutamine is the preferred inotropic agent for patients with cardiogenic shock. This intravenous inotropic agent has activity at both the β_1- and β_2-adrenergic receptors, and causes increased cardiac contractility, increased heart rate, and (at high doses) peripheral vasoconstriction. Intravenous vasodilators such as nitroprusside and nitroglycerin may also be used to reduce systemic vascular resistance and increase cardiac output, provided the patient has sufficient blood pressure to tolerate these agents.

Unfortunately, although the treatments described above for cardiogenic shock may help to stabilize the patient, they have not been shown to improve survival. Early revascularization, on the other hand, does appear to improve survival in selected patients. Emergent percutaneous coronary intervention is clearly superior to thrombolytic therapy for patients with cardiogenic shock: thus, in centers appropriately equipped, emergent catheterization and revascularization are the treatments of choice. In other centers, consideration should be given to placement of an intra-aortic balloon pump and transfer to a center that can perform urgent percutaneous coronary intervention.

Right ventricular myocardial infarction

Right ventricular infarction is a frequent complication of inferior wall MI, and is almost always caused by proximal occlusion of the right coronary artery. The diagnosis should be suspected in patients with inferior wall MI and unsuspected hypotension, particularly when it occurs after small doses of nitrates. Patients usually will have jugular venous distension, but the lungs will be clear unless significant left ventricular infarction is present as well. A right sided electrocardiogram should be performed in all patients with inferior wall MI; ST-segment elevation of 0·1 mV or more in V_4R is sensitive and specific for the diagnosis of right ventricular infarction (Figure 6.7). The hemodynamic profile of right ventricular infarction includes elevated right sided filling pressures with reduced cardiac output, findings similar to those of pericardial tamponade. In patients without electrocardiographic evidence of right ventricular infarction, therefore, echocardiography (or placement of a pulmonary artery catheter) is indicated to distinguish between these two diagnoses.

The hemodynamic derangements of right ventricular infarction can be improved by administration of intravenous fluids such as normal saline; many liters of fluid may be required to achieve hemodynamic stability. Short-term morbidity and mortality are increased in patients with right ventricular MI as compared with those with inferior wall MI alone, but in patients who stabilize the prognosis for full recovery of right ventricular function is good.

Free wall rupture

Rupture of the left ventricular free wall is the most catastrophic mechanical complication of acute MI, with mortality rates greater than 90%. Patients present with pericardial tamponade and cardiogenic shock, and the terminal rhythm is usually pulseless electrical activity. Incomplete free wall rupture can lead to formation of a pseudoaneurysm. In this situation, the rupture site is sealed by hematoma and the pericardium itself, and when the thrombus organizes a pseudoaneurysm cavity is formed. In contrast to a true aneurysm, in which the wall is composed of myocardial tissue, the

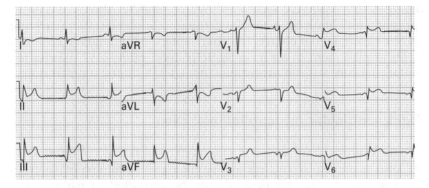

Figure 6.7 Right ventricular infarction. ST-segment elevation is present in the inferior leads (II, III, and aVF), indicating inferior myocardial infarction. Right sided precordial leads demonstrate ST-segment elevation in lead V₄R, which is indicative of right ventricular involvement

wall of the pseudoaneurysm is composed of thrombus and pericardium but no myocardial tissue.

Septal rupture

Rupture of the interventricular septum causes an acute ventricular septal defect, with left to right flow across the defect (Figure 6.8).[19] Congestive heart failure usually develops over hours to days (depending on the size of the defect), associated with a harsh holosystolic murmur that may resemble the murmur of acute mitral regurgitation. Either Doppler echocardiography or insertion of a pulmonary artery catheter can be used to confirm the diagnosis. If a significant increase ("step-up") in the oxygen saturation is seen between the right atrium and the right ventricle, then the presence of ventricular septal defect is likely.

Acute mitral regurgitation

Acute mitral regurgitation following acute MI is caused by ischemic dysfunction or frank rupture of a papillary muscle. This complication is more common following inferior MI because the posteromedial papillary muscle typically has a single blood supply from the right coronary artery, whereas the anterolateral papillary muscle has dual supply from the left anterior descending and circumflex arteries. As opposed to cardiac rupture, this complication can occur with

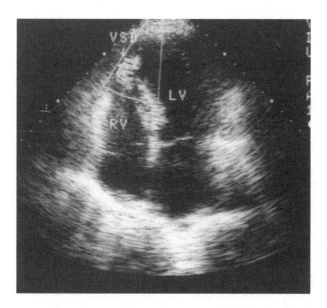

Figure 6.8 Ventricular septal rupture complicating acute myocardial infarction. Four chamber echocardiographic view demonstrating color flow traversing across the ventricular septal defect (VSD) from the left ventricle (LV) to the right ventricle (RV). From Armstrong and Feigenbaum[19]

relatively small, but well localized, infarctions. The presentation is similar to septal rupture, with a new holosystolic murmur classically present in the setting of acute pulmonary edema and cardiogenic shock. As blood pressure falls, the murmur may disappear entirely. Doppler echocardiography is particularly helpful in distinguishing between acute mitral regurgitation and septal rupture.

Ventricular tachycardia and ventricular fibrillation

Ventricular tachycardia is common in patients during the first hours and days after MI, and does not appear to increase the risk for mortality if the arrhythmia is rapidly terminated. Ventricular tachycardia occurring after 24–48 hours, however, is associated with a marked increase in mortality. Monomorphic ventricular tachycardia is usually due to a re-entrant focus around a scar, whereas polymorphic ventricular tachycardia is more commonly a function of underlying ischemia, electrolyte abnormalities, or drug effects.

Ventricular fibrillation is felt to be the primary mechanism of arrhythmic sudden death. In patients with acute MI, the vast majority of episodes of ventricular fibrillation occur early (<4–12 hours) after infarction. Similar to sustained ventricular tachycardia, late ventricular fibrillation occurs more frequently in patients with severe left ventricular dysfunction or congestive heart failure, and is associated with a poor prognosis. Patients with ventricular fibrillation, or sustained ventricular tachycardia associated with symptoms or hemodynamic compromise should be cardioverted emergently. Underlying metabolic and electrolyte abnormalities must be corrected, and ongoing ischemia should be treated. Lidocaine remains effective for the treatment of symptomatic ventricular tachycardia or ventricular fibrillation, but should rarely be used as a prophylactic measure. Intravenous amiodarone may be a particularly effective antiarrhythmic agent in the setting of acute MI because it also has antianginal properties.

Bradyarrhythmias

Bradyarrhythmias are common following acute MI, and may be due either to increased vagal tone or to ischemia/infarction of conduction tissue. Sinus bradycardia and Mobitz type I (Wenkebach) second-degree atrioventricular block are usually the result of stimulation of cardiac vagal receptors on the inferoposterior surface of the left ventricle. As a result, these generally benign rhythms are seen most often with inferior MI. If severe bradycardia is seen (heart rate <40–50 beats/min) or if bradycardia leads to hypotension, then intravenous atropine should be given. Temporary pacing is rarely required unless there is hemodynamic or electrical instability. In contrast to Mobitz type I block, Mobitz type II block is seen less frequently but can progress suddenly to complete heart block; therefore, a temporary pacemaker should be inserted.

Compete heart block following MI is an indication for a temporary pacemaker. The long-term implications of complete heart block depend on the infarct location. With inferior MI the effect is usually transient, and so a permanent pacemaker is rarely required. With anterior MI complete heart block is usually due to extensive infarction that involves the bundle branches, and as a result the atrioventricular block is usually permanent. Mortality is extremely high, and permanent pacing should be performed unless there are contraindications.

Left ventricular aneurysm

A true left ventricular aneurysm is a discrete "out pouching" of a thinned, dyskinetic, myocardial segment. As opposed to a

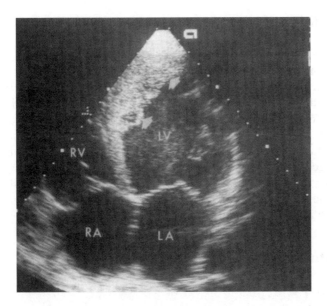

Figure 6.9 Mural thrombus complicating acute anterior myocardial infarction. Four chamber echocardiographic view showing the mural thrombus delineated by arrows. LA, left atrium; LV, left ventricle; RA, right atrium; RV, right ventricle. From Armstrong and Feigenbaum[19]

pseudoaneurysm, the wall of a true aneurysm contains cardiac and fibrous tissues, the neck is broad based, and the risk for rupture is small. Although rupture is rare, aneurysms are still associated with increased morbidity and mortality. The dyskinetic aneurysm segment is frequently lined with thrombus and may be a source for arterial embolus; in addition, the scarred aneurysm tissue may be a source for malignant ventricular arrhythmias. Long-term oral anticoagulation is often indicated to prevent mural thrombus and systemic embolization, but surgery is only indicated for intractable congestive heart failure or arrhythmias.

Left ventricular mural thrombus

Left ventricular mural thrombus occurs in approximately 40% of patients with Q-wave anterior MI. Although echocardiography can detect mural thrombus in many cases (Figure 6.9),[19] patients with large anterior MI remain at risk for systemic embolization even if no thrombus is seen. Intravenous heparin, followed by coumadin for 3–6 months, is indicated to prevent embolic complications in patients with large anterior MI who are candidates for long-term anticoagulation.

Pericarditis

Fibrinous pericarditis may occur in the first few weeks following transmural infarction, and is often confused with recurrent angina or infarction. The pain of pericarditis is usually pleuritic, positional, and often radiates to the shoulder. A pericardial friction rub may be present. Aspirin should be given, but non-steroidal anti-inflammatory agents should be avoided because they may prevent normal healing of the infarct. Patients with Dressler's syndrome have pericardial pain, generalized malaise, fever, elevated white blood cell count, elevated erythrocyte sedimentation rate, and pericardial effusion. This syndrome occurs several weeks to several months following MI and is felt to be immunologically mediated.

Case studies

Case 6.1

A 75-year-old man presents to the hospital complaining of 2 hours of severe substernal chest discomfort, radiating to the jaw. The pain began while the patient was lying in bed, and has been unrelieved by three sublingual nitroglycerin tablets. He feels nauseous and lightheaded, but is not dyspneic.

Examination. Physical examination: the patient appeared diaphoretic lying flat in bed. No abnormalities of skin, nail beds, or oral mucosa. Pulse: 36 beats/min. Blood pressure: 88/50 mmHg in right arm. Jugular venous pulse: 12 cm. Cardiac impulse: normal. First heart sound: normal. Second heart sound: split normally on inspiration. No added sounds or murmurs. Chest examination: normal air entry, no rales or rhonchi. Abdominal examination: Soft abdomen, no tenderness, and no masses. Normal liver span. No peripheral edema. Femoral, popliteal, posterior tibial, and dorsalis pedis pulses: all normal volume and equal. Extremities: all cool. Carotid pulses: normal, no bruits. Optic fundi: normal.

Investigations. His electrocardiogram is shown in Figure 6.10.

Questions

1. Which of the following statements is not correct regarding the patient's current condition? (A) The initiating event was rupture of an atherosclerotic plaque. (B) The patient is suffering an acute inferoposterior ST-segment elevation MI. (C) The patient probably has a subtotal occlusion of his right coronary or circumflex coronary artery. (D) The patient is at high risk because of his

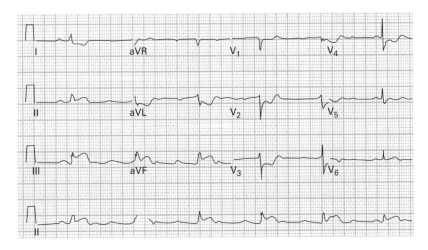

Figure 6.10 Electrocardiogram for Case 6.1. (See text for details)

advanced age, prior coronary disease, and low blood pressure. (E) Activated platelets play a critical role in the pathophysiology of this disorder.

2. Which of the following therapies would not be appropriate for this patient? (A) Immediate reperfusion therapy with primary percutaneous coronary intervention or fibrinolytic therapy. (B) Aspirin. (C) Intravenous unfractionated heparin. (D) Intravenous β-blocker. (E) Temporary ventricular pacing.

3. Which of the following diagnostic tests should not be performed routinely in this patient? (A) Serial measurement of cardiac enzymes. (B) A right sided electrocardiogram to assess for the possibility of right ventricular infarction. (C) Coronary angiography following fibrinolytic therapy. (D) Echocardiography. (E) Measurement of fasting lipids.

4. Following placement of a transcutaneous pacemaker, the patient is administered fibrinolytic therapy and becomes free of chest pain 60 min later, with a stable heart rate and blood pressure. Six hours later, the patient develops severe dyspnea. Physical examination at that time reveals wet rales three-quarters of the way up both lung fields, and a new holosystolic murmur at the left lower sternal border. Which of the following complications are most likely? (A) Ventricular free wall rupture with pericardial tamponade. (B) Ventricular pseudoaneurysm. (C) Rupture of the interventricular septum with creation of an acute ventricular septal defect. (D) Acute mitral regurgitation due to papillary muscle ischemia or infarction. (E) Either C or D.

5. Which of the following tests or procedures is indicated to diagnose and treat this patient? (A) Doppler echocardiography. (B) Placement of a pulmonary artery catheter to measure oxygen saturations in the right atrium and right ventricle. (C) Placement of an intra-aortic balloon pump. (D) Urgent surgery. (E) All of the above.

Answers

Answer to question 1 C. ST-segment elevation MI is caused by complete thrombotic occlusion of an epicardial coronary artery, whereas subtotal occlusion typically leads to non-ST-segment elevation ACS. For this reason, fibrinolytic therapy is beneficial in patients with ST-segment elevation MI but not in those with non-ST-segment elevation ACS.

Answer to question 2 D. The rhythm demonstrated on the electrocardiogram is complete heart block. In the setting of inferior MI, this is likely to be due to reflex increase in vagal tone or ischemia to the atrioventrciular node. Temporary pacing is indicated but the patient is unlikely to require placement of a permanent pacemaker. With anterior MI, the prognosis of complete heart block is much more ominous. β-Blockers are contraindicated because they further block atrioventricular nodal function.

Answer to question 3 C. Serial cardiac enzymes should be measured to confirm the diagnosis of myocardial infarction, to assess infarct size, and to monitor the success of reperfusion therapy. A right sided electrocardiogram is indicated for all patients with inferior MI to assess for right ventricular involvement. This patient has clear lungs and elevated jugular venous pressure, which are suggestive of right ventricular infarct. Routine assessment of left ventricular function should be performed after MI, but in stable patients this measurement can wait for around 5–7 days to minimize the effects of "stunning" on the measurement of left ventricular function. Measurement of fasting lipids should be performed to identify which patients should be treated with statins. Following successful fibrinolysis, routine coronary angiography is not indicated unless patients have significant left ventricular dysfunction, recurrent ischemia, or a positive predischarge exercise test.

Answer to question 4 E. The clinical presentation of acute congestive heart failure and a new holosystolic murmur suggests either acute mitral regurgitation or a ventricular septal defect. Ventricular free wall rupture typically presents with sudden collapse, and a ventricular pseudoaneurysm is usually noticed incidentally during cardiac imaging procedures.

Answer to question 5 E – all of the above. Doppler echocardiography is the simplest technique to distinguish between acute mitral regurgitation and ventricular septal defect (see Figure 6.8). In addition, a significant increase in the oxygen saturation between the right atrium and right ventricle suggests that oxygenated blood is moving from the left ventricle to the right ventricle across a ventricular septal defect. Placement of an intra-aortic balloon pump may be a lifesaving measure to stabilize patients with these complications while a surgical team is mobilized.

Case 6.2

A 71-year-old woman has had intermittent chest discomfort for 3 days. While watching her grandson's graduation she develops severe resting chest pain that lasts for several hours, and she is now short of breath. Her past history is significant for hypertension and non-insulin-dependent diabetes, and she has smoked cigarettes for many years.

Examination. Physical examination: the patient appeared to be suffering significant pain. Pulse: 114 beats/min, regular. Blood pressure: 170/95 mmHg in right arm. Respiratory rate: 28/min. Jugular venous pulse: 8 cm. Cardiac impulse: normal. First heart sound: normal. Second heart sound: split normally on inspiration. Third heart sound present. Chest examination: rales one-quarter of the way up the lung fields. Abdominal examination: soft abdomen, no tenderness, and no masses. Normal liver span. No peripheral edema. Femoral, popliteal, posterior tibial, and dorsalis pedis pulses: all normal volume and equal. Carotid pulses: normal, no bruits. Optic fundi: normal.

Investigations. Her admission electrocardiogram demonstrates 1·5 mm ST depressions in leads V_2–V_6.

Questions

1. Which of the following therapies is not indicated at this time? (A) Intravenous β-blockers. (B) Oral diltiazem. (C) Intravenous morphine. (D) A chewed aspirin. (E) Low molecular weight heparin.
2. Following the initiation of aspirin, low molecular weight heparin, β-blockers, and nitroglycerin, the patient becomes pain-free and the ST depressions resolve. Cardiac enzymes are sent from a sample of blood collected 8 hours after the onset of chest pain.

Which of the following statements are true? (A) An elevated creatinine kinase (CK)-MB or troponin T would suggest a diagnosis of non-ST-segment elevation myocardial infarction. (B) If the enzymes are elevated then no further testing for cardiac markers should be performed. (C) There is no need to check cardiac enzymes because the diagnosis of ACS is already known from the history and electrocardiography. (D) At this time point, 8 hours after the onset of symptoms, one would expect myoglobin but not CK-MB or troponin to be elevated. (E) If the troponin is elevated but CK-MB is normal, then this suggests that the troponin elevation is a "false positive".

3. The CK-MB is elevated to three times the upper limit of normal, and cardiac troponin I is elevated to 10 times the upper limit of normal. The patient has three further episodes of chest pain on medical therapy. Which of the following statements about an early invasive (cardiac catheterization and revascularization) versus early conservative (medical therapy with catheterization reserved for treatment failures) strategy is true for this patient? (A) Because of the patient's advanced age and female sex, an early conservative strategy is preferable. (B) An early invasive strategy is indicated for all patients with suspected ACS. (C) The patient is at high risk for adverse events because of her advanced age, ST changes, elevated cardiac markers, the presence of congestive heart failure, and recurrent ischemic symptoms, and an early invasive strategy is likely to be beneficial. (D) The patient should be treated with a glycoprotein IIb/IIIa inhibitor and, if she has no further episodes of chest pain, discharged home. (E) Statin therapy is not indicated if she is managed with an invasive approach.

Answers

Answer to question 1   B. Aspirin, β-blockers, and heparin (either unfractionated heparin or low molecular weight heparin) are indicated as initial therapy for this patient with non-ST-segment elevation ACS. Morphine would be expected to be particularly effective in relieving both chest pain and dyspnea. Diltiazem is contraindicated in the presence of congestive heart failure.

Answer to question 2   A. Elevated cardiac biomarkers in the setting of typical anginal pain and dynamic ST changes are diagnostic of non-ST-segment elevation MI. However, it is still important to perform serial measurements to confirm a typical rise and fall in the cardiac marker curve so that accurate timing of the infarct can be performed. This is particularly important in patients who have stuttering chest pain over several days, such as the one discussed here. Although the diagnosis of ACS is established, the presence and degree of cardiac biomarker elevation is important for prognostic purposes and to help select between therapies. At 8 hours, one would expect all of the markers (myoglobin, CK-MB, and troponins T and I) to be elevated (see Figure 6.5). Finally, low level troponin elevations in the absence of CK-MB elevation are indicative of microinfarction and are associated with an increased risk for adverse events.

Answer to question 3 C. Although controversy exists as to the superiority of an early invasive or early conservative approach in non-ST-segment elevation ACS, for patients at high risk an early invasive approach is generally preferred. Elderly women frequently receive less intensive care, despite the fact that they may be at particularly high risk. Glycoprotein IIb/IIIa inhibitors are most beneficial when combined with an early invasive approach. Finally, statin therapy is clearly indicated for patients following revascularization. Figure 6.3 shows an angiogram that is representative of non-ST-segment elevation ACS.

References

1 Cannon CP. Optimizing the treatment of unstable angina. *J Thromb Thrombolysis* 1995;2:205–18.
2 Libby P. Molecular bases of the acute coronary syndromes. *Circulation* 1995;91: 2844–50.
3 de Lemos JA, Cannon CP Stone PH. Acute myocardial infarction. In: Rosendorff C, ed. *Essential cardiology*. Philadelphia: WB Saunders, 2001:463–501.
4 Davies MJ. The pathophysiology of acute coronary syndromes. *Heart* 2000;83: 361–6.
5 Antman EM, Braunwald E. Acute myocardial infarction. In: Braunwald E, Libby P, Zipes D, eds. *Heart disease. A textbook of cardiovascular medicine, 6th ed*. Philadelphia: W.B. Saunders Company, 2001:1114–218.
6 Antman EM. General hospital management. In: Julian DG, Braunwald E, eds. *Management of acute myocardial infarction*. London: W.B. Saunders Ltd., 1994:29–70.
7 Antman EM, Tanasijevic MJ, Thompson B, *et al*. Cardiac-specific troponin I levels to predict the risk of mortality in patients with acute coronary syndromes. *N Engl J Med* 1996;335:1342–9.
8 Wu A. *Cardiac markers*. Totowa: Humana Press Inc., 1998.
9 Fibrinolytic Therapy Trialists' (FTT) Collaborative Group. Indications for fibrinolytic therapy in suspected acute myocardial infarction: collaborative overview of early mortality and major morbidity results from all randomised trials of more than 1000 patients. *Lancet* 1994;343:311–22.
10 The TIMI-IIIB Investigators. Effects of tissue plasminogen activator and a comparison of early invasive and conservative strategies in unstable angina and non-Q-wave myocardial infarction. Results of the TIMI IIIB trial. *Circulation* 1994;89:1545–56.
11 Antiplatelet Trialist' Collaboration. Collaborative overview of randomised trials of antiplatelet therapy – I: prevention of death myocardial infarction and stroke by prolongued antiplatelet therapy in various categories of patients. *BMJ* 1994; 308:81–106.
12 Oler A, Whooley MA, Oler J, Grady D. Adding heparin to aspirin reduces the incidence of myocardial infarction and death in patients with unstable angina. A meta-analysis. *JAMA* 1996;276:811–15.

13 CAPRIE Steering Committee. A randomised, blinded, trial of clopidogrel versus aspirin in patients at risk of ischaemic events (CAPRIE). *Lancet* 1996;**348**:1329–39.
14 The PRISM-PLUS Trial Investigators. Inhibition of the platelet glycoprotein IIb/IIIa receptor with tirofiban in unstable angina and non-Q-wave myocardial infarction. *N Engl J Med* 1998;**338**:1488–97.
15 The Pursuit Trial Investigators. Inhibition of platelet glycoprotein IIb/IIIa with eptifibatide in patients with acute coronary syndromes. *N Engl J Med* 1998;**339**: 436–43.
16 Antman EM, Cohen M, Radley D, *et al*. Assessment of the treatment effect of enoxaparin for unstable angina/non-Q-wave myocardial infarction. TIMI 11B-ESSENCE meta-analysis. *Circulation* 1999;**100**:1602–8.
17 ACE Inhibitor Myocardial Infarction Collaborative Group. Indications for ACE inhibitors in the early treatment of acute myocardial infarction: systematic overview of individual data from 100,000 patients in randomized trials. *Circulation* 1998;**97**:2202–12.
18 Yusuf S, Sleight P, Pogue J, Bosch J, Davies R, Dagenais G. Effects of an angiotensin-converting-enzyme inhibitor, ramipril, on cardiovascular events in high-risk patients. The Heart Outcomes Prevention Evaluation Study Investigators. *N Engl J Med* 2000;**342**:145–53.
19 Armstrong WF, Feigenbaum H. Echocardiography. In: Braunwald E, Libby P, Zipes D, eds. *Heart disease: a textbook of cardiovascular medicine, 6th ed*. Philadelphia: W.B. Saunders Company, 2001:160–236.

7: Chronic ischemic heart disease

RAO H NASEEM, MICHAEL L MAIN,
JOHN D RUTHERFORD

During myocardial ischemia an imbalance occurs between myocardial oxygen supply and demand. Because the heart is an aerobic organ and relies almost exclusively on oxidation of substrates for the generation of energy, it can develop only a small oxygen debt. The oxygen supply to the myocardial cells falls, with anaerobic glycolysis and lactate production. The common clinical symptom associated with anaerobic metabolism is an uncomfortable sensation in the chest, usually brought on by effort, called angina pectoris.

Myocardial oxygen supply

Supply of oxygen to the myocardium depends on the oxygen carrying capacity of the blood and the rate of coronary blood flow. Oxygen carrying capacity of the blood is determined by the hemoglobin content and systemic oxygenation, and in the absence of anemia or lung disease it remains fairly constant.

Coronary artery blood flow is determined by the perfusion pressure into the artery and the resistance to flow by the vessel. Coronary blood flow (CBF) is directly proportional to the perfusion pressure (P) and is inversely proportional to coronary vascular resistance (R; CBF = P/R). The systolic flow of blood in the coronary arteries is reduced by compression of the contracting myocardium. Therefore, the coronary arteries have maximal flow during diastole, and the perfusion pressure is approximately the aortic diastolic pressure.

In the coronary circulation the major resistance to flow comes from the resistance arterioles, in accordance with Poiseuille's law, which states that resistance increases by a power of four as the vessel radius decreases. The large conductance arteries (epicardial arteries) govern the quantity of blood arriving at the resistance vessels. Coronary vascular resistance is modified by extravascular compressive forces, autoregulation, metabolic regulation, neural and neurotransmitter control, as well as humoral endothelial factors.

Myocardial oxygen demand

The three major determinants of myocardial oxygen consumption or demand are:

- ventricular wall (myocardial) tension, or wall stress
- heart rate
- contractility (the inotropic state, or force of myocardial contraction).

Myocardial wall tension is the tangential force acting on ventricular fibers, tending to pull them apart, which necessitates an opposing expenditure of energy. Wall tension is approximated by the formula of Laplace, which states that in a case of an idealized thin wall spherical shell:

$$\text{Wall stress} = (P \times r)/2h$$

where P is the transmural pressure, r is radius of the sphere, and h is the wall thickness. Increased left ventricular filling (for example volume overload states such as mitral or aortic regurgitation) increases the ventricular radius, raises the wall tension, and thus oxygen consumption. Conversely, any physiologic or pharmacologic maneuver that decreases left ventricular filling and size (for example blood loss, nitrate therapy) decreases wall tension and myocardial oxygen consumption. Circumstances that increase pressure in the left ventricle (aortic stenosis, hypertension) increase wall tension, and conditions that decrease ventricular pressure reduce it (vasodilator therapy). Finally, wall tension is inversely proportional to ventricular wall thickness. In a hypertrophied heart the force is spread throughout a greater mass that has a lower wall tension, and oxygen consumption per gram of tissue is less than in a heart with thin walls. Therefore, when ventricular hypertrophy develops (for example chronic pressure overload of aortic stenosis), it can serve a compensatory role in reducing oxygen consumption.

Heart rate is a very important determinant of myocardial oxygen demand. As heart rate increases, the number of cardiac contractions and the amount of adenosine triphosphate (ATP) consumed per min increases, and oxygen requirements rise. Conversely, slowing heart rate (for example, with β-blocker therapy) reduces ATP utilization and oxygen consumption. Following an inotropic stimulus, the change in myocardial oxygen consumption depends on the extent to which wall tension is reduced (as a consequence of reduction in heart size) and the degree of augmentation of contractility.

In the absence of heart failure drugs that stimulate myocardial contractility will elevate myocardial oxygen consumption because heart size, and therefore wall tension, are not reduced substantially and do not offset the influence of increased contractility. Negative inotropic agents such as β-blockers may decrease myocardial oxygen consumption.

Angina

History

Heberden's initial description of angina being accompanied by "a sense of strangling and anxiety" is still relevant, although other adjectives are frequently used to describe this distress, including "vice-like", "suffocating", "crushing", "heavy", and "squeezing". The patient may not interpret these symptoms as pain. The site of the discomfort is usually retrosternal, but radiation of the discomfort often occurs and is usually projected to the left shoulder, neck, jaw, and ulnar distribution of the left arm. Radiation to the same areas on the right side and to the epigastric area also occurs. Less commonly, pain is referred to the left scapular region of the back.

Typically angina pectoris begins gradually, and reaches a maximum intensity over a period of minutes before dissipating. It is usually provoked by activity and is relieved within minutes by rest or use of nitroglycerin. Patients with angina prefer to pause, rest, sit, or stop walking during episodes. Angina may be precipitated by less activity following a large meal or by cold weather. Severity of angina is assessed by the circumstances associated with its occurrence (Table 7.1).[1]

Characteristics that are not suggestive of angina are fleeting, momentary chest pains described as "needle jabs" or "sharp pains"; discomfort that is aggravated or precipitated by breathing, or by a single movement of the trunk or arm; or a pain that is localized to a very small area, or that is reproduced by pressure on the chest wall.

A careful history should uncover risk factors that predispose to coronary artery disease. In general, angina pectoris will tend to occur in males who are older than 40 years and females older than 50 years, a history of cigarette smoking is common, and the presence of diabetes mellitus, hypertension, hypercholesterolemia, or peripheral arterial disease is highly relevant (Table 7.2).[2] Similarly, a prior history of myocardial infarction, or a family history of myocardial infarction or sudden death in a male parent or sibling before 55 years, or a female parent or sibling before 65 years is very important.

Table 7.1 Severity of angina (Canadian Cardiovascular Society)

Angina class	Features
I	Angina does not occur with ordinary physical activity. Angina occurs only with strenuous or prolonged exertion
II	Slight limitation in ordinary activity. Angina occurs with rapid walking on level ground or up inclines or steps
III	Marked limitation of ordinary physical activity. Angina occurs when walking
IV	Inability to carry out even mild physical activity without angina, which also may occur briefly at rest

From Campeau[1]

Table 7.2 Pretest likelihood of coronary artery disease according to age, sex, and symptoms

Age (years)	No symptoms (%)		Non-anginal pain (%)		Typical angina (%)	
	M	F	M	F	M	F
35–45	4	1	11	3	81	45
45–55	8	2	21	7	91	68
55–65	11	5	28	13	94	84
65–75	11	11	28	17	94	95

F, female; M, male. From Diamond[2]

Physical examination

Inspection

Inspection of the eyes may reveal a corneal arcus (the size of a corneal arcus appears to correlate positively with age and levels of cholesterol and low-density lipoproteins), and examination of the skin may show xanthomas (cholesterol-filled nodules), which are found either subcutaneously or over tendons in patients with hyperlipoproteinemia. Eruptive xanthomas are tiny yellowish nodules that are 1–2 mm in diameter on an erythematous base, which may occur anywhere on the body and are found in association with hyperchylomicronemia and therefore in patients with type 1 hyperlipoproteinemia (familial hyperchylomicronemia) and type 5 hyperlipoproteinemia (severe elevation in triglyceride levels associated with obesity, a fat-rich diet, and poorly controlled diabetes). Patients with xanthoma tendinosum (i.e. nodular swelling of the tendons, especially of the elbows, extensor surfaces to the hands, and Achilles' tendons) usually have type 2 hyperlipoproteinemia (genetic disorder of low-density lipoproteins).

Blood pressure

Blood pressure may be chronically elevated or may rise acutely (along with heart rate) during an angina attack. Changes in blood pressure may precede (and precipitate) or follow (and be caused by) angina.

Pulses

Patients with arterial disease may exhibit abnormalities of the arterial pulses (diminished or absent radial, brachial, carotid, femoral, popliteal, dorsalis, or posterior tibial pulses), bruits of the carotids or abdomen, or a palpable abdominal aortic aneurysm.

Venous insufficiency

The presence of venous insufficiency, particularly of the legs, evidence of prior stripping, or ligation of varicose veins is important to record because this may limit the choice of conduits for coronary revascularization.

Cardiac palpation

Abnormalities of cardiac palpation such as left ventricular heave or lift, which are characterized by sustained outward movement of an area that is larger than the normal apex, might suggest ventricular hypertrophy, whereas displacement of the cardiac apex laterally and downward might suggest left ventricular enlargement.

Auscultation

A fourth heart sound (generated when augmented atrial contraction generates presystolic ventricular distension) can be seen with left ventricular hypertrophy of aortic stenosis or systemic hypertension. A fourth heart sound can also be associated with myocardial ischemia (during angina or acute myocardial infarction) because the atrial "booster pump" is needed to help fill the relatively stiff, ischemic ventricle. Evidence of cardiac failure may be found with elevation in jugular venous pressure, a chest examination revealing rales, an enlarged or congested liver, and the presence of peripheral edema.

Electrocardiogram

The resting electrocardiogram is normal in approximately half of patients with chronic angina pectoris. The most common abnormalities are non-specific ST-T changes with, or without, evidence of prior transmural myocardial infarction manifested by pathologic Q waves. Conduction disturbances such as left bundle branch block, or left anterior fascicular block, can be seen in patients with chronic stable angina and may suggest impairment in left ventricular function reflecting multivessel disease and prior myocardial damage. Left ventricular hypertrophy on the electrocardiogram in patients with chronic stable angina usually suggests the presence of underlying hypertension.

Diagnosis of coronary artery disease

History

The diagnosis of angina pectoris is made by taking an accurate history. Exercise electrocardiography is of limited value in predicting the presence or absence of coronary artery disease after other easily obtainable clinical data have been taken into account. These include age, history of myocardial infarction, history of cigarette smoking, elevated cholesterol, and the presence (or absence) of electrocardiographic Q waves indicating prior infarction. However, the recording of an electrocardiogram during and after exercise – especially if angina is precipitated – is valuable in assessing the severity and prognosis of coronary artery disease. Adding an imaging modality to the stress electrocardiogram adds to the predictive value of the test.

Bayes' theorem

Bayes' theorem describes a method of calculating probabilities, and in clinical cardiology the method is used routinely during stress testing analyses.[3] The pretest likelihood of coronary artery disease in an individual being tested, and the sensitivity and specificity of the less than perfect stress test being used are incorporated into a post-test probability of coronary artery disease being present. Therefore, non-invasive procedures that are used to try to detect coronary artery disease yield probability estimates of the presence of disease rather than a categorical "yes or no" answer.

Issues to consider regarding stress testing are as follows.

- There is a large discrepancy in the predictive value of stress tests in symptomatic versus asymptomatic subjects. In an asymptomatic 50-year-old male a "positive" electrocardiographic exercise stress test result consisting of 1 mm ST-segment depression has a very low probability of being associated with coronary artery disease. However, a "positive" result consisting of symptoms typical of angina and ST-segment depression of 2 mm or greater has a very high probability of reflecting coronary artery disease.
- Bayes' theorem indicates that, although the reliability of a less than perfect test is defined by sensitivity and specificity, a test cannot be adequately interpreted without reference to the prevalence of disease in the population under study (pretest likelihood of disease). Details of the history, including the environment or country of origin, age, history of myocardial infarction, history of cigarette smoking, elevated cholesterol, and the presence (or absence) of electrocardiographic Q waves indicating prior infarction, all help to define the pretest probability of disease.
- In a given population, a finite proportion of normal persons, defined by test specificity, will manifest an abnormal (false positive) response. Therefore, the predictive value of a positive test is diminished in part by the proportion of normal subjects in the population being studied (Table 7.3).[3]
- The pretest likelihood of coronary artery disease changes dramatically according to age, sex, and symptoms (see Table 7.2).
- A negative test has a low predictive value in a population with high prevalence of disease, whereas it has a high predictive value in a population with low prevalence of disease.
- Changes that develop during a stress test do not provide a "yes or no" statement regarding the presence of coronary artery disease, but rather provide a probability based on a continuum of risk.

Stress testing

Exercise electrocardiogram

In a patient with a chest pain syndrome the monitoring of symptoms and recording of electrocardiograms during and after exercise is useful for assessing the probability of the presence significant of coronary artery disease. The presence of a critical obstruction in one or more coronary arteries is suggested by certain

Table 7.3 Relation of predictive value to the prevalence of disease in a population

	Total	Positive test	Negative test
Disease prevalence 85%			
With disease	850	739	111
Without disease	150	54	96
Total	1000	793	207
Predictive value		739/793 = 93% (predictive value of positive test)	96/207 = 46% (predictive value of negative test)
Disease prevalence 2%			
With disease	20	17	3
Without disease	980	353	627
Total	1000	370	630
Predictive value		17/370 = 5% (predictive value of positive test)	627/630 = 99% (predictive value of negative test)

Assumptions of this particular calculation are as follows. The disease prevalence is assumed to be 85% (Florida retirement community) and 2% (recruits in a military base nearby) in two different populations. The test to be performed is single-photon emission computed tomography during exercise, and the literature reports that the test has an 87% sensitivity and a 64% specificity. Definitions: the "predictive value" of a positive test is the probability that a patient has disease given a positive test outcome (i.e. number of patients with disease/total number of patients with a positive test); the "sensitivity" of a test is the probability that a patient with disease will have a "positive" test (i.e. number of patients with disease with a "positive" test/total number of patients with disease tested); and the "specificity" of a test is the probability that a patient without disease will have a "negative" test (i.e. the number of patients without disease with a "negative" test/total number of patients with disease tested). Adapted from Epstein[3]

symptomatic and electrocardiographic responses during exercise testing.

The presence of typical anginal chest pain alone, in the absence of ST-segment electrocardiographic changes, has a high predictive value for the detection of coronary artery disease. If typical anginal chest discomfort occurs during the test associated with 1 mm or more ST-segment depression (of horizontal or downsloping nature), then the predictive value for the detection of coronary artery disease is 90%. If greater than 2 mm ST-segment depressions coexist with typical angina, then this is virtually diagnostic of significant coronary artery disease.

An exercise test associated with a drop in systolic blood pressure during exercise below the pre-exercise value (in the absence of known major ventricular dysfunction) has an 80% predictive value for the detection of significant coronary artery disease.

Table 7.4 Metabolic equivalents for exercise

METs	Description
1	Resting
2	Level walking 2 mph
4	Level walking 4 mph
<5	Poor prognosis; usual limit immediately after a myocardial infaction, peak cost of basic activities of daily living
10	Prognosis with medical therapy as good as revascularization therapy
13	Excellent prognosis regardless of other exercise responses
18	Elite endurance athletes

A metabolic equivalent (MET) is a unit of sitting resting oxygen uptake, or 3·5 ml/kg per min oxygen uptake. From Fletcher et al.[4]

Exercise test predictors of multivessel coronary artery disease include exercise-induced hypotension, ST-segment changes of greater than 2 mm, a low work load capacity (Table 7.4),[4] or a limited duration of exercise (which reflects the functional state of the left ventricle) and persistent ST-segment depressions. In outpatients with suspected coronary artery disease, treadmill exercise scores incorporating the presence or absence of symptoms of angina, the duration of exercise, and the maximal ST-segment deviation during or after exercise can help clinicians to predict long-term survival.[5]

Because the standard exercise stress test relies on ischemia-related changes on the electrocardiogram, the test is less useful in patients with abnormal electrocardiographic changes at baseline (for example left bundle branch block). In addition, there are times when a patient is unable to exercise because of physical limitations or deconditioning. The solution to these problems has been a combination of pharmacologic stress testing with various imaging modalities for the diagnosis of coronary artery disease.

Stress echocardiography

Stress echocardiography demonstrates myocardial ischemia by detection of stress-induced wall motion abnormalities on comparison of prestress and poststress images. The echocardiographer assesses wall thickness before and usually immediately after stress. This can be technically very difficult and is unreliable in patients with poor "echocardiographic windows". Echocardiography may be combined with exercise or non-pharmacologic stressors such as dobutamine, dipyridamole, and adenosine. Stress echocardiography is a useful adjunct to the standard electrocardiographic exercise test, and provides a more sensitive, and specific, form of testing to detect coronary artery disease. When stress echocardiographic and nuclear tests are compared, the sensitivities are similar (85% and 87%, respectively), but the echocardiographic test has more specificity (77% versus 64%) and therefore higher discriminatory capabilities.[6]

Radionuclide methods

Thallium scintigraphy allows visualization of myocardial perfusion at rest and during exercise. Agents administered intravenously, such as thallium-201, are extracted efficiently by the myocardium and transported across the cell membrane by the sodium–potassium ATPase pump. As with potassium, initial thallium extraction into the myocardium is affected by myocardial viability. Thallium is normally taken up by healthy myocardial cells, but regions of myocardial ischemia or infarction cannot take up the radionuclide and appear as "cold spots" when imaged by a γ camera. During the exercise test, thallium-201 is injected intravenously at maximal exertion and an image of the heart is obtained. If a cold spot is detected, this suggests the presence of either reversible ischemia or a previous (non-reversible) infarction. To differentiate these, a repeat image is taken several hours later. If the cold spot "fills in" then a region of transient ischemia has probably been provoked by exercise, whereas if the cold spot remains unchanged then a previous infarction is likely.

This technique is approximately 85–90% sensitive and 60–70% specific for the diagnosis of coronary artery disease.[6] However, perfusion imaging scans are expensive and should be restricted to application in patients with an abnormal baseline electrocardiogram that precludes interpretation during a standard exercise test, or to improve testing sensitivity in patients with an equivocal treadmill test. Expertise and excellent equipment are required for optimal results. In patients who are unable to exercise, pharmacologic agents such as intravenous dipyridamole, adenosine, and dobutamine can be used as stressors.

Prognostic importance of ventricular function and extent of coronary artery disease

In randomized trials using angiographic criteria for the evaluation of patients with chronic stable angina pectoris, the two most important prognostic variables are:

- left ventricular systolic function (usually expressed as left ventricular ejection fraction) and
- the severity and extent of coronary artery disease.

Although these two factors are synergistic, the degree of left ventricular dysfunction is a more important determinant of prognosis than is the extent and severity of coronary artery disease. The adverse influence of impaired ventricular function is greater in patients with severe, multivessel coronary artery disease. Therefore, in patients with chronic stable angina who have clinical indicators of impaired ventricular function (for example excessive breathlessness on exertion, a fourth heart sound or cardiac failure evident on clinical examination, electrocardiographic evidence of a prior myocardial infarction, or chest x ray evidence of an enlarged heart or pulmonary congestion) an echocardiogram should be performed to assess ventricular function (most readily accomplished non-invasively by either two-dimensional echocardiography or radionuclide ventriculography). If left ventricular function is abnormal at rest, then coronary angiography should be performed.

If left ventricular function is normal then some form of stress testing should be performed (treadmill exercise testing, radionuclide ventriculography at rest and during exercise, or perfusion imaging scans with exercise or pharmacologic stressors). If as a result of this there is evidence of significant exercise- or stress-induced ischemia or left ventricular dysfunction, then coronary angiography should be performed. On the other hand, a trial of medical therapy is reasonable if a stress protocol is completed that is equivalent to or greater than completion of stage 3 of a Bruce protocol treadmill test (approximately 10 METs) without evidence of significant exercise-induced ischemia or left ventricular dysfunction.

If this approach is used the results of coronary arteriography will lead to logical management choices. For all patients with significant (>60% diameter narrowing) left main coronary artery disease coronary artery surgery is advised. For most patients with significant (>70% diameter narrowing) three vessel coronary disease, revascularization is usually advised (coronary surgery more frequently than percutaneous transluminal coronary angioplasty [PTCA]). This is because major randomized trials have shown that coronary artery revascularization, with its known procedural risks, on balance will improve survival as compared with medical therapy in these patients (Figure 7.1).[7]

With significant two vessel disease the options of revascularization surgery, PTCA, and medical therapy are considered.[8] Either coronary artery surgery or PTCA is usually advised in patients with moderate angina pectoris and/or inducible ischemia, or a critical obstruction in the proximal left anterior descending coronary artery associated with a significant obstruction of one other major vessel. Again, for this category of patients, from a prognostic viewpoint revascularization is likely to result in improved survival.[7] In these patients PTCA represents an intermediate therapy between medical therapy and

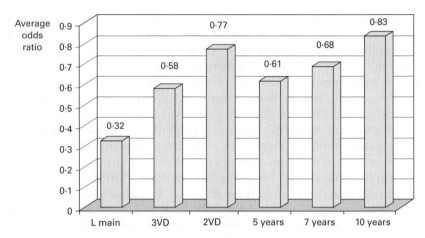

Figure 7.1 Mortality: coronary artery bypass grafting versus medical treatment. The 10-year mortality results of the randomized trials assessing medical treatment versus coronary artery surgery are displayed as average odds ratio (OR) of survival for patients with left main (L main), three vessel (3VD), and two vessel (2VD) coronary artery disease at 5 years, and for all patients at 5, 7, and 10 years. A ratio of 1·0 indicates a similar benefit for a patient whether treated medically or with surgical revascularization. A ratio of less than 1·0 indicates a survival benefit for patients treated with revascularization (versus medical treatment), which is seen for all categories of patients. The survival benefit for patients with L main (68% reduction in mortality) and 3VD (42% reduction in mortality) was greater than that for patients with 2VD (23%). Over time (5, 7, and 10 years) the mortality benefits of surgery declined compared with medical therapy because of the known attrition of coronary artery bypass grafts. Adapted from Yusuf et al.[4]

revascularization surgery. PTCA is a less traumatic revascularization procedure than surgery, and it is associated with a short hospital stay and convalesence. However, the relief from angina is less complete and approximately 33% of patients need to be revascularized within 1 year (Figures 7.2 and 7.3). For other categories of significant two vessel coronary artery disease survival outcomes are similar with medical or revascularization therapy, although revascularization is recommended in patients who, despite appropriate medical therapy, have symptoms that limit household, daily, or recreational activities.

In patients with significant one vessel coronary artery disease, the decision regarding coronary artery surgery, PTCA, or medical therapy is made individually.[9] Either PTCA or coronary artery surgery is favored in these patients when the results of non-invasive testing indicating extensive inducible ischemia, poor functional capacity, and the presence of a critical (>70% diameter narrowing) obstruction. Finally, revascularization is considered for symptomatic relief in any patient

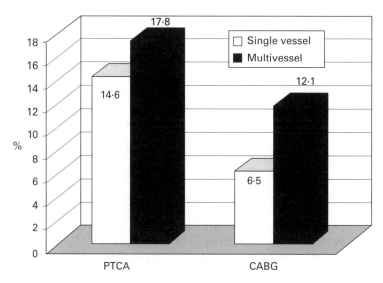

Figure 7.2 Angina recurrence in 1 year. Results of a meta-analysis comparing recurrence of class II (or greater) angina within 12 months of percutaneous transluminal coronary angioplasty (PTCA) and coronary artery bypass grafting (CABG) in patients with single and multivessel disease. For patients with single and multivessel disease relief of angina was more complete following CABG. For definition of class II angina, see Table 7.1. Adapted from Pocock et al.[5]

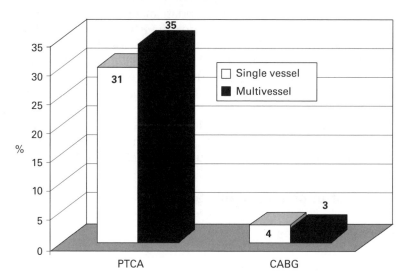

Figure 7.3 Revascularization within 1 year. Results of a meta-analysis of need for revascularization within 12 months of percutaneous transluminal coronary angioplasty (PTCA) and coronary artery bypass grafting (CABG) in patients with single and multivessel disease. For patients with single and multivessel disease need for revascularization was dramatically less following CABG. Adapted from Pocock et al.[5]

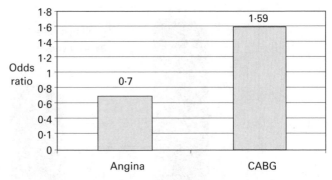

Figure 7.4 Percutaneous transluminal coronary angioplasty (PTCA) versus medical treatment. An analysis of PTCA versus medical treatment in patients with non-acute coronary heart disease shows the odds ratio (OR) of developing angina or requiring revascularization by coronary artery bypass grafting (CABG) during a follow up period of 6–57 months. An OR of 1·0 would suggest no difference in treatment effect between PTCA and medical therapy. An OR of less than 1·0 indicates an advantage of PTCA (less angina during follow up) and an OR of more than 1·0 (increased need for CABG during follow up) indicates a disadvantage of PTCA as compared with medical therapy. Adapted from Bucher et al.[6]

whose normal daily working, household, or recreational activities are limited by angina, despite an appropriate medical regimen. An analysis of randomized controlled trials comparing PTCA with medical therapy in patients with non-acute coronary heart disease showed that, during a follow up ranging from 6 to 57 months, relief of angina was more complete following PTCA, but the need for revascularization with coronary artery bypass grafting was substantially greater than in patients treated medically (Figure 7.4).[9] The authors concluded that PTCA should be reserved for patients whose symptoms are not well controlled with medical therapy but attention was drawn to the substantial need for repeat revascularization after PTCA.

Treatment of chronic stable angina

General measures

General measures include:

- an attempt to attain ideal body weight (weight reduction may raise the threshold for or may even abolish angina)
- discontinuation of smoking (the risk for myocardial infarction and sudden death is higher in smokers)

- achievement of excellent blood pressure and diabetes control
- performance of the equivalent of regular, brisk walking exercise for 30–40 min three or four times a week.

Medical therapy

In patients with chronic stable angina the secondary prevention measures of aspirin therapy and effective low-density lipoprotein (LDL) lowering have both been shown to reduce mortality and prevent acute myocardial infarction. Therapy with nitrates, β-blockers and calcium channel blockers will reduce symptoms of angina and improve exercise performance, but have not been clearly shown to reduce mortality or prevent myocardial infarction in these patients.

Aspirin

Aspirin (81–325 mg) daily is advisable in patients with chronic stable angina without contraindications to this drug. Reduction in platelet aggregability appears to reduce the risks for myocardial infarction and sudden death in this population.[10]

Lipid lowering

The secondary prevention lipid lowering trials[11–13] provide convincing evidence that effective LDL lowering improves survival and reduces cardiovascular morbidity in patients with coronary artery disease. In all patients with known coronary artery disease the combination of diet, exercise, and drugs is used to try to achieve concentrations of total cholesterol of 200 mg/dl (5·2 mmol/l) and LDL-cholesterol of 100 mg/dl (2·6 mmol/l) or lower. There is also evidence that, compared with revascularization by PTCA, an aggressive lipid lowering strategy employed as part of medical therapy in patients with one or two vessel coronary artery disease avoids future ischemic events at least equally effectively.[14] However, symptomatic relief of angina is not as good.

Nitrates

The action of nitrates is to relax vascular smooth muscle. The vasodilator effects of nitrates appear to be predominant in the venous circulation (reducing ventricular preload, and therefore myocardial wall tension and oxygen requirements). In addition they have some vasodilator effects on the systemic and coronary arteries. Nitrate therapy in the form of sublingual nitroglycerin, long-acting oral nitrates, and transdermal nitrate preparations reduces the frequency of silent and symptomatic myocardial ischemia in patients with angina.[15] The term "nitrate tolerance"[16] refers to the attenuation or loss of nitrate effects when such agents are administered as frequent doses of long-acting preparations, as continuous delivery systems (intravenous infusions or transdermal patches), or as long-acting sustained release preparations, all of which produce constantly maintained "therapeutic" plasma levels. In order to minimize tolerance, dosing regimens must be planned so that "nitrate free" intervals of 8–10 hours are achieved. The prophylactic use of sublingual nitroglycerin, taken before anticipated physical activity that would normally provoke angina, is usually very effective in achieving symptom relief but is underutilized.

β-Adrenergic blocking agents

These agents cause competitive inhibition of the effects of neuronally released and circulating catecholamines on β-adrenoreceptors. β-Blockade reduces myocardial oxygen consumption primarily by slowing heart rate (especially during activity or excitement) and by reducing afterload or wall stress and cardiac contractility. Although the "resting" heart rate is an important vital sign, it is important for the clinician to assess the efficacy of the prescribed β-blocker on heart rate during exercise or physical activity when sympathetic activity is heightened. In general, the goal is to reduce resting heart rate to 50–60 beats/min, and with moderate exercise an increase of less than approximately 30 beats/min is expected with optimal therapy. Most β-blockers act to some extent on both β_1-receptors (myocardium) and β_2-receptors (vascular smooth muscle and bronchial muscle). Because of this, we believe that a history of asthma, or wheezing, should be an absolute contraindication to their use because effective heart rate control can usually be achieved with other agents, such as the calcium channel blockers diltiazem and verapamil. Studies indicate that for the treatment of angina pectoris the use of a β-blocker, at a maximally tolerated dose, confers as much benefit as the combination of a β-blocker and a calcium channel blocker. However, if a patient remains symptomatic despite a maximally tolerated dose of β-blocker, then the addition of a calcium channel blocker will reduce the frequency of anginal attacks and improve exercise performance.[17,18]

Calcium channel blockers

Calcium channel blockers are a heterogeneous group of compounds that inhibit calcium ion movement through slow channels in cardiac and smooth muscle membranes by non-competitive blockade of voltage-sensitive L-type calcium channels. There are three major classes of calcium channel blockers: the dihydropryidines (of which nifedipine is the prototype), the phenyl alkylamines (of which verapamil is the prototype), and the modified benzothiazepines (of which diltiazem is the prototype). Calcium channel blockers reduce myocardial oxygen demand by reducing preload, wall stress (reducing blood pressure), and contractility and heart rate (verapamil and diltiazem), and by increasing coronary perfusion and minimizing coronary vasospasm. It is not clear that the addition of a β-blocker to diltiazem or verapamil improves antianginal efficacy,[17] although the combination of a β-blocker with a dihydropyridine such as nifedipine does.

Revascularization therapy

Percutaneous transluminal coronary angioplasty (PTCA), with or without stent placement, offers relief of symptoms in patients with coronary artery disease. Randomized trials to date have shown no difference in prognosis when percutanous revascularization is compared with coronary artery bypass surgery.[8] However, revascularization surgery provides greater relief of symptoms during the first 2 or 3 years following the procedure, with less need for a second revascularization procedure (see Figures 7.2 and 7.3).[8]

Single vessel coronary artery disease

PTCA with stent placement is an excellent form of treatment for symptom relief in patients with significant, single vessel coronary artery disease. Revascularization by PTCA appears to be superior to medical therapy in patients with single vessel coronary artery disease for relief of symptoms, improved quality of life, and improved exercise duration. However, as compared with medical therapy, patients treated with PTCA appear to show a greater need for subsequent revascularization by coronary artery bypass grafting (CABG).[9] PTCA does not appear to offer a survival benefit in patients with single vessel coronary artery disease, and does not reduce the incidence of recurrent myocardial infarction. Special consideration is usually given to patients with significant proximal left anterior descending coronary artery stenosis. Percutaneous revascularization with stent placement is the most widely used treatment option for such lesions. However, CABG with an internal mammary artery graft provides the best long-term revascularization results, with less need for further revascularization. CABG does not decrease mortality or recurrent myocardial infarction in patients with proximal left anterior descending stenoses as compared with PTCA or medical therapy.[19] The decision regarding treatment in patients with proximal left anterior descending disease needs to be individualized based on the type of lesion, comorbid conditions, and an informed decision by the patient.

In summary, single vessel coronary artery disease involving the proximal left anterior descending coronary artery is usually treated with revascularization. For all other single vessel coronary artery disease, the decision to treat medically or to recommend revascularization therapy is usually based on symptoms and on whether the patient has responded to medical therapy.

Multivessel coronary artery disease

Patients with significant left main coronary artery stenosis should undergo surgical revascularization to improve their long-term mortality. In patients with stable angina pectoris, normal left ventricular function, and either three vessel disease or a severe proximal left anterior descending coronary artery stenosis and involvement of one other major vessel, revascularization appears superior to medical therapy from a prognostic view point. Provided patient selection is appropriate and the risks associated with revascularization are within the usual expected range, then survival is improved.[7]

Cardiac surgical vascularization has an advantage over both PTCA and medical therapy in patients with significant three vessel disease and moderately impaired ventricular function (left ventricular ejection fraction 35–50%), whether symptoms exist or not. Surgical revascularization appears to confer the greatest advantage in those patients with diabetes mellitus, the most severe anginal symptoms, the most severe left ventricular dysfunction, and the most extensive coronary artery disease. Although the risk associated with surgery is higher in such patients, their chance of long-term survival is still improved.

In the treatment of chronic stable angina it has been shown that aspirin and effective low-density lipoprotein lowering reduce mortality and recurrent myocardial infarction. Each of the three major classes of therapeutic agents prescribed to provide symptomatic relief (nitrates, β-blockers, and calcium channel blockers) have been shown to reduce angina and to improve ability to exercise, but they have not been conclusively shown to reduce morbidity or mortality. In addition to historical information about the patient and of risk factors, assessment of left ventricular function and knowledge of the patient's response to some form of stress testing are required to determine whether continued medical therapy or coronary angiography, with a view to revascularization, should be considered. The goals of revascularization are to provide relief from angina or to improve survival.

Case studies

Case 7.1

A 54-year-old male presents with a 2 week history of cough and shortness of breath on exertion. For three nights he has been unable to lie flat because of breathlessness. Twelve years earlier he was treated for testicular seminoma with orchiectomy, radiation to the abdomen and chest, and chemotherapy (doxorubicin, cyclophosphamide, and vincristine). He was diagnosed as having type 2 diabetes 12 years ago. He also has hyperlipidemia, and recent measurements are as follows: total cholesterol 242 mg/dl (6·2 mmol/l), triglycerides 379 mg/dl (4·3 mmol/l), low-density lipoprotein cholesterol 123 mg/dl (3·2 mmol/l), high-density lipoprotein (HDL)-cholesterol 43 mg/dl (1·1 mmol/l), and total cholesterol/HDL ratio 5·6 (normal <5·0). His brother and sister have a history of premature onset coronary artery disease. He is a non-smoker.

Examination. Physical examination: the patient appeared slightly breathless at rest. Pulse: 100 beats/min, normal character. Blood pressure: 115/80 mmHg in right arm. Jugular venous pulse: 8 cm. Cardiac impulse: displaced laterally. First heart sound: normal. Second heart sound: split normally on inspiration. Fourth heart sound at apex. Chest examination: normal air entry, bibasilar rales. Abdominal examination: soft abdomen, no tenderness, and no masses. Normal liver span. No peripheral edema. Femoral, popliteal, posterior tibial, and dorsalis pedis pulses: all normal volume and equal. Carotid pulses: normal, no bruits. Optic fundi: normal.

Investigations. Electrocardiogram (Figure 7.5). Chest *x* ray (Figure 7.6).

Questions

1. What does the electrocardiogram show?
2. What does the chest *x* ray film show?
3. What is the differential diagnosis?

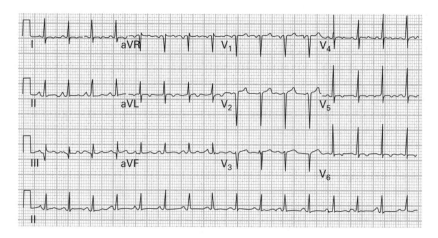

Figure 7.5 Electrocardiogram of the patient described in Case 7.1. (See text for details)

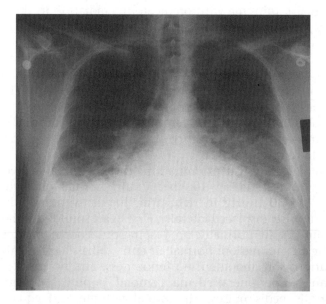

Figure 7.6 Chest x ray film of the patient described in Case 7.1. (See text for details)

4. What therapy should the patient be started on?
5. What further tests would you order?
6. What would you recommend to the patient? Should he continue medical therapy or will you recommend coronary artery revascularization?

7. What is myocardial contractile reserve?
8. What are the different descriptions of ischemic myocardial dysfunction?
9. How can one determine whether there is viable myocardium?

Answers

Answer to question 1 The electrocardiogram shows normal sinus rhythm at 96 beats/min; poor R wave progression from V_1 to V_3, possibly due to a remote anterior myocardial infarction; a Q wave in III; and T-wave inversions in leads I, aVL, V_5, and V_6. These findings could be consistent with prior infarction and ongoing anterolateral myocardial ischemia or evolving non-Q-wave myocardial infarction. The shape of the ST-T changes in leads I, aVL, V_5, and V_6 could also be consistent with left ventricular hypertrophy.

Answer to question 2 The chest x ray film shows cardiomegaly, a right chest effusion, and pulmonary vascular markings consistent with heart failure.

Answer to question 3 The patient presents with cough and shortness of breath and has clinical findings consistent with heart failure, including sinus tachycardia, elevated jugular venous pressure, a displaced cardiac impulse, a fourth heart sound, bilateral chest rales, and a chest x ray film showing cardiomegaly, an effusion, and pulmonary congestion. He has a family history of premature coronary disease, and has diabetes and hyperlipidemia. The electrocardiogram suggests possible prior infarction (Q wave lead III and poor R wave progression in anterior chest leads) with anterolateral ischemia and/or left ventricular hypertrophy. Because of the history of chemotherapy 12 years ago, congestive cardiomyopathy caused by doxorubicin is also possible. The anthracyclines (including doxorubicin) are the chemotherapeutic agents most widely recognized as causing cardiotoxicity, but many other agents may cause cardiac pathology. The cumulative dose of doxorubicin administered is the most important risk factor for the development of cardiomyopathy, and at doses greater than 400 mg/m^2 this risk increases substantially. The patient may have both doxorubicin-induced cardiomyopathy and coronary artery disease contributing to heart failure.

Answer to question 4 The patient was digitalized, given diuretics, and stabilized on a regimen of digoxin 0·25 mg/day, furosemide 40 mg/day, captopril 25 mg four times daily, aspirin 325 mg/day, and glyburide 10 mg/day.

Answer to question 5 The patient had serial cardiac enzymes taken, which showed no evidence of an evolving myocardial infarction. A two-dimensional echocardiogram taken after hospital admission showed severely depressed left ventricular function, with a left ventricular diastolic diameter of 5·2 cm (normal range 3·5–6·0 cm) and end-systolic diameter of 4·0 cm (normal range 2·1–4·0 cm), without evidence of ventricular hypertrophy. Regional wall motion abnormalities were noted, with dyskinesis and akinesis of the anterior myocardium and akinesis of the septal region. The inferior region of the heart was not adequately imaged. These findings are consistent with a dilated heart with severely reduced systolic function. The regional wall motion abnormalities suggest coronary artery disease, ischemia, and/or infarction, although they may also be seen with dilated cardiomyopathy.

The cumulative amount of myocardial damage accrued is the most important determinant of prognosis for any acute or chronic coronary syndrome. Because this relatively young male patient presents with heart failure and has documented severely reduced left ventricular systolic function, his prognosis is poor. He has major risk factors for premature coronary artery disease. In this situation, after stabilization and treatment of his heart failure, it is important to define his coronary anatomy, and determine whether ischemia is at least partly responsible for his cardiac dysfunction and whether revascularization might potentially improve his prognosis and his systolic cardiac function.

The patient was discharged from hospital after 7 days, and arrangements were made for him to have an elective cardiac catheterization in 2 weeks. When he was admitted for this procedure he said that, although he felt much better taking his new medications and that his breathing had improved so that he could lie flat in bed, he had noticed chest tightness and shortness of breath on three occasions during mild physical activity.

Cardiac catherization. Left ventricular ejection fraction: 30%. Moderate mitral regurgitation was noted at the time of LV angiography. Pressures (in mmHg): left ventricle 90/20; mean pulmonary wedge 8; pulmonary artery 24/14. Left anterior descending coronary artery: 90% proximal stenosis, and serial 50% and 70% stenoses in its mid-portion. Circumflex coronary artery: 40% stenosis. First obtuse marginal branch of circumflex coronary artery: 40% stenosis. Right coronary artery: serial stenoses of 50% and 50% in its mid-portion.

Answer to question 6 The patient has severe proximal coronary disease of the left anterior descending coronary artery, and moderate disease of the circumflex and right coronary arteries associated with significant cardiac dysfunction (left ventricular ejection fraction 30%, moderate mitral regurgitation). The echocardiographic appearances of the anterior wall of the heart show akinesis and dyskinesis. This then is a symptomatic patient (chest tightness corresponding to angina, and breathlessness corresponding to heart failure and possibly ischemia) with moderate to severe cardiac dysfunction and multivessel coronary disease, including a proximal left anterior descending coronary artery stenosis. For survival or prognostic reasons, revascularization would be contemplated provided it was felt that there was viable myocardium suitable for revascularization.

Answer to question 7 Myocardial contractile reserve is the ability of dysfunctional but viable myocardium to exhibit improvement in function following an inotropic stimulus (such as post-extrasystolic potentiation or infusion of a sympathomimetic amine [dobutamine] or exercise). The regional function of the myocardium is typically observed using echocardiography or nuclear imaging at baseline and during or immediately after the stimulus.

Answer to question 8 There are two common descriptors of ischemic myocardial dysfunction.

Stunned myocardium is "prolonged, but temporary, post-ischemic ventricular dysfunction without irreversible myocyte damage".[20] Typically, a brief period of acute ischemia followed by restoration of coronary perfusion results in prolonged contractile dysfunction. Minutes of ischemia may result in hours or days of postischemic ventricular dysfunction. The features of stunned myocardium include abnormal systolic and diastolic dysfunction, viable myocardium that exhibits contractile reserve, and the absence of myocyte necrosis with routine microscopy. The pathogenesis of stunning after reperfusion is believed to involve either oxidant stress after generation of reactive oxygen species or transient calcium overload during reperfusion with decreased responsiveness of the contractile machinery to calcium, or a combination of both. Myocardial stunning is observed in humans following acute myocardial infarction with early reperfusion, with unstable angina, coronary vasospasm, after percutaneous transluminal coronary angioplasty, with exercise-induced ischemia, and after open heart surgery or cardiac transplantation.

Hibernating myocardium is a term used for "severe, prolonged, cardiac dysfunction secondary to chronic ischemia associated with viable though poorly contractile, myocardium".[21,22] The features of hibernating myocardium include abnormal systolic and diastolic dysfunction; the dominant clinical features may be cardiac failure without overt symptomatic or electrocardiographic evidence of ischemia; the myocardium is viable and exhibits contractile reserve with reversible dysfunction, and the ventricular dysfunction will persist as long as myocardial perfusion is inadequate. There is debate over whether the pathogenesis involves reduced flow or normal flow with reduced coronary artery vasodilator reserve.

Answer to question 9 In the patient under discussion the presentation with symptoms of heart failure and angina and clinical signs of heart failure raise the possibility of "hibernating" myocardium. In order to determine whether the patient had viable or ischemic myocardium (that might benefit from revascularization) rather than infarcted or scarred myocardium (non-viable; that would not benefit from revascularization) a stress perfusion imaging scan was ordered.

The patient exercised on a treadmill according to the Bruce protocol. The test was terminated at 7·3 min (mid-stage III) because of angina. The patient's heart rate had increased from 84 to 136 beats/min and his blood pressure from 100/67 to 166/62 mmHg, achieving a work load of 8·3 METs. His resting electrocardiogram showed poor R-wave progression consistent with an anterior myocardial infarction. During exercise he developed 2 mm downsloping ST-segment depression in leads II, III and aVF, and 2 mm ST-segment elevation in leads V_2–V_3, progressing to 3·5 mm ST-segment depression inferolaterally in recovery. The stress test was positive for angina and ST-segment change at a moderate level of activity. Qualitative analysis of the perfusion tomograms demonstrated a large, primarily reversible anterior, apical, and septal defect with abnormal wall motion on gated images (Figure 7.7).

These findings were thought to be consistent with severe ischemia in the left anterior descending coronary artery distribution associated with moderately depressed left ventricular systolic dysfunction and "hibernating" myocardium. It was recommended that the patient undergo revascularization surgery. Within 2 weeks he underwent coronary artery bypass grafting with an internal mammary artery graft applied to the left anterior descending artery, and saphenous vein grafts to the second diagonal, obtuse marginal, and right coronary arteries. He recovered uneventfully, his postoperative echocardiogram showed an improvement in left ventricular function ("mildly depressed"), and he was discharged from hospital taking aspirin 81 mg/day, pravastatin 20 mg/day, glyburide, metformin, and vitamin E. He resumed his normal life and, although asymptomatic, he requested a stress test 41 months later to monitor his progress. He exercised on a Bruce protocol for 9 min (10 METs) and the test was terminated for fatigue and dyspnea. His heart rate increased from 100 to 165 beats/min and his blood pressure from 120/75 to 150/90 mmHg. He had 1·5 mm ST-segment depression in leads II, III, aVF, V_5,

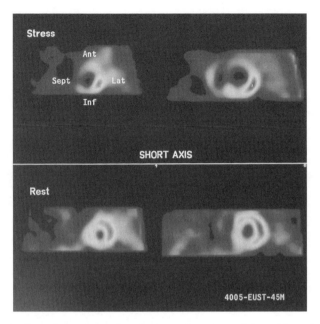

Figure 7.7 Qualitative analysis of perfusion tomograms of the patient described in Case 7.1. (See text for details)

and V_6. His poststress nuclear study showed a left ventricular ejection fraction of 45%, anteroseptal hypokinesis, and a mild, reversible septal defect. He continued on medical therapy.

Case 7.2

A 44-year-old male, warehouse worker is hit accidentally in the chest by a broom. He has prolonged chest pain unrelieved by sublingual nitroglycerin and is admitted to hospital. His past history reveals that over an 18 month period he has had four or five emergency room visits with brief episodes of chest pain developing while he has played "pick up" basketball or lifted weights. During the past month he has had four episodes of chest pain associated with leg tingling, palpitations, darkened vision, and loss of consciousness. He is participating in an alcohol abuse rehabilitation program, he has an active 80 pack-year smoking history, and has had pulmonary tuberculosis in the past.

Examination. Physical examination: the patient appeared normal and had mild chest discomfort. Pulse: 70 beats/min, normal character. Blood pressure: 130/80 mmHg in right arm. Jugular venous pulse:

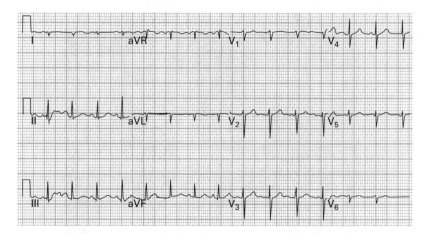

Figure 7.8 Electrocardiogram of the patient described in Case 7.2. (See text for details)

normal. Cardiac impulse: normal. First heart sound: normal. Second heart sound: split normally on inspiration. No added sounds or murmurs. Chest examination: normal air entry, no rales or rhonchi. Abdominal examination: soft abdomen, no tenderness, and no masses. Normal liver span. No peripheral edema. Femoral, popliteal, posterior tibial, and dorsalis pedis pulses: all normal volume and equal. Carotid pulses: normal, no bruits.

Investigations. Electrocardiogram taken on admission to hospital: normal sinus rhythm at 93 beats/min. Normal intervals, and no significant ST-T changes (Figure 7.8). An electrocardiogram taken 7 months earlier was the same.

Questions

1. What treatment and investigations should be initiated?
2. What is your interpretation of the two event strips shown in Figure 7.9, recorded continuously in three leads (from above down the leads are I, aVF, and V₁)?
3. What is the probable diagnosis?
4. Should he have further investigations and what therapy should be initiated?

Answers

Answer to question 1   The patient is treated symptomatically with analgesia because there is no evidence of myocardial ischemia

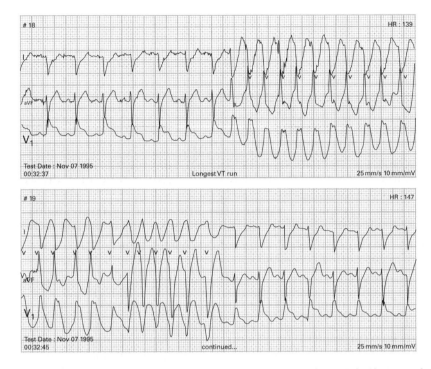

Figure 7.9 Holter recording from the patient described in Case 7.2. (See text for details.) HR, heart rate

following an incident provoked by chest trauma. A series of cardiac enzymes are drawn and are normal. Two further electrocardiograms taken over the first 18 hours are normal. Because of the impressive history of "four episodes of chest pain associated with leg tingling, palpitations, darkened vision, and loss of consciousness", a Holter monitor is ordered (see Figure 7.9). The patient notes in the diary that at the time of the illustrated recording he feels chest pain, nausea, and dizziness.

Answer to question 2 In the top strip, seven beats of normal sinus rhythm are followed by a wide complex, regular tachycardia of a different morphology (and probable dissociation of P waves and QRS complexes), which is self-limiting after 23 beats when normal sinus rhythm continues (bottom strip). Correlation of this rhythm with the patient's diary suggests symptomatic, ventricular tachycardia. Close inspection of the third lead (V₁) during the seven beats of normal sinus rhythm shows approximately 3–4 mm of ST-segment elevation.

Answer to question 3   In 1959 Prinzmetal described a variant form of angina pectoris.[23] The pain, which was identical to angina with respect to location, occurred when the subject was at rest or during normal activities, and did not appear to be precipitated by increased cardiac work. Arrhythmias, often ventricular, occurred in about half of the described cases during the peak of the attack but the electrocardiogram remained unchanged during mild attacks or during the early phase of severe attacks. At the peak of severe attacks, ST elevations (with reciprocal depressions) were noted in the distribution of a large coronary artery. It was thought that the transient nature of the attacks was due to an increase in vascular tone of a diseased epicardial coronary artery.

It was subsequently shown that Prinzmetal's variant angina is associated with a primary decrease in myocardial oxygen supply caused by an increase in coronary vascular tone or "spasm". Death may occur during the attacks as a result of myocardial infarction or ventricular arrhythmias. Patients with the condition may have normal stress tests (or stress may occasionally provoke an attack). Variant angina may be idiopathic, associated with manipulation of a cardiac catheter, or occur in patients with classic angina. Nitrates are used for symptomatic relief, and chronic administration of calcium channel blockers has been shown to provide symptomatic relief and to control attacks. Since β-blocking drugs might theoretically allow unopposed α-receptor mediated coronary artery vasoconstriction to occur, which could aggravate coronary vasospasm, they are usually avoided if the diagnosis is made. In patients without significant, or critical, coronary artery stenoses demonstrated at the time of coronary angiography, medical therapy is pursued. If the symptoms persist despite medical therapy, then revascularization of significant stenoses may be undertaken with periprocedure (and long-term) treatment with nitrates and calcium channel blockers. In these patients the efficacy of revascularization is unpredictable.

The patient had typical symptoms of angina (his presentation after being struck by a broom handle was fortuitous), associated with palpitations and episodes of brief loss of consciousness. His Holter monitor and diary showed symptomatic, self-limiting episodes of ventricular tachycardia associated with transient ST-segment elevations, with normal electrocardiograms on other occasions. It was thought his most likely diagnosis was variant angina.

Answer to question 4   He is a 44-year-old male with an active 80 pack-year history of smoking, symptoms of angina, episodes of angina associated with ST elevations, reflecting "transmural ischemia", and ventricular tachycardia. Therefore, coronary angiography is indicated. He was started on aspirin and a calcium channel blocker (verapamil slow release 180 mg/day). Cardiac catheterization: normal left ventricular angiography with an ejection fraction of 67%, left ventricular pressure 112/5 mmHg. Coronary anatomy – left main: normal; left anterior descending: minor irregularities; first diagonal: 25% stenosis; first obtuse marginal: 25% stenosis; right coronary: 50% lesion in proximal third; posterior descending coronary artery: 50% lesion. The overall impression was "non-critical" coronary artery disease. After 4 days of treatment in hospital, he remained asymptomatic, telemetry revealed no arrhythmias, and before discharge he performed a Bruce protocol exercise test to a level of 10 METs when he was asymptomatic, and electrocardiography showed no ST changes or arrhythmias.

Three weeks later while washing dishes he developed severe chest pain, shortness of breath, leg tingling, loss of consciousness, and incontinence. When the emergency ambulance arrived he was found conscious with chest pain. He was readmitted to hospital, his electrocardiograms were initially normal, and his cardiac enzymes were normal. His medications were increased to aspirin 325 mg/day, isosorbide dinitrate 30 mg three times daily and verapamil slow release 240 mg twice daily. In hospital over several days he had occasional chest pain associated with ST elevations and sinus tachycardia on telemetry. He had one episode of asymptomatic ventricular tachycardia with ST elevations. After considerable debate, he accepted the recommendation of placement of an implantable defibrillator. He remained well taking his medications with the implantable defibrillator for 6 months, and subsequently did not return for follow up.

References

1 Campeau L. Grading of angina pectoris. *Circulation* 1976;**54**:522–3.
2 Diamond GA. A clinically relevant classification of chest discomfort. *J Am Coll Cardiol* 1983;**1**:574.
3 Epstein SE. Implications of probability analysis on strategy used for noninvasive detection of coronary artery disease. Role of single or combined use of exercise electrocardiographic testing, radionuclide cineangiography and myocardial perfusion imaging. *Am J Cardiol* 1980;**46**:491–9.
4 Fletcher GF, Froelicher VF, Hartley LH, Haskell WL, Pollock ML. Exercise standards. A statement for health professionals from the American Heart Association. *Circulation* 1990;**82**:2286–322.
5 Mark DB, Shaw L, Harrell FE, *et al*. Prognostic value of a treadmill exercise score in outpatients with suspected coronary artery disease. *N Engl J Med* 1991;**325**:849–53.
6 Fleischmann KE, Hunink MGM, Kuntz KM, Douglas PS. Exercise echocardiography or exercise SPECT imaging? A meta-analysis of diagnostic test performance. *JAMA* 1998;**280**:913–20.
7 Yusuf S, Zucker D, Peduzzi P, *et al*. Effect of coronary artery bypass graft surgery on survival: overview of 10-year results from randomised trials by the Coronary Artery Bypass Graft Surgery Trialists Collaboration. *Lancet* 1994;**344**:563–70.
8 Pocock SJ, Anderson RA, Rickards AF, *et al*. Meta-analysis of randomised trials comparing coronary angioplasty with bypass surgery. *Lancet* 1995;**346**:1184–9.

9 Bucher HC, Hengstler P, Schindler C, Guyatt GH. Percutaneous transluminal coronary angioplasty versus medical treatment for non-acute coronary heart disease: meta-analysis of randomised controlled trials. *BMJ* 2000;**321**:73–7.

10 Ridker PM, Manson JE, Gaziano M, Buring JE, Hennekens CH. Low-dose aspirin therapy for chronic stable angina. *Ann Intern Med* 1991;**114**:835–9.

11 Scandinavian Simvastatin Survival Study Group. Randomised trial of cholesterol lowering in 444 patients with coronary heart disease: the Scandinavian Simvastatin Survival Study (4S). *Lancet* 1994;**344**:1383–9.

12 Sacks FM, Pfeffer MA, Moye LA, *et al*. The effect of pravastatin on coronary events after myocardial infarction in patients with average cholesterol levels. *N Engl J Med* 1996;**335**:1001–9.

13 LIPID Study Group, The Long-term Intervention with Pravastatin in Ischaemic Disease. Prevention of cardiovascular events and death with pravastatin in patients with coronary heart disease and a broad range of initial cholesterol levels. *N Engl J Med* 1998;**339**:1349–57.

14 Pitt B, Waters D, Brown WV, *et al*. Aggressive lipid-lowering therapy compared with angioplasty in stable coronary artery disease. *N Engl J Med* 1999;**341**:70–6.

15 Pepine CJ. Daily life ischemia and nitrate therapy. *Am J Cardiol* 1992;**70**:54B–63B.

16 Packer M. What causes tolerance to nitroglycerin? The 100 year old mystery continues. *J Am Coll Cardiol* 1990;**16**:932–5.

17 Packer M. Combined beta-adrenergic and calcium entry blockade in angina pectoris. *N Engl J Med* 1989;**320**:709–18.

18 Strauss WE, Parisi AF. Combined use of calcium-channel and beta-adrenergic blockers for the treatment of chronic stable angina. Rationale, efficacy and adverse effects. *Ann Intern Med* 1988;**109**:570–81.

19 Hueb WA, Bellotti G, De Oliveira SA, *et al*. Five-year follow-up of the Medicine, Angioplasty, or Surgery Study (MASS): a prospective, randomized trial of medical therapy, balloon angioplasty, or bypass surgery for single proximal left anterior descending coronary artery stenosis. *Circulation* 1999;**100(suppl)**:II107–13.

20 Kloner RA, Bolli R, Marban E, Reinlib L, Braunwald E. Medical and cellular implications of stunning, hibernation, and preconditioning: an NHLBI workshop. *Circulation* 1998;**97**:1848–67.

21 Braunwald E, Rutherford JD. Reversible ischemic dysfunction: evidence for the "hibernating myocardium". *J Am Coll Cardiol* 1986;**8**:1467–70.

22 Rahimtoola SH. Concept and evaluation of hibernating myocardium. *Annu Rev Med* 1999;**50**:75–86.

23 Prinzmetal M, Kennamer R, Merliss R, Wada T, Bor N. Angina pectoris. I. A variant form of angina pectoris. *Am J Med* 1959;**27**:375–88.

8: Arrhythmias

DAVID J KESSLER, RICHARD L PAGE

The spectrum of arrhythmias, which range from benign extra beats to fatal ventricular fibrillation, are reviewed and discussed.

Normal sinus rhythm

Normal sinus rhythm is usually defined as rates of 60–100 beats/min, although it is normal to have heart rates below 50 beats/min at rest or during sleep. Because atrial activation originates in the high right atrium, the surface electrocardiogram shows an upright P wave in leads I and aVF. In some patients, the dominant atrial pacemaker at rest is located elsewhere in the atria, resulting in an atrial rhythm with an unusual P-wave axis; this finding is not clinically important.

Bradycardia and conduction disturbances

Sinus node dysfunction

Sinus bradycardia, defined as a sinus rhythm of less than 60 beats/min, is recognized as regular P waves followed by a QRS complex. Causes of sinus bradycardia include the following: carotid sinus pressure (or hypersensitivity); the Valsalva maneuver; vomiting and other vagal stimulation; myocardial infarction, especially when it occurs in the inferior distribution; sepsis; increased intracranial pressure; hyperkalemia; hypoxemia; hypothermia; and hypothyroidism. In addition, several drugs can slow the sinus rate, including the β-adrenergic and calcium channel blocking agents, and digoxin. Finally, sinus bradycardia is common in well conditioned athletes.

Sinus pause or arrest refers to an abrupt absence of P waves; etiologies include many of the causes of sinus bradycardia, specifically degenerative fibrosis of the sinus node, acute myocardial infarction, myocarditis, digitalis toxicity, stroke, and increased vagal tone. The most common etiology for a pause on the electrocardiographic monitor is a premature atrial beat that is blocked in the atrioventricular (AV) node; the abnormal P wave is often buried in the T wave and is not recognized.

The term "sick sinus syndrome" (also called "tachy-brady syndrome") refers to sinus node dysfunction occurring in combination with intermittent atrial arrhythmias. Aging, with fibrosis of the sinus node, is thought to be the underlying mechanism.

Symptoms related to sinus node dysfunction include fatigue, presyncope, and syncope. Rarely, ventricular arrhythmias can result from sinus arrest. Following elimination of reversible causes of symptomatic sinus node dysfunction, the principal therapy for symptomatic patients is placement of a permanent transvenous cardiac pacemaker. On the other hand, if sinus bradycardia or dysfunction is asymptomatic, then pacing is not necessary.

Atrioventricular block

AV conduction disturbances are classified by the degree of conduction from the atria to the ventricles; these distinctions are meaningful in terms of the anatomic site of block, the mechanism, and the prognosis.

First-degree AV block refers to prolonged conduction. There is always a 1:1 relationship between P waves and QRS complexes, but the PR interval is increased (>0·2 seconds).

Second-degree AV block refers to intermittent conduction, resulting in more P waves than QRS complexes. In Mobitz type I second-degree AV block, the PR interval gradually prolongs until block of one P wave occurs; the next P wave is conducted with a shorter PR interval. The AV block in Mobitz type I usually occurs in the AV node, and results from conditions similar to those that cause sinus nodal slowing. Vagal influence, drugs, and inferior myocardial infarction are particularly common. Importantly, the prognosis is good because of the presence of subsidiary pacemakers in the AV junction below the level of block. In Mobitz type II AV block, the PR interval is fixed until block suddenly occurs; the block occurs below the AV node (in the His bundle), and typically is accompanied by other evidence of infranodal conduction delay (bundle branch block). Type II second-degree AV block frequently results from myocardial infarction or other cardiomyopathy. The risk for progression to complete heart block with a slow ventricular rate is significant with Mobitz type II block, and so permanent pacing is recommended.

Third-degree (or "complete") heart block refers to no conduction between the atrium and the ventricle. The atrial and ventricular rates are entirely independent, so that the PR interval is random. The ventricular rate may be sufficiently slow to cause syncope, or may approach a normal rate and cause no symptoms (Figures 8.1 and 8.2). Etiologies are similar to those for second-degree AV block. Pacemaker therapy is recommended for symptomatic patients and no evidence of a reversible cause; recent studies suggest that a permanent pacemaker

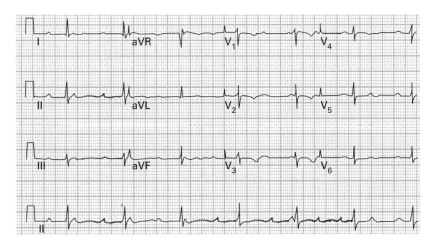

Figure 8.1

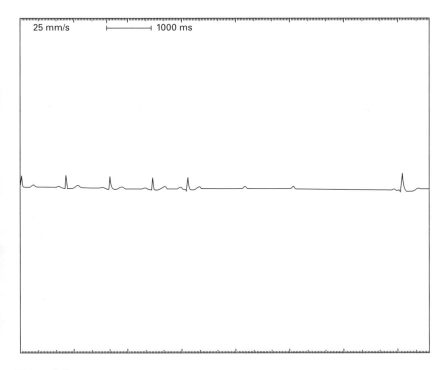

Figure 8.2

should be placed, even for asymptomatic patients with complete heart block.[1]

When heart block complicates myocardial infarction, prognosis depends on the level of block. Inferior myocardial infarction may be accompanied by exaggerated vagal tone that causes type I second-degree or third-degree AV block; this usually resolves spontaneously and does not require permanent pacing. In contrast, prognosis is poor when anterior myocardial infarction is complicated by type II second-degree or third-degree heart block; even if normal conduction returns, permanent pacing is recommended.

Supraventricular arrhythmias

The term "supraventricular" refers to arrhythmias in which the atrium or AV node is involved in the tachycardia focus or circuit.[1]

Atrial fibrillation

Atrial fibrillation (AF) is the most common arrhythmia encountered in clinical practice. It is characterized by fibrillation of the atria with an irregularly irregular ventricular response, typically in the range of 120–160 beats/min (Figure 8.3). It occurs most commonly in older patients, and may be associated with conditions that affect cardiac function (hypertension, heart failure [systolic or diastolic], coronary artery disease, valvular heart disease), obstructive pulmonary disease, hyperthyroidism, post-thoracic surgery, pericarditis, and concurrent infection. The presence of AF is associated with an increased risk for death in men and women.[2] Lone AF may occur in structurally normal hearts.

Although AF is occasionally asymptomatic, more frequently symptoms include palpitations, breathlessness, and dyspnea. Heart failure may result from AF in patients with valvular disease or with systolic or diastolic left ventricular dysfunction. However, the major risk associated with AF is neurologic. The lack of synchronous atrial contraction results in blood stasis and clot formation within the left atrium, which can embolize, causing transient or permanent neurologic impairment.

Clinical signs of AF include an irregularly irregular pulse and absent a waves in the jugular venous pulse, whereas other physical findings will depend on the patient's underlying heart condition and function. Signs of congestive failure (jugular venous distension, rales, a third heart sound gallop, and peripheral edema) may be present. Signs of rheumatic disease include murmurs or an opening snap associated

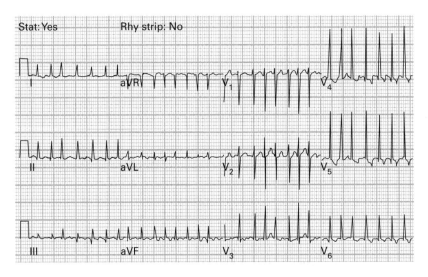

Figure 8.3

with mitral stenosis. There may also be signs of pulmonary hypertension or obstructive pulmonary disease.

The electrocardiogram demonstrates a chaotic baseline with irregularly irregular R–R intervals. A regular ventricular response in the presence of AF suggests digitalis toxicity or complete heart block. The QRS is usually narrow. Wide QRS complexes may suggest chronic or tachycardia-related bundle branch delay, or pre-excitation (see Atrioventricular re-entrant tachycardia and Wolff–Parkinson–White syndrome, below). A wide complex beat that results from a "long–short" pattern of QRS activation is called an Ashman beat; this is a normal phenomenon and relates to unequal refractoriness of the left and right bundles. Ashman beats are often mistaken for ventricular ectopy.

The management of AF depends on symptoms and duration of the arrhythmia.[3] Unstable patients, defined by hemodynamic compromise, uncontrollable angina, or congestive heart failure, should undergo immediate direct current cardioversion. Reversible causes of AF (such as thyrotoxicosis) should be identified and treated. Otherwise, therapy should be directed at four goals: ventricular rate control, restoration of sinus rhythm, maintenance of sinus rhythm, and reduction in risk for stroke.

Initial management of the patient with a rapid ventricular response is rate control with an AV nodal blocking agent. Intravenous β-blockers (esmolol or metoprolol) or calcium channel blockers (diltiazem or verapamil) may be used. Although digoxin has traditionally been used as a first line agent, its slow onset of action and lower efficacy in hyperadrenergic states makes it less attractive than other agents. AV nodal blocking agents are not usually efficacious in converting AF to sinus rhythm.

The underlying cause and duration of AF should be addressed because this will affect anticoagulation and timing of cardioversion. The risk of an embolic cerebrovascular accident following cardioversion is about 0·3–0·8% in anticoagulated patients, versus 5–7% in patients who have not been anticoagulated. Higher risk patients include those with prior embolism, mechanical valve prosthesis, and mitral stenosis. AF with a duration of less than 2 days, occurring in a structurally normal heart, can usually be safely cardioverted without prior anticoagulation. For episodes of longer or uncertain duration, the patient should be anticoagulated with warfarin (target International Normalized Ratio 2–3) for 3 full weeks before and 4 weeks after cardioversion. Transesophageal echocardiography may be used to identify clot in the left atrium or appendage, and the absence of abnormalities may facilitate the decision to cardiovert a patient without pretreatment with anticoagulants.

The decision to attempt cardioversion depends on several factors, including chronicity of AF, symptoms, and cardiac abnormalities. Although duration greater than 12 months and left atrial enlargement are risk factors for recurrence of AF, at least one attempt at conversion is usually justified.

Membrane stabilizing agents may cause "pharmacologic" cardioversion of AF and are used to stabilize the atrium after electrical cardioversion. They include the Vaughan Williams class 1A (procainamide, disopyramide, quinidine), class IC (flecainide, propafenone), and class III (sotalol, amiodarone) drugs. The efficacy of these agents in maintaining sinus rhythm at 1 year ranges from 30% to 80%, and the use of any one agent must be balanced against its side effect profile.

The class IA agents slow conduction to a minor degree and prolong the QT interval; excessive QT prolongation may result in polymorphic ventricular tachycardia (torsades de pointes) and so patients should be monitored carefully during initiation of therapy. A meta-analysis of randomized trials with quinidine demonstrated an increase in mortality associated with the drug.[4] Other side effects of type 1A agents include nausea, diarrhea (quinidine), anticholinergic symptoms (disopyramide), and a lupus-like syndrome (procainamide).

The class IC agents flecainide and propafenone slow intracardiac conduction, resulting in PR and QRS prolongation on the electrocardiogram. These agents are well tolerated and their efficacy is similar to that of quinidine and sotalol. Flecainide has been shown to increase the risk for sudden death in patients with prior infarction and ventricular ectopy, and both drugs may cause proarrhythmia. In general, these agents are not administered as first line therapy in patients with structural heart disease.

Sotalol, as a class III agent, works primarily by prolonging the action potential duration, and as such may cause substantial QT interval prolongation and torsades de pointes. It also causes substantial slowing of the sinus rate. The β-blocking properties of sotalol cause intolerance in patients with lung disease, bradycardia, and heart failure.

Amiodarone is considered a class III agent but shares properties with the other antiarrhythmic drug classes. It has many potential side effects, including thyroid and liver abnormalities, skin discoloration, corneal microdeposits, bradycardia, and pulmonary fibrosis. However, in low doses it is relatively well tolerated and effective in maintaining sinus rhythm.

Dofetilide is a class III agent that selectively blocks the potassium channel. It is effective in persistent AF, and has been used safely in high risk patients with careful inpatient monitoring. It is only used by approved physicians in approved facilities. It is mainly excreted by the kidneys, and concomitant administration is contraindicated with verapamil, ketoconazole, cimetidine, trimethoprim–sulfamethoxazole, prochlorperazine, and megestrol.

The algorithm for utilizing these agents developed by European and North American cardiologists serving on the Task Force for Practice Guidelines was updated in 2001 (Table 8.1).

A systematic approach to therapy for the patient with AF and a well controlled ventricular response includes anticoagulation with warfarin (target International Normalized Ratio 2–3) for at least 3 weeks. During this time, rate control is maintained with a β-blocker or calcium channel blocker, or digoxin. After 3 weeks, a membrane stabilizing agent (usually class I) is initiated, typically during electrocardiographic monitoring. If this does not cause conversion, then direct current cardioversion is performed. After sinus mechanism is restored and maintained, the membrane stabilizing agent is continued. Warfarin therapy is continued for at least 4 weeks. If the patient reverts back to AF following successful cardioversion to normal sinus rhythm, then the process may be repeated with another antiarrhythmic agent. If a patient has reverted to AF in spite of therapeutic levels of one or more antiarrhythmic agents, then management of chronic AF with rate control becomes the goal of

Table 8.1 Choice of antiarrhythmic agent for atrial fibrillation

	What is the condition of the heart			
Choice	Normal	Coronary disease	Left ventricular hypertrophy	Heart failure
First line	Propafenone, flecainide, sotalol	Sotalol, dofetilide	Propafenone	Amiodarone, defetilide
Second line	Class IA agents	Amiodarone	Amiodarone	

therapy. Again, long-term anticoagulation is recommended in nearly all patients. If rate control cannot be achieved pharmacologically, then radiofrequency catheter ablation of the AV junction with implantation of a permanent ventricular pacemaker is a reasonable option. Finally, surgically and catheter mediated "maze" procedures that are designed to stabilize the atrium and maintain sinus rhythm are under clinical investigation.

Atrial flutter

Atrial flutter is characterized by a regular atrial rhythm of approximately 300 beats/min; the "flutter P waves" are due to atrial re-entry and have a sawtooth pattern in inferior electrocardiographic leads. The typical P wave morphology may be difficult to identify at ventricular rates of 150 beats/min (2:1 conduction), but is quite apparent at higher degrees of AV block. Higher degree block in atrial flutter is often related to AV nodal blocking drugs or intrinsic conduction system disease.

The causes of atrial flutter are similar to those responsible for AF. The physical examination may reveal "flutter waves" in the jugular venous waveform. Symptoms are also similar to those seen with AF, although the higher heart rate (150 beats/min, with 2:1 block) may precipitate more pronounced hemodynamic compromise. Rarely, atrial flutter will conduct in a 1:1 manner to the ventricles and precipitate presyncope or syncope.

Management issues for atrial flutter are analogous to those for AF: rate control, conversion, maintenance of sinus rhythm, and anticoagulation. Rate control is often more difficult in patients with atrial flutter than in those with AF, and blocking to an AV ratio of greater than 2:1 may require a combination of AV nodal blocking drugs. With respect to the risk for thromboembolic complications with atrial flutter, a prudent approach is to treat AF and atrial flutter in the same way (especially because patients with atrial flutter frequently also have AF). We advocate anticoagulation for 3 weeks before and 4 weeks after cardioversion. Drugs to stabilize the atrium are identical to those used in AF. Direct current cardioversion is performed similarly, although less energy is required (50–100 J versus 200 J for AF). Unlike AF, atrial flutter can also be terminated by overdrive pacing of the atrium. This is accomplished by placing a pacing electrode transvenously to the right atrium; alternatively, atrial pacing can be performed using a transesophageal electrode. Once cardioversion has been accomplished, chronic maintenance therapy with an atrial stabilizing agent is continued in a manner similar to the management of AF.

When conversion from atrial flutter cannot be maintained, then one can consider chronic rate control with AV nodal blocking drugs or AV junction ablation with pacemaker (as with AF). In pure atrial flutter the catheter mediated procedure for atrial stabilization is quite effective, with success reported in excess of 80% in well selected populations, and radiofrequency ablation may be considered.[5]

Atrial tachycardia

Atrial tachycardia (AT), also referred to as ectopic or automatic atrial tachycardia, is due to spontaneous depolarization of an ectopic site within the atria. This ectopic site gives a P wave that is different from that seen during normal sinus rhythm. It may be sudden in onset and termination, or it may exhibit a "warm-up" phenomenon with gradual onset. AT accounts for 5–10% of supraventricular arrhythmias and occurs typically in the setting of structural heart disease. Drug therapy consists of AV nodal blocking agents and atrial stabilizing drugs. Radiofrequency catheter ablation can offer permanent cure, and ablation of the AV node with pacemaker placement will eliminate symptoms in refractory cases.

Multifocal atrial tachycardia

Multifocal atrial tachycardia occurs in the setting of decompensated lung disease, often with hypoxia and acid–base or electrolyte disturbances. It is defined by an atrial tachycardia with at least three different P wave morphologies and PR intervals. This irregular rhythm may be mistaken for AF, although close inspection demonstrates discrete P waves. Treatment to improve respiratory status is important, and either verapamil or diltiazem may be used to help control the arrhythmia.

Sinus nodal re-entrant tachycardia

This tachycardia can mimic sinus tachycardia in that the P wave is identical to that seen during sinus rhythm. Unlike sinus tachycardia, it is a re-entrant rhythm that starts and stops abruptly. The symptoms are similar to those seen with atrial tachycardia. Treatment with β-blockers and calcium channel blockers can reduce the recurrence of the rhythm, and radiofrequency catheter ablation may offer a cure.

Atrioventricular nodal re-entrant tachycardia

AV nodal re-entrant tachycardia (AVNRT) is responsible for approximately 60% cases of paroxysmal supraventricular tachycardia (PSVT; also referred to as "PAT" and "SVT"). These arrhythmias have a narrow QRS complex, paroxysmal onset and termination, and ventricular rates between 150 and 250 beat/min (Table 8.2). In the typical form of AVNRT, the electrical impulse travels down the "slow" pathway of the AV node and re-enters back up the "fast" pathway. This results in a tachycardia with P waves that are either buried within or occur just before or after the QRS complex. An R' in electrocardiogram lead V_1 that is only present during tachycardia represents the superimposed P wave and is diagnostic (Figure 8.4). In the atypical form of AVNRT (<5%), the re-entry circuit is reversed (down the "fast" and back up the "slow") and the P wave occurs substantially after the QRS (so-called "long RP tachycardia"). AVNRT occurs in structurally normal hearts with a slight preponderance in women, and increases in incidence with age. Clinically, the patient presents with palpitations, breathlessness, and neck pounding. There may be no precipitating factor. Presyncope and syncope are uncommon, but may occur early following onset.

AVNRT may be terminated using vagal maneuvers such as carotid massage and Valsalva; these techniques yield transient block in the slow pathway of the AV node and terminate re-entry. Adenosine, an endogenous nucleoside, represents the best drug option for conversion to sinus rhythm, and is effective in over 90% of cases.[6] This drug causes transient AV block when administered as an intravenous bolus injection. The drug may cause transient breathlessness and anxiety, but this resolves promptly due to the very short half-life (<2 seconds). Alternatively, intravenous verapamil injection is effective but does not work as quickly. For chronic therapy, calcium channel blockers, β-blockers, and digoxin reduce the frequency of recurrence. Membrane stabilizing agents are also effective for chronic therapy but are second line agents. Finally, radiofrequency catheter ablation is effective in curing AVNRT in over

Table 8.2 Differential diagnosis of narrow complex regular tachycardia

Rhythm	P wave
Sinus tachycardia	Normal
Sinus nodal re-entrant tachycardia	Normal
Atrial tachycardia	Variable
Atrial flutter	Sawtooth (2:1)
Atrioventricular nodal re-entrant tachycardia	Inverted (superimposed on QRS)
Atrioventricular re-entrant tachycardia	Inverted (superimposed on QRS)

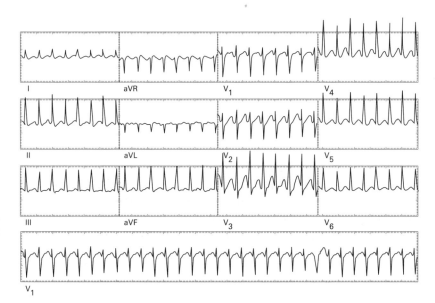

Figure 8.4

90% of patients; it is associated with rare side effects and is now offered as first line therapy in many centers.

Atrioventricular re-entrant tachycardia and Wolff–Parkinson–White syndrome

AV re-entrant tachycardia (AVRT) is the second most common paroxysmal supraventricular tachycardia, accounting for about 30%

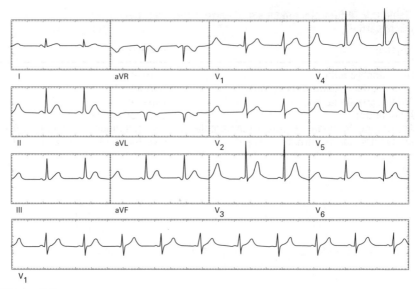

Figure 8.5

of supraventricular tachycardias. The mechanism involves activation of the ventricles using the normal conduction system and re-entry to the atria via an accessory AV pathway (Kent bundle). Accessory pathways are congenital, and may occur in the left or right AV ring or septum. Most commonly, AVRT occurs in patients with Wolff–Parkinson–White (WPW) syndrome. WPW syndrome is defined by a short PR interval, QRS prolongation during sinus rhythm (due to slurring of the upstroke called a δ wave), and symptoms during tachycardia (Figure 8.5). The prolonged QRS in sinus rhythm is caused by pre-excitation of the ventricle down the accessory pathway. During orthodromic tachycardia, the QRS is narrow: anterograde activation of the ventricles occurs down the AV node, whereas retrograde activation of the atria is via the accessory pathway. In some patients with AVRT, the accessory pathway functions only in the retrograde direction; this allows AVRT but gives no evidence of pre-excitation during sinus rhythm.

The electrocardiogram during AVRT may appear identical to that of AVNRT, although the P wave, if visible, occurs distinctly after the QRS (instead of being fused with the QRS complex). The differential diagnosis of regular supraventricular tachycardias and the clues from the P wave are summarized in Table 8.2. The rate of AVRT tends to be slightly faster, and may show alternation in the QRS amplitude or R–R

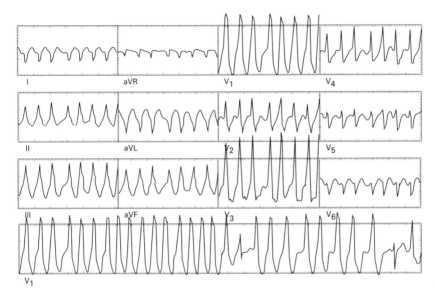

Figure 8.6

interval (QRS or cycle length alternans). The prevalence of the WPW pattern in the general population is 1–3/1000, but less than half of patients with the WPW pattern have tachycardia. WPW syndrome occurs primarily in structurally normal hearts, but there is an association with Ebstein's anomaly and mitral valve prolapse.

Patients with WPW syndrome are also at risk for wide complex tachycardia due to either AF (with conduction down the accessory pathway) or antidromic AVRT (reversal of the usual re-entrant circuit of AVRT, with anterograde activation of the ventricle down the accessory pathway and retrograde activation of the atria via the AV node; Figure 8.6). Antidromic AVRT is quite rare, but pre-excited AF is not uncommon and can cause syncope and even sudden death. Pre-excited AF is recognized by an irregularly irregular wide complex rhythm that may also have occasional narrow beats.

Patients with AVRT present with symptoms of palpitations, chest discomfort, dyspnea, and light-headedness, and rarely true syncope. There is frequently a history of palpitations dating back to childhood. Rarely, a patient presents with sudden cardiac death due to pre-excited AF and subsequent ventricular fibrillation. WPW syndrome should always be considered in the differential diagnosis of a young person resuscitated from sudden death.

The acute management for AVRT is similar to that for AVNRT and is aimed at AV nodal block to terminate paroxysmal supraventricular tachycardia. If vagal maneuvers are not successful, then adenosine is the drug of choice. Alternatively, intravenous verapamil may be administered. On the other hand, if the patient presents with a wide complex tachycardia (pre-excited AF), then AV nodal blocking drugs are contraindicated because they can accelerate the tachycardia by facilitating conduction down the accessory pathway. For pre-excited AF, procainamide is the drug of choice because it blocks conduction in the accessory pathway and may terminate AF.

Chronic medical management for patients who have AVRT but no pre-excitation is similar to that for patients with AVNRT, and any AV nodal blocking drug may be effective. When there is a δ wave present, drugs that impair accessory pathway conduction are indicated (quinidine, procainamide, disopyramide, flecainide, propafenone, sotalol). AV nodal blocking agents are not recommended in the presence of a δ wave because of the potential for accelerating the ventricular response to AF. Alternatively, radiofrequency catheter ablation has become a first line option. In more than 90% of cases a single procedure confirms the mechanism of the paroxysmal supraventricular tachycardia and allows ablation of the accessory pathway.

Ventricular arrhythmias

Monomorphic ventricular tachycardia

Ventricular tachycardia is defined by three or more consecutive QRS complexes of ventricular origin at a rate of over 100 beat/min; "sustained" ventricular tachycardia is defined as lasting greater than 30 seconds or causing hemodynamic compromise. Monomorphic ventricular tachycardia has a uniform morphology and cycle length; conversely, polymorphic ventricular tachycardia is variable in morphology and cycle length.

Over 90% of monomorphic ventricular tachycardia is associated with ischemic heart disease, and is secondary to re-entry in the border zone of a previous myocardial infarction. Monomorphic ventricular tachycardia also occurs in the setting of dilated cardiomyopathy, hypertrophic cardiomyopathy, infiltrative diseases (sarcoid or right ventricular dysplasia), and in the patient who has undergone surgery for congenital heart disease. In addition, monomorphic ventricular tachycardia is occasionally seen in the setting of a structurally normal heart.

The patient with a sustained, regular wide complex tachycardia may present with minimal symptoms, or may experience chest pain, dyspnea, presyncope, syncope, or sudden death. A bedside diagnosis of monomorphic ventricular tachycardia versus supraventricular tachycardia is useful for both acute and chronic management (Box 8.1). The clinical history is critical; prior infarction, coronary disease, or coronary risk factors are all suggestive that a wide complex tachycardia is ventricular tachycardia. Likewise, a history of heart failure or severe hypertension may suggest cardiomyopathy as the etiology of ventricular tachycardia.

Box 8.1 Differential diagnosis of wide complex tachycardia

Ventricular tachycardia
Supraventricular tachycardia: abberancy; fixed intraventricular delay/bundle branch block
Pre-excited supraventricular tachycardia

Patients with ventricular tachycardia are usually hypotensive, but a normal blood pressure does not exclude the diagnosis. Intermittent cannon a waves of the jugular venous waveform and variability in the first heart sound both are consistent with dissociation of atrial and ventricular contraction, and thus suggest the diagnosis of ventricular tachycardia.

Although a number of diagnostic schemes have been published for evaluation of the 12-lead electrocardiogram, a few simple guidelines will help confirm the diagnosis of ventricular tachycardia (as opposed to aberrant supraventricular tachycardia; Box 8.2). AV dissociation is the only finding that is diagnostic of ventricular tachycardia. This is demonstrated by P waves during the tachycardia that march through at a slower rate, or the presence of capture or fusion beats. A capture beat is an early, narrow complex beat originating in the atrium. A fusion beat is seen when the sinus impulse causes a QRS complex that is a combination of the ventricular tachycardia complex and the narrow QRS (Figure 8.7).

Box 8.2 Wide complex tachycardia: criteria for ventricular tachycardia

Atrioventricular dissociation: P waves marching through tachycardia; fusion complexes; capture beats
Absence of RS in all chest leads (V_1–V_6)
QRS morphology: left bundle branch block pattern (monophasic downward in V_1) – >0·16 seconds; right bundle branch block pattern (monophasic upward in V_1) – >0·14 seconds
R/S ratio in V_6 <1 (mostly negative QRS complex in V_6)

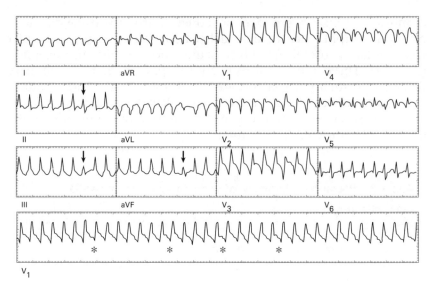

Figure 8.7

The unstable patient with a wide complex tachycardia should undergo immediate direct current cardioversion. If the patient is without hemodynamic compromise or angina, then pharmacologic management is appropriate. The first drug of choice for suspected ventricular tachycardia is lidocaine. If the patient is stable and the diagnosis is in doubt (especially if pre-excited AF is considered), then intravenous procainamide is preferred. If drug therapy is unsuccessful, then cardioversion with synchronized direct current counter-shock (as low as 50 J) is indicated.

After conversion of a wide complex tachycardia has been accomplished, evaluation of the electrocardiogram during sinus rhythm can assist in diagnosis. For example, a δ wave or a bundle branch block similar in morphology to the QRS during tachycardia would suggest a supraventricular origin of the arrhythmia. Following cardioversion of ventricular tachycardia, a patient is observed in a monitored setting and myocardial infarction ruled out. Continued intravenous therapy with lidocaine or procainamide should be considered if the patient was unstable with the ventricular tachycardia.

After infarction has been excluded in the patient with monomorphic ventricular tachycardia, work up for etiology is initiated. Echocardiography is used to assess for the presence of structural heart disease such as infarction, dilated or hypertrophic cardiomyopathy, congenital anomalies, or valvular abnormalities. Patients with coronary risk factors should undergo cardiac catheterization to assess coronary anatomy, and revascularization if indicated. In patients with structurally normal hearts and monomorphic ventricular tachycardia with a left bundle branch block pattern, cardiac magnetic resonance imaging is useful to assess for right ventricular dysplasia. Exercise testing may demonstrate exercise-related ventricular tachycardia. A 24-hour ambulatory (Holter) monitor will quantify the amount of spontaneous ventricular arrhythmias. Clinical electrophysiology study is indicated to confirm the diagnosis and guide therapy.

At electrophysiology study, about 95% of patients with sustained ventricular tachycardia and coronary disease will have their clinical ventricular tachycardia induced by programmed electrical stimulation. This is useful to confirm the diagnosis and to determine whether the patient's ventricular tachycardia may be terminated by overdrive pacing. If the ventricular tachycardia is pace terminable, then the patient may be a candidate for an implantable cardioverter–defibrillator (ICD) with antitachycardia pacing. Traditional management of ventricular tachycardia included serial electrophysiology studies that evaluated the response to one or more antiarrhythmic drugs. The Multicenter Unsustained Tachycardia Trial tested the hypothesis whether antiarrhythmic therapy guided by electrophysiology testing could reduce the risk for arrhythmic death and cardiac arrest in patients with coronary artery disease, reduced cardiac function (left ventricular ejection fraction of 40% or less), and non-sustained ventricular tachycardia.[7] It was found that electrophysiology guided pharmacotherapy conferred no survival benefit, and ICD implantation reduced total mortality and arrhythmic death or cardiac arrest. As an alternative to invasive electrophysiology testing, Holter guided therapy can be considered. Antiarrhythmic agents used for chronic treatment of sustained ventricular tachycardia include quinidine, procainamide, disopyramide, flecainide, propafenone, moricizine, sotalol, and amiodarone. In selected cases, if the ventricular tachycardia is tolerated hemodynamically and is unifocal in origin, then radiofrequency ablation may be effective.

In recent years the ICD has become a mainstay of therapy for patients with hemodynamically significant ventricular tachycardia or sudden cardiac death.[8] The Antiarrhythmics Versus Implantable Defibrillators trial randomly assigned patients resuscitated from ventricular fibrillation or sustained ventricular tachycardia to ICD implantation or antiarrhythmic drugs (mainly amiodarone).[9] It found that ICDs were more effective than antiarrhythmic therapy in reducing arrhythmic cardiac death. ICD implantation has been simplified by the introduction of improved lead systems that are placed transvenously and by reduction in the size of the generator. Newer devices offer both low output cardioversion shocks and antitachycardia pacing to terminate ventricular tachycardia.

In patients with non-ischemic cardiomyopathy and sustained ventricular tachycardia, electrophysiology study is successful in reproducing the clinical ventricular tachycardia in only about 60% of patients. Thus, electrophysiology study may not be useful in diagnosis and guidance of therapy. On the other hand it may be useful to assess for pace terminability of the rhythm, in order to guide selection of ICD if syncope or sudden cardiac death has occurred. Additionally, about 5–10% of patients with a dilated cardiomyopathy and sustained ventricular tachycardia will have a bundle branch re-entrant ventricular tachycardia that is amenable to cure by radiofrequency ablation of the right bundle branch.

There are several ventricular tachycardias that occur in structurally normal hearts. Most commonly, the ventricular tachycardia originates in the right ventricular outflow tract and has a left bundle branch morphology and inferior axis (negative QRS in lead V_1 and positive in leads II, III, and aVF). Salvos of ventricular tachycardia may be almost constant ("repetitive monomorphic ventricular tachycardia"). Episodes of ventricular tachycardia are often exercise-related and suppressed by β-blockers or calcium channel blockers. Another ventricular tachycardia that occurs in structurally normal hearts, known as idiopathic left ventricular tachycardia, originates at the base of the posterior papillary muscle; during ventricular tachycardia the electrocardiogram has a right bundle branch and left axis pattern (positive in V_1, I, and L; negative in F). This rhythm is responsive to verapamil and most antiarrhythmic agents. In addition to being responsive to drug therapy, both right ventricular outflow tract ventricular tachycardia and idiopathic left ventricular tachycardia are amenable to radiofrequency ablation for permanent cure.

Ventricular tachycardia in what appears to be a normal heart may in fact be caused by right ventricular dysplasia. Structurally, there is focal or diffuse fatty infiltration and thinning of the right ventricle. These abnormalities may not be apparent on echocardiogram or cause minor abnormalities on right ventriculogram, but are best visualized with magnetic resonance imaging. Often there may be several different ventricular tachycardia morphologies, all originating from the right ventricle. Because of the risk of sudden cardiac death and the difficulty of suppression or ablation, ICD therapy is usually recommended.

Polymorphic ventricular tachycardia

Polymorphic ventricular tachycardia (PMVT), like monomorphic ventricular tachycardia, may occur in the settings of ischemic and non-ischemic cardiomyopathy. At times, monomorphic ventricular tachycardia will degenerate to PMVT. Likewise, PMVT may degenerate to ventricular fibrillation. The diagnosis is usually obvious, although pre-excited atrial fibrillation in the setting of two or more accessory AV pathways may resemble PMVT.

The mechanism responsible for PMVT is diagnosed according to the presence or absence of QT prolongation on the electrocardiogram during sinus rhythm. In the absence of QT prolongation, PMVT is treated in a similar manner to poorly tolerated monomorphic ventricular tachycardia or ventricular fibrillation. In the presence of QT prolongation, PMVT is called "torsades de pointes".[10] The mechanism for torsades de pointes is believed to be "after-depolarizations" that occur during the prolonged plateau phase of the cardiac action potential. It is recognized in two distinct situations: acquired and congenital. Acquired QT prolongation typically is due to medication toxicity and/or electrolyte abnormalities (such as quinidine or sotalol, and low potassium or low magnesium). Treatment is directed at correcting the precipitating factor and increasing the heart rate with isoproterenol or pacing. Congenital long QT may occur spontaneously or may be inherited in two distinct syndromes. The Jervell–Lange–Nielson syndrome is an autosomal recessive trait and is associated with deafness. The Romano–Ward syndrome is an autosomal dominant trait and is associated with normal hearing. Patients may present with syncope, sudden cardiac death, or simply a family history of sudden cardiac death. They commonly develop arrhythmias during periods of increased adrenergic tone such as fright, exertion, and stress. Management of these patients includes β-blockers, pacemaker therapy, stellate ganglion blockade or resection, and implantation of an ICD.

Ventricular fibrillation and sudden cardiac death

Ventricular fibrillation (VF) is recognized on the electrocardiogram as a coarse undulating baseline without other electrical activity (Figures 8.8 and 8.9). VF often occurs in the same setting as ventricular tachycardia (other than for the "normal heart" ventricular tachycardias) and can result from degeneration of ventricular tachycardia. In addition, primary VF may be a consequence of acute ischemia.

The patient who experiences VF loses consciousness within seconds. If cardiopulmonary resuscitation is not initiated and the arrhythmia persists, irreversible neurologic injury will result within minutes. The first treatment is immediate direct current defibrillation. If the first three shocks do not result in conversion, then direct

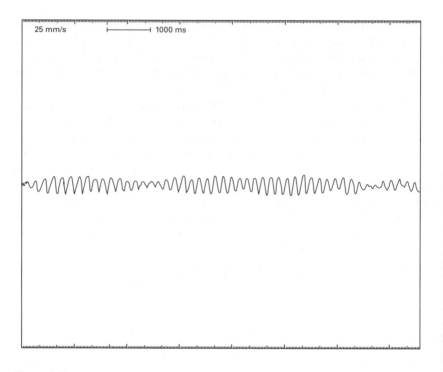

25 mm/s   ⊢―――⊣ 1000 ms

Figure 8.8

current shocks are repeated following epinephrine (adrenaline), then lidocaine, then bretylium.

In spite of improved life support training and paramedic availability, only one patient in three survives out-of-hospital arrest. VF resulting from a reversible cause, such as ischemia, does not require further evaluation or therapy. In the absence of a reversible cause, survivors of cardiac arrest are at high risk for recurrence. VF is typically evaluated by invasive electrophysiology study. The finding of monomorphic ventricular tachycardia implies that ventricular tachycardia may have caused VF. The provocation of VF is a non-specific response, but is significant if the pacing protocol to induce the rhythm is not aggressive. In the past, drug therapy was guided by the serial electrophysiology studies. Recently the use of the ICD has replaced drug therapy in most cases. In addition, empiric amiodarone therapy may improve survival in patients with VF.

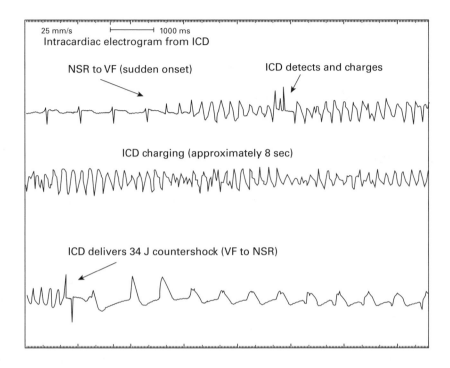

Figure 8.9

Case studies

Case 8.1

A 60-year-old man presents with a 4 day history of palpitations, accompanied by intermittent chest pain; presently, he is pain free. He has a past medical history of hypertension, for which he takes enalapril and furosemide, but has no previous cardiac history.

Examination. Physical examination: blood pressure 150/90 mmHg, pulse 130 beats/min (irregular); respiratory rate 20/min. Neck examination: no thyromegaly or bruits. Cardiovascular examination: no elevation in jugular venous pressure; normal (but irregular) first and second heart sounds. The lungs are clear, and there is no peripheral edema.

Investigations. Laboratory data: normal. Chest x ray: mildly enlarged cardiac silhouette, but no effusions or peripheral vascular redistribution. Electrocardiogram: see Figure 8.3.

Questions

1. What is the diagnosis?
2. What questions should be addressed in order to manage this patient?
3. How would you manage this patient over the first 24 hours?
4. How would you manage this patient subsequently?

Answers

Answer to question 1 The electrocardiogram demonstrates atrial fibrillation with a rapid ventricular response. The chest discomfort may represent angina that has been provoked by rapid atrial fibrillation over the past 4 days.

Answer to question 2 One should investigate for conditions associated with the development of atrial fibrillation, such as hypertension, valvular heart disease, hypertrophic heart disease, coronary artery disease, cardiomyopathy, pulmonary disease, and hyperthyroidism. In particular, we need to know whether he has a history of rheumatic heart disease, risk factors for toxic cardiomyopathies such as alcoholism or drug ingestion, and conditions that predispose him to pulmonary hypertension, including smoking and other exposures. Risk factors for coronary artery disease should be explored. The electrocardiogram does not suggest prior myocardial infarction but demonstrates left ventricular hypertrophy. The chest pain will need to be investigated.

Answer to question 3 The patient should be admitted to a telemetry unit, with rate control and anticoagulation being the two main issues to address. Rate control may be achieved with intravenous β-blockade or calcium channel blockade. Digoxin, long a mainstay of acute therapy, is generally not as effective acutely as these other agents. A ventricular response of less than 100 beats/min should be achieved as soon as possible. The atrial fibrillation has probably persisted for 4 days, which places the patient at increased risk for stroke if cardioversion is performed. Therefore, if rate control is achieved and the patient remains pain free, then we would recommend rate control and anticoagulation acutely. We recommend initially anticoagulating the patient with intravenous heparin.

An echocardiogram should be performed to assess for left ventricular dysfunction, atrial enlargement, valvular heart disease, and atrial thrombus. Thyroid function and arterial blood gas tests (to assess for pulmonary embolus) should be performed. Most clinicians would rule out myocardial infarction with serial cardiac enzymes, although acute myocardial infarction is rarely a cause of atrial fibrillation.

Answer to question 4   Patients with atrial fibrillation of duration greater than 48 hours who tolerate the rhythm after rate control has been established should be anticoagulated for 3 weeks before attempted cardioversion, and for at least 4 weeks following cardioversion. A negative transesophageal echocardiogram, excluding overt intracardiac clots, may lead to consideration of immediate cardioversion without preceding anticoagulation in a patient in whom there is a contraindication to anticoagulation or a special reason for prompt cardioversion.

After anticoagulation with warfarin for 3 weeks, cardioversion can be attempted. This can be performed in the absence of an atrial stabilizing agent or after loading with intravenous procainamide or another class I or III agent by mouth. One advantage of administering an antiarrhythmic agent is that the drug alone will occasionally convert the atrial fibrillation; if an antiarrhythmic drug has been administered, it is often continued for 6–12 weeks and then withdrawn.

Alternative antiarrhythmic agents may be introduced if atrial fibrillation recurs, but if reasonable efforts at maintenance of sinus rhythm fail then rate control becomes the goal of therapy.

Chronic anticoagulation is recommended for patients with chronic or paroxysmal atrial fibrillation who have no contraindication to warfarin. The only exceptions are patients with "lone" atrial fibrillation who are younger than 60 years and are without hypertension, valvular disease, congestive failure, or a history of embolus.

One other issue in this patient is the chest pain. If he remains pain free following control of the ventricular response to atrial fibrillation, one could defer exercise testing until after sinus rhythm has been restored.

Case 8.2

A 51-year-old man presents to the emergency room complaining of palpitations and light-headedness.

Examination. Vital signs are as follows: blood pressure 90/60 mmHg, pulse 220 beats/min; respiratory rate 20/min.

Investigations. Electrocardiogram: see Figure 8.7.

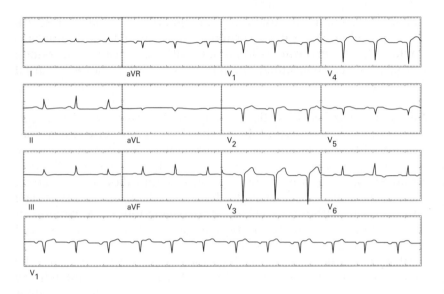

Figure 8.10

Questions

1. What is the differential diagnosis?
2. Further history reveals the patient has no known cardiac history, but he does smoke and has a cholesterol level of 210 mg/dl (5·4 mmol/l). How would you manage him over the next 24 hours?
3. Myocardial infarction is excluded in the patient; however, the electrocardiogram (Figure 8.10) during sinus rhythm shows evidence of an old anteroseptal myocardial infarction. The echocardiogram shows anterior hypokinesis, left ventricular ejection fraction of approximately 35%, and no valvular abnormalities. Cardiac catheterization shows three vessel disease. The coronary care unit attending physician recommends coronary artery bypass grafting but would like your advice before referring him to the cardiothoracic surgeon. What advice would you give?

Answers

Answer to question 1 The electrocardiogram (see Figure 8.7) shows a wide complex tachycardia. The primary differential diagnosis is between supraventricular tachycardia with aberrant conduction and ventricular tachycardia. The patient's age and presence of any risk factors for coronary artery disease would support a diagnosis of ventricular tachycardia. Application of the criteria listed in Box 8.2 assist in the diagnosis. Most importantly, P waves marching through the rhythm (stars on the electrocardiogram) and a fusion beat (seventh beat of each panel, designated by the arrow) provide the diagnosis of ventricular tachycardia.

Answer to question 2 Once the diagnosis is established, cardioversion is necessary. Precordial thump, with defibrillator available in case ventricular fibrillation results, may be successful. Because the rhythm is well tolerated, pharmacologic conversion with lidocaine or procainamide may be tried. If this is unsuccessful or if the patient is unstable, then direct current cardioversion is performed (using sufficient sedation).

The patient should be admitted to the coronary care unit, and myocardial infarction ruled out with serial cardiac enzymes and electrocardiograms. An echocardiogram should be done to assess cardiac ejection fraction and wall motion. Empiric β-blockade, which would be effective in the setting of myocardial infarction as well as some ventricular tachycardias, may be started. If the patient is to be monitored closely with readily available defibrillation equipment, then prophylactic therapy with lidocaine or procainamide may be withheld until further electrophysiologic evaluation unless the rhythm is incessant.

Answer to question 3 Several issues should be addressed. First, it is important to understand that monomorphic ventricular tachycardia is always significant, and in the presence of coronary artery disease is almost always due to re-entry at the border of a prior myocardial infarction. One should not assume that revascularization will eliminate the substrate for ventricular tachycardia. This is in contrast to polymorphic ventricular tachycardia that occurs in the setting of an acute myocardial infarction, which is an acute ischemic rhythm and does not require further evaluation.

Second, the timing of electrophysiologic evaluation needs to be addressed. In general, revascularization should be performed first, followed by programmed electrical stimulation. A patient with coronary disease and clinical ventricular tachycardia will have the rhythm inducible in about 90–95% of cases. Serial antiarrhythmic therapy, with response to programmed stimulation as an end-point, may be attempted. If adequate suppression of the arrhythmia is not achieved, then implantation of an ICD with antitachycardia pacing capabilities should be recommended. In the past, the ICD leads were often placed at the time of surgery; however, with the development of non-thoracotomy ICD lead systems, this is no longer necessary nor recommended.

Case 8.3

A 44-year-old man presents to the emergency room with sudden onset of palpitations and presyncope.

Examination. Blood pressure: 90/60 mmHg. Pulse: >200 beat/min.

Investigations. Electrocardiogram: see Figure 8.4.

Questions

1. What is the differential diagnosis?
2. How would you treat this rhythm acutely?
3. While you are evaluating the patient, he spontaneously develops another rhythm (see Figure 8.6). What is the rhythm and how should it be treated acutely?
4. Following cardioversion with procainamide, an electrocardiogram is obtained (see Figure 8.6). What are your recommendations at this point?

Answers

Answer to question 1   The electrocardiogram shows a narrow complex tachycardia at a rate of almost 200 beats/min, representing supraventricular tachycardia. Inspection of leads V_1, II, and III reveal retrograde P waves just past the QRS complex. The differential diagnosis includes atrioventricular re-entrant tachycardia (AVRT) and atrioventricular nodal re-entrant tachycardia (AVNRT). Atrial tachycardia, sinus tachycardia, or sinus nodal re-entrant tachycardia are less likely because the P wave is closer to the preceding QRS complex rather than the following one (see Table 8.2).

Clues to distinguishing between AVRT and AVNRT can be derived from the history and physical examination. Patients with AVNRT will often note neck pounding, and cannon a waves may be seen on physical examination. This is due to almost simultaneous contraction of the atrium and ventricle, leading to atrial contraction against a closed atrioventricular valve.

Answer to question 2   The tachycardia is probably due to re-entry, and so therapy is directed at terminating conduction in one limb of the circuit. Vagal maneuvers, including carotid massage and Valsalva, may be effective in converting the rhythm. Pharmacologic agents including adenosine, which provides brief but profound atrioventricular nodal block, and verapamil (which is slower in action but nearly as effective) will usually convert the rhythm to sinus.

Answer to question 3 As in Case 8.2, we are faced with the differential diagnosis of a wide complex tachycardia. In this example, the irregular rhythm suggests atrial fibrillation, with the wide complex due to pre-excitation down an accessory atrioventricular connection (Wolff–Parkinson–White [WPW] syndrome). Unlike the situation with the presenting paroxysmal supraventricular tachycardia, nodal blocking drugs are contraindicated; such agents could accelerate the ventricular response and (especially in the case of verapamil) could cause hemodynamic collapse. The treatment of choice is intravenous procainamide, which prolongs refractoriness in the accessory pathway and slows the ventricular response. In addition, procainamide may yield conversion to sinus rhythm because of its atrial stabilizing properties. If conversion is not spontaneous after administration of procainamide, or if hemodynamic compromise should occur, then direct current cardioversion should be performed without delay. Occasionally, pre-excited atrial fibrillation will cause ventricular fibrillation and hemodynamic collapse, which also requires immediate cardioversion.

Answer to question 4 The electrocardiogram shows sinus rhythm with pre-excitation, confirming the diagnosis of the WPW syndrome. This patient has demonstrated a very rapid ventricular response (shortest pre-excited RR interval 230 ms) during atrial fibrillation. Data suggest that patients with WPW syndrome and a pre-excited R–R interval of less than 250 ms are at increased risk of sudden death (presumably due to degeneration of atrial fibrillation to ventricular fibrillation). Although WPW syndrome can be treated with antiarrhythmic medications, electrophysiology study and radiofrequency catheter ablation is the best option for primary therapy.

Case 8.4

You are asked to see a 74-year-old woman on the surgical service. She has enjoyed excellent health but admits to increased fatigue over the past 2 months. The elective resection of a squamous cell tumor on her forehead was postponed because an abnormal electrocardiogram was obtained (see Figure 8.1). Her past medical history is significant for hypertension. She takes hydrochlorothiazide and aspirin daily.

Investigations. Laboratory studies: normal. Echocardiogram: normal left ventricular function, chambers, and valves. There is no evidence of myocardial infarction by history, electrocardiograms, or serum cardiac isoenzyme analysis.

Questions

1. What is her rhythm?
2. What is the etiology of her rhythm?
3. How would you treat this patient?

Answers

Answer to question 1 The electrocardiogram (see Figure 8.1) demonstrates sinus rhythm with complete heart block (third-degree heart block). Analysis of the electrocardiogram reveals more P waves than QRS complexes, and there is no relationship between P waves and QRS complexes. Of note, the ventricular escape is a wide complex at a rate of 45 beats/min. The sinus heart rate is 85 beats/min.

Answer to question 2 Complete heart block may be due to a variety of causes, including acute myocardial infarction, medications (digoxin, verapamil, β-blockers, class I antiarrhythmic agents, or amiodarone), and progressive fibrosis of the conduction system; in some cases it is congenital. Medications need to be excluded as a cause of the heart block in this patient. Interestingly, many patients with congenital complete heart block are indeed asymptomatic despite low ventricular escape rates, but frequently have decreased exercise tolerance. In this patient, however, acquired complete heart block secondary to fibrosis of the conduction system is more likely because of the wide complex escape (as opposed to congenial heart block, which is typically associated with a narrow QRS complex) and the recent onset of symptoms. The acquired nature of the heart block is confirmed by examination of a routine electrocardiogram recorded 10 months earlier (Figure 8.11), which showed sinus rhythm with right bundle branch block and left anterior fascicular block.

Answer to question 3 Because the patient has complete heart block associated with symptoms, most physicians would implant a permanent pacemaker, and would do so before allowing even minor

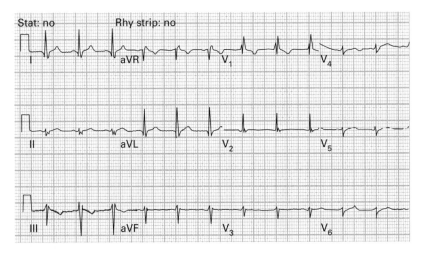

Figure 8.11

elective surgery. Indications for permanent pacing include nearly all cases of complete or type II second-degree atrioventricular block, in addition to most cases of well documented symptomatic bradycardia without reversible cause. This patient should receive a dual chamber pacemaker, which will allow atrioventricular synchrony (sensed P waves will prompt paced ventricular beats).

Case 8.5

A 60-year-old woman in a cardiology clinic complains of syncope. She has a history of paroxysmal atrial fibrillation and hypertension. Her medications include quinidine, digoxin, warfarin, and enalapril.

Examination. Her physical examination reveals an irregularly irregular pulse at 80 beats/min, a 1/6 systolic ejection murmur, clear lung fields, and no peripheral edema.

Investigations. Serum chemistries: normal. Electrocardiogram: atrial fibrillation with a ventricular response of 102 beats/min. Echocardiogram: mild concentric left ventricular hypertrophy, 1+ mitral regurgitation, left atrial size 4·0 cm (normal range 1·9–4·0 cm), and preserved left ventricular function.

Questions

1. How would you manage this patient?
2. On the first hospital day the rhythm converts to sinus. That night a rhythm strip is obtained (see Figure 8.2). How does your management proceed?
3. What type of pacemaker would you implant?

Answers

Answer to question 1   There are a number of causes of syncope, but in this patient one must consider arrhythmias as a primary culprit. Specifically, two possibilities include quinidine associated syncope secondary to torsades de pointes, or tachycardia–bradycardia syndrome. Because sinus mechanism is not maintained, there is no reason to continue the quinidine. The patient should be admitted to a telemetry unit and ruled out for myocardial infarction. An echocardiogram should be obtained because of both atrial fibrillation and syncope.

Answer to question 2   The electrocardiogram shows sinus rhythm slowing and then pausing for 2·3 seconds; at the same time, transient complete heart block is seen with two blocked P waves (resulting in a total pause of 4·6 seconds). A pause during sleep in excess of 3 seconds is occasionally seen in patients without syncope; however, in this setting, the pause represents a reasonable explanation for her syncope.

It is possible that an atrioventricular nodal blocking agent such as digoxin contributed to the pause. Nevertheless, the digoxin (and perhaps increased atrioventricular nodal blockade) is necessary because the ventricular response during atrial fibrillation is not adequately slowed at times (rate of 102 beats/min on arrival). Therefore, a pacemaker would be recommended.

Answer to question 3   The appropriate type of pacemaker is a complex issue in this patient. Although she has failed quinidine, she has maintained sinus rhythm for some period of time while taking an antiarrhythmic. The patient will need to remain hospitalized for discontinuation of warfarin, and initiation of heparin until pacemaker placement. During this time, it is reasonable to initiate therapy with a new atrial stabilizing agent such as propafenone. If she maintains sinus rhythm, then it is reasonable to implant a dual chamber device. There is some evidence that dual chamber pacing helps to prevent the onset of atrial fibrillation.

Case 8.6

A 60-year-old woman collapses suddenly while at work as a custodian in a hospital, and is promptly defibrillated from the rhythm shown in Figure 8.8. Her history reveals that there was no pain or palpitations preceding the event. The past medical history is significant for a dilated cardiomyopathy secondary to hypertension, and paroxysmal atrial fibrillation. A cardiac catheterization 1 year earlier revealed normal coronary arteries, left ventricular ejection fraction of 20%, and minimal mitral regurgitation. Medications on admission were captopril, furosemide, and digoxin.

Questions

1. What is your initial management?
2. The patient's electrocardiogram shows underlying left bundle branch block (unchanged from prior electrocardiograms); over the next 24 hours there are no abnormalities in serum chemistries, and myocardial infarction is excluded. How do you manage her now?
3. At electrophysiologic study there is no inducible tachycardia. Comment on this and how you would further manage the patient.
4. A defibrillator is implanted. At a routine 2 month check up, the patient states that she has been asymptomatic. Interrogation of the device shows the sequence shown in Figure 8.9. What is your interpretation? What would you do next?

Answers

Answer to question 1   This patient has been resuscitated from sudden cardiac death (ventricular fibrillation). She should be admitted to the coronary care unit, and although a cardiac catheterization showed normal coronaries most physicians would rule out myocardial infarction by serial enzymes and electrocardiography over the next 24 hours. Additionally, serum electrolytes, digoxin level, and arterial blood gases are helpful to exclude hypokalemia or hyperkalemia, calcium or magnesium derangements, digitalis toxicity, or pulmonary embolus as possible etiologies of the primary arrest. Ventricular fibrillation can be due to acute ischemia, electrolyte abnormalities, degeneration of torsades de pointes (in this case from pause dependent or acquired QT prolongation), or a primary event.

The use of prophylactic lidocaine or procainamide infusion over the first 24–48 hours is generally unnecessary if the patient is to be monitored in a coronary care unit setting where rapid cardioversion may be performed.

Answer to question 2   Given the normal coronary arteries previously and the absence of myocardial infarction now, ventricular fibrillation secondary to acute ischemia is less likely; this is probably a primary event. An electrophysiologic study is recommended, with several specific questions to answer. Electrophysiologic study will demonstrate whether sinus pauses cause pause-dependent ventricular tachycardia leading to ventricular fibrillation (rare), or whether ventricular tachycardia (that precipitates ventricular fibrillation) can be induced by programmed stimulation. In about 5–10% of patients with dilated cardiomyopathy a special form of ventricular tachycardia, namely bundle branch re-entry, may be induced. This ventricular tachycardia is readily treated by radiofrequency catheter ablation.

Answer to question 3   Electrophysiologic study is less sensitive in patients with dilated cardiomyopathy, as opposed to patients with coronary artery disease. Specifically, clinical ventricular tachycardia can only be induced in about 60% of patients with non-ischemic cardiomyopathy as compared with more than 90–95% of those with coronary artery disease. Given this and the greater than 25% chance of recurrent sudden death in the next 12 months, we would recommend implantation of a cardioverter–defibrillator. An important point to emphasize is that electrophysiologic study in patients with dilated cardiomyopathy is helpful to assess for ventricular tachycardia, which may be ablated or potentially pace terminated by an implantable cardioverter–defibrillator. Electrophysiologic study is not as useful for serial drug testing or assessing prognosis because of relatively low sensitivity and reproducibility.

Answer to question 4   The strip is obtained from the stored electrogram (in the device memory) from the endocardial lead. It shows spontaneous onset of ventricular fibrillation, a detection notation (arrow), a charge time of about 8 seconds, reconfirmation of the rhythm, and internal defibrillation with 34 J to normal sinus rhythm.

The single recurrence of ventricular fibrillation is not uncommon and generally does not warrant a change in therapy; in fact, it confirms that our therapy was appropriate. However, if shocks become frequent then one would add an antiarrhythmic medication in an attempt to reduce the frequency of shocks.

References

1 Kusumoto FM, Goldschlager N. Cardiac pacing (medical progress). *N Engl J Med* 1996;**334**:89–98.

2 Benjamin EJ, Wolf PA, D'Agostino RB, Silbershatz H, Kannel WB, Levy D. Impact of atrial fibrillation on the risk of death: the Framingham Heart Study. *Circulation* 1998;**98**:946–52.

3 Pritchett ELC. Management of atrial fibrillation. *N Engl J Med* 1992;**326**:1264–71.

4 Coplen SE, Antman EM, Berlin JA, Hewitt P, Chalmers TC. Efficacy and safety of quinidine therapy for maintenance of sinus rhythm after cardioversion. A meta-analysis of randomized control trials. *Circulation* 1990;**82**:1106–16.

5 Morady F. Drug therapy: radio-frequency ablation as treatment for cardiac arrhythmias. *N Engl J Med* 1999;**340**:534–44.

6 Camm AJ, Garratt CJ. Adenosine and supraventricular tachycardia. *N Engl J Med* 1991;**325**:1621–9.

7 Buxton AE, Lee KL, Fisher JD, *et al.* A randomized study of the prevention of sudden death in patients with coronary artery disease. *N Engl J Med* 1999; **341**:1882–90.

8 Gregoratus G, Cheitlin MD, Conill A, *et al.* ACC/AHA Guidelines for implantation of cardiac pacemakers and antiarrhythmia devices: a report of the ACC/AHA Taskforce on Practice Guidelines (Committee on Pacemaker Implantation). *J Am Coll Cardiol* 1998;**31**:1175–206.

9 The Antiarrhythmics Versus Implantable Defibrillators Investigators. A comparison of antiarrhythmic drug therapy with implantable defibrillators in patients resuscitated from near-fatal ventricular arrhythmias. *N Engl J Med* 1997;**337**: 1576–83.

10 Smith WM, Gallagher JJ. "Les Torsades de Pointes": an unusual ventricular arrhythmia. *Ann Intern Med* 1980;**93**:578–84.

9: Sudden cardiac death and resuscitation

ROBERT C KOWAL

Sudden cardiac death, defined as death occurring within 1 hour of symptom onset in a person otherwise not suffering from an imminently fatal condition, claims the lives of over 250 000 people each year in the USA.[1] Cardiac arrest, the lethal cessation of cardiac pump function in the absence of rapid intervention, occurs in an additional 500 000 hospitalized patients.[2] Because of the large number of sudden cardiac deaths, attempts are being made to identify patients who are at risk for this fatal event and to initiate cost effective preventive measures. The highest risk patients, who are either survivors of cardiac arrest or patients with coronary artery disease, depressed left ventricular systolic function, and inducible ventricular tachycardia, represent only a minority (10–15%) of sudden cardiac death victims (Figure 9.1). The majority of sudden cardiac death victims occur in lower risk populations at frequencies of 1 or 2 per 1000 with absent or minimal warning before death.

Risk factors for sudden cardiac death

The majority of patients suffering sudden cardiac death have coronary artery disease, and risk factors for the two entities are similar.[3] Hypertension, hyperlipidemia, obesity, diabetes mellitus, and an elevated resting heart rate are all risk factors for sudden cardiac death, and in combination dramatically increase an individual's risk. Studies of sudden cardiac death victims in North America and Europe show that a family history of sudden cardiac death is an independent risk factor.[4] The presence of left ventricular hypertrophy from any cause, interventricular conduction delay manifest on a 12-lead electrocardiogram, and frequent premature ventricular contractions associated with depressed left ventricular systolic function are all associated with increased risk for sudden death.[5] Heavy drinking, lifestyles associated with "high stress",[6] and tobacco use all may increase the risk for sudden cardiac death. Although regular exercise appears to reduce the risk for events caused by coronary artery disease, sudden vigorous exertion appears to trigger sudden cardiac death. The proarrhythmic influence of increased sympathetic tone associated

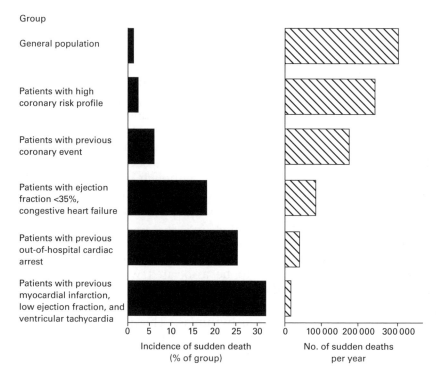

Figure 9.1 Risk for sudden cardiac death versus the yearly incidence of sudden cardiac death by risk group. Note that most deaths occur in the lowest risk population. Adapted with permission from Myerburg and Castellanos[1]

with coronary artery disease or cardiac dysfunction may partly account for this. In certain inherited conditions associated with sudden cardiac death, specific activities have been found to be triggers of arrhythmia; for example, with some hereditary long QT syndromes activities such as swimming or sudden arousal caused by the ringing of a telephone or alarm clock may trigger arrhythmic events.

Cardiac disorders predisposing to sudden cardiac death

Coronary artery disease is found in 70–85% of people suffering sudden cardiac death or resuscitated cardiac arrest.[7] Upward of 50% of persons with sudden cardiac death appear to have an unstable coronary lesion, such as plaque rupture, observed at autopsy.[6] In 20–25% of victims, sudden cardiac death is the first manifestation of coronary artery disease and at least 50% of victims have evidence of prior recognized or "silent" myocardial infarction. The presence of acute myocardial ischemia due to plaque rupture or an imbalance between supply of and demand for oxygen can increase susceptibility to polymorphic ventricular tachycardia or ventricular fibrillation.

In patients with prior myocardial infarction, abnormal electrical conduction in ischemic or scarred myocardium can provide a substrate for re-entrant ventricular tachycardia. In addition to these common associations, the presence of certain rare congenital coronary anomalies, predominantly those in which the left coronary artery traverses between the aorta and the pulmonary artery, are also associated with increased risk for sudden cardiac death. Finally, although coronary vasospastic syndromes typically carry a benign prognosis, in some patients coronary vasospasm may increase the risk for non-sustained, and sustained, polymorphic ventricular tachycardia.[4,6]

Cardiomyopathies unassociated with coronary artery disease are found in some individuals suffering sudden cardiac death, and fast or slow heart rhythms appear to be associated with death in many patients with dilated cardiomyopathy.[8] Patients with infiltrative and infectious cardiomyopathies such as sarcoidosis and Chagas' disease are also prone to ventricular arrhythmias.[4] The risk and incidence of sudden death associated with cardiomyopathy increases with worsening degrees of congestive heart failure, but the absolute number of persons suffering sudden cardiac death is greater in patients with mild to moderate symptoms. This creates the challenge of identifying other prognostic indicators of sudden death.

Some inherited cardiomyopathies increase the risk for sudden cardiac death even in the absence of depressed left ventricular systolic function. Hypertrophic cardiomyopathy is a genetically heterogeneous disorder in which single gene mutations, in a variety of protein components of the sarcomere, lead to abnormal myocyte growth and possibly asymmetric left ventricular hypertrophy associated with obstruction to ventricular outflow.[9] These molecular, cellular, and physiologic abnormalities act together to create an environment susceptible to ventricular tachycardia/ventricular fibrillation. Within the population of patients with hypertrophic cardiomyopathy, sudden death is more likely to occur in those with severe ventricular hypertrophy, early age of presentation, a family history of sudden cardiac death, and a history of prior syncope or a hypotensive response during exercise testing. In addition, molecular genetic analysis has demonstrated mutations in certain genes (for example, that encoding β-myosin heavy chain) carry a significantly greater likelihood of sudden cardiac death than do others.[10] Also, within a given gene, mutations in region of close proximity can result in profoundly differing propensities toward sudden cardiac death.

Arrhythmogenic right ventricular cardiomyopathy, or dysplasia, is a condition that is characterized by fibro-fatty infiltration mainly of right ventricular myocardium, associated with increased likelihood of re-entrant ventricular tachycardia and sudden cardiac death. Fifty percent of cases are inherited; two genetic loci have been identified, and the gene at one of those loci has been identified as the ryanodine receptor, highlighting the importance of calcium homeostasis in myocardial electrical stability.

Patients with congenital heart disease and acquired valvular disease are at increased risk for sudden cardiac death.[1] Congenital and acquired aortic valve stenosis, transposition of the great vessels, pulmonary arterial malformations, and tetralogy of Fallot are all associated with an increased risk of sudden cardiac death.[11] Patients with arrhythmias associated with Wolff–Parkinson–White syndrome are susceptible to sudden cardiac death caused by degeneration of rapid atrial fibrillation to ventricular fibrillation if they have a rapidly conducting accessory pathway (capable of conducting with ventricular coupling of 250 ms or less).

A variety of inherited disorders with normal cardiac structure but associated with increased risk for sudden cardiac death due to ventricular tachycardia/ventricular fibrillation have been elucidated.[4,6,12] The common feature of these conditions is mutations in genes that encode ion channels, typically leading to abnormalities in myocyte repolarization. The best characterized is hereditary long QT syndrome (LQTS). Initially described by Romano and Ward, patients with this syndrome can have variable prolongation of the QT interval and propensity to develop torsades de pointes (polymorphous ventricular tachycardia), as well as hereditary deafness and seizures. The LQTS is a heterogeneous disorder with several known mutations of different chromosomes, which each confer different risks for cardiac events. These mutations lead to defective repolarization with increased early after-depolarizations and torsades de pointes ventricular tachycardia. Four of the affected genes encode subunits of either the delayed or rapidly rectifying potassium currents, and the fifth encodes the gene for SCN5A, a sodium channel that has roles in both myocyte depolarization and repolarization.[4]

Finally, mutations in the gene encoding SCN5A have also been identified in patients with degenerative conduction system disease, placing them at risk for complete heart block and bradycardic arrest.

Reversible causes of sudden cardiac death

A variety of reversible factors appear to increase the propensity for sudden cardiac death.[4,6] Myocardial ischemia can produce significant local drops in tissue pH as well as elevations in extracellular potassium to 10–15 mEq/l (10–15 mmol/l) and increased intracellular calcium

Table 9.1 Medications that can prolong the QT interval

State/drug type	Examples	State/drug type	Examples
Antiarrhythmics		Antihistamine	Astemazole
Class I	Dysopiramide		Terfenadine
	Procainamide		Diphenhydramine
	Quinidine	GI prokinetic	Cisapride
Class III	Sotalol	Psychoactive	Chloral hydrate
	Amiodarone		Haloperidol
Class IV	Bepridil		Lithium
Antibiotic	Erythromycin		Phenothiazines
	Trimethoprim–sulfamethoxazole		Tricyclic antidepressants
Antifungal	Fluconazole	Miscellaneous	Amantadine
	Itraconazole		Indapamide
	Ketoconazole		Probucol
Antiparasitic	Chloroquine		Tacrolimus
	Halofantrine		Vasopressin
	Mefloauine	Electrolytes	Hypokalemia
	Pentamidine		Hypocalcemia
	Quinine		Hypomagnesemia

GI, gastrointestinal

levels. These changes can lead to abnormal automaticity and triggered activity in ventricular myocytes. Decompensated heart failure with associated myocardial stress can also lead to increased intracellular calcium loads. The associated neurohormonal changes in the renin–angiotensin, endothelin, and sympathetic nervous systems can all contribute to induction of lethal ventricular arrhythmia in heart failure and other stress response situations. Finally, a variety of medications can lead to repolarization abnormalities, increasing the likelihood of torsades de pointes, in otherwise normal hearts (Table 9.1).

Resuscitation of cardiac arrest

The likelihood of survival from cardiac arrest is low, especially when ventricular bradyarrhythmias or asystole are the cause.[1] Most effort has been directed toward the resuscitation of victims of the more common ventricular tachyarrhythmias. The American Heart Association developed a multifaceted approach toward the care of patients with out-of-hospital cardiac arrest.[13] The links of this "chain of survival" involve rapid activation of emergency medical systems, rapid restoration of sinus rhythm via direct current defibrillation, maintenance of circulation, and supportive medical care (Box 9.1).[14]

Box 9.1 Summary of the Americal Heart Association protocol for the management of sudden cardiac death due to ventricular fibrillation (VF) and pulseless ventricular tachycardia (VT)

Basic cardiopulmonary resuscitation and defibrillation

1. Check responsiveness of patient
2. Activate emergency response system
3. Call for a defibrillator
4. Primary ABCD survey
   A (Airway) Open the airway
   B (Breathing) Provide positive-pressure ventilations
   C (Circulation) Give chest compressions
   D (Defibrillation) Assess for and shock VF/pulseless VT up to three times if necessary (200 J, 200–300 J, 360 J or biphasic equivalent)
   Is there a rhythm after three shocks?
   If persistent or recurrent VF/VT exists then ...

More advanced cardiopulmonary resuscitation and defibrillation

4a. Secondary ABCD survey
   A (Airway) Place airway device as soon as possible
   B (Breathing) Confirm airway device placement
   C (Circulation) Establish intravenous access, identify rhythm and monitor, administer appropriate drugs
   D (Differential diagnosis) Identify and treat reversible causes
4b. I mg of epinephrine intravenously every 3–5 min
   or
   40 U of vasopressin intravenously once
4c. Resume attempts to defibrillate
5. Consider antiarrhythmics (amiodarone, lidocaine, magnesium, procainamide)
6. Resume attempts to defibrillate

Adapted with permission from Kern et al.[14]

Instrumental to the success of such a program has been widespread training of both medical and lay personnel in the use of cardiopulmonary resuscitation. The combination of chest compression, in order to preserve some degree of circulation, and ventilation is beneficial over short periods of time in preserving survival until emergency care is available. Novel methods of chest compression and decompression are continually being developed.

The single most important factor leading to cardiac arrest survival is rapid restoration of sinus rhythm via defibrillation in cases of ventricular tachycardia/ventricular fibrillation. Mortality increases by 10% with every minute of cardiopulmonary resuscitation alone in the absence of restored sinus rhythm. Overall survival from ventricular tachycardia/ventricular fibrillation arrest depends primarily on time to successful shock delivery.[13] Unfortunately, access to defibrillation is a limiting factor. This has led to the development of portable defibrillators operated by trained emergency medical system personnel, and automated external defibrillators (AEDs) designed to be employed by non-traditional operators.[15] Initial success with such an approach was observed in Seattle, where survival from cardiac arrest improved from 19% to 30% when firefighters used AEDs while waiting for emergency medical personnel to arrive. Further success was recently demonstrated on commercial aircraft, where AED use led to a 40% survival in patients with ventricular fibrillation[16]; and in casinos, where their use yielded 59% survival. In the latter study, if shock delivery occurred within 3 min of witnessed arrest, survival improved to 74%. Currently, larger scale studies of public access defibrillation with AEDs are ongoing.

In cases in which initial defibrillation fails to convert life-threatening rhythms, supportive medical care can be used in conjunction with ongoing cardiopulmonary resuscitation. The initial recommended drug in resuscitation of ventricular tachycardia/ventricular fibrillation has traditionally been epinephrine (adrenaline), which in animal models produces vasoconstriction in order to preserve perfusion pressure. Recently, the option of replacing epinephrine with vasopressin was introduced, stemming from the results of a single study showing its efficacy in cardiac arrest. This agent may have a theoretical advantage over epinephrine by reducing the proarrhythmic influence of catecholamines. Owing to the benefit of early administration of amiodarone, this agent is now the first line antiarrhythmic drug, followed by lidocaine or procainamide if clinically indicated.[14]

Prevention of sudden cardiac death

Survivors of cardiac arrest have a 20–35% risk of recurrence in the year following their initial event, and so secondary prevention is a high priority in these patients. Initial strategies aimed at antiarrhythmic drug therapy guided by Holter monitoring or electrophysiologic studies, or empiric use of amiodarone did not influence long-term survival. β-Blocker therapy modestly reduces overall mortality after myocardial infarction. In the Antiarrhythmics Versus Implantable Defibrillators trial, survivors of cardiac arrest or hemodynamically unstable ventricular tachycardia were randomly assigned to receive either guided antiarrhythmic drug therapy or implantable cardioverter–defibrillator (ICD) therapy.[17] The group receiving ICDs had a 39% reduction in mortality as compared with

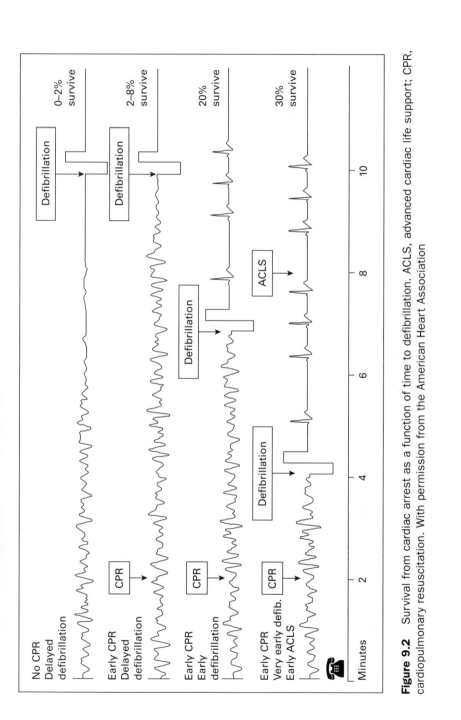

Figure 9.2 Survival from cardiac arrest as a function of time to defibrillation. ACLS, advanced cardiac life support; CPR, cardiopulmonary resuscitation. With permission from the American Heart Association

the drug therapy arm. That trial did not enrol patients with presumed reversible causes of cardiac arrest such as ischemia, electrolyte abnormalities, and use of QT-prolonging drugs, but ICD therapy may also be warranted in such patients.[4]

The high mortality due to cardiac arrest observed in another high risk group, those with depressed left ventricular systolic function due to coronary artery disease and associated frequent ventricular ectopy, has led to attempts at primary prevention of sudden cardiac death. Initial approaches with antiarrhythmic drugs, predominantly class 1C agents to suppress such ectopy, led to increased mortality in treated patients. The Multicenter Automatic Defibrillator Implantation Trial[18] and the Multicenter Unsustained Tachycardia Trial[19] both examined similar patients, randomly assigning those with inducible ventricular tachycardia (following ventricular programmed electrical stimulation) to either ICD versus antiarrhythmic drug and/or placebo. These studies showed a 33–57% reduction in mortality in the groups receiving ICD therapy. Some evidence also supports the use of amiodarone in primary prevention of sudden cardiac death in patients with non-ischemic heart failure.

The success of primary prevention of sudden cardiac death with ICDs in patients with coronary artery disease, depressed left ventricular systolic function, and inducible ventricular tachycardia has led to the expanded use of ICDs in other high risk patients with hypertrophic cardiomyopathy, LQTS, and Brugada syndromes. However, adequate prediction of sudden cardiac death risk remains lacking for the vast majority of lower risk patients.

Conclusion

The mortality from sudden cardiac death remains a large problem, and survival from cardiac arrest remains low. However, the development of widespread emergency systems of rapid response as well as the expanded use of AEDs and novel supportive measures may improve survival in out-of-hospital arrest victims.

References

1   Myerburg RJ, Castellanos A. Cardiac arrest and sudden cardiac death. In: Braunwald, ed. *Heart disease: a textbook of cardiovascular medicine*. Philadelphia, PA: WB Saunders, 1997:742–9.
2   Eisenberg MS, Mengert TJ. Primary care: cardiac resuscitation. *N Engl J Med* 2001; **344**:1304–13.
3   Kannel WB, Schatzkin A. Sudden death: lessons from subsets in population studies. *J Am Coll Cardiol* 1985;**5(suppl)**:141B–9B.

4   Spooner PM, Albert C, Benjamin EJ, *et al.* Sudden cardiac death, genes and arrhythmogenesis: consideration of new population and mechanistic approaches from a National Heart, Lung and Blood Institute workshop, parts I and II. *Circulation* 2001;**103**:2361–4, 2447–52.

5   Bigger JT. Relation between left ventricular dysfunction and ventricular arrhythmias after myocardial infarction. *Am J Cardiol* 1986;**57**:8B–14B.

6   Zipes DP, Wellens HJJ. Sudden cardiac death. *Circulation* 1998;**98**:2334–51.

7   Hinkle LE, Thaler HT. Clinical classification of cardiac deaths. *Circulation* 1982;**65**:447–64.

8   Stevenson WG, Stevenson LW, Middlekauff HR, Saxon LA. Sudden death prevention in patients with advanced ventricular dysfunction. *Circulation* 1993;**88**:2953–61.

9   Spirito P, Seidman CE, McKenna WJ, Maron BJ. The management of hypertrophic cardiomyopathy. *N Engl J Med* 1997;**336**:775–85.

10 Marian AJ, Roberts R. Molecular genetic basis of hypertrophic cardiomyopathy; genetic markers for sudden cardiac death. *J Cardiovasc Electrophysiol* 1998;**9**:88–9.

11 Gatzoulis MA, Till JA, Somerville J, Redington AN. Mechanoelectrical interaction in tetralogy of Fallot: QRS prolongation relates to right ventricular size and predicts malignant ventricular arrhythmias and sudden death. *Circulation* 1995;**92**:231–7.

12 Priori SG, Barhanin J, Hauer RNW, *et al.* Genetic and molecular basis of cardiac arrhythmias: impact on clinical management parts I and II. *Circulation* 1999;**99**:518–28.

13 American Heart Association. Guidelines 2000 for cardiopulmonary resuscitation and emergency cardiovascular care. *Circulation* 2000;**102(suppl)**:I1–I384.

14 Kern KB, Halperin HR, Field J. New guidelines for cardiopulmonary resuscitation and emergency cardiac care: changes in the management of cardiac arrest. *JAMA* 2001;**285**:1267–9.

15 Takata TA, Page RL, Joglar JA. Automated external defibrillators: technical considerations and clinical promise. *Ann Intern Med* 2001;**135**:990–8.

16 Page RL, Joglar JA, Kowal RC, *et al.* Automated external defibrillator use aboard a U.S. airline. *N Engl J Med* 2000;**343**:1210–6.

17 The Antiarrhythmics Versus Implantable Defibrillators (AVID) Investigators. A comparison of antiarrhythmic-drug therapy with implantable defibrillators in patients resuscitated from near-fatal ventricular arrhythmias. *N Engl J Med* 1997;**337**:1576–84.

18 Moss AJ, Hall WJ, Cannom DS, *et al.* Multicenter Automatic Defibrillator Implantation Trial Investigators. Improved survival with an implanted defibrillator in patients wit coronary disease at high risk for ventricular arrhythmia. *N Engl J Med* 1996;**335**:1933–44.

19 Buxton AE, Lee KL, Fisher JD, Josephson ME, Prystowsky EN, Hafley G. A randomized study of the prevention of sudden death in patients with coronary artery disease. Multicenter Unsustained Tachycardia Trial Investigators. *N Engl J Med* 1999;**341**:1882–90.

10: Heart failure and cardiac transplantation

CLYDE W YANCY JR

A definition of congestive heart failure (CHF) should incorporate two major points: the presence of a specific cardiac disease and a mismatch of cardiac performance for a given cellular/metabolic requirement. This is manifested as a clinical syndrome of impaired cardiac output, with evidence of increased ventricular filling pressures due to a cardiac illness. An even simpler definition can be reached: any condition that causes overt cardiac dysfunction resulting in impaired exercise capacity is consistent with the diagnosis of heart failure.

Epidemiology

In North America the prevalence of CHF is 2% in the general population, with an increasing incidence of over 500 000 new cases per year. Beyond age 45 years, the incidence of CHF doubles with each decade. For those who are older than 70 years the incidence of CHF is nearly 10%. The increase in persons affected with CHF has been associated with large increases in healthcare expenditure, and it is the leading cause of hospitalization for persons over the age of 65 years. The inpatient costs alone are in the range of several billion dollars.

The annual mortality rate ranges from 10% to greater than 70% depending on severity. For those patients with impaired ventricular function, but without overt symptoms/signs of reduced cardiac output or volume overload, the average annual mortality is 5–10%. Class I symptomatology implies that the patient is able to function adequately at most normal levels of exertion. Only with extensive effort and/or exercise does that individual become symptomatic. Class I patients have an annual mortality risk of 15%. Class II symptomatology implies that the patient is only comfortable at rest, and during mild to moderate levels of activity, and annual mortality risk in this class is approximately 30%. Class III patients are comfortable only at rest or with mild activity. The annual mortality risk for these patients is 50%. For those patient who have symptoms at rest (i.e. class IV), the annual mortality risk is greater than 70% (Table 10.1).

Of patients with CHF, 50% die suddenly (i.e. symptoms precede death by less than 1 hour). These events may be due to ventricular

Table 10.1 Annual mortality risks associated with various New York Heart Association functional classes

Functional classification of cardiovascular disability	Annual mortality risk (%)
Asymptomatic LV dysfunction	<5
NYHA class I	5–10
NYHA class II	30
NYHA class III	50
NYHA class IV	>70

Definitions of New York Heart Association (NYHA) functional classes are as follows. Class I: patients with cardiac disease but without resulting limitations in physical activity; ordinary physical activity does not cause undue fatigue, palpitation, dyspnea, or anginal pain. Class II: patients with cardiac disease resulting in slight limitation in physical activity; they are comfortable at rest; ordinary physical activity results in fatigue, palpitation, dyspnea, or anginal pain. Class III: patients with cardiac disease resulting in marked limitation in physical activity; they are comfortable at rest; less than ordinary physical activity causes fatigue, palpitation, dyspnea, or anginal pain. Class IV: patients with cardiac disease resulting in inability to carry on any physical activity without discomfort; symptoms of cardiac insufficiency or of the anginal syndrome may be present even at rest; if any physical activity is undertaken, discomfort is increased. LV, left ventricular

arrhythmias, high grade atrioventricular block, asystole, or "pulseless electrical activity", and other patients die as a result of progressive pump dysfunction or the consequences of either pulmonary or systemic emboli.

Even though CHF is a common illness, it should not be treated as a "routine" diagnosis. It is imperative that the severity of the diagnosis be established and that the patient be made aware of the associated prognosis. For younger patients this may prompt consideration of heart transplantation, whereas for older patients with multiple diseases this may prompt a more conservative management strategy.

Etiologies

Ischemic heart disease

Coronary artery disease is the leading cause of congestive heart failure. Of those patients who undergo heart transplantation, 55% have an etiology of end-stage ischemic heart disease. A diligent search for evidence of coronary artery disease should be considered in all patients who present with new onset congestive heart failure. For those patients without angina or prior myocardial infarction, the history may be sufficient. If significant positive risk factors are discovered, then a more aggressive work up may be indicated. Those patients with CHF and a prior history of a myocardial infarction, but without active angina, should undergo either a physiologic or pharmacologic stress test with the concomitant use of an imaging modality. A positive evaluation would warrant cardiac catheterization. Finally, for the patient with CHF and clinical evidence of ischemia, such as active angina, an aggressive work up is warranted, including cardiac catheterization and subsequent revascularization, if appropriate. Patients with an ischemic etiology of CHF have a much poorer prognosis than do those with a non-ischemic etiology, possibly because of the risk for reinfarction and/or the increased risk for cardiac arrhythmias.

Hypertensive heart disease

The Framingham database tabulated the incidence of a number of cardiovascular illnesses by prospectively following an index population from 1949 through the mid-1980s. Heart failure was a common illness. Of those affected by CHF, 75% had an antecedent history of hypertension. Hypertension is associated with heart failure via several mechanisms: it is a risk factor for coronary artery disease; it causes left ventricular hypertrophy, which in turn causes a decrease in ventricular compliance otherwise known as diastolic dysfunction; and the left ventricle is a target for end-organ damage because of the effects of hypertension. Recent data have suggested that the concomitant presence of left ventricular hypertrophy with varying degrees of coronary artery disease leads to a synergistic effect on mortality; for example, single vessel disease with left ventricular hypertrophy may have a worse prognosis than multivessel coronary disease without left ventricular hypertrophy.

Cardiomyopathies

Three major classes of cardiomyopathy are recognized, with numerous etiologies (Figure 10.1)[1]: dilated cardiomyopathy, hypertrophic cardiomyopathy, and restrictive cardiomyopathy.

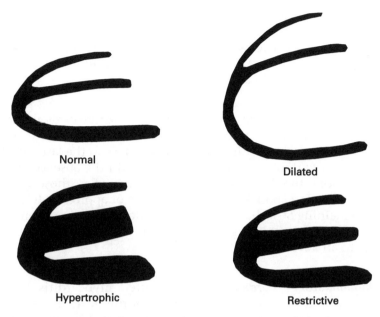

Figure 10.1 Anatomic classification of cardiomyopathy. Dilated cardiomyopathy has increased left and right ventricular chambers and thin walls. Hypertrophic cardiomyopathy demonstrates thickened walls with predominant septal thickening. Restrictive cardiomyopathy has smaller ventricular cavities and thick walls. Reprinted with permission from Hosenpud and Greenberg[1]

Dilated cardiomyopathy

This is the most common primary cardiomyopathy. The etiology of this muscle disease is usually unknown. Familial cases do exist. There appears to be a higher incidence among men. Its course may be indolent, with a 5–10 year period before the development of symptoms of CHF. Cardiac complications include serious arrhythmias, (ventricular tachycardia) and embolic phenomena arising from the severely hypocontractile ventricle with stagnant blood flow. Pathology demonstrates massive hearts with globular configuration and cellular disarray. The echocardiogram can be particularly helpful in establishing anatomy and ventricular size.

Causes of dilated cardiomyopathy are discussed below.

Alcoholic cardiomyopathy Alcohol consumption may be a factor in 20–30% of dilated cardiomyopathies. The drug acts as a negative inotrope and may thus limit cardiac performance. If alcohol consumption can be completely discontinued, then there may be recovery in ventricular performance. For those patients with an alcohol-induced cardiomyopathy, continued drinking results in a 4 year mortality in excess of 50%. For those abstaining, the 4 year mortality is under 10%. Atrial dysrhythmias are commonly associated with alcoholic heart disease.

Postpartum cardiomyopathy Postpartum or peripartum cardiomyopathy is a poorly understood, uncommon condition characterized by the onset of cardiac failure with no identifiable cause in the last month of pregnancy or within 5 months after delivery, in the absence of heart disease before the last month of pregnancy. For those patients affected, there is a spontaneous recovery rate of approximately 50%.[2] Of the remaining 50%, half will have chronically impaired ventricular function and the remaining half will need cardiac transplantation or referral to an advanced treatment facility.

Postinflammatory cardiomyopathy Acute myocarditis is an uncommon but important inflammation of the heart that may lead to permanent damage to the left ventricle. It is presumably mediated by a viral inflammation. The classic virus is coxsackie B. Adenovirus has also been associated with acute myocarditis. A typical viral prodrome may precede the clinical illness, often by weeks. Patients will usually become acutely and severely ill. Endomyocardial biopsy may provide confirmatory information. Some patients may show improvement with supportive therapy and some recovery in ventricular function. The use of immunosuppressive therapy has not led to dramatic improvement.

Hypertrophic cardiomyopathy

Hypertrophic cardiomyopathy is an important cause of heart failure due to diastolic dysfunction. It is relatively infrequent and can be familial. The pathology is classic, with myocardial cells noted for their "whirls and swirls" appearance with disarray of cells. The gross pathology demonstrates heterogeneity of regional hypertrophy and often septal hypertrophy that is disproportionate. This pathology creates a subaortic stenosis (idiopathic subaortic stenosis, idiopathic hypertrophic subaortic stenosis), which may be responsible for a gradient from the left ventricular apex to the left ventricular outflow tract. Because of this pathology, any procedure, maneuver, or event that increases ventricular size or diminishes contractility will decrease the outflow tract obstruction. A particular concern regarding hypertrophic cardiomyopathy is its association with sudden cardiac death in the younger patient. Because the majority of recorded events have taken place during vigorous activity, patients who are found to have obstructive cardiomyopathy are often advised to refrain from competitive sports or physically intense activities.

Restrictive cardiomyopathy

This is usually an acquired condition with scarring and fibrosis of the endocardium. Frequently, an endomyocardial biopsy is indicated to rule out infiltrating causes of restrictive ventricular function, such as amyloidosis, hemachromatosis, or sarcoidosis. Atrial fibrillation and a requirement for chronic anticoagulation typically complicate the management. Restrictive physiology is often associated with volume overload, and diuretic therapy is often required. Left ventricular systolic performance is usually preserved such that inotropic drugs and vasodilators are not indicated.

Valvular heart disease

Both obstructive and regurgitant valvular lesions can be associated with the development of CHF, which is potentially reversible. End-stage aortic stenosis with a major increase in left ventricular afterload may be associated with a significant reduction in left ventricular ejection fraction and increases in left ventricular filling pressures. The presence of aortic stenosis as a cause of CHF may be difficult to diagnose, especially in the elderly, and an echocardiogram is particularly helpful. Those patients found to have CHF due to aortic stenosis can experience a dramatic improvement in CHF if successful aortic valve replacement can be achieved. Once the valvular lesion is corrected, the left ventricular hypertrophy regresses and normal contractility is restored. Conversely, prognosis is poor in patients with symptomatic aortic stenosis complicated by CHF who are treated medically, with survival of 2 years or less.

Aortic regurgitation may also lead to CHF due to chronic volume overload of the left ventricle (i.e. excessive preload). Wall stress increases because there is both ventricular dilatation and hypertrophy, but the hypertrophy does not compensate for the left ventricular dilatation. Even with successful surgery there may be little or no recovery in ventricular function.

Mitral regurgitation often leads to CHF because of volume overload. Wall stress is increased substantially, with little compensatory increase in ventricular wall thickness. The development of heart failure symptoms in a patient with significant mitral regurgitation usually suggests advanced ventricular dysfunction. Surgical replacement of the mitral valve may actually result in deterioration in ventricular function. The concepts of wall stress are based on the law of Laplace, which states the following:

$$\text{Wall stress} = (P \times r)/2h$$

where P is transmural pressure, r is the sphere radius (in this case left ventricular radius), and h is the left ventricular wall thickness.

Increased left ventricular filling, as occurs in volume overload states such as mitral or aortic regurgitation, increases the ventricular radius, and raises wall tension and thus oxygen consumption. Conversely, any physiologic or pharmacologic maneuver that decreases left ventricular filling and size such as blood loss or nitrate therapy decreases wall tension, and hence myocardial oxygen consumption. Circumstances that increase pressure development in the left ventricle (aortic stenosis, hypertension) increase wall tension, and conditions that decrease ventricular pressure reduce it (vasodilator therapy). Finally, wall tension is inversely proportional to ventricular wall thickness. In a hypertrophied heart the force is spread throughout a greater mass that has a lower wall tension and oxygen consumption per gram of tissue than does a heart with thin walls. Thus, when ventricular hypertrophy develops (for example, in chronic pressure overload of aortic stenosis), it can serve a compensatory role in reducing oxygen consumption. In a setting in which ventricular hypertrophy is sufficient to equalize the effects of left ventricular dilatation and/or increased intraventricular pressures, wall stress remains normal and intrinsic ventricular function is unaffected. This is the case with aortic stenosis, but not with aortic regurgitation, mitral regurgitation, or chronic hypertension.

Other causes of congestive heart failure

A host of other illnesses have been associated with impaired ventricular function. Direct toxicity to the heart can occur from the use of adriamycin (an antimetabolite chemotherapeutic agent) or external radiation. Chest wall trauma, either blunt injury or penetrating injury, can damage the heart directly and lead to CHF. Illicit drug use with amphetamines and sympathomimetics (for example, cocaine) can be directly toxic to the heart. Diabetes can lead to a well described diabetic cardiomyopathy that is characterized by diffuse small vessel coronary artery disease, and both systolic and diastolic abnormalities. Thyroid disorders can be particularly toxic to the heart, with hypothyroidism leading to reduced ventricular contractility and pericardial effusions. Hyperthyroidism is associated with an unusual syndrome known as high output heart failure, in which cardiac flow is more than adequate but intraventricular filling pressures are elevated. Significant atrial arrhythmias are known to occur in the setting of hyperthyroidism.

Where does one begin to construct a differential diagnosis for CHF? How does one decide which diagnoses are most likely? The direction of the differential diagnosis and subsequent work up is based on the original history, physical examination, and clinical presentation, and common illnesses should be considered first. Therefore, focus on a careful evaluation for coronary artery disease and on evidence of prior myocardial infarction, hypertensive heart disease, valvular heart disease, and dilated cardiomyopathy. In particular, those illnesses that may be associated with a reversible cause of CHF need to be pursued. Carefully explore prior alcohol exposure, pregnancy history, recent viral prodromes, and evidence of hypothyroidism or hyperthyroidism. The history and physical examination, along with basic laboratory results, electrocardiograms, and x ray films, will dictate any additional work up. An echocardiogram for the patient with new onset CHF is essential.

Pathophysiology of congestive heart failure

Basic mechanisms

If illness results in a significant loss of cardiac myocytes, then CHF will ensue and the prognosis can be quite poor. Cardiac muscle cells, or cardiac myocytes, contain contractile units known as sarcomeres. The sarcomeres are anchored at Z lines and consist of a series of thick (myosin) and thin (actin) filaments. The actin filaments, along with tropomyosin molecules, run in a double helix. The tropomyosin is associated with a troponin complex, which serves as the regulatory protein for actin and myosin contraction. Myosin is responsible for contraction via hydrolysis of high energy phosphates because of its role as an adenosine triphosphate (ATP)ase (Figure 10.2).[1]

The process of myocyte contraction, or excitation–contraction coupling, is initiated with calcium entry in the myocyte. The presence of calcium allows the regulatory troponin complex to convert inactive myosin to active myosin ATPase. The hydrolysis of high energy phosphate bonds generates the energy required for the appropriate interdigitation of actin and myosin, such that cardiac contraction occurs.

Calcium homeostasis is important in preserving normal ventricular function. Ordinarily, calcium enters the myocyte in response to cellular excitation. This process is mediated by the release of catecholamines from sympathetic stimulation. These endogenous

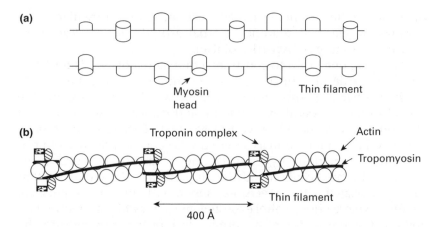

Figure 10.2 Thick and thin filaments. **(a)** Heads of the thick myosin filaments face the thin filament and contain the enzymatic centers to combine with actin. **(b)** The interaction of troponin and tropomyosin controls the binding of actin and myosin. Reprinted with permission from Hosenpud and Greenberg[1]

catecholamines interface with adrenergic receptors (β-receptors) that then cause a conformational change in calcium channels, thus allowing for calcium entry within the cell. Regulatory proteins known as G proteins (both stimulatory and inhibitory) determine the degree to which the activation of adrenergic receptors results in calcium entry. The presence of increased cytosolic calcium leads to a calcium triggered release of calcium from the sarcoplasmic reticulum. It is this release of calcium within the myocyte that initiates excitation–contraction coupling, and it is the active and avid reuptake of calcium that facilitates myocyte relaxation.

In heart failure several sites of disordered calcium handling may be present. Downregulation of the β-receptors has been described and results in attenuation of the neurohormonal response to sympathetic stimulation. Basic disorders of the G proteins may attenuate entry of calcium into the myocyte despite maximal adrenergic stimulation. Calcium released from the sarcoplasmic reticulum to initiate excitation–contraction coupling may not be actively sequestered back into the sarcoplasmic reticulum. This may cause impairment of cardiac relaxation, which is clinically evident as diastolic dysfunction. Eventually, stores of calcium in the sarcoplasmic reticulum are depleted and myocyte contractility is reduced, which is clinically evident as systolic dysfunction. Mitochondria do not usually serve as a store for calcium, but in heart failure mitochondria absorb excess cytosolic calcium that is not resorbed by the sarcoplasmic reticulum. However, this only uncouples the electron transport chain, which is a major source of ATP generation, thus restricting availability of high

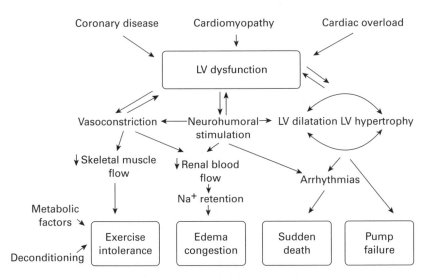

Figure 10.3 Interaction of various pathophysiologic mechanisms that lead to heart failure. Note the central role of neurohormonal stimulation. LV, left ventricular. Reprinted with permission from Hosenpud and Greenberg[1]

energy phosphate compounds for myocyte contraction. One or more of these sites of disordered calcium handling is responsible for the cellular dysfunction in cardiac contraction and relaxation, which is responsible for the heart failure syndrome. All treatment strategies designed to improve left ventricular contraction do so by increasing the available supply of intracellular calcium, and drugs that impede the delivery of calcium to the myocyte are associated with negative inotropic properties.

Neurohormonal compensatory mechanisms

Vasoeffector neurohormonal systems defend against intravascular volume shifts (Figure 10.3).[1] These systems act to preserve regional blood flow, maintain blood pressure, and restore intravascular volume in the event of hemorrhage or volume depletion. CHF results in chronic stimulation of these systems, perpetuating heart failure and injuring myocytes.

With reduced cardiac output and diminished effective arterial blood volume, baroreceptors increase sympathetic stimulation. Evidence supporting the presence of a stimulated sympathetic nervous system in CHF comes from elevated circulating levels of norepinephrine (noradrenaline) and increased sympathetic nerve traffic. The high concentration of norepinephrine at the synaptic cleft results in downregulation of adrenergic or β-receptors. The increased circulating levels of norepinephrine are also directly toxic to the myocardium, and result in myocardial ischemia and arrhythmias. The most significant effect, however, is the increase in peripheral vasomotor tone, or vasoconstriction, which contributes substantially to an increase in impedance to ventricular ejection known as afterload. Further impairment in left ventricular systolic function ensues, with a reduction in cardiac output and additional baroreceptor mediated stimulation of the sympathetic nervous system, thus creating a cycle of worsening heart failure.

Activation of the sympathetic nervous system also results in decreased renal blood flow, decreased glomerular filtration rate, and an increase in tubular reabsorption of sodium. These effects lead to the production of renin, which initiates stimulation of the renin–angiotensin system. The renin–angiotensin system is both systemic and local (i.e. tissue sites of angiotensin II production). In either circumstance, renin acts on angiotensinogen to produce angiotensin I. The latter is acted upon by angiotensin-converting enzyme to produce angiotensin II, which then circulates and interfaces with angiotensin II receptors. It is the union of effector hormone and receptor (i.e. angiotensin II/angiotensin II receptor complex) that mediates vasoconstriction, cellular hypertrophy, and release of aldosterone, which results in sodium and water retention via renal tubular mechanisms. Once again, the vasoconstrictor influences are profound and contribute further to increased ventricular afterload and further impairment in ventricular function. The sodium and water retention leads directly to an increase in blood volume and ultimately to an increase in ventricular end-diastolic pressures. Increased circulating levels of angiotensin II are directly toxic to the myocardium and are associated with arrhythmias. The overall effects of stimulation of the renin–angiotensin–aldosterone system are vasoconstriction, volume overload, myocardial hypertrophy, and cardiac arrhythmias, all of which perpetuate the heart failure syndrome.

Endothelin, another vasoconstricting hormone, is also released in heart failure. It is released from endothelial cells in response to norepinephrine. The degree of release is related most closely to the increase in intracardiac filling pressures. Arginine vasopressin is released from the posterior pituitary in response to hyperosmolar states and causes an increase in free water absorption. It also has vasoconstrictor properties and is a negative inotrope. In heart failure it is not released in response to hyperosmolarity, but rather in response to the effects of angiotensin II stimulation of the pituitary.

Along with the release of these vasoconstricting substances, there is the counterregulatory release of endogenous vasodilators.

288

Atrial natriuretic peptide is a hormone that is released directly from the atria. Its effects are to cause vasodilatation and sodium and water excretion. It is released in response to atrial stretch. Therefore, it serves as a counterregulatory response to sympathetic stimulation and renin–angiotensin–aldosterone activation. Because the overall vasomotor tone in heart failure is vasoconstriction, the vasodilatory effects of atrial natriuretic peptide are presumed to be weak. However, the emerging understanding of natriuretic peptides lends itself well to newer diagnostic and therapeutic strategies.

Endothelial derived relaxing factor is derived from the vascular endothelium and causes vascular smooth muscle cell vasodilatation. Its production appears to be related to blood flow such that in states of decreased flow (i.e. CHF) less endothelial derived relaxing factor is produced. A new area of investigation in heart failure focuses on cytokines that may play a role in CHF. Currently interleukin-1, interleukin-6, and tumor necrosis factor have been identified as being stimulated in CHF.

The degree of neurohormonal activation in heart failure can be determined from the degree of hyponatremia. The serum sodium concentration is inversely related to the degree of neurohormonal activation, such that high levels of renin, angiotensin II, aldosterone, and plasma norepinephrine are associated with serum sodium levels below 137 mEq/l (137 mmol/l), and even below 130 mEq/l (130 mmol/l). In fact, serum sodium below 130 mEq/l (130 mmol/l) is among the most serious adverse prognostic indicators in CHF.

Hemodynamic mechanisms of heart failure

The Frank–Starling law of the heart states that the velocity of cardiac contraction is a direct function of the end-diastolic volume or the diastolic stretch on the sarcomere (Figure 10.4).[1] Preload is the clinical assessment of the degree of stretch on the sarcomere, which is usually determined by the end-diastolic filling pressure. The end-diastolic pressure is most significantly affected by the degree of volume expansion due to sodium and water retention and by the inherent stiffness of the ventricle, known as ventricular compliance. For the same degree of distending volume, a pliable left ventricle will generate lower filling pressure than a stiff ventricle. The clinical expression of increased preload is atrial hypertension, given that atrial pressures are generally equivalent to their corresponding ventricular end-diastolic pressure in the absence of mitral or tricuspid stenosis. Increased preload of the right ventricle results in increased central venous pressures, which results in hepatomegaly, splanchnic congestion, ascites, and edema. Increased preload of the left ventricle results in increased left

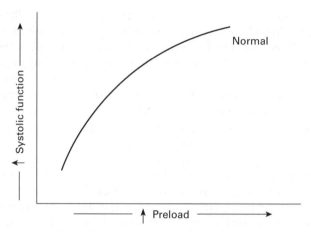

Figure 10.4 Frank–Starling law of cardiac contraction. Systolic function varies directly as preload increases. Reprinted with permission from Hosenpud and Greenberg[1]

atrial pressures, pulmonary venous hypertension, and pulmonary congestion (for example, dyspnea on exertion, orthopnea, etc.).

Ventricular afterload is the summation of forces that the ventricle must overcome to eject its contents. As such, it is a complex entity that encompasses systolic blood pressure, systemic arterial vasoconstriction, compliance or elasticity of the great vessels, and wall stress. Increased ventricular afterload leads to a decrease in left ventricular systolic function for varying degrees of ventricular dysfunction (Figure 10.5a).[1] Conversely, a reduction in left ventricular afterload via the use of vasodilators will result in improvement in left ventricular systolic function (Figure 10.5b).

In general, any clinical evidence of right and/or left atrial hypertension is an indication for diuretic therapy, given that it suggests increased preload. Diuresis should not, however, be too vigorous. Based on the Frank–Starling law, diuresis to the point that the patient is on the ascending limb of the Starling curve is deleterious because it is associated with decreased cardiac contractility, diminished stroke volume, and decreased cardiac output. Although symptoms of excessive afterload are less obvious clinically, the impact of reduced left ventricular afterload is so substantial that vasodilator therapy should always be considered in patients with left ventricular systolic dysfunction.

Diastolic heart failure

Nearly 40% of patients presenting with heart failure have normal systolic function but abnormal diastolic function due to cardiac

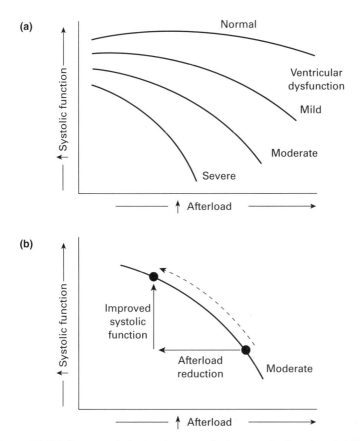

Figure 10.5 Influence of afterload on ventricular systolic function. **(a)** For varying degrees of left ventricular (LV) systolic dysfunction, increasing afterload causes a progressive decrease in systolic function. This is most striking for severe ventricular dysfunction. **(b)** A reduction in afterload is associated with improved systolic function (i.e. systolic function varies inversely with afterload). Reprinted with permission from Hosenpud and Greenberg[1]

diseases associated with impaired ventricular relaxation or left ventricular filling (Box 10.1, Figure 10.6).[1] The most common form of diastolic dysfunction is due to decreased ventricular compliance as a result of increased stiffness. This is classically seen in hypertrophied states, such as chronic hypertension or hypertrophic cardiomyopathy. Impaired ventricular filling may also result from mitral stenosis or pericardial diseases. Because diastole is composed of at least two phases, namely passive and active filling (the latter being the result of atrial systole), diastolic dysfunction is an abnormality not only of ventricular filling but also of atrial contraction. Atrial arrhythmias, especially atrial fibrillation, may lead to heart failure or exacerbate heart failure via less efficient ventricular filling during the active

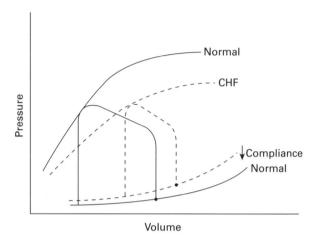

Figure 10.6 Pressure–volume curves for normal heart function and heart failure. The curve shifts to the right, which is indicative of systolic dysfunction, and upward because of diastolic dysfunction. Reprinted with permission from Hosenpud and Greenberg[1]

phase of diastole. Restoration of atrial synchrony may be among the most effective therapies for symptomatic heart failure.

Box 10.1 Causes of heart failure due to diastolic dysfunction

Abnormal cardiac relaxation, for example myocardial ischemia and cardiac hypertrophy (hypertension)

Abnormal ventricular compliance (higher filling pressures are required to fill a "stiffer" or "less elastic" ventricle), for example restrictive and hypertrophic cardiomyopathies

Abnormal atrial contraction: the presence of atrial fibrillation or atrioventricular asynchrony adds to diastolic dysfunction, especially if there is abnormal cardiac relaxation or compliance

---

Evaluation of the patient with congestive heart failure

With a careful clinical history and examination, including an electrocardiogram and chest x ray film, the diagnosis of heart failure can be made. With the addition of basic laboratory data and an echocardiogram, the etiology and prognosis can usually be determined (Table 10.2). There must be evidence from the history that the cardiac performance is insufficient for the needs of that patient.

Table 10.2 Evaluation of the heart failure patient

Aspect of evaluation	Details
History	Establish diagnosis; identify underlying heart disease; assess symptoms of right and left heart failure; establish severity of CHF
Physical examination	Assess vital signs; look for jugular venous distension; chest examination to establish absence or presence of pulmonary congestion; identify S_3, S_4, murmurs; identify ascites, hepatomegaly; identify edema
Laboratory database	Sodium, potassium, creatinine, blood urea nitrogen, hemoglobin, thyroid function tests
Electrocardiogram	Look for atrial fibrillation; left ventricular hypertrophy, Q waves
Chest x ray	Establish heart size, pulmonary congestion
Echocardiogram	Cardiac dimensions and function, cardiac anatomy, valvular lesions
Right heart catheterization*	Assess hemodynamics, monitor therapy
Endomyocardial biopsy*	Evaluate causes of acute heart failure or restrictive cardiomyopathy
Coronary arteriography*	Evaluate CAD
Stress perfusion imaging*	Evaluate CAD
Cardiopulmonary stress testing*	Determine aerobic capacity; predict survival in pretransplant patients

*Data acquisition for advanced heart failure. CAD, coronary artery disease; CHF, congestive heart failure; $S_{3/4}$, third/fourth heart sound

Table 10.3 Summary of symptoms in congestive heart failure

Left heart failure symptoms	Right heart failure symptoms
Dyspnea on exertion	Lower extremity swelling
Orthopnea	Abdominal fullness
Paroxysmal nocturnal dyspnea	Increasing girth
Nocturnal cough	Right upper quadrant discomfort
Pulmonary edema	Weight gain

The usual symptoms that one pursues relate to volume overload, diminished cardiac output, and symptomatic arrhythmias. Right sided heart failure results in clinical evidence of increased central venous pressures. One looks for weight gain, visible edema, bloating, increasing abdominal girth, and abdominal pain from splanchnic congestion or hepatic swelling (Table 10.3). Left sided heart failure results in clinical evidence of pulmonary venous congestion. One looks for abnormal dyspnea. Dyspnea on exertion accompanies pulmonary venous hypertension. Orthopnea implies slightly greater pulmonary venous hypertension, with discomfort and dyspnea noted in a recumbent position. Paroxysmal nocturnal dyspnea is a more severe form of symptomatology, with the patient awakened with episodic symptoms of heart failure. The most severe clinical expression of left heart failure is overt pulmonary edema, with rest breathlessness, cough, and blood tinged or pink sputum production (see Table 10.3).

History

In order to discover the presence of any prior or underlying cardiac disease responsible for the ventricular dysfunction, pertinent questions include those pertaining to the following: risk factors for coronary artery disease, prior myocardial infarction, current angina, prior bypass surgery or other revascularization, hypertension, known valvular heart disease, prior valve surgery, recent pregnancy if applicable, alcohol intake, known thyroid disease, or any suspicious family history of heart failure. A relatively recent onset of symptoms should prompt questions regarding an antecedent viral prodrome or toxin exposure. Irrespective of socioeconomic status, no history is complete without a query regarding illicit drug exposure.

Physical examination

The physical examination identifies signs that are consistent with the diagnosis of heart failure. Weight is important as a baseline to use to monitor the effects of therapy. The presence of tachypnea and the use of accessory muscles of respiration should raise the question of dyspnea and thus place CHF in the differential diagnosis. A resting tachycardia is an important finding of left ventricular dysfunction if all other reasonable causes of tachycardia can be ruled out. A low volume, thready pulse is consistent with a severely reduced cardiac output. A narrow pulse pressure is indicative of a severely reduced cardiac index (i.e. <2·5 l/min per m^2) and supports the diagnosis of systolic dysfunction. An important finding is that of an alternating weak and strong beat, known as pulsus alternans, which has been shown to be associated with poor ventricular function. Hypotension due to heart failure alone is usually consistent with poor ventricular function. If patients have hypertension and symptoms of CHF, then they typically have some degree of diastolic dysfunction or diastolic heart failure.

Jugular venous pulse

The level of the jugular venous pulse (JVP) allows estimation of the filling pressure of the right heart (i.e. the central venous filling pressure.[3] It is elevated with heart failure, hypervolemia, conditions that reduce compliance (or increase "stiffness") of the right ventricle, constrictive pericarditis, and obstruction of the superior vena cava. To assess the JVP the right internal jugular vein is usually examined with the patient in a supine position, their back, head, and neck inclined at a 30–45° angle. In the absence of obesity the pulsations of the jugular veins are transmitted to the skin. The maximal height of the JVP above the heart, with the patient lying at 45°, closely reflects mean right atrial pressure. A perpendicular plane is extended from the highest point at which the jugular venous pulsation is seen to the sternal angle. The height from the sternal angle is measured. Because the right atrium is approximately 5 cm below the sternal angle, 5 cm is added to the height of the JVP seen above the sternal angle. This approximates jugular venous pressure in centimeters of water. The upper limit of normal for JVP is 4 cm above the sternal angle or a central venous pressure of 9 cm. With a patient sitting in a 90° upright position any visible venous waveform is abnormally elevated. In some patients, with severe elevation in right heart filling pressures, the patient will need to sit upright so that the pulses can be visualized and the right atrial pressure estimated.

Auscultation

Percussion of the chest may identify pleural effusions, which are not uncommon in chronic heart failure. Auscultation is necessary to identify evidence of pulmonary venous congestion. The classic finding is the presence of rales (fine noises that resemble the sound of Velcro® being released); however, the presence of clear lungs should not steer one away from the diagnosis of heart failure if it is otherwise clinically supported.

Inspection of the precordium may reveal a hyperdynamic ventricle. The point of maximal cardiac impulse should be sought with palpation. Normally, it is a discrete impulse that is transient and occurs with the first heart sound (S_1). In heart failure it may be a diffuse and/or sustained impulse that is due to ventricular dilatation.

An important auscultatory finding is the presence of a third heart sound (S_3), which is a mid-diastolic sound best heard with the stethoscope "bell" applied lightly with the patient in the left lateral decubitus position. The S_3 occurs during the rapid filling phase of the ventricle, occurring after closure of the aortic and pulmonary valves, and coinciding with the wide ascent of the atrial pressure pulse. In children, young adults, and women during pregnancy an S_3 may be a normal finding. An abnormal S_3 may be generated if the ventricle is dysfunctional (heart failure) or if there is an increase in flow during the rapid filling phase of the ventricles (mitral and tricuspid regurgitation). An S_3 at the lower left sternal border that is accentuated with inspiration is a right sided S_3 and is consistent with right ventricular dysfunction.

The fourth heart sound (S_4) is probably never a normal finding. It is a late diastolic (or presystolic) sound and is generated within the ventricle during the atrial filling phase. Active atrial systole is required to generate an S_4 and the sound is not heard in patients with atrial fibrillation when coordinated atrial contraction is absent. An S_4 is typically generated in situations in which the ventricle is "stiff" or "non-compliant", and augmented atrial contraction is needed to fill the ventricle appropriately. Such situations include left ventricular hypertrophy associated with hypertension or aortic valve stenosis; right ventricular hypertrophy associated with pulmonary hypertension or pulmonary stenosis; and acute myocardial ischemia with a stiff, non-compliant left ventricle. When these sounds originate from the left ventricle they are best heard with the patient in the left lateral decubitus position, applying the bell of the stethoscope lightly to the cardiac apex. When the sounds originate from the right ventricle they may be best heard at the left lower sternal edge with the patient supine, and may be accentuated by inspiration.

In order to properly identify S_3 or S_4, it is best first to identify S_1 correctly. This is best accomplished by simultaneously palpating the right carotid artery upstroke and listening to the heart sounds. The heart sound that corresponds with the carotid upstroke is S_1. A low intensity additional sound noted just before S_1 represents an S_4 gallop. A louder sound present at the apex of the heart occurring after S_1 and S_2 is an S_3 gallop. No murmur is pathognomonic for heart failure; however, the presence of atrioventricular valvular regurgitation is consistent with ventricular dilatation, with stretch of the valvular annulus and subsequent AV leak (i.e. either mitral or tricuspid insufficiency).

Abdominal examination

The abdominal examination may reveal overt ascites, a dramatic consequence of central venous pressure elevation or hepatomegaly. A positive hepatojugular reflux may expose early clinical evidence of right heart failure. Edema is due to the abnormal presence of excess extracellular fluid, caused by an imbalance of Starling forces at the capillary–interstitium interface. Forces that keep fluid within the intravascular space include extrinsic pressure from the extravascular space and the oncotic pressure of intravascular fluids. Forces that cause fluid to exit from the intravascular space include the hydrostatic pressure of intravascular volume and laxity of gap junctions between

Table 10.4 Summary of clinical signs of congestive heart failure

Left heart failure signs	Right heart failure signs
Rales, crackles	Jugular venous distension
S_3 gallop	Tricuspid regurgitation
S_4 gallop	Right sided S_3 gallop
Mitral insufficiency	Hepatomegaly
Displaced, diffuse point of	Ascites
maximal impulse	Edema: ankle, pretibial, sacral
Pulsus alternans	

$S_{3/4}$, third/fourth heart sound

vessel endothelial cells. These latter forces that result in the exit of fluid from the intravascular space predominate in heart failure and result in the formation of edema. In the average adult, edema formation is usually indicative of at least 5–10 lb of excess extravascular volume. Therefore, even "mild" amounts of edema should be considered to be a major clinical problem.

When assessing for the presence of edema, remember to assess the dependent sites. A patient in bed with the lower extremities elevated may have little or no ankle edema. However, that same patient will have marked sacral edema. Not infrequently one can find evidence of edema in the upper thighs, abdominal wall, scrotum, chest wall, and eyelids (Table 10.4).

Investigations

Laboratory assessment

The laboratory assessment should include electrolytes, especially serum sodium, creatinine, blood urea nitrogen, hematology, and thyroid function tests. Hyponatremia is related to the degree of neurohormonal activation. The presence of concomitant renal insufficiency will either suggest an alternative etiology for the volume overload state or pharmacotherapeutic limitations. Patients with severe anemia may have easily provocable ischemic heart disease. Both hyperthyroid and hypothyroid states are associated with heart failure. Repeatedly, multivariate analyses of survival characteristics in heart failure demonstrate that cardiomegaly on a plain film chest radiograph is predictive of a poor prognosis. The standard definition of cardiomegaly on chest radiograph is a cardiothoracic ratio greater than 0·55 (or heart diameter/thoracic diameter >0·55).

Electrocardiogram

Although the electrocardiogram does not reveal any definitive findings of heart failure, it will reveal concurrent or pre-existing cardiac disease. Pathological Q waves, poor R wave progression, or resting ST/T wave abnormalities are all indicative of ischemic heart disease. Left ventricular hypertrophy may suggest chronic hypertension, valvular heart disease, or cardiomyopathy. The presence of atrial arrhythmias reveals additional therapeutic interventions that will be necessary.

Echocardiogram

The echocardiogram is perhaps the most useful adjunctive test in the assessment of newly diagnosed heart failure. Left ventricular dimensions are readily measured; the distinction between left ventricular systolic dysfunction and diastolic dysfunction can be made; mitral and tricuspid regurgitation are assessed; and anatomic features consistent with a dilated, restrictive, ischemic, or a hypertrophic cardiomyopathy may be identified.

Resting radionuclide ventriculogram

The resting radionuclide ventriculogram is a useful non-invasive tool for assessing ventricular function in a quantitative manner, and a test done with exercise will provide information about cardiac functional reserve.

Cardiac catheterization

In advanced heart failure or challenging clinical situations, invasive hemodynamics using diagnostic right heart catheterization to measure the filling pressures and cardiac output allows definitive assessment of hemodynamics and more aggressive medical therapy guided by hemodynamic responses. Classic systolic heart failure is characterized by a cardiac index below 2·5 l/min per m^2 and a pulmonary capillary wedge pressure greater than 18 mmHg. Successful therapy of severe heart failure guided by hemodynamic therapy results in a cardiac index of 2·5–3·0 l/min per m^2 and a pulmonary capillary wedge pressure below 15 mmHg, while maintaining a systolic blood pressure in excess of 80 mmHg.

Endomyocardial biopsy

Endomyocardial biopsy is infrequently indicated. It is most helpful in establishing the absence or presence of inflammation associated with acute myocarditis and in resolving the etiology of restrictive cardiomyopathies. It is a much more common procedure in transplanted patients, in whom frequent assessments for rejection occur.

Stress testing

In patients with an indeterminate risk for coronary artery disease, use of a stress (either physiologic or pharmacologic) perfusion imaging evaluation can be helpful in determining whether more aggressive evaluation for coronary artery disease is indicated. Coronary arteriography is indicated whenever there is any question of clinically important coronary artery disease.

The quantitative assessment of exercise capacity using direct measure of gas exchange during treadmill or bicycle exercise can be very useful. Cardiopulmonary stress testing determines the maximal delivery of oxygen to exercising muscles, allowing a precise evaluation of aerobic capacity and indirectly reflecting the maximal cardiac output or reserve. The expected normal range of oxygen uptake for untrained individuals is 2–3 l O_2/min. The very fit athlete is able to consume 3–4 l O_2/min or greater. In patients with severe heart failure, the maximal oxygen consumption is below 1 l O_2/min. When indexed to body weight, normal oxygen consumption is 25–35 ml/kg per min; in those who are fit it is greater than 40 ml/kg per min whereas in the presence of heart failure below 20 ml/kg per min. Within the group with heart failure, those patients with a maximal oxygen consumption below 15 ml/kg per min demonstrate the poorest 1 year survival and are candidates for cardiac transplantation.

Therapy for congestive heart failure

An algorithm for the management of CHF is presented in Table 10.5.

Improved survival, decreased hospitalizations, and improved exercise capabilities are all possible with current therapy for heart failure.[4] Heart failure is characterized by both hemodynamic and neurohormonal alterations, and drug therapy is targeted at mechanisms that perpetuate the syndrome (neurohormonal responses) and those that generate the overt symptoms of heart failure (hemodynamic abnormalities; Table 10.6).

An appropriate adjustment in lifestyle is the correct first step in any treatment algorithm for heart failure.[5] Restricted sodium intake is imperative if edematous states are to be controlled. Patients should be instructed to avoid added salt to their diets and to adhere to a 2000 mg

Table 10.5 Treatment algorithm for congestive heart failure

Step	Details
1 Initial presentation	General measures of sodium and fluid restriction; β-blockers and ACE inhibitors; titrate to target doses Diuretics if volume overloaded Work up for reversible etiologies Assess nature of cardiac disease Evaluate left ventricular function Add in therapy if LVEF <30%
2 Persistent symptoms	Additional sodium and water restrictions Titrate ACE inhibitors to maximal dose At least triple therapy with diuretics, β-blockers, ACE inhibitors and/or spironolactone; consider addition of direct vasodilators Add digoxin in patients in NYHA class III or IV If the etiology of CHF is ischemic, then is the patient a candidate for high risk revascularization?
3 Refractory to step 2	Inpatient evaluation is warranted Change diuretics to intravenous route Proceed with right heart catheterization to define hemodynamics and adjust therapy Consider parenteral therapy with intravenous vasodilators and inotropes
4 Refractory to step 3	Evaluate prognostic characteristics: LVEF (<20%) Serum [Na^+] (<135 mEq/l [<135 mmol/l]) Presence of ventricular arrhythmias Exercise capacity (maximal O_2 consumption <15 ml/kg per min) Cardiac size (left ventricular diastolic dimension >6 cm) Hemodynamic profile (cardiac index <2·0 l/min per m^2; PCWP >18 mmHg) Uncorrectable ischemia If the prognosis is poor, then determine transplant candidacy or experimental protocol participation

ACE, angiotensin-converting enzyme; LVEF, left ventricular ejection fraction; NYHA, New York Heart Association; PWCP, pulmonary capillary wedge pressure

sodium intake or less. Because of the increased drive for thirst in CHF (via elevated vasopressin levels), patients may ingest free water to excess and potentially exacerbate problems with hyponatremia. For all patients, a restriction of fluids to 2000 ml/day is advisable. If significant hyponatremia is present then the fluid restriction may be cut to 1500 ml/day or less. Avoidance of alcohol, an important negative inotrope, is mandatory even if alcohol is not suspected as the

Table 10.6 Mechanisms of heart failure and appropriate therapeutic interventions

Mechanism of heart failure	Therapeutic intervention
Depressed cardiac output	Digoxin and other inotropes
Neurohormonal activation	Neurohormonal antagonists
RAAS	ACE inhibitors, spironolactone
SNS	β-Blockers
Sodium and water retention	Diuretics; venodilators
Vasoconstriction	Direct vasodilators

ACE, angiotensin-converting enzyme; NYHA, New York Heart Association; RAAS, renin–angiotensin–aldosterone system; SNS, sympathetic nervous system

responsible etiology for heart failure. Bed rest prescriptions are limited only to the most severely ill patients. Otherwise, patients are encouraged to remain physically active.

Digoxin

In patients with chronic heart failure and abnormal systolic function, digoxin (when added to diuretics and angiotensin-converting enzyme inhibitors) reduces the rate of hospitalizations and reduces admissions for worsening heart failure, but it does not reduce overall mortality.[6] The molecular target for cardiac glycosides is the Na^+/K^+-ATPase (or sodium pump), which works to maintain a high extracellular $[Na^+]$ and a high intracellular $[K^+]$. Inhibition of this pump allows an increase in the intracellular $[Na^+]$. At a separate site on the sarcolemma, a passive Na^+/Ca^{2+} exchange occurs, resulting in an increase in intracellular $[Ca^{2+}]$. Drugs that increase the delivery of Ca^{2+} are associated with enhanced contractility. By this mechanism there is an increase in left ventricular ejection fraction, stroke volume, and cardiac output. Digoxin decreases heart rate and decreases the rate response to atrial fibrillation. Also, in patients with heart failure digoxin has been shown to cause a decrease in sympathetic nerve traffic.

Digoxin is indicated in the management of all patients with heart failure due to systolic dysfunction and is particularly useful if concomitant atrial arrhythmias are present. It is given initially as a loading dose of 0·75–1·0 mg over a 24-hour interval. Maintenance therapy is then given as 0·125–0·375 mg/day. Because the drug is excreted by the kidneys, patients with renal insufficiency will require an adjustment in maintenance therapy based on measurements of serum drug levels. A potential problem is the narrow therapeutic window, with a therapeutic range of 0·8–1·4 ng/dl. The drug is extensively protein bound and exhibits significant drug–drug interactions. In particular, concomitant use of amiodarone, quinidine, verapamil, or coumadin demands close attention to the serum digoxin level. Any acute change in renal function should also prompt a quick re-evaluation of the serum digoxin level.

Digoxin toxicity is an important clinical problem. The diagnosis is based on evidence of increased cardiac rhythm automaticity and/or newly developed conduction abnormalities (i.e. high grade atrioventricular block). Virtually every cardiac dysrhythmia has been associated with digoxin toxicity. Therefore, any significant change in the cardiac rhythm should raise the issue of digoxin toxicity. The pathognomonic arrhythmia is paroxysmal atrial tachycardia with variable degrees of atrioventricular block. In the setting of hypokalemia, digoxin toxicity may occur even with normal digoxin levels. The treatment of digoxin toxicity is based on the severity of the episode. Withholding therapy and correcting any electrolyte abnormalities may be all that is necessary for milder cases. If high grade atrioventricular block is present, a temporary transvenous pacemaker may be required. For digoxin induced life-threatening arrhythmias digoxin antibodies may be administered.

Diuretics

The use of diuretics is recommended in all patients with CHF who have evidence of fluid retention.[5] Diuretics are easy to administer, well tolerated, and relatively inexpensive. They increase sodium and water excretion from the kidney, acting at various sites in the nephron (Table 10.7). Thiazide diuretics act on the proximal convoluted tubule to block sodium reabsorption. Thiazide diuretics and thiazide-like diuretics (for example metolazone) also act on the distal convoluted tubule to block sodium reabsorption. Thiazide diuretics have a fairly modest effect, are used in mild heart failure, and are ineffective if creatinine clearance is reduced. A number of metabolic abnormalities are associated with thiazide use, including hyperglycemia, hypokalemia, hyperuricemia, and hyperlipidemia.

Loop diuretics are so-called because they act on the thick ascending limb of Henle to block the active reabsorption of chloride (Figure 10.7).[7] This blocks sodium reabsorption because sodium is transported with chloride at this site. These drugs cause a vigorous diuresis and represent the diuretics of choice in heart failure. There are three loop diuretics commonly used for heart failure: furosemide, bumetamide, and torsemide. Furosemide and bumetamide are quite similar in

Table 10.7 Use of diuretics in heart failure

Agent	Initial dose (maximal dose)	Adverse effects
Thiazide and thiazide-like		
Hydrochlorothiazide	25 mg/day (50 mg/day)	Hypokalemia, hyperglycemia, hyperuricemia
Metolazone	5 mg/day (10 mg/day)	Prolonged effects; erratic absorption; hypokalemia, hypomagnesemia, hyperuricemia
Loop diuretics		
Furosemide	10 mg/day (240 mg twice/three times daily)	Hypokalemia, hyperglycemia, hyperuricemia; high frequency hearing loss at high doses
Bumetamide	0·5 mg/day (10 mg/day)	Same
Torsemide	50% of usual furosemide dose given daily	Same
Potassium-sparing		
Spironolactone	25 mg/day (50 mg/day)	Hyperkalemia (with ACE inhibitor); rash; gynecomastia
Triamterene	100 mg twice daily (300 mg/day)	Hyperkalemia

ACE, angiotensin-converting enzyme

efficacy but have different pharmacokinetics, such that 40 mg furosemide is equivalent to 1 mg bumetamide. The onset of action is within 1 hour of oral administration and the duration may be up to 4–6 hours. The drugs are usually given once daily. More severely ill patients will require more frequent administration, up to every 6 hours.

To exert their effect, loop diuretics must be secreted into the proximal tubule to act on the loop of Henle. Therefore, drug delivery is dependent on renal blood flow. This is clinically important because a "threshold dose" of the loop diuretic must be administered before diuresis will be observed. Additionally, as renal function worsens, the diuretic dose will again need to be increased to continue to realize the same diuretic efficacy. Skill at administering loop diuretics will result in quick and effective relief of symptoms in decompensated states of CHF. When giving furosemide for the first time, start with a low dose (i.e. 20 mg) and observe the resultant diuresis. The drug should be

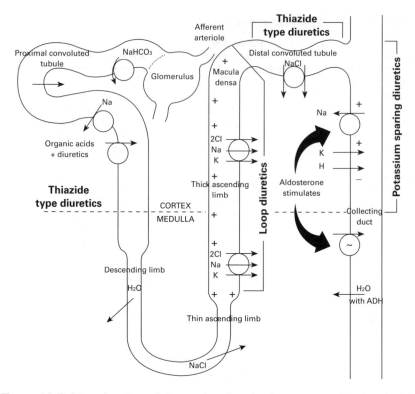

Figure 10.7 Site of action of the major diuretic drug groups. Reprinted with permission from Crawford[7]

readministered every 1–2 hours at progressively increasing doses until the desired effect is achieved. The dose at which such an effect occurs represents the maintenance dose, which should then be readministered every 8–24 hours depending on the clinical severity of volume overload.

Potential adverse effects of loop diuretics include hypokalemia, hyperuricemia, and prerenal azotemia. The latter stimulates additional renin production that actually increases neurohormonal activation in heart failure, which is an undesirable consequence. Diuretics should be given to the extent that symptoms of congestion are relieved; however, excessive diuresis should be avoided.

Metolazone is a thiazide-like diuretic that blocks sodium reabsorption in the distal convoluted tubule (see Figure 10.7). It exerts profound diuretic efficacy when given with a loop diuretic. This combination can effectively create a diuresis even in refractory cases. In clinical practice, metolazone is given before the administration of the loop diuretic. The response to metolazone is somewhat unpredictable and the effects can last for several days. The major concern with metolazone use is the degree of hypokalemia that can ensue after combination therapy. Reductions in the serum potassium concentration to below 3·0 mEq/l (<3·0 mmol/l) are not uncommon and can be life-threatening. It is preferable to initiate therapy with metolazone on an inpatient basis with frequent assessment of [K⁺]. If it is started on an outpatient basis, then the patient will need to return frequently within the first week to follow changes in potassium.

Potassium-sparing diuretics are helpful primarily because they preserve potassium by blocking its excretion into the collecting duct (see Figure 10.7). None of these diuretics are particularly potent and are almost always given in combination with loop diuretics. They work via two mechanisms: direct antagonism of aldosterone with the competitive antagonist spironolactone; and direct inhibition of sodium transport with triamterene or amiloride, thus preventing potassium excretion into the collecting duct. Care is to be taken when these drugs are given, especially if potassium supplementation is continued and if the patient is on angiotensin-converting enzyme inhibitors. The risk of dangerous hyperkalemia is real. Careful and frequent monitoring of serum potassium levels is required after these drugs are initiated. Other potential adverse effects of potassium-sparing diuretics include gynecomastia and hirsutism, both of which are seen with spironolactone use.

In patients with severe heart failure already treated with loop diuretics, angiotensin-converting enzyme inhibitors, and in most cases digoxin, the addition of spironolactone 25 mg/day reduced the risk for death and the frequency of hospitalization for heart failure.[8] The incidence of serious hyperkalemia was minimal.

Vasodilators

Direct vasodilators are those that act directly on the peripheral and central vasculature, and they are either predominantly venodilators or arterial vasodilators, or have mixed properties. Nitrates act directly on smooth muscle vasculature through production of cyclic guanosine monophosphate, which reduces entry of calcium into the vascular smooth muscle cell. To exert their action, they must first be reduced to nitric oxide. Nitrates cause predominant venodilatation, which reduces central venous pressures and pulmonary artery pressures. There is also a mild dilatation in arterial beds, which can be associated with a fall in peripheral vascular resistance. The usual drug given is oral isosorbide dinitrate in doses of 10–60 mg every 6–8 hours. An 8–10 hour nitrate-free interval every 24 hours reduces the inevitable tolerance that occurs with continuous dosing.

Isosorbide dinitrate administration results in decreases in pulmonary capillary wedge pressure, mean pulmonary artery pressure and right atrial pressure, and increases in stroke volume and cardiac output. Side effects include headaches and dizziness, and can limit the maximal dose that can be given.

Hydralazine is a direct vasodilator that causes predominant arterial vasodilatation and has a poorly understood mechanism of action. It has a short half-life but it is at least partly metabolized by acetylation, and patients who are "slow acetylators" may be much more sensitive to its administration. When used in heart failure, hydralazine causes a decrease in systemic and pulmonary vascular resistance and an increase in cardiac output, with only minor increases in sympathetic activity. The drug is given at a dose of 25–100 mg every 6–8 hours, and a dose of 75 mg every 6–8 hours is the preferred dose. When combined with isosorbide dinitrate survival improved in the first Veterans Administration Heart Failure Trial.[9] Side effects include headache, dizziness, gastrointestinal symptoms, and rarely a drug-induced lupus condition with arthralgias and skin rash.

Angiotensin-converting enzyme inhibitors

Angiotensin-converting enzyme (ACE) inhibitors are both indirect vasodilators (by reducing angiotensin II) and neurohormonal antagonists. These drugs inhibit the conversion of angiotensin I to angiotensin II by inhibition of the converting enzyme (Figure 10.8).[7] The result of this inhibition is a reduction in vasoconstriction and a reduction in aldosterone release. The impact of this therapeutic intervention in heart failure is profound. In the Cooperative North Scandinavian Enalapril Survival Study, reported in 1987, patients with class IV heart failure were randomly assigned to receive either digoxin and diuretics alone, or digoxin, diuretics and enalapril.[10] In patients randomized to enalapril there was a reduction in mortality of 40% at 6 months and 27% at 1 year (Figure 10.9).[7] Since then it has become evident that in patients with symptomatic CHF a variety of ACE inhibitors reduce mortality and hospitalization for heart failure, with the greatest benefits seen in patients with the lowest ejection fraction.[11] ACE inhibitor therapy is indicated for all patients with CHF unless there is a compelling contraindication. Furthermore, ACE inhibitor therapy is increasingly recommended for patients with asymptomatic left ventricular systolic dysfunction, whether they have a history of myocardial infarction or not.[5]

In general, the drugs are initially administered in low doses and titrated to the target and/or maximal doses. The dose titration needs to proceed cautiously in the elderly, patients with borderline blood

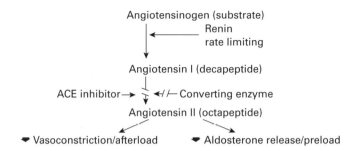

Figure 10.8 Effect of angiotensin-converting enzyme inhibition on the renin–angiotensin–aldosterone system. Reprinted with permission from Crawford[7]

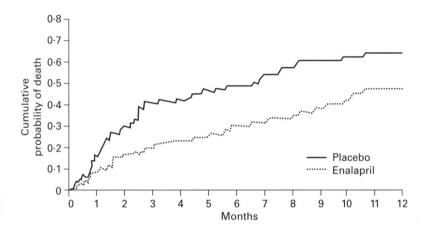

Figure 10.9 Cooperative North Scandinavian Enalapril Survival Study results in patients with class IV congestive heart failure. Patients on digoxin, diuretics, and enalapril had a significantly better 12 month survival than did patients on digoxin and diuretics alone. Reprinted with permission from *N Engl J Med*[10]

pressure, and those with pre-existing renal insufficiency. A special population is that group of patients with hyperkalemia (usually due to a type IV renal tubular acidosis). Careful observation of the potassium concentration is required. Even in patients with normal potassium levels, the potassium concentration may still rise when ACE inhibitor therapy is initiated. Hypotension is a particularly difficult issue in ACE inhibitor therapy. Because of the mandate to achieve targeted total doses in order to realize similar survival benefits as those seen in the major trials, it is important not to have therapy limited by hypotension. Reflecting back on the principles of vasodilator therapy, hypotension can be avoided by initiating therapy at the flat portion of the Starling curve. This may require a reduction in the diuretic dose or even a "diuretic holiday" for 1 or 2 days in order to introduce ACE inhibitors. A slow upward titration will also increase the likelihood that targeted doses will be reached.

Adverse reactions include the development of an ACE inhibitor-induced cough; this is mediated by bradykinins, which are increased with ACE inhibition. No specific therapy is effective in relieving cough. Patients either cope with antitussives or discontinue therapy. Less frequently, development of angioneurotic edema, drug eruptions, and rarely drug-induced neutropenia occur. ACE inhibitors are contraindicated in pregnancy.

Several points regarding ACE inhibitor therapy for heart failure should be remembered.

- ACE inhibitors are indicated in all patients with heart failure and left ventricular systolic dysfunction.
- Therapy should mimic that of the major survival trials in terms of dose and agent selected.
- ACE inhibitors should not be suspended or discontinued because of hypotension unless the patient is symptomatic. This is because of the interrelationship between blood pressure (BP), cardiac output (CO) and systemic vascular resistance (SVR), which is defined by BP = CO × SVR. Even though ACE inhibitors and other vasodilators decrease SVR, the corresponding increase in CO offsets any drop in BP unless the patient is volume depleted.

Angiotensin II receptor antagonists

These agents competitively inhibit the receptors for angiotensin II, and there is a lack of associated cough because there is no effect on bradykinins. The weight of evidence suggests that these agents should be considered in patients being treated with digitalis, diuretics, and a β-blocker who cannot tolerate an ACE inhibitor because of cough or angioedema.[5]

β-Blockers

Activation of the sympathetic nervous system adversely influences the course of chronic heart failure. Until relatively recently, it was thought that β-adrenoreceptor antagonists were contraindicated in heart failure because of their negative inotropic effects. However, it has emerged that several β-blockers (carvedilol,[12] bisoprolol, and extended release metoprolol) improve mortality and quality of life, and reduce hospitalization in patients with mild to moderate (New York Heart Association class II or III) heart failure.[13] Initiation of this therapy requires individualized drug dosing and very careful clinical monitoring.

Additional therapy for congestive heart failure

Electrolyte supplementation is frequently required in patients on significant diuretic doses. Potassium supplementation is most frequently required but can cause gastrointestinal irritation. The usual supplemental dose required is 20–120 mEq/day (20–120 mmol/day). If higher doses are required, then concomitant use of a potassium-sparing diuretic should be considered. Hypokalemia may be difficult to correct without first correcting hypomagnesemia, because Mg^{2+} is a cofactor for the Na^+/K^+-ATPase pump. Magnesium supplementation is difficult because serum measures do not accurately reflect magnesium stores. The oral supplements are poorly absorbed, which also makes repletion difficult. If renal function is normal, then the dose of magnesium is 14 mEq (14 mmol) three to four times daily.

Anticoagulants are often given to patients with marked impairment in systolic function, or dilated cardiomyopathy to protect against the development of formation of mural thrombus and possible systemic embolization, which may result in strokes or pulmonary emboli.[14] Certainly, anticoagulants should be given to patients at highest risk (i.e. those with multiple risk factors for emboli [atrial fibrillation, mitral valve disease] or prior embolic events). Warfarin sodium is the preferred agent and should be given to adjust the International Normalized Ratio to 2·0.

Amiodarone is a class III antiarrhythmic that has shown some promise in small trials of heart failure patients. It causes a slower heart rate and mild vasodilatation, and suppresses arrhythmias, but it does not reduce the incidence of sudden death or prolong survival.[15]

Many patients with heart failure require care in a critical care setting where parenteral agents are used. The available agents include the following:

- intravenous nitroglycerin, which causes preload reduction
- intravenous nitroprusside, which reduces afterload
- dobutamine, which stimulates cardiac contractility and increases cardiac output
- dopamine, which at low doses improves renal blood flow; at moderate doses it stimulates cardiac contractility, and at higher doses it causes systemic vasoconstriction and raises blood pressure
- milrinone, which causes vasodilatation and augmented cardiac output by inhibiting phosphodiesterase.

Cardiac transplantation

Advances in candidate selection, surgical techniques, postoperative care, immunosuppression, surveillance for rejection, and avoidance of severe infection has resulted in dramatic improvements in survival since the introduction of cardiac transplantation in 1968. One year survival rates now average 80%, and in selected centers the 1 year survival exceeds 90%. Five year survival is approximately 70%. The major limitation to cardiac transplantation is the availability of donor organs, and not every patient who can benefit from cardiac transplantation will receive a heart. The task for transplant committees is to decide who are the best candidates for this limited resource (Box 10.2).

Box 10.2 Heart transplantation

When to refer for transplantation?
Left ventricular ejection fraction $<<0\cdot20$
Class IV congestive heart failure
Intractable arrhythmias that are not amenable to other therapy
Refractory ischemia despite efforts at revascularization
Poor exercise capacity by objective criteria
Marked hyponatremia
Fluctuating renal/hepatic function
Contraindications
Severe comorbidities
Intrinsic renal, hepatic, or pulmonary disease
Severe peripheral vascular disease
Insulin-dependent diabetes with end-organ complications
Recent stroke
Recent pulmonary infarction
Active infection or malignancy
Psychosocial instability

Case studies

Case 10.1

A 43-year-old male executive with positive risk factors for coronary artery disease including obesity, hypertension, smoking, and hyperlipidemia presented acutely with substernal chest pain. The character of the pain was consistent with angina pectoris. The patient is an active, 20 pack-year smoker, with hypertension treated for 5 years with calcium channel blockers and hyperlipidemia. Blood pressure was 160/90 mmHg 3 months previously.

Examination. Physical examination: the patient appeared morbidly obese (305 lb [138·6 kg]). Height: 68 inches (172·7 cm). No abnormalities of skin, nail beds, or oral mucosa. Pulse: 92 beats/min, normal character. Blood pressure: 110/70 mmHg in right arm. Jugular venous pulse: normal. Cardiac impulse: normal. First heart sound: normal. Second heart sound: split normally on inspiration. Fourth heart sound present. No murmurs. Two component friction rub heard. Chest examination: normal air entry, no rales or rhonchi. Abdominal examination: soft abdomen, no tenderness, and no masses. Normal liver span. No peripheral edema. Femoral, popliteal, posterior tibial, and dorsalis pedis pulses: all normal volume and equal. Carotid pulses: normal, no bruits.

Investigations. Chest x ray: cardiomegaly with clear lung fields. Electrocardiogram: 2 mm flat ST depression in leads I, aVL, V_5, V_6; T-wave inversions in leads V_4–V_6. Electrolytes: potassium 3·6 mEq/l (3·6 mmol/l); creatinine 1·9 mg/dl (168 µmol/l); glucose 165 mg/dl (9·1 mmol/l). Serial cardiac enzymes: creatinine kinase-MB 79–96–54 units (normal range 0–3). Echocardiogram: inferolateral hypokinesis; mild mitral regurgitation; left ventricular dimension 5·8 cm (normal <5·5 cm); left ventricular septum 1·6 cm; left ventricular posterior wall 1·5 cm (normal <1·1 cm); small pericardial effusion; left ventricular ejection fraction 0·27. Exercise stress test: the patient exercised for 12 min on a modified Bruce protocol to peak heart rate 140 beats/min, peak systolic blood pressure 190 mmHg, MET level 6·5 (consistent with peak oxygen consumption of 23 ml/kg per min). No anginal symptoms or ST-T changes on electrocardiogram during exercise.

Hospital day 5. The patient is ambulating and is asymptomatic, with normal vital signs and cardiac examination, except for presence of a fourth heart sound on auscultation.

Questions

1. What diagnosis or diagnoses are applicable? (A) Congestive heart failure. (B) Pericarditis. (C) Q-wave myocardial infarction. (D) Non-Q-wave myocardial infarction. (E) A and C. (F) B and D. (G) A, B, and C.
2. Based on the diagnosis and clinical course, what would be the best medical regimen at the time of discharge? (A) The patient is not ready for discharge; additional procedures need to be done. (B) Aspirin, lipid lowering therapy, and calcium channel blocker (nifedipine). (C) β-blocker (propanolol). (D) Aspirin, ACE inhibitor, β-blocker, and lipid lowering medication. (E) No medical therapy is indicated.
3. Which of the following findings confirm the diagnosis of CHF in this case? (A) Left ventricular ejection fraction below 0·30.

(B) Dilated left ventricle. (C) History of hypertension. (D) All of these. (E) None of these.
4. Is this patient a candidate for eventual heart transplantation? (A) Yes – he has reduced left ventricular function with an ejection fraction under 0·30 and reduced exercise capacity, with an estimated maximal oxygen consumption below 30 ml/kg per min. (B) No – his clinical course is inconsistent with the indications for transplantation.

Answers

Answer to question 1 F. This patient has had a non-Q-wave myocardial infarction complicated by pericarditis. The electrocardiographic findings rule out a Q-wave myocardial infarction. The diagnosis of an acute myocardial infarction is confirmed by the diagnostic enzyme pattern. Pericarditis is confirmed by the presence of a pericardial friction rub and a small pericardial effusion.

The important concept arising from this question is that the diagnosis of CHF cannot be made on the basis of an abnormal measure of left ventricular function. The left ventricular ejection fraction is reduced and suggests a poor prognosis, but is not sufficient for the diagnosis of CHF. Remember that, for the diagnosis of CHF to be confirmed, there must be both evidence of ventricular dysfunction and evidence of symptoms due to ventricular dysfunction. This patient has asymptomatic left ventricular dysfunction after a myocardial infarction.

Answer to question 2 D. Asymptomatic left ventricular dysfunction following myocardial infarction represents a newly appreciated area of left ventricular dysfunction that is clinically important. Patients with left ventricular dysfunction after myocardial dysfunction go on to develop eventual CHF, recurrent myocardial infarction, and premature death. The use of ACE inhibitors in this group of patients has been associated with an improvement in survival, a reduced likelihood of development of heart failure, and a reduced rate of recurrent myocardial infarction. β-Blockers and aspirin are indicated after myocardial infarction. The addition of lipid lowering therapy is specific for this patient, given the history of a significant but untreated hyperlipidemia.

There is no indication for most types of calcium channel blockers after myocardial infarction, and their routine use is usually contraindicated, especially in patients with known pulmonary congestion and ventricular dysfunction. This is probably due to their negative inotropic properties.

Based on this patient's benign clinical course, a cardiac catheterization after myocardial infarction is not indicated.

Answer to question 3   E. Again, this patient does not have CHF but rather has asymptomatic left ventricular dysfunction. All of the descriptors are valid, including depressed left ventricular function, dilated left ventricle, and prior history of hypertension, but again the lack of symptoms prevents one from making a diagnosis of heart failure.

Answer to question 4   B. The data listed in A are not indications for heart transplantation. A maximal oxygen consumption greater than 20 ml/kg per min is consistent with a good short-term prognosis and does not suggest that transplantation is indicated. Similarly, heart transplantation is not done on the basis of a depressed left ventricular ejection fraction alone.

Case 10.2

A 21-year-old gardener with no prior history of cardiac disease or positive risk factors presented after 6 weeks of a persistent complaint of a "cold". He describes the onset of a severe flu-like illness that caused him to miss 4 days of work 6 weeks ago. He recovered partially after bed rest and fluids, but had a persistent cough. He attempted to return to work after 1 week but had cough and fatigue. He saw a nurse practitioner who diagnosed bronchitis and pleurisy based on a productive cough and basilar rhonchi. Two weeks of oral antibiotics did not resolve his symptoms. He once again stopped work and visited an internist. A work up for mononucleosis and Epstein–Barr virus was instituted, and the antibiotics were changed to erythromycin to cover atypical pneumonias. A CD4 count was borderline normal. The patient had one homosexual encounter 2 years ago. After 2 more weeks of malaise, cough, and fatigue, the patient developed difficulty sleeping and vague abdominal discomfort. He then presented to a university hospital emergency room where he was evaluated by a senior medical student. He did not use tobacco or alcohol, and had no prior illnesses.

Examination. Physical examination: the patient appeared seriously ill. Extremities cool. Pulse: 120 beats/min, with pulsus alternans. Blood pressure: 80/60 mmHg. Jugular venous pulse: 12 cm at 45°. Parasternal lift. First heart sound: normal. Second heart: normal. Third and fourth heart sounds were present, along with a grade 3/6 mitral holosystolic murmur. Chest examination: diffuse crackles to mid-chest. Abdominal examination: soft abdomen, liver span 16 cm. No peripheral edema. Femoral and popliteal pulses: all palpable and equal. Carotid pulses: normal, no bruits.

Investigations. Chest *x* ray: markedly enlarged cardiac shadow; blunted costophrenic angles; enlarged pulmonary arteries; diffuse pan-lobar infiltrates in an alveolar pattern. Electrocardiogram: sinus tachycardia, biatrial overload, prominent voltage, diffuse non-specific ST-T wave changes. Laboratory tests: hemoglobin 12 g/dl (120 g/l), sodium 131 mEq/l (131 mmol/l), creatinine 2·2 mg/dl (194 µmol/l), aspartate aminotransferase 125 U/l (2·1 µkat/l; normal range 0–0·58 µkat/l), alanine aminotransferase 100 U/L (1·7 µkat/l), alkaline phosphatase 235 U/l (Normal range 30–120 U/l); total bilirubin 2·1 mg/dl (36 µmol/l; normal range 5·1–17 µmol/l); thyroid function tests normal. Echocardiogram: severe depression of left ventricular systolic function, left ventricular diastolic diameter 8·2 cm (normal <6 cm), left ventricular ejection fraction 0·15, dilated left atrium, moderately severe mitral insufficiency, moderate tricuspid insufficiency, estimated right ventricular systolic pressure 56 mmHg. Right heart catheterization: cardiac output 2·8 l/min (normal >4·0 l/min), right atrium 20 mmHg (normal 2–10 mmHg), right ventricle 60/20 mmHg (normal range 15–30/2–10 mmHg), pulmonary artery 60/35 mmHg (normal range 15–30/5–10 mmHg), wedge pressure 33 mmHg (normal 5–14 mmHg), mixed venous saturation 49% (normal >60%), systemic vascular resistance 1428 dynes·s/cm^5 (143 kPa·s/l). Endomyocardial biopsy: normal myocardial cells with sparse interstitial inflammatory infiltrate.

Hospital day 3. For the first 2 hospital days the patient was treated with oral medications while undergoing the hospital evaluation outlined above. He remained uncomfortable throughout the first 48 hours. The patient awoke with nausea and extreme malaise. His blood pressure was 65 mmHg. He had a witnessed syncopal episode with telemetry demonstrating a wide complex tachycardia at 175 beats/min. Emergent direct current cardioversion was required twice. The patient was transferred to intensive care unit. A right heart catheter was placed, with findings identical to those noted above.

Hospital day 20. After intensive medical therapy the patient was recovering well. He became ambulatory. His blood pressure was 116/70 mmHg and his heart rate was 68 beats/min. His cardiac examination was normal. Repeat echocardiography revealed a left ventricular ejection fraction 0·25 with a small apical shadow, consistent with a ventricular clot. Three months later, echocardiography demonstrated an ejection fraction of 0·54. One month later he returned to his usual employment.

Questions

1. The diagnosis of CHF was not originally suspected because of which of the following? (A) The patient had no clinical evidence of heart disease at the onset of his illness. (B) The patient's demographics were atypical for the diagnosis of heart

failure. (C) No signs or symptoms of heart failure were present at the onset of his illness. (D) The diagnosis of CHF can be difficult to discriminate from atypical pneumonia. (E) A and C. (F) B and D.

2. At the time of hospital presentation, this patient had CHF of what severity? (A) Class I. (B) Class II. (C) Class III. (D) Class IV. (E) The patient did not have CHF at the time of presentation.

3. The diagnostic right heart catheterization revealed which hemodynamic profile? (A) Increased preload. (B) Decreased afterload. (C) Increased afterload. (D) Normal cardiac index. (E) A and C. (F) B and D. (G) None of the above.

4. The hemodynamic findings are consistent with which of the following? (A) Septic shock. (B) Cardiogenic shock. (C) Hypovolemic shock.

5. Regarding the dramatic decompensation on day 3, which of the following statements is correct? (A) Ventricular tachycardia is an unexpected complication. (B) The presence of ventricular tachycardia represents a serious negative prognostic factor. (C) This patient should be treated with antiarrhythmic agents indefinitely in view of this life-threatening episode of ventricular tachycardia.

6. What is the best therapy at the time of transfer to the intensive care unit? (A) Oxygen, high dose oral diuretics, high dose dopamine, and broad spectrum antibiotics. (B) Dobutamine titrated to a cardiac index greater than 2·5 l/min per m^2, and parenteral diuretics, oxygen, lidocaine, and intravenous nitroprusside. (C) High dose steroid therapy, intravenous immune globulin, and norepinephrine.

Answers

Answer to question 1 F. This patient had CHF probably due to acute myocarditis. Because he does not represent the usual patient affected with CHF and because upper respiratory illnesses are so common in his age range, the diagnosis of heart failure was missed. This is a frequent occurrence in daily practice. The evidence for heart failure was present in the beginning, with cough and fatigue as well as the resting tachycardia. In this case, the diagnosis of CHF was not made even though symptoms were present.

Answer to question 2 D. By the time this patient was admitted the diagnosis of heart failure was obvious and he was critically ill. The presence of symptoms at rest is consistent with class IV CHF, which carries a 70% 1 year mortality.

Answer to question 3 E.

Answer to question 4 B. A review of the hemodynamic profile demonstrates severe left ventricular dysfunction. The cardiac output is severely depressed. The preload is markedly increased, given the pulmonary capillary wedge pressure of 33 mmHg and the central venous pressure of 20 mmHg. The afterload is also increased, based on a calculated systemic vascular resistance in excess of 1400 dynes·s/cm^5. The profile of severely reduced cardiac output and increased filling pressures with a markedly elevated peripheral resistance is consistent with the diagnosis of cardiogenic shock.

Answer to question 5 B. For patients with heart failure the incidence of ventricular arrhythmias approaches 75% and the presence of complex ventricular rhythm disturbances, including ventricular tachycardia, approaches 50%. Ventricular tachycardia is an expected complication of severe heart failure. Despite the prevalence of ventricular arrhythmias in heart failure, no data as yet suggest that medical therapy can modify the rate of death due to sudden cardiac events. Antiarrhythmic therapy is not necessarily indicated on a chronic basis. Nevertheless, when serious ventricular arrhythmias complicate CHF, the prognosis is noted to be quite poor.

Answer to question 6 B. At the time of transfer to the intensive care unit, this patient is seriously ill having just been resuscitated from a cardiac arrest. The right heart catheterization confirms poor ventricular function. The goal of management is to improve the cardiac output, reduce the elevated filling pressures, provide supplemental oxygen, and initiate prophylactic therapy for ventricular arrhythmias. The addition of nitroprusside is of benefit because of its vasodilator properties and ability to reduce afterload.

The choices listed in A are not inappropriate except for the use of oral diuretics. In a critically ill patient with evidence of central venous pressure elevation and elevated liver function tests consistent with a congested liver, it is unwise to continue to administer oral agents that will have an unpredictable absorption and therefore an unpredictable response.

The biopsy evidence of acute myocarditis suggests that immunosuppressive therapy may be of benefit to resolve this acute inflammatory process. The available data demonstrate that the spontaneous recovery rate from such an illness is as high as 40–50%, which is identical to the recovery rate seen with immunosuppressive therapy but without the toxicity of steroids. Supportive care remains the best option for patients with acute onset CHF, even if myocarditis is biopsy proven.

Case 10.3

A 69-year-old woman with a longstanding history of essential hypertension presents to the primary care clinic for routine evaluation. She initially denied any specific complaints at the present time. On further questioning she notes that she has had an unexplained weight gain. She also describes frequent episodes of fatigue, which she attributes to "old age". She is unable to take her evening walk without resting halfway through. Her family thinks she is well and simply needs to rest more frequently. Past history: a 20 year history of documented hypertension, intermittent compliance with medications, and no history of stroke or renal disease; overweight by 30 lb (13·6 kg) for 30 years; and an active 13 pack-year history of smoking. Current medications: verapamil 80 mg three times daily and hydrochlorothiazide 75 mg/day.

Examination. Physical examination: the patient appeared normal. Pulse: 96 beats/min, normal character. Blood pressure: 170/95 mmHg. Jugular venous pulse: normal. Cardiac impulse: displaced laterally, diffuse. First heart sound: normal. Second heart sound: split normally on inspiration. No added sounds or murmurs. Chest examination: normal air entry, fine basilar crackles. Abdominal examination: soft abdomen, liver tender to palpation, no masses. Normal liver span. Trace ankle edema. Carotid pulses: normal, no bruits.

Investigations. Chest x ray: clear lung fields, cardiothoracic ratio of 0·65. Electrocardiogram: sinus tachycardia, left atrial overload, left ventricular hypertrophy. Laboratory findings: hemoglobin 10 g/dl (100 g/l), creatinine 2·9 mg/dl (256 µmol/l), potassium 3·5 mEq/l (3·5 mmol/l), glucose 160 mg/dl (8·9 mmol/l).

Questions

1. Does this patient have CHF? (A) Yes – she has a known history of hypertension. (B) No – there is no assessment of ventricular function to establish the diagnosis of CHF. (C) No – she has poorly controlled hypertension. (D) Yes – she has probable hypertensive heart disease and symptoms of volume overload. (E) There are insufficient data to make the diagnosis.
2. What is the next most appropriate step in the evaluation? (A) Evaluation for coronary artery disease. (B) Echocardiogram. (C) Both A and B. (D) Neither A nor B – all of the data needed are available already.
3. What is the mortality risk over the next year based on the severity of her illness at the present time? (A) 5%. (B) 10–15%. (C) 30%. (D) 70%.

4. She seeks a second opinion and undergoes a diagnostic cardiac catheterization. Results: left ventricular ejection fraction 0·35, diffuse mild global hypokinesis, left ventricular end-diastolic pressure 35 mmHg; normal coronary arteries. Based on these findings, what is her major pathology? (A) Systolic dysfunction. (B) Diastolic dysfunction. (C) Both A and B. (D) Neither A nor B. (E) None of these – she has a primary idiopathic dilated cardiomyopathy.

5. Based on the current diagnosis, which of these regimens would represent the best medical therapy? (A) Captopril 6·25 mg three times daily, furosemide 10 mg twice daily, and digoxin 0·37 mg/day. (B) Verapamil 240 mg three times daily and hydrochlorothiazide 100 mg/day. (C) Coumadin 10 mg/day, nifedipine 60 mg three times daily, metolazone 2·5 mg/day, bumetamide 1 mg/day, and potassium chloride 10 mEq/day (10 mmol/day). (D) Enalapril 10 mg twice daily, furosemide 40 mg twice daily, digoxin 0·25 mg every other day, and potassium chloride 10 mEq/day (10 mmol/day). (E) She needs to be referred for consideration of cardiac transplantation.

Answers

Answer to question 1   D. The diagnosis of heart failure is made with hypertensive heart disease (lengthy history of hypertension and left ventricular hypertrophy with cardiomegaly) and CHF symptoms.

Answer to question 2   C. This is a newly appreciated diagnosis of heart failure. Therefore, an assessment of ventricular function is indicated to determine the etiology and extent of left ventricular dysfunction. It is appropriate to evaluate for coronary artery disease because this remains the most common cause of heart failure. Moreover, this patient has a number of important risk factors, including hypertension, smoking, obesity, and lack of postmenopausal estrogen therapy.

Answer to question 3   C. This patient has symptoms consistent with class III heart failure. Although these patients are ambulatory and comfortable at rest, they carry a very worrisome prognosis over the short term.

Answer to question 4   C. Given that this patient has had longstanding hypertension, the diagnosis of a primary cardiomyopathy cannot be made. The left ventricular systolic function is depressed based on a left ventricular ejection fraction below 0·40, and the diastolic function is similarly impaired on the basis of an elevated left ventricular end-diastolic pressure. As a consequence, this patient has both systolic and diastolic dysfunction. This is a common observation in patients who have heart failure due to chronic hypertension.

Answer to question 5   D. This patient has several contraindications to cardiac transplantation in view of her advanced age and renal insufficiency. She has not yet had an appropriate trial of medical therapy that might result in substantial improvement in her symptoms. The choice of appropriate medical therapy for patients with heart failure is a critical question. Option A includes a subtherapeutic dose of an ACE inhibitor and daily administration of high dose digoxin therapy, which is not likely to be well tolerated in this patient with renal insufficiency. Option B includes high dose calcium channel blocker therapy, which, although intriguing because of the diastolic dysfunction, is not indicated because the known negative inotropic action of this drug will probably exacerbate heart failure. Thiazide diuretics are not likely to be effective, even in high doses, in a patient with renal insufficiency. Option C includes the use of anticoagulants, which are not routinely indicated unless the risk for clot formation is exaggerated because of atrial fibrillation, mitral valve disease, or known prior emboli. Even though nifedipine is a vasodilator, its negative inotropic action once again makes it a suboptimal choice in the management of heart failure. Only option D includes an appropriate dose of ACE inhibitor, reduced dose of digoxin, loop diuretic, and modest potassium supplementation.

Case 10.4

A 37-year-old woman 2 years postpartum presents for evaluation of dyspnea. She describes a normal pregnancy and a benign postpartum course immediately after delivery. She now notes that it is much more difficult for her to complete her tasks at work. She previously rode a stationary bike 30 min a day three times per week. She now has too much fatigue. She has recently experienced stress in her married life because she is always tired. She twice noted over the past month that she has nearly passed out. Past history: no illnesses or surgery; she drinks two to three glasses of wine nightly and smokes one or two cigarettes two or three times per week. Family history: a distant cousin died suddenly at age 31 years; no autopsy was conducted. Medications: oral contraceptives.

Examination. Physical examination: the patient had dusky lips. Pulse: 96 beats/min, normal character. Blood pressure: 90/70 mmHg in right arm. Jugular venous pulse: >15 cm with 'v' waves. Cardiac impulse: parasternal lift. First heart sound: normal. Second heart sound: loud. Third heart sound: louder with inspiration. 3/6 holosystolic murmur at lower left sternal edge. Chest examination: normal air entry, no rales or rhonchi. Abdominal examination: liver enlarged and pulsatile. Trace peripheral edema.

Investigations. Chest x ray: enlarged main pulmonary arteries with oligemia of the lung fields; diminished retrosternal air space. Electrocardiogram: sinus tachycardia; right atrial overload; axis of (+)120°. Prominent RSR' in leads V_1–V_3. Anterior ST depression with T-wave inversion.

Questions

1. The differential diagnosis includes which of the following? (A) CHF. (B) Primary pulmonary hypertension. (C) Atrial septal defect. (D) A and B. (E) A and C. (F) All of these.
2. The next most appropriate step in the work up would be which of the following? (A) Work up for mediastinal tumors based on the abnormal x ray film. (B) Echocardiogram and right heart catheterization. (C) Left heart catheterization. (D) Connective tissue disease work up. (E) A and C. (F) B and D.
3. After another near syncopal episode she returned and was admitted. A Swan–Ganz catheter was placed and demonstrated the following findings: pulmonary artery pressure 90/45 mmHg, pulmonary capillary wedge pressure 6 mmHg, cardiac output 3 l/min, right atrial pressure 20 mmHg, right atrial oxygen saturation 58%, pulmonary artery oxygen saturation 61%. The most appropriate therapy for this patient includes which of the following? (A) Captopril 75 mg three times daily, furosemide 80 mg/day, and potassium chloride 20 mEq/day (20 mmol/day). (B) Digoxin 0·25 mg/day and furosemide 20 mg/day. (C) Nifedipine 60 mg every 6 hours, hydrochlorothiazide 50 mg/day, and coumadin 5 mg/day.
4. After 2 years she began to fail on the above medical therapy. She is placed on oxygen at 4 l/min and a continuous prostacyclin infusion. Which is the most appropriate treatment option? (A) Surgical repair of congenital heart disease. (B) Heart transplantation evaluation. (C) Heart lung transplant evaluation. (D) Lung transplantation evaluation.

Answers

Answer to question 1 F. All of the choices comprise an appropriate differential diagnosis for a young patient who presents with dyspnea and evidence of at least right ventricular dysfunction. Adult forms of congenital heart disease are uncommon but should be considered in atypical cases, especially in the younger patient. This patient has evidence of right heart failure and pulmonary hypertension. The history of progressive dyspnea in a young woman is associated with this diagnosis. The examination contains impressive evidence for right heart dysfunction: "v" waves consistent with tricuspid regurgitation; a prominent second heart sound consistent with prominent closure of the pulmonic valve; a parasternal lift due to right ventricular pressure or volume overload and a right sided third hear sound consistent with right ventricular dilatation; tricuspid insufficiency; hepatomegaly; and peripheral edema.

Answer to question 2 F. The retrosternal fullness on chest *x* ray film does not represent a mediastinal tumor but rather right ventricular enlargement, which is otherwise difficult to observe on a chest radiograph. A left heart study is not indicated based on minimal if any risk factors being present. The diagnosis of pulmonary hypertension needs to be confirmed or ruled out. An echocardiogram allows one to confirm the extent of right ventricular disease and to estimate non-invasively the pulmonary artery pressure. It also is quite useful in evaluating adult congenital heart disease. The right heart catheterization is the definitive study in this case. The diagnosis of primary pulmonary hypertension cannot be established until connective tissue disorders have been ruled out.

Answer to question 3 C. The right heart catheterization confirms the diagnosis of primary pulmonary hypertension. Left heart failure may be associated with striking elevations in pulmonary artery pressure but with associated elevations in pulmonary capillary wedge pressure. The finding of a normal wedge pressure with near systemic pulmonary artery pressures confirms the diagnosis. The measured oxygen saturations are not consistent with a left to right shunt and effectively rule out the common adult congenital heart diseases. The best available medical therapy at present for primary pulmonary hypertension includes calcium channel blockers, gentle diuretics, and anticoagulation.

Answer to question 4 D. The use of prostacyclin (a prostaglandin that causes vasodilatation) is an effective strategy for relief of symptoms in patients with primary pulmonary hypertension who have failed high dose calcium channel blocker therapy. Lung transplantation is the last treatment option after all medical attempts have failed. Even though this patient has evidence of right ventricular dysfunction, it appears that successful lung transplantation for this illness relieves the afterload on the right ventricle and normal function returns. A heart–lung transplant is therefore not indicated.

The 1 year survival for heart–lung transplantation is approximately 50%. A heart transplantation alone does not solve the problem with pulmonary hypertension. In fact, patients cannot receive a heart transplant until significant pulmonary hypertension not due to left heart failure has been ruled out. The available data have revealed that patients with pulmonary hypertension, that is fixed, do not do well with heart transplantation even if overt heart disease is the major pathology. The heart transplant work up for all potential recipients includes a right heart catheterization for this reason. A lung transplantation is the only way to prolong survival once the patient has reached the point of continuous prostacyclin infusion.

References

1 Hosenpud JD, Greenberg BH. *Congestive heart failure. Pathophysiology, diagnosis, and comprehensive approach to management*. New York: Springer-Verlag, 1994.
2 Felker GM, Thompson RE, Hare JM, *et al*. Underlying causes and long-term survival in patients with initially unexplained cardiomyopathy. *N Engl J Med* 2000; **342**:1077–84.
3 Cook DJ, Simel DL. Does this patient have abnormal central venous pressure? *JAMA* 1996;**275**:630–4.
4 Report of the American College of Cardiology/American Heart Association Task Force on Practice Guidelines. Guidelines for the Evaluation and Management of Heart Failure. *Circulation* 1995;**92**:2764–84.
5 Hunt SA, Baker DW, Chin MH, *et al*. ACC/AHA Guidelines for the Evaluation and Management of Chronic Heart Failure in the Adult: executive summary: a report of the American College of Cardiology/American Heart Association Task Force on Practice Guidelines. *J Am Coll Cardiol* 2001;**38**:2101–13.
6 The Digitalis Investigation Group. The effect of digoxin on mortality and morbidity in patients with heart failure. *N Engl J Med* 1997;**336**:525–33.
7 Crawford M. *Cardiology clinics: congestive heart failure*, vol 12. Philadelphia: WB Saunders, 1994.
8 Pitt B, Zannad F, Remme WJ, *et al*. The effect of spironolactone on morbidity and mortality in patients with severe heart failure. *N Engl J Med* 1999;**341**:709–17.
9 Cohn JN, Johnson G, Ziesche S, *et al*. A comparison of enalapril with hydralazine-isosorbide dinitrate in treatment of chronic congestive heart failure. *N Engl J Med* 1991;**325**:303–10.
10 The CONSENSUS Trial Study Group. Effects of enalapril on mortality in severe congestive heart failure. *N Engl J Med* 1987;**316**:1429–35.
11 Garg R, Yusuf S, for the Collaborative Group on ACE Inhibitor Trials. Overview of randomized trials of angiotensin-converting enzyme inhibitors on mortality and morbidity in patients with heart failure. *JAMA* 1995;**273**:1450–6.
12 Frishman WH. Carvedilol. *N Engl J Med* 1998;**339**:1759–65.
13 Califf RM, O'Connor CM. β-Blocker therapy for heart failure. The evidence is in, now the work begins. *JAMA* 2000;**283**:1335–7.
14 Baker DW, Wright RF. Management of heart failure. IV. Anticoagulation for patients with heart failure due to left ventricular systolic dysfunction. *JAMA* 1994;**272**:1614–18.
15 Singh SN, Fletcher RD, Fisher SG, *et al.*, for the Survival Trial of Antiarrhythmic Therapy in Congestive Heart Failure Trial. Amiodarone in patients with congestive heart failure and asymptomatic ventricular arrhythmia. *N Engl J Med* 1995; **333**:77–82.

11: Congenital heart disease

M ELIZABETH BRICKNER

Congenital heart disease occurs in fewer than 1% of all live births. Although the majority of cases are diagnosed in childhood, patients may not present until adulthood. Improvements in both medical therapy and surgery have also resulted in an increasing number of patients with congenital heart disease surviving into adulthood. The present discussion focuses on the types of congenital heart disease that may present for the first time in adulthood.[1-4]

Left to right shunts

Atrial septal defects

Atrial septal defects account for 5–10% of all congenital heart defects and are more common in females than males (2:1 female : male ratio). There are three common anatomic types (Figure 11.1). Ostium secundum defects are located in the middle portion of the interatrial septum and are the most common type (70%). Ostium primum defects (15%) are located in the inferior portion of the interatrial septum and are often associated with abnormalities of the mitral and tricuspid valves (clefts) that may result in significant valve regurgitation. Sinus venosus atrial septal defects (10–15%) are located in the superior portion of the interatrial septum, at the junction of the superior vena cava and the right atrium. Partial anomalous pulmonary venous drainage is commonly associated with sinus venosus defects, and usually involves drainage of one (but occasionally both) of the right pulmonary veins into the superior vena cava or right atrium. Sinus venosus defects may be associated with ectopic atrial rhythms.

Atrial septal defects result in continuous left to right flow across the interatrial septum, and the size of the defect and the difference in compliance between the pulmonary and systemic circulations determine the magnitude of the shunt. The resulting volume overload of the right atrium and right ventricle leads to enlargement of those chambers. Atrial septal defects are usually asymptomatic in childhood and early adulthood, and may not be diagnosed. With increasing age, symptoms of fatigue, exercise intolerance, palpitations, and exertional dyspnea become more common.

The cardinal finding on physical examination is a widely split second heart sound (S_2) that does not vary with respiration (i.e. fixed splitting) because of delay in pulmonary valve closure in patients with

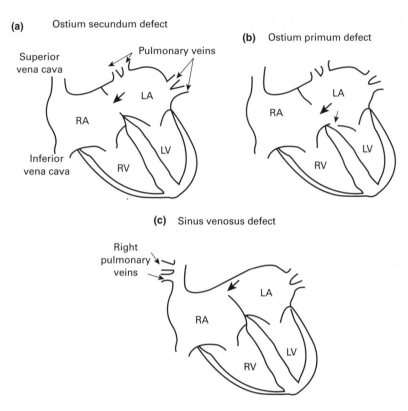

(a) Ostium secundum defect

Superior vena cava

Pulmonary veins

LA

RA

Inferior vena cava

RV

LV

(b) Ostium primum defect

LA

RA

RV

LV

(c) Sinus venosus defect

Right pulmonary veins

LA

RA

RV

LV

Figure 11.1 Anatomic types of atrial septal defects. **(a)** Ostium secundum defect with normal pulmonary venous connections. **(b)** Ostium primum defect with an abnormal mitral valve (cleft in anterior mitral leaflet). **(c)** Sinus venosus defect with associated partial anomalous pulmonary venous drainage (right pulmonary veins draining into the superior vena cava). LA, left atrium; LV, left ventricle; RA, right atrium; RV, right ventricle

normal pulmonary pressures and low pulmonary vascular resistance. A parasternal lift due to a prominent, hyperdynamic right ventricular impulse may be palpated. A mid-systolic ejection murmur over the pulmonic area is invariably present, and is caused by increased blood flow across the pulmonic valve. (Flow across the atrial septal defect itself does not cause a murmur.) If the shunt is large the increased flow across the tricuspid valve may result in a mid-diastolic rumbling murmur at the lower left sternal border.

Over time, in response to the increased pulmonary blood flow, pulmonary vascular resistance and pulmonary pressures may increase. As pulmonary hypertension develops, the physical examination findings change. Splitting of S_2 becomes narrower as pulmonary pressures increase and the pulmonary component of S_2 (P_2) becomes louder. As pulmonary vascular resistance increases, the magnitude of the left to right shunt decreases and the pulmonary flow murmur also decreases. As the pulmonary vascular resistance rises, predominant right to left shunting may ensue with resulting hypoxia, cyanosis, and clubbing (Eisenmenger physiology).

Classic electrocardiographic findings in an uncomplicated ostium secundum atrial septal defect include right axis deviation, right ventricular hypertrophy, and incomplete right bundle branch block. This delay in right ventricular activation may be due either to volume overload or to actual conduction delay in the right bundle. Electrocardiographic evidence of right ventricular hypertrophy may be present as well. Left axis deviation suggests an ostium primum atrial septal defect and an ectopic atrial rhythm suggests the presence of a sinus venosus type of defect. The chest x ray film in an uncomplicated atrial septal defect demonstrates cardiomegaly, with enlargement of the right atrium and ventricle and increased pulmonary vascular markings ("plethora") indicative of increased pulmonary blood flow. Enlargement of the main pulmonary arteries may be seen.

The diagnosis of an atrial septal defect can be made by echocardiography, which demonstrates enlargement of the right atrium and ventricle, the location and size of the defect, and the direction of the intracardiac shunt. Ostium secundum and ostium primum defects can usually be seen by transthoracic echocardiography, whereas only 50% of sinus venosus defects can be seen using this technique. Transesophageal echocardiography is a superior technique for demonstrating the sinus venosus type of defects. Cardiac catheterization is another technique for diagnosing atrial septal defects. A "step-up" in oxygen saturation due to left to right shunting across the defect is demonstrated by taking blood samples proximal to the shunt (from the vena cavae) and distal to the shunt (from the right ventricle or pulmonary artery). The ratio of pulmonary to systemic blood flow (Q_p/Q_s) can be calculated from these oxygen saturation data to determine the size of the shunt. Cardiac catheterization also allows measurement of pulmonary pressures and pulmonary vascular resistance. In older patients, coronary angiography is also performed to diagnose concomitant coronary artery disease.

Eisenmenger's syndrome (pulmonary hypertension with reversed or bidirectional shunt at atrial, ventricular, or aortopulmonary level) is an uncommon complication of atrial septal defects, and occurs in fewer than 10% of longstanding cases appearing in adulthood. More commonly, patients with untreated atrial septal defects develop right heart failure and atrial arrhythmias as a consequence of volume overload of the right ventricle. In these patients symptoms usually develop by the fourth or fifth decade of life.

Prophylaxis for bacterial endocarditis is not required for atrial septal defects unless valvular defects are also present. Closure of the defect is recommended for all atrial septal defects of significant size (pulmonary to systemic flow ratio >2:1) unless pulmonary vascular resistance is prohibitively high. In addition to surgical closure, there are percutaneous devices that can be can be used in suitable candidates. With a pulmonary to systemic vascular resistance ratio of greater than 0·7, surgery is associated with increased morbidity and mortality, and shunt closure is almost always contraindicated. Surgery should be done as early as possible after the defect is detected. Closure before age 40 years may allow normal cardiac size and function to return, whereas closure in older patients is often associated with residual right heart failure and atrial arrhythmias. Transcatheter closure of small to moderate size defects represents a new option for some patients, although long-term results are not available and direct comparisons with surgical outcomes have not been conducted.

Ventricular septal defects

Ventricular septal defects are among the most common forms of congenital heart disease (20–30% of all defects) and are more common in males. Ventricular septal defects may involve the membranous septum (70%), the muscular septum (25%), the supracristal region (involving the annuli of the aorta and pulmonary artery; 5%), or the inlet portion of the septum (under the mitral and tricuspid valves; Figure 11.2). Both perimembranous and muscular types of ventricular septal defects may close spontaneously (as many as 50%), usually within the first year of life.

Because ventricular septal defects usually produce a loud murmur, they are commonly detected in childhood. Small defects result in small shunts and are usually asymptomatic. Moderate to large defects result in volume overload of the left atrium and left ventricle, and are associated with symptoms such as poor exercise tolerance and congestive heart failure. These larger defects are usually diagnosed in childhood. With larger shunts, pulmonary pressures and pulmonary vascular resistance may be elevated. With severe pulmonary hypertension, shunt reversal occurs (Eisenmenger's syndrome). When ventricular septal defects are discovered in adulthood, they are usually small (an incidental finding) or the patient has had prior surgery or has developed a complication related to the defect.

The physical examination, electrocardiographic, and chest x ray findings depend on the size of the ventricular septal defect and the amount of pulmonary hypertension. With small defects (<0·5 cm^2), the small left to right shunt does not result in significant volume overload to the heart. The left to right shunt across the defect causes a palpable thrill and a loud, holosystolic murmur that is heard best along the left sternal border. The S$_2$ is normal. The electrocardiogram and chest x ray

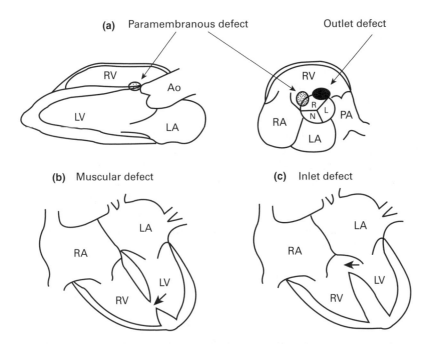

Figure 11.2 Anatomic types of ventricular septal defects. **(a)** Paramembranous defects are located beneath the aortic valve, adjacent to the tricuspid valve. Outlet defects are related to both the aortic and pulmonary valves. **(b)** Muscular defect. **(c)** Inlet defect, underlying the mitral and tricuspid valves. Ao, ascending aorta; L, left coronary cusp of aortic valve; LA, left atrium; LV, left ventricle; N, non-coronary cusp; PA, pulmonary artery; R, right coronary cusp of aortic valve; RA, right atrium; RV, right ventricle

film are normal. With defects of moderate size (0·5–1·0 cm²) volume overload of the left atrium and left ventricle occurs. A systolic thrill and holosystolic murmur are again present and a mid-diastolic rumble can be heart over the mitral area, indicating increased blood flow across the valve. Left ventricular hypertrophy is seen on the electrocardiogram, and pulmonary plethora (increased pulmonary vascular markings) is seen on the chest x ray film. With large defects (>1·0 cm²) left sided third heart sound (S₃) and fourth heart sound (S₄) are usually present, in addition to a palpable thrill and systolic and diastolic murmurs. Signs of pulmonary hypertension may be present as well, with a palpable parasternal lift due to right ventricular pressure overload and a loud P₂ on auscultation. At this stage the electrocardiogram demonstrates biventricular hypertrophy and the chest x ray film shows frank cardiomegaly in addition to pulmonary plethora. With development of irreversible pulmonary hypertension and shunt reversal (Eisenmenger's syndrome), the murmurs and systolic thrill disappear, the S₂ (P₂) becomes narrow or even single, and cyanosis and clubbing appear. The electrocardiogram now demonstrates pure right ventricular hypertrophy. The chest x ray film may now show dilated main pulmonary arteries and small, "pruned" distal pulmonary vessels with relative oligemia of the vascular markings.

The diagnosis of a ventricular septal defect can be made by transthoracic echocardiography, which demonstrates the location and size of the defect and the direction of the shunt. With moderate to large shunts, left atrial and ventricular enlargement is seen. Transesophageal echocardiography is needed only for patients with technically inadequate transthoracic imaging. Cardiac catheterization is also used to diagnose left to right shunting associated with ventricular septal defects by demonstrating a "step-up" between the right atrium and the pulmonary artery, or by demonstrating contrast shunting from the left to right ventricle. The ratio of pulmonary to systemic blood flow (Q_p/Q_s) is calculated to determine the size of the shunt and pulmonary pressures and pulmonary vascular resistance is also calculated. If pulmonary vascular resistance is markedly elevated (>70% of systemic vascular resistance), then shunt closure is contraindicated.

The development of severe pulmonary hypertension with shunt reversal causing cyanosis (Eisenmenger's syndrome) is a dreaded complication of ventricular septal defects, occurring in 10–25% (more commonly than with atrial septal defects). In patients with ventricular septal defects, this syndrome usually presents in the first or second decade of life. Despite severe disease, survival to early adulthood is common. Infective endocarditis is another complication in patients with ventricular septal defects. The tricuspid valve, or the right ventricular endocardium itself, where the turbulent left to right "jet" strikes, is usually involved. Other acquired complications include the development of aortic regurgitation and subaortic stenosis.

When a ventricular septal defect is diagnosed it is important to assess the magnitude of the shunt and the degree of pulmonary vascular disease. Surgical closure is recommended for significant left to right shunts (pulmonary to systemic flow ratio 2:1). If significant pulmonary hypertension is suspected, then cardiac catheterization is necessary to measure pulmonary vascular resistance. As for all shunt lesions, significant pulmonary vascular disease (pulmonary vascular resistance to systemic vascular resistance ratio greater than 0·7) is a contraindication to shunt closure because it is likely to result in acute right heart failure and death. Prophylaxis for bacterial endocarditis is required for all ventricular septal defects, regardless of their size. Continued antibiotic prophylaxis is also recommended for any patients with a residual ventricular septal defect after surgical closure.

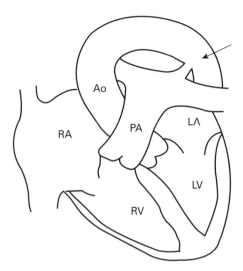

Figure 11.3 Patent ductus arteriosus. Ao, ascending aorta; LA, left atrium; LV, left ventricle; PA, pulmonary artery; RA, right atrium; RV, right ventricle

Patent ductus arteriosus

The ductus arteriosus is a normal part of the fetal circulation, connecting the pulmonary trunk and the descending aorta just distal to the left subclavian artery so that most of the fetal right ventricular output bypasses the unexpanded lungs and travels to the placenta where oxygenation occurs. Persistence of this communication after birth is referred to as a patent ductus arteriosus (Figure 11.3). It is more common in females than in males (3:1) and may be seen in association with maternal rubella, and pulmonary disease in infants and in premature infants. A patent ductus arteriosus produces hemodynamic changes that are similar to those seen with ventricular septal defects. The left to right shunt produces a volume load on the left heart, and the magnitude of the shunt depends on the size of the ductus and the pulmonary vascular resistance.

The clinical manifestations of a patent ductus arteriosus depend on the size of the shunt. Patients with a small shunt are asymptomatic, whereas large shunts can result in recurrent pulmonary infections, poor exercise tolerance, exertional dyspnea, and congestive heart failure. A large ductus can cause compression of the recurrent laryngeal nerve, resulting in hoarseness.

The classic finding on physical examination is a "machinery-type" continuous murmur (for example, a murmur that persists throughout systole and continues past the second heart sounds) at the left upper sternal border. With a small ductus, the remainder of the physical examination is normal, as are the electrocardiogram and the chest *x* ray findings. With moderate to large shunts, the precordium is hyperactive, peripheral pulses are bounding (due to rapid run-off through the ductus), and a diastolic rumble is heard across the mitral valve, indicating an increased volume of blood flow. The pulmonary component of S_2 is usually increased. The electrocardiogram demonstrates left ventricular hypertrophy and may show right ventricular hypertrophy as well. Cardiomegaly with pulmonary plethora is seen on the chest *x* ray.

As with other shunts, pulmonary vascular disease may develop resulting in Eisenmenger's syndrome. If the Eisenmenger physiology is present, then S_2 is loud and single, and the continuous murmur and the mitral diastolic murmur are no longer heard. Differential cyanosis may be present (cyanosis of the lower extremities) as desaturated blood from the right to left shunt enters the descending aorta through the ductus. The upper extremities, perfused by unshunted blood, will be acyanotic.

The diagnosis of an uncomplicated patent ductus arteriosus can be made by transthoracic echocardiography, which demonstrates continuous left to right shunting from the aorta to the pulmonary artery. At cardiac catheterization the shunt can be diagnosed by demonstrating an oxygen "step-up" in the pulmonary artery or by demonstrating contrast shunting from the aorta to the pulmonary artery.

The presence of a patent ductus increases the risk for infective endocarditis, and with significant shunts it increases the risk for heart failure and Eisenmenger's syndrome. Severe pulmonary vascular obstruction may cause calcification, aneurysmal dilatation, or rupture of the ductus. Closure of the shunt is recommended for all patients except those with Eisenmenger physiology and elderly patients. Quantitation of the shunt size is not important in determining the need for shunt closure. In general, surgical ligation or division of the ductus has a low operative mortality and morbidity, although complications such as damage to the recurrent laryngeal nerve, the phrenic nerve, or the thoracic duct can occur. Newer, non-surgical options for closure of the patent ductus arteriosus include "button" devices, "double umbrella" occluders, and spring coils. These various devices can be placed percutaneously with low complication rates and may become the procedure of choice for selected patients.

Obstructive lesions

Aortic stenosis

Congenital abnormalities of the aortic valve can result in a valve that is obstructive at birth or may develop progressive obstruction

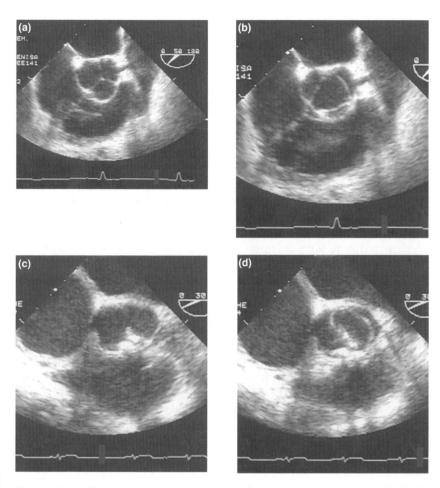

Figure 11.4 Transesophageal echocardiographic images of a normal aortic valve and a bicuspid aortic valve. A normal aortic valve in **(a)** closed and **(b)** open position, and a bicuspid aortic valve in **(c)** closed and **(d)** open position

over time. Aortic valve stenosis may be due to bicuspid valves or unicuspid valves. Unicuspid valves are inherently stenotic and symptoms present in infancy and childhood. Bicuspid aortic valves occur in 1–2% of the general population, more commonly in males than in females. The bicuspid aortic valve has only two cusps (usually of unequal size), rather than three normal cusps (Figure 11.4). In 50% of cases, a raphe or false commissure is seen on the larger of the two leaflets. Bicuspid valves are usually not inherently stenotic and may function normally throughout life. In some patients, progressive fibrosis and calcification of the cusps occurs, resulting in progressive aortic stenosis. Bicuspid valves commonly exhibit some degree of aortic regurgitation that may be progressive over time, and infective endocarditis is common in patients with bicuspid aortic valves and is a major cause of aortic regurgitation. Bicuspid aortic valves are also associated with coarctation of the aorta, dilatation of the aortic root, and an increased risk for aortic dissection.

Patients with bicuspid aortic valves are usually asymptomatic but may present with symptoms if the valve is dysfunctional. Patients with mild aortic stenosis are usually asymptomatic but patients with moderate to severe aortic stenosis may present with angina, syncope, or symptoms of heart failure. Typically, patients present with symptomatic aortic stenosis in their 40s or 50s, whereas patients with degenerative aortic stenosis typically present at an older age.

The physical examination, electrocardiogram, and chest x ray findings in patients with congenital aortic stenosis are similar to those seen in patients with acquired forms of aortic stenosis, except that bicuspid valves are frequently associated with an ejection click. Echocardiography can document valve anatomy and quantitate the severity of stenosis. Cardiac catheterization is also used to quantitate the severity of stenosis. The management of congenital aortic stenosis in adults is similar to that for patients with acquired forms of aortic stenosis, and intervention is indicated for symptomatic patients. Valve replacement is required for most patients but balloon valvuloplasty is an option for a few patients with stenotic valves that are relatively pliable and non-calcified. All patients with bicuspid aortic valves require prophylaxis against bacterial endocarditis.

Pulmonic stenosis

Obstruction of the right ventricular outflow tract can occur at the level of the valve, in the infundibulum (below the valve), or above the valve. Valvular stenosis accounts for approximately 90% of cases of pulmonic stenosis and is commonly associated with survival into adulthood. Infundibular stenosis is usually associated with tetralogy of Fallot or other congenital malformations.

Symptoms depend on the severity of the stenosis. Patients with trivial (peak gradient <25 mmHg) or mild stenosis (peak gradient 25–50 mmHg) are usually asymptomatic. With more significant stenosis, fatigue and exertional dyspnea are common. Syncope can also occur. Symptoms of right ventricular failure can occur with severe stenosis (peak gradient >75–100 mmHg). Right to left shunt with central cyanosis can occur if there is an associated atrial septal defect or patent foramen ovale in the presence of severe pulmonic stenosis.

On physical examination, a parasternal lift may be palpated due to right ventricular pressure overload, and a systolic ejection murmur is heard along the left sternal border. With mild stenosis, the murmur peaks early, a systolic ejection click is often heard, and P_2 is usually normal. A systolic thrill along the left sternal border may be present with mild degrees of stenosis but is more common with moderate to severe obstruction. With increasing degrees of obstruction, the systolic murmur peaks later, the ejection click often disappears, and P_2 becomes softer and delayed. With severe pulmonic stenosis one may find a prominent "a" wave in the jugular venous pulse and a right ventricular S_4. As the severity of pulmonic stenosis increases the electrocardiogram progresses from normal to right axis deviation and right ventricular hypertrophy, and eventually a right ventricular strain pattern develops as well. The chest x ray film usually demonstrates normal heart size and poststenotic dilatation of the main pulmonary artery.

Echocardiography demonstrates thickened pulmonary valve leaflets with limited mobility. The pressure gradient can be determine by Doppler techniques, and associated lesions such as interatrial shunts can also be detected. At cardiac catheterization, the pressure gradient between the right ventricle and the pulmonary artery can be measured. Balloon valvuloplasty can also be performed at the time of catheterization and is recommended as the initial therapy for symptomatic patients with moderate to severe stenosis. Balloon valvuloplasty achieves reductions in gradient that are comparable to those achieved by surgery, but with lower morbidity and mortality rates. Surgery is reserved for patients with other associated lesions that require repair or for those in whom balloon valvuloplasty is not successful. No intervention is required for asymptomatic patients with mild to moderate stenosis.

Coarctation of the aorta

Coarctation of the aorta accounts for approximately 8% of all congenital heart disease. It is more common in males than in females (ratio 2:1) and is commonly seen in association with Turner's syndrome (gonadal dysgenesis in phenotypic women with primary amenorrhea, short stature, and multiple congenital abnormalities). Bicuspid aortic valves are seen in approximately half of all patients with coarctation of the aorta. Other obstructive lesions of the left heart (mitral stenosis, subaortic stenosis, aortic stenosis) are also associated with coarctation of the aorta. As many as 20% of cases of coarctation are undetected in childhood, presenting either in adolescence or adulthood. In adults, a ridge, or web, of tissue causing obstruction to flow is present in the aorta just distal to the left subclavian artery (Figure 11.5). Collateral circulation to the lower body is usually well developed and patients are often asymptomatic (collaterals may be palpated in the posterior intercostal spaces).

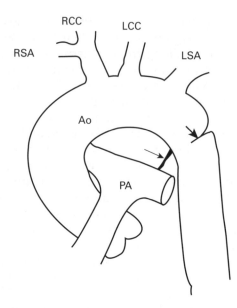

Figure 11.5 Coarctation of the aorta (postductal type). The area of obstruction is located distal to the left subclavian artery (LSA), near the ligamentum arteriosum (fine arrow). Ao, aorta; LCC, left common carotid artery; PA, pulmonary artery; RCC, right common carotid artery; RSA, right subclavian artery. (Thick arrow shows site of coarctation of the aorta)

Coarctation of the aorta should be suspected in a young adult who presents with hypertension.

Patients are hypertensive with a higher blood pressure in the arms than in the legs (>20 mmHg). Simultaneous palpation of the radial and femoral arteries reveals the femoral pulses to be diminished and delayed. Pulses in the lower extremities are decreased or even absent. On cardiac auscultation, an aortic ejection click and increased intensity of the aortic component of S_2 (A_2) may be heard, with a bicuspid aortic valve. Murmurs may arise from an associated bicuspid aortic valve, from the coarctation itself, or from collateral arterial flow. A systolic ejection murmur is commonly heard and a diastolic murmur of aortic insufficiency may be detected. A localized systolic murmur over the spine can be heard at the site of the coarctation. Bruits secondary to collateral flow may be heard both anteriorly (flow through the internal mammary arteries) and posteriorly (flow through the intercostal arteries). If right arm pulses are intact but left arm pulses are absent, then the coarctation is proximal to or at the level of the left subclavian artery.

The electrocardiogram may be normal (in up to 20%) but left ventricular hypertrophy is common. On chest x ray, the heart size is normal or only mildly enlarged. The ascending aorta may appear dilated (suggesting a bicuspid aortic valve). A "three" sign may be seen, caused by a dilated left subclavian artery above the coarctation and poststenotic dilatation of the aorta below the coarctation. Rib notching is seen in the posterior aspect of the fourth to eighth ribs in older children and adults as a result of erosion of the rib margins by enlargement of the intercostal arteries.

The diagnosis of coarctation of the aorta can best be confirmed by magnetic resonance imaging, which can demonstrate the anatomy and assess the degree of obstruction. Echocardiography is also useful, particularly in children, in whom the area of coarctation may be directly visualized. Color Doppler can demonstrate turbulent flow across the obstruction and the pressure gradient can be measured by Doppler. Cardiac catheterization also provides excellent anatomic and hemodynamic definition. The pressure gradient across the coarctation can be measured. The lesion itself can be demonstrated by angiography.

Identification and correction of coarctation of the aorta is important because the median survival for patients with uncorrected coarctation of the aorta is in the mid-30s. Complications of coarctation include left ventricular failure due to longstanding hypertension, endocarditis (occurring either on the associated bicuspid valve or at the site of the coarctation), dissecting aortic aneurysm, and rupture of the aorta. Rupture or dissection most commonly occurs in the third or fourth decade of life with an increased risk during pregnancy. Stenosis or regurgitation of the associated bicuspid aortic valve can also occur.

Intervention is recommended when a significant gradient (>30–50 mmHg) is present. Options include surgical correction and balloon aortoplasty. Surgical repair can be achieved with resection and end-to-end anastomosis, use of the left subclavian artery as a patch, or use of a Dacron patch. Long-term survival after surgical repair depends on the age at the time of repair, with best results seen with repair in infancy and the shortest survival times reported with repair after age 40 years. Persistent hypertension is common postoperatively, and appears to be related to increased age at the time of repair. Balloon aortoplasty is an alternative to surgery that appears to be most appropriate for infants and children, and may be useful in the setting of postoperative restenosis.

Cyanotic congenital heart disease

Tetralogy of Fallot

Tetralogy of Fallot accounts for approximately 10% of all congenital heart disease and is the most common cyanotic defect presenting in

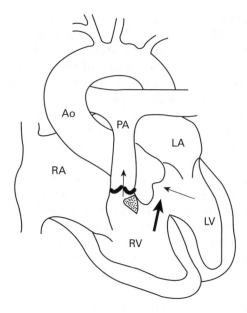

Figure 11.6 Tetralogy of Fallot with left aortic arch (normal orientation). A large non-restrictive ventricular septal defect with an overriding aorta is shown. Obstruction to right ventricular outflow is present (both valvular pulmonic stenosis and infundibular stenosis in this example) with decreased flow into the pulmonary artery. Flow across the ventricular septal defect is predominantly right to left. Right ventricular hypertrophy is present. Ao, aorta; LA, left atrium; LV, left ventricle; PA, pulmonary artery; RA, right atrium; RV, right ventricle

adulthood (Figure 11.6). The four components of tetralogy are a large ventricular septal defect, overriding of the aorta, obstruction of the right ventricular outflow tract, and right ventricular hypertrophy. The ventricular septal defect is large and non-restrictive, which results in equalization of right and left ventricular pressures. Obstruction of the right ventricular outflow tract may occur at the level of the infundibulum (50%), at the level of the pulmonic valve (isolated valvular stenosis in 10%), or at multiple levels within the right ventricular outflow tract and pulmonary artery. The pathophysiology and clinical presentation depend on the degree of right ventricular outflow tract obstruction. In the classic form of tetralogy with significant stenosis of the outflow tract, pulmonary blood flow is diminished and pulmonary pressures are low to normal. A significant right to left shunt is present, its magnitude determined by the ratio of pulmonary to systemic vascular resistance. Patients present with cyanosis and exertional dyspnea. Cyanotic "spells" occur in infants but are not seen in adults.

In contrast to the classic form of tetralogy of Fallot, mild degrees of obstruction across the right ventricular outflow tract are associated with increased pulmonary blood flow and a small to moderate left to right shunt across the ventricular septal defect. In this form, the patient is acyanotic (so-called "pink tetralogy") and is usually asymptomatic. However, over time progression of the right ventricular outflow tract obstruction usually occurs, resulting in development of cyanosis and symptoms.

On physical examination in classic tetralogy of Fallot, cyanosis and clubbing are present. In the jugular venous pulse "a" and "v" waves are prominent, and a parasternal lift due to right ventricular pressure overload may be felt. The S_2 is usually single (inaudible pulmonary component). A systolic ejection murmur is heard along the sternal border caused by the outflow tract obstruction, with the intensity and duration of the murmur directly related to the severity of obstruction. A systolic thrill secondary to the outflow tract obstruction may also be noted. If there is significant collateral circulation to the lungs from the bronchial arteries, then continuous murmurs may be heard in the chest. The electrocardiogram demonstrates right axis deviation and right ventricular hypertrophy. On chest x ray, the heart size is small to normal and is classically "boot-shaped". Pulmonary vascular markings are decreased with "oligemia" of the lung fields. A right sided aortic arch is seen in 25% of cases.

While most patients with tetralogy of Fallot present with cyanosis in infancy, some patients may survive to adulthood in the unoperated state. Symptoms typically worsen with increasing age as the degree of right ventricular obstruction increases. In addition to complaints of cyanosis and exercise limitations, patients also develop complications associated with cyanotic heart disease, including erythrocytosis, hyperviscosity, coagulation abnormalities, gout, stroke, brain abscess, and infective endocarditis.

The diagnosis of tetralogy of Fallot can be made by echocardiography or cardiac catheterization. Echocardiography demonstrates right ventricular hypertrophy, the ventricular septal defect, the overriding aorta, and the level and severity of right ventricular outflow tract obstruction. Cardiac catheterization is required if surgical correction is being considered. The ventricular septal defect with right to left shunting is demonstrated on ventriculography, and the degree of right ventricular outflow tract obstruction can be measured. In addition, coronary angiography is performed to exclude the possibility of anomalous coronary arteries (seen in 10%).

All patients with tetralogy of Fallot require bacterial endocarditis prophylaxis. Surgical correction with patch closure of the ventricular septal defect and relief of right ventricular outflow tract obstruction is performed to provide relief of symptoms and improve survival. Relief of right ventricular outflow tract obstruction may involve pulmonary valvotomy, enlargement of the pulmonary artery annulus with a prosthetic patch, and resection of infundibular stenosis; in some cases it requires a prosthetic conduit to bypass the obstruction. Surgical correction in uncomplicated forms of tetralogy of Fallot can be performed with a mortality rate of approximately 5% and results in good long-term survival. Postoperatively, patients need to be followed carefully because they are at risk for arrhythmias and conduction disorders, recurrent right heart obstruction, pulmonic insufficiency, right ventricular dysfunction, and complications associated with prosthetic patches, valves, or conduits.

Eisenmenger' syndrome

In patients with left to right shunts and increased pulmonary blood flow, progressive histologic changes may occur in the pulmonary vascular bed as a consequence of the increased pulmonary blood flow and pressure. These histologic changes occur predominantly in the small muscular arteries, ultimately resulting in irreversible pulmonary hypertension and elevation in pulmonary vascular resistance, a condition referred to as pulmonary vascular obstructive disease. The initial changes (largely reversible) consist of medial hypertrophy, intimal proliferation, and fibrosis. The later stages (irreversible) consist of dilatation and thinning of the vessel wall, development of plexiform lesions within the lumen of the vessels, and fibrinoid necrosis of the arteries. As pulmonary vascular resistance approaches or exceeds systemic vascular resistance, the shunt flow becomes bidirectional or predominantly right to left. The term "Eisenmenger's syndrome" is used to describe patients with shunt reversal due to severe pulmonary vascular disease.

The pathologic changes that occur in the pulmonary vascular bed begin in childhood but may not result in symptoms until late childhood or early adulthood. Symptoms usually occur earlier with large shunts at the level of the aorta or ventricle and later with shunts at the atrial level. Patients commonly present with complaints of exertional fatigue and dyspnea as well as cyanosis. Recurrent episodes of hemoptysis may occur due to *in situ* thrombosis of small pulmonary arteries, recurrent pulmonary emboli with infarction, or hemorrhage from plexiform lesions within the pulmonary vessels. Occasionally, patients may present with massive hemoptysis due to rupture of a pulmonary artery. Exertional angina may occur because of right ventricular ischemia. Exercise can also result in syncope by causing a reduction in systemic vascular resistance, increased right to left shunting, and decreased cerebral oxygenation. Syncope or sudden death also occur as the result of arrhythmias. Arrhythmias may result in rapid clinical deterioration. Right heart failure is a late complication of pulmonary vascular obstructive disease and is more commonly seen in older patients.

Patients with significant right to left shunting have chronic hypoxemia, stimulating erythropoietin production and resulting in an elevated red blood cell mass (erythrocytosis). Marked erythrocytosis can result in symptoms of hyperviscosity (headache, myalgias, paresthesias, blurry vision, dizziness, and exertional dyspnea). The increase in red cell turnover can result in calcium bilirubinate gallstones, placing patients at risk for acute cholecystitis. Patients may develop anemia secondary to iron deficiency (most commonly) or folate or vitamin B_{12} deficiency, a diagnosis that can easily be missed in a patient who presents with hemoglobin within the "normal" range. The development of iron deficiency is detrimental in these patients because iron deficiency results in increased blood viscosity, which can worsen hyperviscosity symptoms. Coagulation abnormalities including factor deficiencies and platelet dysfunction also occur, placing patients at risk for both thrombotic and hemorrhagic complications. Brain abscess is an uncommon complication, resulting from paradoxic embolism of infected material. Patients frequently develop impaired renal function. Impaired excretion of uric acid resulting in hyperuricemia is common and is a marker of underlying renal dysfunction.

The predominant finding on physical examination is central cyanosis and clubbing, as well as evidence of pulmonary hypertension. If Eisenmenger's syndrome is due to a patent ductus arteriosus, cyanosis and clubbing will be limited to the lower extremities ("differential cyanosis"). Signs of pulmonary hypertension include prominent "a" wave in the jugular venous pulse, a parasternal lift due to right ventricular pressure overload, a prominent (and often palpable) P_2, and murmurs of tricuspid and pulmonic regurgitation. Other murmurs are not present (for example, the classic murmurs of a ventricular septal defect or patent ductus arteriosus are absent). The chest x ray film demonstrates dilatation of the central pulmonary arteries with "pruning" of the distal vessels. Cardiomegaly is not usually seen. The electrocardiogram shows right axis deviation, right atrial overload, and right ventricular hypertrophy.

Echocardiography is useful in demonstrating a right ventricular pressure overload pattern, estimating the severity of pulmonary hypertension, and demonstrating the underlying cardiac defect. Cardiac catheterization is extremely important in evaluating patients with possible Eisenmenger's syndrome. In addition to demonstrating the underlying structural abnormality, it is necessary to assess the severity of pulmonary hypertension and to assess for the reversibility of the elevated pulmonary vascular resistance. In most laboratories, measurements of flow, pulmonary pressures, and pulmonary vascular resistance are made on room air and during the administration of 100% oxygen.

Therapy for Eisenmenger's syndrome is fairly limited. Surgical closure of the shunt is not an option because this is associated with a high operative mortality. Combined heart and lung transplantation or lung transplantation with repair of the cardiac defect may be an option for severely symptomatic patients.

Medical management involves attempts to prevent many of the known complications of Eisenmenger's syndrome. Endocarditis prophylaxis is mandatory. Anemia should be diagnosed and treated. Anticoagulants and antiplatelet agents should be avoided. Other medications to be avoided include vasodilators, drugs that increase uric acid levels, and oral contraceptives (increased risk for thrombosis). Some effective form of birth control is extremely important because of the high risk of both fetal and maternal mortality in pregnant women with Eisenmenger's syndrome. Intrauterine devices should be avoided because of the risk of infection. Permanent sterilization by tubal ligation is preferred.

Phlebotomy can be performed to decrease red blood cell mass but should not be done solely on the basis of the hematocrit. Phlebotomy is indicated for patients with "decompensated erythrocytosis" – moderate to severe symptoms of hyperviscosity with an unstable, increasing hematocrit level. Phlebotomy should be done with simultaneous replacement of intravascular volume because hypovolemia can precipitate hemodynamic collapse in these patients.

Case studies

Case 11.1

A 22-year-old female is referred for evaluation of a newly discovered murmur. She is in the 16th week of her first pregnancy. She has no significant past medical history, and no previous history of heart disease. She describes a normal childhood with no exercise limitations. Currently, she complains of some fatigue and dyspnea that she attributes to her pregnancy. She denies chest pain, palpitations, orthopnea, or syncope. Her only medication is a prenatal vitamin. Family history and social history are non-contributory.

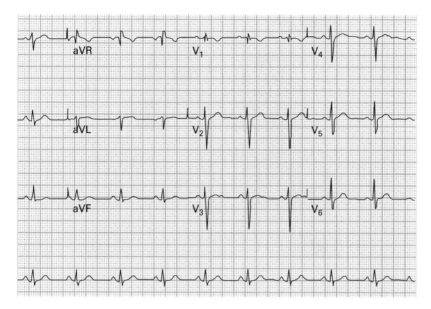

Figure 11.7 Electrocardiogram demonstrating normal sinus rhythm, right axis deviation, and incomplete right bundle branch block

Examination. Physical examination: the patient appeared normal. No abnormalities of skin, nail beds, or oral mucosa. Pulse: 74 beats/min. Blood pressure: 100/60 mmHg in right arm. Jugular venous pulse: normal. Cardiac impulse: normal apical impulse. Parasternal lift. First heart sound normal. Second heart fixed, wide split, P_2 of normal loudness. Grade 3/6 crescendo/decrescendo murmur at left sternal border. Chest examination: normal air entry, no rales or rhonchi. Abdominal examination: soft abdomen, no tenderness, and no masses. Normal liver span. No peripheral edema. Femoral, popliteal, posterior tibial, and dorsalis pedis pulses: all normal volume and equal. Carotid pulses: normal, no bruits. Optic fundi: normal.

Investigations. Electrocardiogram: Figure 11.7.

Questions

1. What further diagnostic tests should be obtained?
2. Can this patient safely continue her pregnancy?
3. Should any special precautions be taken during her pregnancy?
4. Should this patient be referred for surgery?
5. What is the chance that her child will have a congenital heart defect?

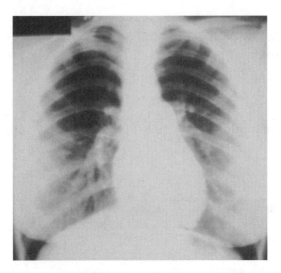

Figure 11.8 Chest *x* ray of a patient with a known ostium secundum atrial septal defect. Pulmonary vascular markings are increased, indicating increased pulmonary blood flow

Answers

Answer to question 1 On the basis of her physical examination, this patient has an uncomplicated atrial septal defect. Her electrocardiogram demonstrates sinus rhythm with right axis deviation and an incomplete right bundle branch block, which is consistent with either a ostium secundum or a sinus venosus atrial septal defect. Although a chest *x* ray would be helpful in confirming the diagnosis by demonstrating cardiomegaly and increased pulmonary vascular markings, it can be deferred in a pregnant woman. (A representative chest *x* ray from a similar, non-pregnant patient is shown in Figure 11.8.) Transthoracic echocardiography should be performed to confirm the presence of the atrial septal defect, assess its location and size, and assess for any other defects. If the transthoracic study is technically inadequate, then a transesophageal echocardiography could be performed to confirm the diagnosis. (Although it is considered a very safe procedure, transesophageal echocardiography usually requires administration of conscious sedation during the procedure, which should be performed with caution in a pregnant woman.) If the echocardiogram confirms the diagnosis of an uncomplicated atrial septal defect, then no further diagnostic work up is required.

Her transthoracic echocardiogram demonstrated a dilated right atrium and right ventricle with evidence of right ventricular volume

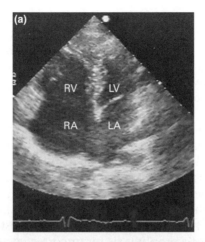

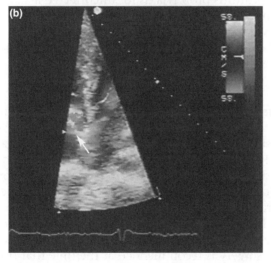

Figure 11.9 Transthoracic echocardiographic images of a large ostium secundum atrial septal defect. **(a)** Apical four chamber view demonstrating large ostium secundum atrial septal defect with right atrial and right ventricular enlargement. **(b)** Left to right shunting of blood across the defect as demonstrated by color Doppler. The arrow indicates flow

overload. A large ostium secundum atrial septal defect with a large left to right shunt was demonstrated (Figure 11.9). No other defects were noted.

Answer to question 2 In general, cardiac lesions that result in a volume overload of the heart, such as left to right intracardiac shunts, are well tolerated during pregnancy. In contrast to uncomplicated left to right shunts, patients with shunt reversal (Eisenmenger's syndrome) have high fetal and maternal mortality, and termination of the pregnancy is usually advised. Because this patient has no evidence of pulmonary hypertension and no evidence of shunt reversal on her physical examination or echocardiogram, she has no contraindications to continuing her pregnancy.

Answer to question 3 She theoretically has an increased potential for paradoxic embolization of venous thrombi through her interatrial communication. However, in natural history studies of atrial septal defects, paradoxic emboli are extremely uncommon. Prophylactic anticoagulation would be risky, has no proven role, and is not recommended. Labor and delivery should be handled routinely, with cesarean section being performed only for obstetric indications. Bacterial endocarditis prophylaxis for uncorrected atrial septal defects is recommended only if there are associated valvular defects and is not necessary for an uncomplicated vaginal delivery. In practice, because the complications of delivery cannot be predicted and the risk associated with antibiotic administration is small, prophylactic antibiotics are often given.

Answer to question 4 If this patient has a significant left to right shunt (pulmonary to systemic flow ratio greater than 2:1) then she should be referred for surgery in the non-pregnant state to decrease the risk for developing right heart failure and atrial arrhythmias in the future. The size of the shunt (trivial, not requiring intervention, or significant, requiring closure) can usually be adequately estimated from the echocardiogram, and Doppler techniques can be used to calculate the shunt ratio. In cases in which the echocardiogram is not diagnostic, cardiac catheterization is performed. For most patients with an atrial septal defect, surgery is recommended at the time that the diagnosis is made. Because the surgery is non-emergent and cardiopulmonary bypass carries a high risk for fetal mortality (as high as 10–20%), surgery should be deferred until after completion of the pregnancy.

Answer to question 5 The incidence of congenital heart disease is approximately 0·5–1% in the general population. The incidence is higher for the offspring of parents who have congenital heart disease and depends on the type of defect in the parent. The fetus of a pregnant woman with congenital heart disease should undergo ultrasonography to examine the heart. Single gene defects, such as Marfan's syndrome, follow the laws of Mendelian genetics, with 50% of offspring affected for dominant genes and 25% affected for recessive genes. For most types of congenital heart disease (including atrial septal defects), the defect appears to be multifactorial. The risk of congenital heart disease in the offspring of parents with multifactorial defects is in the range of 2–5%.

Case 11.2

A 19-year-old female presents for evaluation of syncope. She has experienced two episodes of syncope, each occurring after attempting to run a short distance. She denies palpitations occurring before or after her syncopal episodes. She frequently experiences chest pain during exertion that subsides with rest. She complains of breathlessness with even mild levels of exertion but states that she has always been short of breath. In childhood she reports an inability to keep up with her playmates and was unable to participate in sports. She has a history of some "heart problem" in early childhood but has not undergone any type of cardiac surgery. She has not seen a physician for many years. She is on no medications and denies use of tobacco or alcohol. There is no family history of heart disease.

Examination. Physical examination: the patient appeared slender and had a dusky appearance to her skin. She has perioral cyanosis. She had clubbing of her hands and feet. Pulse: 88 beats/min, regular, normal character. Blood pressure: 110/70 mmHg in right arm. No changes in her blood pressure or pulse upon standing. Jugular venous pulse: 9 cm with prominent "a" waves. Cardiac impulse: right parasternal heave. First heart sound: normal. Second heart sound: loud and single. Ejection click in the left upper sternal border. Chest examination: normal air entry, no rales or rhonchi. Abdominal examination: soft abdomen, no tenderness, and no masses. Normal liver span. No peripheral edema. Femoral, popliteal, posterior tibial, and dorsalis pedis pulses: all normal volume and equal. Carotid pulses: normal, no bruits. Optic fundi: engorged retinal veins.

Investigations. Electrocardiogram: Figure 11.10. Chest *x* ray: Figure 11.11. Arterial saturation: 75%. Hemoglobin: 21 g/dl (210 g/l). Hematocrit: 62%.

Questions

1. What type of congenital heart disease is most likely in this patient? What is the next step in diagnosis?
2. What is the correct diagnosis? Should cardiac catheterization be performed?
3. What is the etiology of this patient's syncope?
4. Is pregnancy contraindicated in this patient and, if so, how should it be prevented?
5. Should phlebotomy be performed?

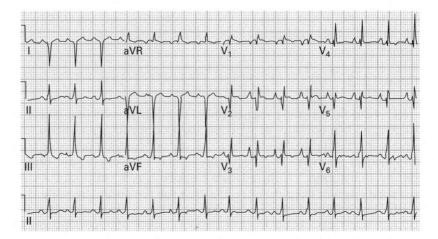

Figure 11.10 Electrocardiogram demonstrating sinus rhythm, biatrial abnormality, right axis deviation, incomplete right bundle branch block, and right ventricular hypertrophy

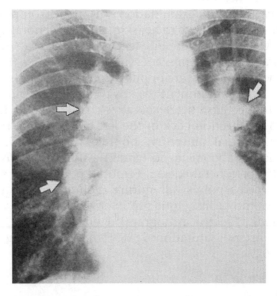

Figure 11.11 Chest *x* ray demonstrating cardiomegaly and dilated main pulmonary artery segments with pruning of peripheral pulmonary vessels (arrows) which is consistent with pulmonary hypertension

Answers

Answer to question 1   The most common forms of cyanotic congenital heart disease in adults are tetralogy of Fallot and Eisenmenger's syndrome. The absence of a murmur excludes the diagnosis of tetralogy

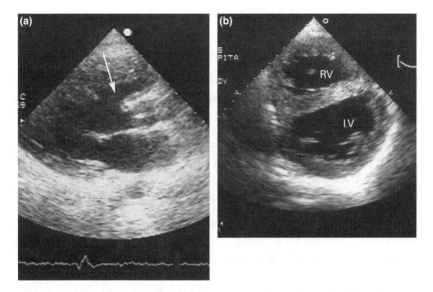

Figure 11.12 Echocardiograms demonstrating Eisenmenger syndrome. **(a)** Transthoracic echocardiogram demonstrating a large ventricular septal defect. **(b)** Right ventricular hypertrophy with flattening of the interventricular septum, consistent with marked right ventricular pressure overload

of Fallot in this patient. By physical examination, this patient has evidence of pulmonary hypertension and cyanosis, which is consistent with Eisenmenger syndrome, although other less common types of congenital heart disease cannot be completely ruled out. An echocardiogram would be the next logical step.

The echocardiogram reveals the following findings: dilated right atrium and ventricle with right ventricular hypertrophy, normal valves, and a large ventricular septal defect with predominant right to left shunting (Figure 11.12). Mild tricuspid and pulmonic regurgitation are present. The estimated right ventricular systolic pressure (calculated from the Doppler velocity of the tricuspid regurgitant jet) is 100 mmHg.

Answer to question 2 This patient has a classic Eisenmenger's syndrome – a large ventricular septal defect with severe pulmonary vascular disease resulting in right to left shunting. Cardiac catheterization should be performed in any patient with suspected Eisenmenger's syndrome in order to confirm the diagnosis and to assess the degree of reversibility of the pulmonary hypertension. Catheterization is mandatory if the diagnosis is uncertain or if a potentially surgically correctable lesion is present. Although pulmonary artery pressure can be estimated using Doppler techniques, the calculation of pulmonary vascular resistance requires cardiac catheterization. Pulmonary pressures and pulmonary vascular resistance should be assessed at rest and after administration of 100% oxygen to assess for any degree of reversibility.

Answer to question 3 In patients with the Eisenmenger's syndrome, syncope is usually caused by one of two mechanisms: cerebral hypoxia or an arrhythmia. In the setting of high, fixed pulmonary vascular resistance, a decrease in systemic vascular resistance such as occurs during or after exercise will result in increased right to left shunting. This results in cerebral hypoxia, which may result in syncope. Arrhythmias may also occur as a complication of right ventricular failure. Sudden death, presumably due to arrhythmias, is the leading cause of death in the Eisenmenger's syndrome. Ambulatory monitoring should be performed in this patient to evaluate for potentially treatable arrhythmias. Likewise, she should be advised to avoid any form of strenuous exercise.

Answer to question 4 Pregnancy is very poorly tolerated in women with Eisenmenger's syndrome, with a maternal mortality ranging from 30% to 50%. Fetal morbidity and mortality is also high, with the degree of risk to the fetus dependent on the degree of maternal cyanosis. In addition to an increased risk for fetal loss, there is also an increased incidence for intrauterine growth retardation, prematurity, and fetal anomalies. This patient should be warned of the risks associated with pregnancy and strongly encouraged to consider permanent sterilization. Other forms of contraception are less reliable and some forms may be contraindicated. Oral contraceptives are contraindicated in patients with cyanotic congenital heart disease because of the increased risk for venous and arterial thrombosis. Depot forms of progesterone via either intramuscular injection (Provera) or slow release implanted capsules (Norplant) offer reliability and may have a lower risk for thromboembolic complications, although their use in patients with congenital heart disease has not been studied. The use of progesterone is contraindicated in patients with congestive heart failure because it causes fluid retention. Intrauterine devices are associated with an increased incidence of pelvic infections, placing patients at risk for bacteremia and endocarditis, and are usually not recommended. Barrier methods are safe in patients with congenital heart disease but have higher failure rates than other forms of contraception.

Answer to question 5 The decision to proceed with phlebotomy should be based on symptoms, not purely on the degree of erythrocytosis. Erythrocytosis may be either compensated (stable hematocrit with minimal or no symptoms) or decompensated (unstable, increasing hematocrit with moderate to severe symptoms of hyperviscosity). This patient has compensated erythrocytosis and should not undergo phlebotomy at this time. Aggressive phlebotomy results in iron deficiency anemia, which can aggravate symptoms of hyperviscosity.

Case 11.3

A 19-year-old male is referred for evaluation of a murmur. He was seen at the college infirmary for an upper respiratory tract infection and a murmur was detected. He was also noted to be hypertensive. He denies any significant past medical history and is on no medications. He does not participate in any organized sports but denies exercise limitations. He denies chest pain, dyspnea, palpitations or syncope.

Examination. Physical examination: the patient appeared normal. No cyanosis, clubbing or edema. Pulse: 68 beats/min, regular. Blood pressure: 157/100 mmHg in both arms. Jugular venous pulse: normal. Cardiac impulse: normal. First heart sound: normal. Second heart sound: split normally on inspiration. Ejection click and fourth heart sound present. Grade 2/6 crescendo/decrescendo murmur heard along left sternal border radiating to upper chest. No diastolic murmur is heard (with the patient sitting up, leaning forward in expiration). Chest examination: normal air entry, no rales or rhonchi. Abdominal examination: soft abdomen, no tenderness, and no masses. Normal liver span. No peripheral edema. Femoral and popliteal pulses: all reduced. Carotid pulses: normal, no bruits. Optic fundi: normal.

Questions

1. What further information should be obtained in the initial evaluation of this patient?
2. What further diagnostic testing should be done?
3. What therapy should be recommended for this patient?
4. Will surgery cure his hypertension?

Answers

Answer to question 1 This young man has significant hypertension, which requires further evaluation. Secondary causes of hypertension should be considered in all patients and should be strongly suspected when hypertension develops before the age of 30 years or after the age of 50 years. Secondary causes of hypertension include renal artery stenosis, coarctation of the aorta, pheochromocytoma, and primary hyperaldosteronism. In a patient of this age, coarctation and renal

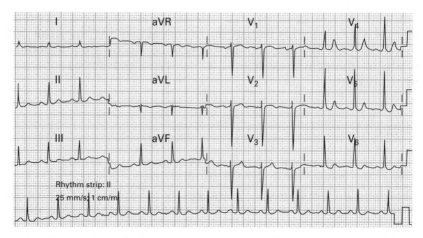

Figure 11.13 Electrocardiogram demonstrating normal sinus rhythm, normal axis, and left ventricular hypertrophy

artery stenosis are the most likely causes. Cocaine or other substance abuse also needs to be considered. Further information that needs to be obtained includes the following: history of any substance abuse, further history to assess for symptoms of a pheochromocytoma (for example headache, sweating, weakness, and weight loss), a funduscopic examination to evaluate for the presence of hypertensive retinopathy, careful auscultation of the abdomen to assess for bruits suggestive of renal artery stenosis, and careful examination of pulses and blood pressure measurement in both upper and lower extremities to rule out coarctation of the aorta.

Further physical findings in this patient include a radial–femoral pulse delay with reduced femoral pulses. No pulses were palpable in the feet, although capillary refill was intact. Repeat blood pressure in both upper extremities were 150/100 mmHg, whereas blood pressure in the left leg was palpable at 80 mmHg systolic. Careful auscultation of the chest and back revealed soft crescendo/decrescendo systolic murmurs over the lateral chest wall, both anteriorly and posteriorly. His electrocardiogram and chest x ray film are shown in Figures 11.13 and 11.14, respectively.

Answer to question 2 This patient has coarctation of the aorta by physical examination. The presence of a systolic ejection click and a systolic ejection murmur suggests the presence of a bicuspid aortic valve as well, although the systolic murmur could be due to large internal mammary artery collateral flow. Options for further evaluation in this patient include echocardiography, magnetic

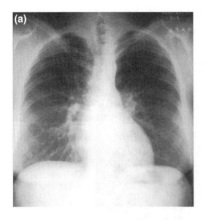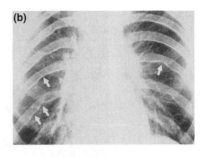

Figure 11.14 **(a)** Chest *x* ray demonstrating normal heart size and pulmonary vascular markings with unusual contour of descending thoracic aorta. **(b)** Rib notching is demonstrated (arrows) in another patient with coarctation of the aorta

resonance imaging, and cardiac catheterization. Transthoracic echocardiography can demonstrate a bicuspid aortic valve and any associated stenosis or regurgitation of the valve. Although transthoracic echocardiography is quite useful in diagnosing coarctation in infants and children, it is less useful in adults because the aortic arch and descending thoracic aorta may not be well visualized in adults. Magnetic resonance imaging is the diagnostic technique of choice for evaluating the aorta, providing excellent anatomic detail and providing an estimation of the pressure gradient across the stenosis. Cardiac catheterization is also an option. The location of the coarctation can be demonstrated by aortography and the pressure gradient across the coarctation can be measured directly.

Magnetic resonance imaging was performed in this patient (Figure 11.15). A pressure gradient of 70 mmHg across the lesion was demonstrated. A transthoracic echocardiogram confirmed the presence of a bicuspid aortic valve with mild aortic insufficiency. Mild left ventricular hypertrophy was present and left ventricular systolic function was normal.

Answer to question 3 Treatment of his coarctation is warranted with either surgery or balloon aortoplasty. Balloon aortoplasty avoids the need for thoracotomy and cardiopulmonary bypass, but carries with it a 10–20% risk for recoarctation and a 5–10% risk for aneurysm formation at the site of the dilatation. Surgery for coarctation of the aorta in adults is usually performed by doing an end-to-end anastomosis. The operative mortality is very low and the risk for

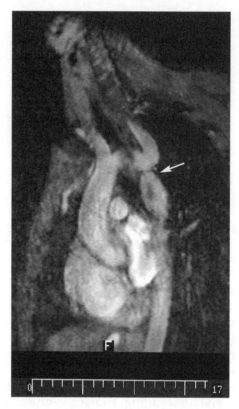

Figure 11.15 Magnetic resonance imaging of the thoracic aorta demonstrating coarctation of the aorta just distal to the left subclavian artery

recoarctation is around 18%. The risk for spinal cord ischemia resulting in paralysis is around 0·4%.

Answer to question 4 Surgical repair of coarctation of the aorta results in normalization in blood pressure in most patients for 5–10 years after operation. During longer follow up the prevalence of hypertension is much greater than in a normal population. Late hypertension is more common in individuals having surgical repair after the age of 20 years. Because of his age, this patient will probably remain hypertensive after correction of his coarctation. The patient's age at the time of repair appears to be the major risk factor for persistent hypertension postoperatively. Many authorities recommend routine exercise testing in the follow up of patients after coarctation repair because they may be normotensive at rest but have a hypertensive response to exercise. The etiology of the persistent hypertension is unclear but is postulated to represent an underlying abnormality of vascular compliance or an alteration in the renin–angiotensin system.

Case 11.4

A 35-year-old female presents to clinic for evaluation of syncope. She has a history of syncope with exertion occurring many times during her life, always precipitated by exertion. Her current episode of syncope occurred while trying to climb a flight of stairs. She reports being told that she had a heart murmur at the age of 1 year and heart surgery was recommended. However, her family declined surgery at that time. She had limited exercise tolerance as a child and was unable to complete school. However, she was able to perform routine household chores until recently, when her dyspnea and fatigue worsened. Her current activity level is minimal because she develops fatigue and dyspnea after walking 20–30 feet. She had two pregnancies in her 20s with one child born prematurely and one spontaneous abortion during the first trimester. She has not had a menstrual period for a year. She is on no medications and has no drug allergies.

Examination. Physical examination: the patient had obvious cyanosis. Her head and neck had a ruddy appearance with perioral cyanosis. She had clubbing of fingers and toes. Respiratory rate: 20/min. Pulse: 90 beats/min, normal character. Blood pressure: 120/90 mmHg in right arm. Jugular venous pulse: normal. Cardiac impulse: right parasternal lift. First heart sound: normal. Second heart sound: single. No added sounds. Loud 3/6 systolic murmur along left sternal border. Chest examination: normal air entry, no rales or rhonchi. Abdominal examination: soft abdomen, no tenderness, and no masses. Normal liver span. No peripheral edema. Femoral, popliteal, posterior tibial, and dorsalis pedis pulses: all normal volume and equal. Carotid pulses: normal, no bruits. Optic fundi: dilated retinal veins.

Investigations. Hemoglobin 21·8 g/dl (218 g/l), hematocrit 61%, room air blood gas pH 7·39, carbon dioxide tension (normal range) 27 mmHg (35–45 mmHg) or 3·6 kPa (4·7–6·0), partial oxygen tension (normal range) 52 mmHg (80–100) or 6·9 kPa (11–13), saturation 88%. Electrocardiogram: Figure 11.16.

Questions

1. What is the most likely diagnosis?
2. What is the next step in the diagnostic work up of this patient?

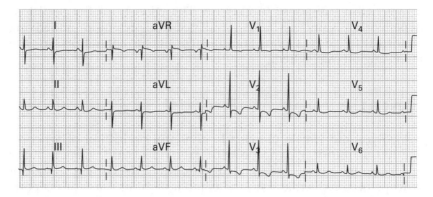

Figure 11.16 Electrocardiogram demonstrating sinus rhythm, a vertical QRS axis, and right ventricular hypertrophy

3. Is this patient a candidate for surgery?
4. After successful repair, what long-term complications might be expected?

Answers

Answer to question 1 The most common causes of cyanosis from congenital heart disease in adults are tetralogy of Fallot and the Eisenmenger's syndrome. The finding of a systolic murmur along the left sternal border and a single second heart sound are most consistent with tetralogy of Fallot. Patients with the Eisenmenger's syndrome typically have no murmurs or murmurs of acquired tricuspid or pulmonic regurgitation.

Answer to question 2 Echocardiography would be the next logical step to confirm the presumed diagnosis of tetralogy of Fallot. Echocardiography can define the cardiac anatomy and function, document the presence and direction of intracardiac shunting, and provide additional hemodynamic information. The echocardiogram in this patient revealed an overriding aorta, a large ventricular septal defect with predominant right to left shunting, severe stenosis of the right ventricular outflow tract (100 mmHg pressure gradient), and right ventricular hypertrophy. These findings are consistent with tetralogy of Fallot (Figure 11.17).

Answer to question 3 This patient probably is a candidate for surgery. Unlike a patient with Eisenmenger physiology, the

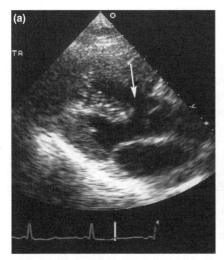 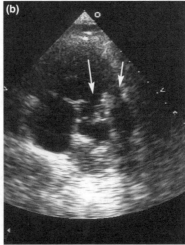

Figure 11.17 (a) Transthoracic echocardiogram of patient with a large ventricular septal defect, overriding aorta, and right ventricular hypertrophy. **(b)** The large ventricular septal defect and marked narrowing of the right ventricular outflow tract

pulmonary circulation has been "protected" in this patient (i.e. the pulmonary pressures will be low) because of the severe subpulmonic stenosis. Thus, the presence of right to left shunting and cyanosis in this patient is not a contraindication to surgery but is actually an indication for surgery. The most important determinant for operability in this patient is the status of her pulmonary arteries (they must be present and of adequate size). Cardiac catheterization should be performed in any patient with tetralogy of Fallot who is being considered for surgery in order to demonstrate the size and anatomy of the pulmonary arteries, to identify any additional sources of pulmonary blood flow, to identify or exclude multiple ventricular septal defects, and to identify anomalous origin of the coronary arteries.

Surgical options include palliative shunts to increase pulmonary blood flow and complete correction with closure of the ventricular septal defect and relief of right ventricular outflow tract obstruction. Complete repair is preferred when possible.

Answer to question 4 Sudden death is reported to occur in as many as 3% of patients with repaired tetralogy of Fallot and is presumed to be caused by malignant ventricular arrhythmias. Both atrial and ventricular arrhythmias are common in patients with repaired tetralogy of Fallot, but a clear relationship between these arrhythmias and risk for sudden death has not been proven. Patients with repaired tetralogy of Fallot often have impaired exercise capacity, which is often due to right ventricular dysfunction. Pulmonary regurgitation is common after tetralogy of Fallot repair and contributes to right ventricular dysfunction. Pulmonic valve replacement is occasionally performed for severe, symptomatic pulmonary regurgitation with right ventricular dysfunction. Reoperation may also be required for residual ventricular septal defects or residual pulmonic stenosis.

References

1 Wilson NJ, Neutze JM. Adult congenital heart disease: principles and management guidelines – part I. *Aust NZ J Med* 1993;**23**:498–503.
2 Wilson NJ, Neutze JM. Adult congenital heart disease: principles and management guidelines – part II. *Aust NZ J Med* 1993;**23**:697–705.
3 Brickner ME, Hillis LD, Lange RA. Congenital heart disease in adults: part I. *N Engl J Med* 2000;**342**:256–63.
4 Brickner ME, Hillis LD, Lange RA. Congenital heart disease in adults: part 2. *N Engl J Med* 2000;**342**:334–42.

12: Valvular disease and infective endocarditis

JOHN A BITTL

The greatest challenge for the clinician caring for patients with valvular heart disease is to decide when to recommend valve surgery. Identifying the optimal timing of surgery demands a clear understanding of the natural history of each valve abnormality and a precise understanding of its pathophysiologic consequences. Although very few randomized trials comparing medical with surgical therapy for valvular heart disease have been reported, important information has come from comparing postoperative survival statistics with the survival rates of medically treated patients. In several conditions such as mitral stenosis and aortic stenosis, it is clear that medical therapy is ineffective in dealing with the primary mechanical abnormality or the secondary compensatory mechanisms. In these conditions, the survival of symptomatic patients treated with surgery is strikingly better than that for medically treated patients. For patients with chronic mitral regurgitation or aortic insufficiency, however, surgery has produced less impressive improvements in survival, although valve replacement may relieve symptoms. Recent studies suggest that valve repair rather than replacement for certain causes of mitral regurgitation results in improved survival, and prophylactic vasodilator therapy for patients with asymptomatic aortic insufficiency prevents left ventricular dilatation and improves event-free survival.

Because no unifying pathophysiologic principles govern the behavior of all valve abnormalities, this chapter contains separate discussions of each type of valvular abnormality and contains a series of decision making algorithms and recommendations based on practice guidelines[1] that can serve as a general guide for the management of the commonest types of valvular heart disease. Although the algorithms contain decision making nodes supported by data from the literature, it must be emphasized that the timing of valve surgery for an individual patient may depend on additional factors not covered in the algorithms, such as the rate of deterioration or the actual etiology of the valvular lesion.

Mitral stenosis

The primary abnormality in mitral stenosis is rheumatic scarring of the mitral valve. The main compensatory mechanism to maintain cardiac output is elevation in left atrial and pulmonary capillary pressures, which results in symptoms of congestive heart failure. The median survival of symptomatic patients treated medically is only 7 years, whereas that for patients treated surgically is greater than 20 years. Decisions about the timing of surgical therapy, or balloon mitral valvuloplasty, are based on the hemodynamic severity of mitral stenosis and functional class.

Etiology and natural history

Rheumatic heart disease is usually the etiology of mitral stenosis, although only 50% of patients provide a clear history of rheumatic fever. Acute, and recurrent, inflammation and pancarditis produce the typical pathologic features of rheumatic mitral stenosis, which include fibrous thickening of the valve leaflets, fusion of the commissures, thickening and shortening of the chordae tendineae, and valve calcification.

Natural history studies reveal the dismal prognosis of patients with symptomatic mitral stenosis treated medically. In the 1940s and 1950s, the mean age at onset of acute rheumatic fever in the UK was 12 years, the average latency period between rheumatic fever and the onset of symptoms of mitral stenosis was 19 years, and the median survival after onset of symptoms was 7 years.[2] In the USA, 58% of patients with only mild symptoms of mitral stenosis were dead 10 years later.[3] Surgical therapy has had an important impact on survival in these patients. In 1947 the technique of closed commissurotomy was developed by Dwight Harken at Peter Bent Brigham Hospital and by Bailey in Philadelphia, and was found to improve survival and quality of life dramatically. In the first 1000 patients treated by Harken with closed commissurotomy, 10 year survival was greater than 80%.[4] With improved surgical techniques the survival of patients with mitral stenosis improved further. In addition to surgical therapy, mechanical treatment of mitral balloon valvuloplasty was first introduced in 1985.[5]

Clinical evaluation

The severity of clinical symptoms in mitral stenosis is related to the reduction in valve area. The normal mitral valve has a physiologic area greater than $4 \cdot 0$ cm^2. When the valve area is reduced to less than $2 \cdot 0$ cm^2 the patient may develop symptoms of pulmonary congestion or experience complications of mitral stenosis. The greater the reduction in valve area, the greater the disability due to elevation in left atrial and pulmonary venous pressures.

As a result of reduction in valve area, left atrial pressure rises in order to maintain normal blood flow across the obstructed valve. Left ventricular pressure remains low or normal in most cases of pure mitral stenosis because the increased resistance to flow across the mitral valve results in decreased left ventricular filling, stroke volume, and cardiac output. This is of particular importance in patients with left ventricular dysfunction. About 20% of patients with pure mitral stenosis have ejection fractions of less than 50%. It must be emphasized that left ventricular dysfunction in pure mitral stenosis is not the result of hemodynamic overload but is probably caused by impaired contractility from pre-existing rheumatic inflammation of the myocardium.

The increase in left atrial pressure in mitral stenosis is transmitted to the pulmonary circulation, resulting in increased pulmonary capillary wedge pressure. This elevation in hydrostatic pressure in the pulmonary vasculature causes transudation of fluid into the interstitium of the lungs and alveoli, causing symptoms of pulmonary congestion.

The elevation in left atrial pressure in mitral stenosis also causes two distinct forms of pulmonary arteriolar hypertension: passive and reactive. Most patients with mitral stenosis exhibit some degree of passive pulmonary hypertension. This increase in pulmonary artery pressure arises to preserve forward flow in the face of increased left atrial and pulmonary venous pressures. Approximately 40% of patients with severe mitral stenosis and chronic elevations in pulmonary venous pressures above approximately 22 mmHg will exhibit reactive pulmonary hypertension with medial hypertrophy and intimal fibrosis of the pulmonary arterioles. Although reactive pulmonary hypertension is considered beneficial by some clinicians, because it impedes blood flow into the engorged pulmonary capillary beds, reduces capillary hydrostatic pressure and thus reduces the degree of pulmonary congestion, reactive pulmonary hypertension in mitral stenosis causes reduced cardiac output and increased right heart pressures. Chronically elevated right heart pressures lead to right ventricular failure, secondary tricuspid regurgitation, and passive hepatic congestion. Additionally, in severe cases of pulmonary hypertension marked elevation in pulmonary pressures leads to the opening of collateral channels between pulmonary and bronchial arteries. Subsequent rupture of one of these vessels can cause hemoptysis.

Thus, the complications of mitral stenosis directly related to the reduction in valve area include the development of congestive heart failure and pulmonary hypertension. Other problems related to the presence but not the severity of mitral stenosis include atrial fibrillation, systemic thromboembolism, pulmonary hypertension, and (rarely) infective endocarditis. Atrial fibrillation is caused by chronic dilatation of the left atrium. Systemic thromboembolism is caused by the formation of the left atrial thrombi in the enlarged left atrium and is usually associated with atrial fibrillation. Patients with mitral stenosis and atrial fibrillation who are not treated with warfarin anticoagulation constitute one of the highest risk groups for systemic thromboembolism, with the incidence of embolic events averaging about 5% per year.

The diagnosis and the assessment of the severity of mitral stenosis begin at the bedside, with examination of the general appearance of the patient. Some patients with chronic low output in advanced stages of mitral stenosis have livedo reticularis of the malar area (the so-called mitral facies). Palpitation of the precordium often reveals a parasternal lift of right ventricular pressure overload in the presence of either passive or reactive pulmonary hypertension. Auscultation discloses a loud or accentuated first heart sound (S_1), if the mitral valve leaflets are flexible, because of the wide closing excursion of the leaflets and the rapidity of the left ventricular pressure rise at the time of closure. An S_1 that is loud but of variable intensity accompanies atrial fibrillation. A normal or soft S_1 raises the questions of the presence of coexisting significant mitral regurgitation, or a heavily calcified immobile mitral valve. Auscultation also reveals a diastolic rumble and an opening snap (OS), with a second heart sound (S_2)–OS interval of 0·06–0·12 seconds, the duration of which is inversely related to severity of mitral stenosis. (The timing of the S_2–OS interval has been suggested by Selzer to be equivalent to the interval between the phonation of two consonants; the intervals of 0·06, 0·08, 0·10, and 0·12 seconds are represented by the combinations of *p-dah*, *p-tah*, *p-bah*, and *p-pah*, respectively.) The diastolic rumble of mitral stenosis is best heard with the patient lying in the left lateral recumbent position with the bell of the stethoscope lightly applied to the point of maximal impulse of the apex of the heart.

Thus, in uncomplicated mitral stenosis with a mobile, flexible but stenosed valve, the clinician should seek a loud S_1, an accentuated pulmonary component of S_2 (P_2), an OS, and a mid-diastolic rumble with presystolic accentuation. The coexisting murmur of tricuspid regurgitation is frequently identified as mitral regurgitation because as the right ventricle dilates it occupies a more leftward orientation, and the "tricuspid area" moves leftward. The intensity of the murmur of tricuspid regurgitation often increases during inspiration.

The auscultatory findings of mitral stenosis raise the differential diagnosis of left atrial myxoma, mitral regurgitation with increased hyperdynamic diastolic transmitral flow, tricuspid stenosis, or aortic regurgitation with an Austin–Flint murmur (the regurgitant jet of blood hits the anterior leaflet of the mitral valve causing vibration and a mid-diastolic murmur).

Non-invasive evaluation

The electrocardiogram may show evidence of left atrial enlargement in the presence of sinus rhythm. As mentioned above, atrial fibrillation may be present. When pulmonary hypertension ensues, right axis deviation or right ventricular hypertrophy may be detectable. The chest radiograph reveals left atrial enlargement, pulmonary vascular redistribution, interstitial edema, and Kerley B lines due to edema within the septae. With the development of pulmonary hypertension, right ventricular enlargement and prominence of the pulmonary arteries also appear.

Doppler echocardiographic evaluation is recommended for all patients with suspected mitral stenosis in order to assess the severity of stenosis, evaluate right ventricular size and function, examine valve morphology and suitability for percutaneous balloon valvuloplasty, evaluate concomitant valve lesions, and re-evaluate patients with changing symptoms and signs.[1] The echocardiographic examination of mitral stenosis may show "doming" of the mitral leaflets, which is a characteristic appearance of the rheumatic deformity associated with thickening, and decreased pliability of the mitral valve, left atrial enlargement, calcification, subvalvular disease, or pulmonary hypertension. Doppler evaluation may show increased transmitral flow velocity, which corresponds to an increased pressure gradient. The measure of peak velocity can be used to estimate mitral valve area from the following relation: mitral valve area = 210/velocity (in m/s). Exercise treadmill testing may reveal evidence of limited effort tolerance. Inability to reach stage three of the Bruce protocol is associated with severe mitral stenosis. The use of transesophageal echocardiography may be considered to determine whether left atrial thrombus is present or absent before contemplated valvotomy or cardioversion, and to improve on inadequate data obtained from transthoracic echocardiography.

Invasive evaluation

Cardiac catheterization is only recommended for symptomatic patients with mitral stenosis who have equivocal findings on non-invasive evaluation, or who are scheduled for balloon mitral valvuloplasty. Coronary arteriography is recommended for patients with angina, those older than 40 years with coronary risk factors, and for patients with other associated significant valvular involvement.

The normal mitral valve area is approximately $4\ cm^2$ in cross-sectional area, and no diastolic gradient exists between pulmonary capillary wedge pressure and left ventricular pressure. When the mitral

Table 12.1 Hemodynamic grades of mitral stenosis

Stage	MVA (cm^2)	Symptoms
Minimal	>2·5	None
Mild	1·4–2·5	Minimal breathlessness on exertion
Moderate	1·0–1·4	Breathless on exertion, orthopnea, PND, with or without pulmonary edema
Severe	<1·0	Resting dyspnea, class IV
Pulmonary hypertension	<1·0	Same as severe plus right ventricular failure

MVA, mitral valve area. From Dalen[6]
PND, paroxysmal nocturnal dyspnea

valve area is reduced to less than 2·0 cm^2 (Table 12.1)[6] the simultaneous measurement of pulmonary capillary wedge pressure and left ventricular pressure reveals a diastolic pressure gradient (Figure 12.1). The gradient between pulmonary capillary wedge pressure and the left ventricle is related to the square of the cardiac output. If cardiac output increases by a factor of two during exercise, for example, then the pressure gradient will increase by a factor of four.[7]

The invasive evaluation of the severity of mitral stenosis is reasonably reliable but depends on the accuracy of the measurements of cardiac output. The substitution of pulmonary capillary wedge pressure for left atrial pressure is generally satisfactory so long as attention is paid to the wave form of the pulmonary capillary wedge tracing. This is to ensure that an over-damped pulmonary artery pressure was not inadvertently obtained. Estimates of valve area from the Gorlin formula are based on the square root of the pressure gradient. Thus, errors incurred in the measurement of the pressure gradient are minimized (see Chapter 3).

When patients undergo invasive evaluation for mitral stenosis, the finding of a normal pulmonary capillary wedge pressure of less than 13 mmHg is an indication for supine bicycle exercise. The increase in cardiac output seen with exercise and its non-linear relation with the transmitral pressure gradient may elicit a sharp rise in pulmonary capillary wedge pressure. This demonstration may thus ensure that the hemodynamic compromise of mitral stenosis is the cause of the patient's symptoms.

Treatment

Important aspects of medical therapy for mitral stenosis include antibiotic prophylaxis against recurrent rheumatic fever. Daily

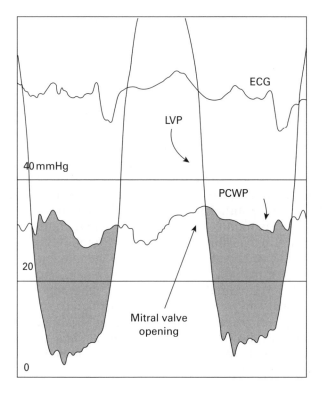

Figure 12.1 Rest hemodynamics in mitral stenosis. The tracings show simultaneous measurement of pulmonary capillary wedge pressure (PCWP) and left ventricular pressure (LVP). Under normal conditions, PCWP and LVP are matched throughout diastole after the time of mitral valve opening. In mitral stenosis the PCWP remains significantly higher than LVP during diastole. The pressure difference, or gradient, is shown as the shaded area. ECG, electrocardiogram

penicillin VK should be considered in patients younger than 35 years. Infective endocarditis prophylaxis at the time of surgical or dental procedures should be recommended in all patients with mitral stenosis.[8,9] Diuretics are useful for volume overload. Digoxin is used only for impaired left ventricular function or for rate control in atrial fibrillation, although calcium channel blockers may be as effective. β-Blockers are used to improve heart rate control and reduce mitral gradient, although this therapy has not been shown to increase exercise tolerance in all patients. Anticoagulation with warfarin is recommended for all patients with paroxysmal or chronic atrial fibrillation or those with a prior embolic event.[1] Patients who develop atrial fibrillation often require emergency treatment for congestive heart failure consisting of diuretic therapy and rate control. Although an attempt at cardioversion is reasonable, patients who develop atrial fibrillation often do not regain their previous level of exercise tolerance on medical therapy alone and require mechanical relief of mitral stenosis.

Surgical therapy

For patients with symptomatic mitral stenosis complicated by mitral regurgitation or valve calcification, either valve replacement or open commissurotomy with valve debridement is ordinarily recommended. The operative mortality is less than 2% and the reoperation rate is less than 10% at 10 years. Mitral valve repair is recommended in patients with functional class III–IV symptoms, moderate or severe mitral stenosis (mitral valve area $\leq 1 \cdot 5$ cm^2) and morphology favorable for repair if percutaneous balloon valvuloplasty is unavailable or if left atrial thrombus is present despite anticoagulants.[1] Mitral valve replacement is recommended in patients not suitable for balloon valvuloplasty or repair, and generally in patients with severe mitral stenosis (mitral valve area $\leq 1 \cdot 0$ cm^2) and severe pulmonary hypertension (pulmonary artery systolic pressure 60–80 mmHg). For patients with pre-existing atrial fibrillation, valve replacement with a more durable mechanical valve is usually more sensible than use of a prosthetic valve because there is a pre-existing need for anticoagulation.

Balloon mitral valvuloplasty

Balloon valvuloplasty was first introduced in 1985 as an alternative to surgical therapy in young patients with pure mitral stenosis.[5] This treatment has demonstrated excellent results for selected patients. The procedure is effective in increasing the valve area from about $0 \cdot 8$ to $2 \cdot 0$ cm^2 in selected patients without mitral regurgitation, calcification, excessive valve thickening, or subvalvular disease.[10]

Predictors of successful dilatation are defined by the echocardiographic evaluation of four characteristics of mitral valve anatomy. Each of those echocardiographic findings (i.e. the degree of valve calcification, leaflet thickening, leaflet immobility, and subvalvular involvement) can be graded on a scale of 0 to 4, yielding a maximum total score of 16. Patients with a prior history of systemic thromboembolism are at increased risk for transseptal catheterization and should not be considered for the procedure unless they have had uninterrupted anticoagulation for 3–6 months and no evidence of left atrial thrombus by transesophageal echocardiography. The risk of restenosis after balloon valvuloplasty is related to several baseline characteristics. Advanced age, presence of valvular calcification, and development of atrial fibrillation are factors associated with decreased survival after valvuloplasty.[11]

Percutaneous balloon mitral valvuloplasty is recommended in patients with New York Heart Association functional class II, III, or IV symptoms, moderate or severe mitral stenosis (mitral valve area ≤1·5 cm²), and a favorable valve morphology in the absence of left atrial thrombus or more than mild mitral regurgitation.[1] Balloon mitral valvuloplasty was compared with closed commissurotomy in a randomized, controlled trial.[12] The mean valve area at baseline was 1·0 cm² in the study group of 40 patients. At follow up 8 months after treatment, the mitral valve area was 1·6 ± 0·6 cm² in the balloon commissurotomy group, and 1·8 ± 0·6 cm² in the surgical closed commissurotomy group. Although one case of severe mitral regurgitation occurred in each group, there was no death, stroke, or myocardial infarction. Balloon mitral valvuloplasty was also compared with open surgical commissurotomy in another randomized, controlled trial.[13] Although the average mitral valve area was identical at baseline in the 60 study patients at about 0·9 cm², the mean mitral valve area 3 years after treatment was 2·3 ± 0·3 cm² for patients treated with mitral valvuloplasty and 1·9 ± 0·3 cm² for patients treated with open surgical commissurotomy.

Timing of mitral valve surgery or valvuloplasty

The timing of mitral valve surgery or valvuloplasty for mitral stenosis depends on two factors, namely functional class and the severity of underlying mitral stenosis (Figure 12.2). Thus, in patients who present with the findings of mitral stenosis, the combination of physical examination and non-invasive evaluation are usually sufficient to define when mechanical treatment is needed. When there are concerns about the reliability about the clinical assessment of functional class, exercise treadmill testing can be very revealing. When additional concerns exist, or the patient has risk factors for coronary artery disease, then cardiac catheterization can be recommended. Patients with evidence of reactive pulmonary hypertension should also undergo mechanical correction of mitral stenosis. It must be emphasized that reactive pulmonary hypertension in mitral stenosis, unlike pulmonary vascular obstructive disease in central cardiac shunts, is an indication for mechanical correction of the underlying valve abnormality. This is because normal or nearly normal pulmonary pressures are usually achieved within a few weeks of successful mechanical correction.

Aortic stenosis

The commonest cause of aortic stenosis is sclerocalcific degeneration of a trileaflet or congenitally bicuspid valve. Although the

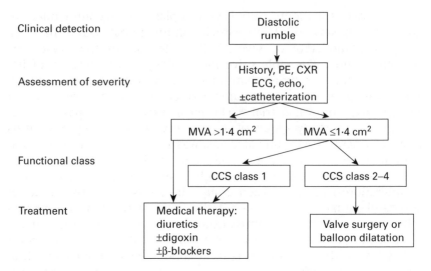

Figure 12.2 Timing of surgery for mitral stenosis. The treatment of patients with mitral stenosis is based on the severity of the underlying valvular abnormality and the functional class of the patient. Although a valve area of $1\cdot4$ cm^2 is arbitrarily selected as the hemodynamic criterion for mechanical relief of mitral stenosis, it should be emphasized that patients may become symptomatic at valve areas as great at $1\cdot8$ cm^2. CCS, Canadian Cardiovascular Society; CXR, chest x ray; ECG, electrocardiogram; echo, Doppler echocardiogram; MVA, mitral valve area; PE, physical examination

compensatory mechanisms of left ventricular hypertrophy and increased left ventricular pressure generation result in long periods of asymptomatic survival for patients with aortic stenosis, gradually worsening stenosis is the rule and survival is severely reduced in medically treated patients with symptoms of angina, syncope, or heart failure. Similar to that for mitral stenosis, the timing of valve replacement in patients with aortic stenosis depends on the hemodynamic severity of aortic stenosis and functional status.

Etiology and natural history

Senile sclerocalcific degeneration affecting a trileaflet valve is the most common type of aortic stenosis seen in adults older than 65˜years. This is the result of cumulative "wear and tear" on an otherwise normal valve. Symptoms generally appear in the seventh or eighth decade of life when degeneration affects a trileaflet valve. Congenital sclerocalcific degeneration of a bicuspid valve may be suspected in the adult patient younger than 60 years. The final pathologic findings of sclerocalcific degeneration include calcification within the fibrosa of the valve cusps that gradually extends toward the surface, ultimately resulting in heaped up or nodular depositions within the valve leaflets.

Before 1970 most cases of aortic stenosis were thought to be caused by rheumatic involvement, but this is now a rare cause of aortic stenosis. When it does occur, rheumatic involvement of the aortic valve is almost always accompanied by rheumatic mitral involvement. Currently, no more than 5% of cases of isolated aortic stenosis are rheumatic in etiology. When rheumatic aortic stenosis is encountered, the pathologic hallmarks include commissural fusion and valve calcification.

In aortic stenosis the ventricle faces increased afterload caused by an obstruction to normal blood flow across the valve during systole. When the valve orifice area is reduced by more than 50% of its normal area, significant elevation in left ventricular pressure is necessary to drive blood into the aorta. It is not unusual to record pressure gradients across the valve of greater than 100 mmHg (Figure 12.3). In aortic stenosis the left ventricle becomes concentrically hypertrophied in response to increased afterload. Although left ventricular hypertrophy serves an important compensatory role in reducing ventricular wall tension, it also reduces the compliance of the ventricle and makes it prone to developing ischemia as hypertrophy outstrips the ability of the coronary arteries to provide adequate perfusion under conditions of increased demand. The resulting elevation in diastolic left ventricular pressure requires the left atrium to fill the "stiff" left ventricle. Whereas left atrial contraction contributes 0–25% of the left ventricular stroke volume in normal individuals, it may contribute as much as 30–40% of the left ventricular stroke volume in aortic stenosis. Thus, left atrial hypertrophy is beneficial, and the loss of atrial contraction (in atrial fibrillation) can abruptly reduce cardiac output.

Although the natural history of asymptomatic aortic stenosis is similar to that for the normal population, the asymptomatic patient should be told to avoid strenuous activities involved in competitive sports. The survival of symptomatic patients with aortic stenosis is poor. Patients with aortic stenosis who experience angina, syncope, congestive heart failure, or atrial fibrillation have median survivals of 5 years, 3 years, 2 years, and 6 months, respectively. The overall 1 year survival is 57% for patients who were found to have severe aortic stenosis but did not undergo surgery because of patient refusal.[14]

Clinical evaluation

The normal aortic valve area is greater than 3.0 cm^2. When the valve area is reduced to less than 1.2 cm^2 a pressure gradient between

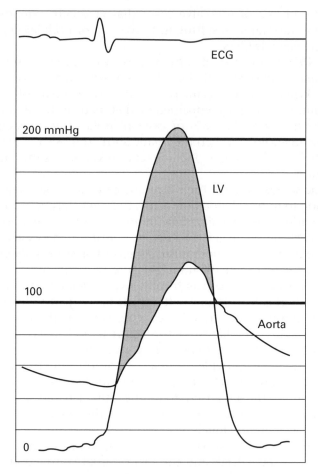

Figure 12.3 Hemodynamic measurements in aortic stenosis. Simultaneous measurement of left ventricular (LV) and central aortic pressures in aortic stenosis shows the characteristic pressure gradient (shaded area). ECG, electrocardiogram

the left ventricle and aorta appears (mild aortic stenosis). If the aortic valve area is reduced to less than 0·7 cm² then critical obstruction is said to be present.

Symptoms of angina, syncope, and congestive heart failure appear relatively late in the natural history of aortic stenosis. The findings of atrial fibrillation and pulmonary hypertension are unusual in aortic stenosis, but occur occasionally late in the natural history. Early in the course of aortic stenosis, the abnormal increase in left atrial pressure occurs mostly at the end of diastole, when the left atrium contracts into the thickened non-compliant left ventricle. As a result, the mean left atrial pressure and the pulmonary venous pressure are not greatly affected in mild cases of aortic stenosis. With progression of the stenosis, however, the left ventricle continues to hypertrophy and may reach the limit of effective ejection caused by insurmountably high afterload. This in turn leads to increased left ventricular end-diastolic volume and pressure, yielding more marked elevations in left atrial and pulmonary pressures, which then produce the symptoms of congestive heart failure.

Aortic stenosis may be associated with angina because myocardial ischemia may be caused by an imbalance between myocardial oxygen supply and demand. Myocardial oxygen demand is increased in two ways. First, the muscle mass of the left ventricle is increased, requiring greater than normal perfusion. Second, wall stress is increased because of elevated systolic ventricular pressure. In addition, aortic stenosis reduces myocardial oxygen supply as the elevated left ventricular diastolic pressure reduces the coronary perfusion pressure gradient between the aorta and the myocardium (particularly in the subendocardium, where intramural pressure is greatest).

Aortic stenosis may lead to syncope during exercise. Although left ventricular hypertrophy allows the ventricle to generate a high pressure and maintain a normal cardiac output at rest, the ventricle cannot significantly increase cardiac output during exercise because of the fixed stenotic aortic orifice. In addition, exercise leads to vasodilatation of the peripheral muscle beds. The vasodilatory response during exercise is enhanced by left ventricular baroreceptor mediated reflex pathways that become activated in the presence of sharp increases in left ventricular wall stress. Thus, vasodilatation and the inability to augment cardiac output contribute to decreased cerebral perfusion pressure and syncope upon exertion.

The physical examination is the most important screening test for aortic stenosis. The carotid arterial pulse rises slowly, and is small and sustained in severe aortic stenosis. The cardiac impulse is unremarkable in uncomplicated aortic stenosis and the S_2 is often single, or soft, because of delay in aortic valve closure. A fourth heart sound (S_4) is often present. Although the presence of an ejection systolic murmur at the base of the heart is the auscultatory hallmark of aortic stenosis, the contour of the carotid upstroke (arterial pulse) reveals more information about the hemodynamic severity of the disease than any of the auscultatory features of pitch, loudness, or timing of a late-peaking, coarse systolic ejection murmur. In many patients, it is challenging to distinguish the systolic murmur of aortic stenosis from that of mitral regurgitation because of radiation of the aortic murmur to the apex (Gallavardin phenomenon). Certain additional clues, however, can establish the source of the murmur. The coexistence of a murmur of aortic insufficiency, the presence of an aortic ejection click, or significant beat to beat variability in the intensity of the systolic murmur strongly favors the diagnosis of aortic stenosis. After the compensatory pause following a premature beat, the combination of increased left ventricular filling and post-extrasystolic potentiation will increase the murmur of aortic stenosis by one or two grades of intensity, whereas the murmur of mitral regurgitation will not change significantly.

Non-invasive evaluation

The chest x ray film may be normal or show left ventricular or ascending aorta prominence. In a young patient, poststenotic dilatation of the ascending aorta may be an important clue to the presence of a congenitally bicuspid valve. The electrocardiogram commonly shows evidence of left ventricular hypertrophy in aortic stenosis, but echocardiography is a more sensitive technique to assess left ventricular wall thickness. The transvalvular gradient can be accurately measured using Doppler echocardiographic analysis. The Doppler measurement assesses the peak instantaneous gradient across the aortic valve, which is the peak gradient measured at any time during the cardiac cycle, usually at the peak of left ventricular systolic pressure at a time when the delayed pressure in the central aorta is still increasing. In patients with atrial fibrillation or any irregularity in the cardiac cycle, for example, the peak instantaneous gradient may also reflect the increased left ventricular filling or post-extrasystolic potentiation of left ventricular contractility, and thus be much greater than the mean gradient measured at cardiac catheterization. Routine exercise treadmill testing is relatively contraindicated in aortic stenosis. In certain "asymptomatic" individuals, however, a carefully performed low level exercise treadmill test may reveal important functional limitations that make the difference between recommending or deferring surgical therapy.

Invasive evaluation

Cardiac catheterization continues to have a useful role in evaluating patients with aortic stenosis, both for confirming the results of non-invasive studies and for assessing the presence of coexisting coronary disease in the elderly population. Hemodynamic measurements at catheterization confirm the severity of aortic stenosis in cases of "intermediate" significance (with a peak instantaneous gradient of 36–64 mmHg by Doppler). Coronary arteriography is also an important part of the evaluation in patients with aortic stenosis who are scheduled for valve surgery, and is recommended in patients with chest pain, decreased left ventricular systolic dysfunction, advanced age and coronary risk factors, and in patients with evidence of ischemia or a history of coronary artery disease.[1] Approximately 30% of patients with aortic stenosis without angina will have angiographic evidence of obstructive coronary artery disease,[15] whereas 30% of those with angina will have no significant coronary disease. Patients undergoing aortic valve replacement may benefit from concurrent coronary artery bypass surgery when coronary artery disease is present.

Treatment

Medical therapy for patients with mild to moderate or asymptomatic aortic stenosis includes close follow up every 6 months. In addition, prophylaxis against infective endocarditis and avoidance of potent vasodilators such as nitroglycerin are important aspects of care for patients with aortic stenosis. The rate of progression of aortic stenosis is unpredictable but the average rate of change is approximately 0·12 cm^2 per year, although up to half of patients under surveillance show no progression over 3–9 years.[1]

Aortic valve replacement is indicated for persons with symptomatic severe aortic stenosis, or patients with severe aortic stenosis undergoing coronary artery bypass surgery or surgery of the aorta or other valves (Figure 12.4).[1] The effect of aortic valve replacement on the natural history of severe aortic stenosis is dramatic. Postoperative survival after valve replacement for aortic stenosis exceeds 75% at 15 years. The left ventricular ejection fraction almost always increases after aortic valve replacement. If impaired left ventricular function is present before surgery, then ejection fraction increases by an average of 10% during the postoperative period. Thus, decreased left ventricular ejection fraction is not considered a contraindication to aortic valve replacement for patients with severe aortic stenosis. A commonly encountered problem, however, is that seen in the patient with low cardiac output, low aortic valve gradient, and severe aortic stenosis (as calculated from the Gorlin formula). Simply stated, a mean valve gradient of less than 30 mmHg is usually not an indication for surgery because the patient either does not have severe aortic stenosis or has such severe impairment in left ventricular function that valve surgery cannot be tolerated.[16]

Balloon valvuloplasty performed for aortic stenosis achieves a mild and transient improvement in hemodynamics. The largest registry for balloon valvuloplasty enrolled more than 600 patients and found a 1 year survival of 57%, which is identical to the natural history of the unoperated disorder in similar patients.[17] The procedure is reserved occasionally as a "bridge" for those patients who are hemodynamically unstable surgical candidates awaiting aortic valve replacement.

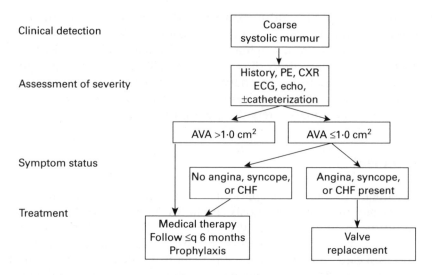

Figure 12.4 Timing of surgery for aortic stenosis. The optimal timing of valve replacement for patients with aortic stenosis depends on the hemodynamic severity of the underlying lesion and the symptomatic status of the patient. AVA, aortic valve area; CHF, congestive heart failure; CXR, chest x ray; ECG, electrocardiogram; echo, Doppler echocardiogram; PE, physical examination

Mitral regurgitation

Mitral regurgitation has many causes. Irrespective of etiology, a portion of left ventricular output is ejected into the low pressure left atrium. Cardiac output may be maintained at rest but is reduced during exercise, resulting in fatigue during exertion. The optimal timing of surgery in mitral regurgitation is complicated and depends on several factors such as the etiology, acuity, and severity of regurgitation; degree of functional impairment; and left ventricular ejection fraction.

Etiology and natural history

Normal functioning of the mitral valve depends on the coordinated action of each of its components including the leaflets, annulus, chordae, papillary muscles, and underlying left ventricular myocardium. Disruption of normal function of any of these components may lead to mitral regurgitation (Box 12.1). In myxomatous degeneration the mitral leaflet tissue or chordae may be redundant, preventing precise coaptation of leaflet edges. In rheumatic deformity of the mitral valve, excessive scarring may shorten the leaflets or chordae, allowing a potential orifice to form during systole. During marked left ventricular dilatation, the geometric orientation of the papillary muscles may pull the leaflet edges away from one another during systole, causing secondary mitral regurgitation.

Box 12.1 Causes of mitral regurgitation

Ischemic heart disease with papillary muscle dysfunction
Myxomatous degeneration (prolapse, Marfan's syndrome)
Infective endocarditis
Rheumatic
Idiopathic hypertrophic subaortic stenosis
Left ventricular dilatation of any cause
Mitral annular calcification
Congenital

In all cases of mitral regurgitation, a fraction of left ventricular blood is ejected into the low pressure left atrium. This reduces left ventricular afterload and improves systolic emptying. The clinical presentation of mitral regurgitation is related to left atrial compliance, and this in turn is related to the acuity of regurgitation. The characteristics of acute mitral regurgitation include a small "unprepared" left atrium with reduced compliance, a high left atrial pressure, a tall "v" wave, pulmonary hypertension, and pulmonary edema (Figure 12.5). In acute mitral regurgitation, forward cardiac output usually falls at the expense of mitral regurgitation (forward cardiac output = total cardiac output – mitral regurgitation), because of preferential ejection of blood from the left ventricle into the low pressure left atrial "sink" at the expense of ejection into the higher pressure aorta. This reduction in forward cardiac output stimulates peripheral baroreceptors to activate the sympathetic nervous system, which produces a reflexive increase in myocardial contractility (increased inotropy), vasoconstriction, and tachycardia. The increase in contractility contributes to supranormal left ventricular emptying, often producing left ventricular ejection fractions greater than 80%. Vasoconstriction and tachycardia, however, may further exacerbate the degree of regurgitation (at the expense of forward output) and further raise left atrial pressure. In acute severe mitral regurgitation a vicious cycle of worsening forward output, worsening regurgitation, and rising left atrial pressures can cause rapid decompensation and pulmonary edema.

The physiologic hallmarks of chronic mitral regurgitation, on the other hand, include a marked increase in left atrial size and compliance,

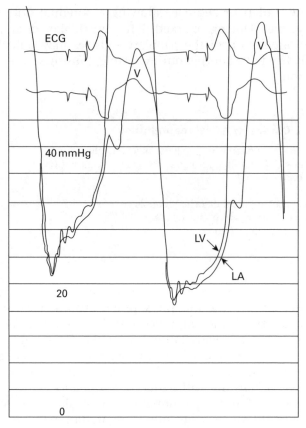

Figure 12.5 Acute mitral regurgitation. Simultaneous measurement of left atrial pressure (LA) and left ventricular pressure (LV) pressure during an episode of acute mitral regurgitation related to ischemic papillary muscle dysfunction. The large systolic "v" wave in the left atrial pressure tracing is caused by the normal return of pulmonary venous flow of blood to the left atrium, the regurgitation of blood from the left ventricle across the incompetent mitral valve, and the rise in end-diastolic pressure in the non-compliant ischemic left ventricle. ECG, electrocardiogram

near normal left atrial pressure, the frequent occurrence of atrial fibrillation and symptoms of fatigue due to low forward cardiac output. The reason that pulmonary congestion is not a consistent feature of chronic mitral regurgitation is that the left atrium dilates and increases its compliance to accommodate large regurgitant volumes from the ventricle without an excessive increase in pressure. Thus, the effects of mitral regurgitation on the pulmonary circulation are minimized. Left atrial dilatation is adaptive as it prevents increases in pulmonary vascular pressures. However, this adaptation occurs at the cost of inadequate forward cardiac output, because the compliant left atrium becomes a preferred low pressure "sump" for left ventricular ejection. Consequently, as progressively larger fractions of blood regurgitate into the left atrium, the main symptoms of chronic mitral regurgitation become those of low forward cardiac output. In addition, chronic left atrial dilatation predisposes the patient to atrial fibrillation.

The natural history of mitral regurgitation depends on its etiology. The natural history of chronic mitral regurgitation caused by rheumatic scarring or myxomatous degeneration is one of very slow progression with survival exceeding 70% at 15 years in medically treated patients. On the other hand, an abrupt worsening in mitral regurgitation in the setting of spontaneous rupture of chordae tendineae, endocarditis, or ischemic heart disease may lead to a life-threatening medical or surgical emergency.

Mitral valve prolapse

Mitral valve prolapse is a common and often asymptomatic billowing of the mitral leaflets into the left atrium during ventricular systole. Other names for this condition include "floppy" mitral valve or myxomatous degeneration. Pathologic findings include enlarged, often redundant valve leaflets with the normal collagen and elastin matrix of the valvular fibrosa, which is fragmented and replaced with loose myxomatous connective tissue. Isolated involvement of the posterior leaflet of the mitral valve is not uncommon. In more severe cases, elongated or ruptured chordae, annular enlargement, and thickened leaflets may be seen. Mitral valve prolapse occurs in about 5% of the normal population and is more common in women. Mitral valve prolapse may be inherited as a primary autosomal dominant disorder with variable penetrance, or may occur as a secondary complication of other heritable diseases of connective tissue such as Marfan's syndrome or Ehlers–Danlos syndrome.

Mitral valve prolapse is often silent, but may manifest as symptoms of palpitations or chest discomfort atypical for angina pectoris. Physical examination may reveal a mid-systolic click and late systolic murmur that is heard best at the apex. The systolic click is believed to correspond to the snapping of an everted leaflet or chordae as the leaflet is forced back through the mitral annulus, whereas the murmur is believed to correspond with regurgitant flow back through the incompetent mitral valve. To make the diagnosis, however, the click and murmur should change characteristically with dynamic auscultation. Maneuvers such as squatting or release of Valsalva that increase the volume of blood in the left ventricle should cause the click and murmur to occur later in the cardiac cycle (closer to S_2). Conversely, if the volume of blood in the left ventricle is decreased by suddenly standing from the squatting position or by the initiation of the Valsalva maneuver, then the click and murmur should occur earlier (closer to S_1). Confirmation of the diagnosis is obtained by echocardiography, which demonstrates posterior displacement of one or both mitral leaflets during systole.

The clinical course of mitral prolapse is almost always uneventful and benign. The most common serious complication is the development of isolated mitral regurgitation, attributed to stretching and elongation of the mitral chordae or leaflets during prolapse. Rupture of a chordae, however, can cause the sudden onset of severe regurgitation. Other rare complications of mitral prolapse include infective endocarditis, peripheral emboli due to microthrombus formation behind the redundant tissue, arrhythmias, and sudden death. The baseline echocardiogram is an excellent screening test for predicting complications of mitral valve prolapse. Patients with thickened leaflets or significant mitral regurgitation are at increased risk for complications of worsening mitral regurgitation, heart failure, or endocarditis.[18] Treatment thus consists of reassurance of those patients without high risk echocardiographic features of the generally benign prognosis, and of re-examination with echocardiography at appropriate intervals, as well as endocarditis prophylaxis, when significant mitral regurgitation or thickened valves are present.

Clinical evaluation

The symptoms of chronic mitral regurgitation, namely fatigue and weakness, are predominantly caused by low cardiac output during exertion. On physical examination, a murmur may be accompanied by a third heart sound (S_3). The physical examination of a patient with mitral regurgitation may reveal an apical holosystolic murmur that radiates to the axilla. There are many exceptions, however, to conventional description of the apical holosystolic murmur radiating to the axilla. For example, when mitral regurgitation is caused by posterior papillary muscle ischemia, the regurgitant jet is directed at the left atrial wall immediately posterior to the aorta, producing a systolic murmur that is best heard radiating to the "aortic" area.

Non-invasive evaluation

The chest radiograph in chronic mitral regurgitation may show ventricular or left atrial enlargement, mitral annular calcification, or pulmonary congestion. The electrocardiogram may show left atrial enlargement, left ventricular hypertrophy, atrial fibrillation, or may be normal.

The Doppler echocardiographic examination is an important part of the clinical evaluation of patients with mitral regurgitation. Not only will the study provide an approximate estimate of the severity of mitral regurgitation, but it may also identify the etiology and provide an estimate of left ventricular function. The echocardiographic estimate of left ventricular ejection fraction is one of the most important determinants of long term survival in mitral regurgitation after mitral valve surgery. Because mitral regurgitation is inherently associated with improved left ventricular emptying caused by reduced afterload, any reduction in ejection fraction reveals a substantial reduction in left ventricular contractility.[19] Echocardiograms are used for surveillance of left ventricular function every 6–12 months in patients who are asymptomatic with severe mitral regurgitation to monitor left ventricular ejection fraction and end-systolic diamensions.

Invasive evaluation

In contrast to the non-invasive assessment of mitral stenosis, the non-invasive assessment of mitral regurgitation is less accurate. For this reason, cardiac catheterization and left ventriculography are required in many patients with symptomatic mitral regurgitation. Cardiac catheterization is useful for defining a possible coronary ischemic (i.e. papillary muscle) cause, grading the severity of mitral regurgitation, assessing left ventricular contractile function, and making a hemodynamic assessment. During left ventriculography a radiocontrast agent is injected into the left ventricle and the severity of mitral regurgitation is judged on the basis of the rapidity and degree to which the left atrium becomes opacified (Table 12.2). Patients with 3+ to 4+ regurgitation have a condition potentially correctable with surgery, whereas those with 1+ to 2+ mitral regurgitation are generally treated with medical therapy.

Hemodynamic measurements may provide insights into the severity of mitral regurgitation and its consequences. Although the height of the "v" wave in the pulmonary capillary wedge tracing provides little information about the severity of mitral regurgitation, elevation in the mean wedge pressure implies that the mitral regurgitation is either acute or associated with left ventricular dysfunction.

Treatment

The use of vasodilators and diuretics in patients with symptomatic mitral regurgitation result in symptomatic improvement by increasing forward flow and reducing the degree of regurgitation.

Table 12.2 Angiographic grades of mitral regurgitation

Grade	Angiographic details
1+	Contrast enters but does not completely opacify the left atrium
2+	Contrast faintly but completely opacifies the left atrium
3+	Contrast completely and quickly opacifies the left atrium equal in intensity to that of the left ventricle
4+	Contrast quickly concentrates in the left atrium to a degree greater than that for the left ventricle, and contrast also enters the pulmonary veins

Mitral valve surgery is recommended for non-ischemic, severe mitral regurgitation in several circumstances (Box 12.2). Most importantly, surgery is reserved for symptomatic improvement in patients with moderately severe (3+) or severe (4+) grades of regurgitation. Patients with acute forms of mitral regurgitation related to endocarditis or chordal rupture are unlikely to stabilize with medical therapy and often require surgery. Patients with impaired left ventricular function, however, have worse postoperative survival than do those with normal left ventricular function. Patients with mitral regurgitation caused by etiologies that are amenable to valve repair such as posterior leaflet redundancy from myxomatous degeneration may have better survival than those who require valve replacement.[20] Thus, a lower threshold for surgical referral should be used for patients with "reparable" valves than for those who will require a valve replacement. The operative mortality rate is about 2–4% for mitral valve repair and about 8–10% for mitral replacement. The 10-year survival rate is about 80% for mitral repair and about 50% for mitral replacement. The differences between valve repair and replacement in postoperative survival cannot be entirely ascribed to surgical technique. Patients who are candidates for valve repair tend to be younger than those who require valve replacement.

Box 12.2 Indications for surgery in severe, non-ischemic mitral regurgitation[1]

Acute, symptomatic mitral regurgitation, in which repair is likely

Patients with New York Heart Association functional class II, III, or IV symptoms, with normal left ventricular function (left ventricular ejection fraction [LVEF] >60% and end-systolic diameter <4·5 cm)

Symptomatic or asymptomatic patients with mild left ventricular dysfunction (LVEF 50–60% and end-systolic diameter 4·5–5·0 cm)

Symptomatic or asymptomatic patients with moderate left ventricular dysfunction (LVEF 30–50% and end-systolic diameter 5·0–5·5 cm)

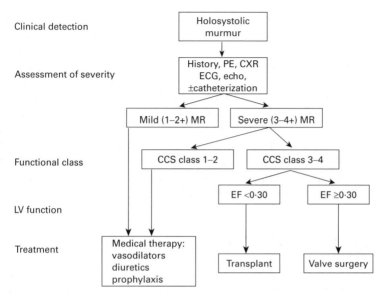

Figure 12.6 Timing of surgery for mitral regurgitation. Decisions about the timing of valve surgery for mitral regurgitation depend on several factors, including the severity of the regurgitation, left ventricular function, and the patient's functional class. Other factors not included in the algorithm include the acuity of mitral regurgitation and the likelihood that repair rather than replacement could be performed, both of these factors increasing referral to surgery. CCS, Canadian Cardiovascular Society; CXR, chest x ray; ECG, electrocardiogram; echo, Doppler echocardiogram; EF, ejection fraction; LV, left ventricular; MR, mitral regurgitation; PE, physical examination

General recommendations for patients with mitral regurgitation according to clinical profiles can be made (Box 12.2 and Figure 12.6). Mitral valve surgery is indicated for patients with severe congestive heart failure, severe mitral regurgitation, and good left ventricular function with ejection fractions greater than 30–40%. Because the ejection fraction falls by an average of 9% after mitral valve repair,[20] preoperative ejection fractions less than about 30% make valve surgery hazardous. For the asymptomatic patient with severe mitral regurgitation and preserved left ventricular function, medical therapy and close follow up are needed. For the "asymptomatic" patient with severe mitral regurgitation and decreasing left function, early symptomatic limitation may be revealed by exercise treadmill testing, and mitral valve surgery should be considered.[19]

Aortic regurgitation

Aortic regurgitation produces left ventricular volume overload but, through the compensatory mechanisms of left ventricular dilatation and hypertrophy, it is well tolerated for years. Unlike the situation for symptomatic aortic stenosis in which surgical therapy has improved survival, the postoperative survival rates of patients undergoing aortic valve surgery for aortic regurgitation are similar to those for patients treated medically. Valve surgery in aortic regurgitation, however, clearly improves symptoms and must be carried out before irreversible left ventricular dysfunction ensues. Recent longitudinal studies suggest that vasodilator therapy can safely delay the time of surgical intervention. Longitudinal follow up studies also show that asymptomatic left ventricular dysfunction is a marker for imminent symptom development and should be an indication for timely surgical therapy, which generally results in recovery in left ventricular function.

Etiology and natural history

There are several causes of aortic regurgitation. Aortic regurgitation may be caused by primary pathology of the valve leaflets as in a congenitally bicuspid valve, destruction of valve tissue in endocarditis, or dilatation of the annulus as in Marfan's syndrome (Table 12.3).

In aortic regurgitation there is abnormal regurgitation of blood from the aorta into the left ventricle during diastole. The main compensatory mechanisms in aortic regurgitation are increased end-diastolic volume and left ventricular hypertrophy. When left ventricular function deteriorates, ejection fraction and stroke volume decrease. The hemodynamic changes and symptoms differ in acute and chronic aortic regurgitation.

In acute aortic regurgitation, the non-dilated, left ventricle cannot accommodate a large regurgitant volume without a marked elevation in left ventricular diastolic pressure, which is transmitted to the left atrium and pulmonary circulation, frequently producing severe dyspnea and pulmonary edema. Rapid aortic diastolic volume run-off into the left ventricle during diastole reduces aortic diastolic pressure. Increased ventricular wall stress (elevated ventricular pressures) and its resulting increase in myocardial oxygen demand, in conjunction with reduced coronary perfusion pressure (myocardial oxygen supply) from the lowered aortic diastolic pressure, can produce complicating ischemia, arrhythmias, or left ventricular dysfunction. Acute, severe aortic regurgitation is usually a surgical emergency, requiring immediate aortic valve replacement.

In chronic aortic regurgitation, the left ventricle undergoes compensatory changes in response to the longstanding regurgitation. Aortic regurgitation results primarily in left ventricular volume overload, but also pressure overload; therefore, the ventricle compensates through dilatation and hypertrophy. Over time, the

Table 12.3 Causes of aortic regurgitation

Etiology	Causes
Valvular	Common
	Endocarditis
	Rheumatic fever
	Less common
	Degenerative aortic valve disease
	Bicuspid valve
	Arthritis and connective tissue disease
	associations: seronegative arthritis,
	ankylosing spondylitis, systemic lupus
	erythematosus, rheumatoid arthritis
Aortic root dilatation	Common
	Hypertension (usually mild aortic
	regurgitation)
	Age-related (degenerative) aortic root
	disease
	Cystic medial necrosis (isolated or with
	classic Marfan's syndrome)
	Less common
	Aortic dissection
	Seronegative arthritis: ankylosing
	spondylitis, psoriatic arthritis, Behçet's
	syndrome, Reiter's syndrome
	Giant cell arteritis
	Relapsing polychondritis
	Syphilitic aortitis
	Polycystic renal disease

dilatation increases the compliance of the left ventricle and allows it to accommodate a large regurgitation volume with less of an increase in diastolic pressure, reducing the pressures transmitted into the left atrium and pulmonary circulation. However, by allowing the aorta to regurgitate an even larger volume of blood into the left ventricle during diastole, left ventricular dilatation also causes aortic (and therefore systemic arterial) diastolic pressure to drop substantially.

Because left ventricular dilatation and hypertrophy are generally adequate to meet the demands of chronic aortic regurgitation, the patient is usually asymptomatic for many years and the natural history of chronic aortic regurgitation is benign. Bland and Wheeler from Massachusetts General Hospital followed 87 patients with free aortic regurgitation (diastolic pressure ≤30 mmHg) and found a 10 year mortality rate of 30% and 20 year mortality rate of 56%.[21] Gradually, however, progressive remodeling of the left ventricle occurs, resulting in myocardial dysfunction. This, in turn, results in decreased forward cardiac output and in an increase in left atrial and pulmonary pressures. At that point, the patient develops the symptoms of congestive heart failure.

Clinical presentation

Many patients with aortic regurgitation are asymptomatic, and the murmur of aortic regurgitation is detected as an incidental finding on careful auscultation during physical examination. If heart failure has ensued, common presenting symptoms include dyspnea on exertion. Physical examination may show bounding, wide pulse pressure, pulses, a hyperdynamic left ventricular cardiac impulse, and a blowing murmur in diastole along the left sternal border (but this may be loudest at the apex in barrel chested or elderly individuals, and louder along the right sternal border in those with dilated ascending aorta). If the aortic regurgitation is moderate, or severe, an associated ejection systolic flow murmur is generated in the absence of aortic stenosis. A rumbling mid-diastolic murmur at the cardiac apex (the Austin–Flint murmur) may be detected and is due to regurgitant blood from the aorta hitting the anterior leaflet of mitral valve. An Austin–Flint murmur is almost always preceded by an S_3 (in contrast to the diastolic apical murmur of significant mitral stenosis).

The combination of a very high left ventricular stroke volume (and therefore high systolic arterial pressure) and a decreased aortic diastolic pressure produces a considerably widened systemic arterial pulse pressure (the difference between arterial systolic and diastolic pressure), which is a hallmark of chronic aortic regurgitation. Many of the associated signs of aortic regurgitation are based on the widened pulse pressure. Duroziez's sign is a to and fro bruit heard over the femoral arteries, de Musset's sign is bobbing of the head, and Quincke's sign is pulsatile blanching of the nail beds.

Non-invasive evaluation

The electrocardiogram may show evidence of left ventricular hypertrophy. The chest radiograph often shows left ventricular prominence or dilatation of the ascending aorta. Doppler echocardiography may show left ventricular hypertrophy and dilatation, a Doppler signal of aortic regurgitation, and diastolic fluttering of anterior mitral leaflet.

Invasive evaluation

Cardiac catheterization is useful for the semiquantitative analysis of aortic regurgitation, using aortography, for evaluation of left ventricular function and for assessment of coexisting coronary artery disease. The grading of the severity of aortic regurgitation is based on a classification similar to that for mitral regurgitation (see Table 12.2).

Treatment

The primary goal of therapy in aortic regurgitation is to prevent irreversible left ventricular enlargement. It is now known that many asymptomatic patients with aortic regurgitation and normal left ventricular function remain clinically stable for years, but a small proportion of patients develop symptoms of left ventricular dysfunction and require operation. Asymptomatic patients with a progressive increase in end-systolic dimension are at high risk for symptomatic deterioration. A timely question remains. Is an increase in end-systolic dimension a firm indication for surgery or merely evidence that the patient will soon develop symptoms and require an operation? There has been concern that a subset of patients will develop irreversible left ventricular dysfunction by the time symptoms arise. A longitudinal view of asymptomatic patients with aortic regurgitation suggests that most patients develop symptoms before or at the time of left ventricular dysfunction. Thus, when patients with significant aortic regurgitation develop an ejection fraction of less than 50% confirmed by repeat echocardiography studies, they will demonstrate symptomatic deterioration soon thereafter. The finding of decreased function is thus a signal to increase the frequency of follow up or to recommend aortic valve surgery.

Several studies have documented that vasodilators can delay the onset of left ventricular dysfunction in patients with aortic regurgitation. Nifedipine, hydralazine, and angiotensin-converting enzyme inhibitors have been shown to reduce left ventricular enlargement and delay the need for aortic valve replacement in patients with aortic insufficiency. Other goals of therapy are to treat underlying congestive heart failure with diuretics, digoxin and vasodilators, and to prevent infective endocarditis. In patients with Marfan's syndrome long term β-blocker therapy is advised to slow the rate of aortic dilatation and to reduce complications.[22]

If aortic valve replacement is carried out after the left ventricle enlargement has been present for more than 3–6 months, then postoperative survival is severely impaired. Based on natural history and surgical series, the following recommendations are made (Figure 12.7).

Aortic valve replacement is recommended for the following:

1. Patients with NYHA functional class III or IV symptoms and preserved left ventricular systolic function, defined as normal ejection fraction at rest (ejection fraction ≥50%).
2. Patients with NYHA functional class II and preserved left ventricular systolic function (ejection fraction ≥50%) but with

Clinical detection

Assessment of severity

Functional class

LV function

Treatment

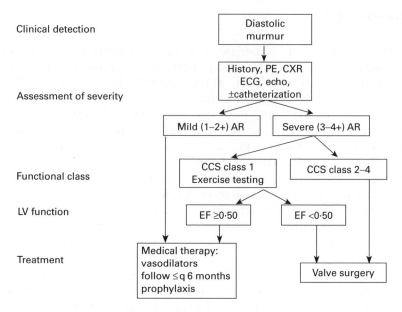

Figure 12.7 Timing of surgery for aortic regurgitation. The timing of surgery depends on the severity of aortic regurgitation, functional class, and left ventricular function. For asymptomatic patients, exercise treadmill testing is very useful to uncover possible effort intolerance and confirm the indication for valve surgery. Valve surgery should be offered to patients with decreasing ejection fractions, as confirmed by repeat testing with echocardiography. Symptomatic patients with moderately severe or severe aortic regurgitation should be sponsored for surgery. AR, aortic regurgitation; CCS, Canadian Cardiovascular Society; CXR, chest x ray; ECG, electrocardiogram; echo, Doppler echocardiogram; LV, left ventricular; PE, physical examination

progressive left ventricular dilation or declining ejection fraction at rest on serial studies or declining effort tolerance during exercise testing.

3. Patients with angina (Canadian class II or greater) with or without coronary artery disease.

4. Asymptomatic or symptomatic patients with mild to moderate left ventricular dysfunction at rest (ejection fraction 25–49%).

5. Patients undergoing bypass surgery or surgery on the aorta or other valves.[1]

For the truly asymptomatic patient, if left ventricular function is normal, the patient should have close follow up at least every 6 months: prophylactic therapy with vasodilators has been recommended.

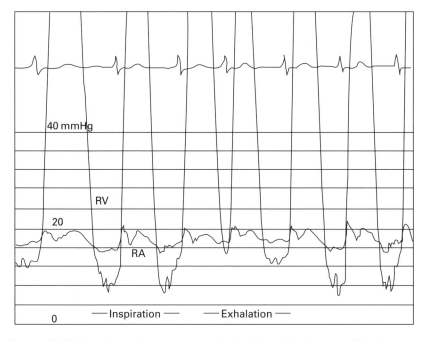

Figure 12.8 Hemodynamic measurements in tricuspid stenosis. Simultaneous measurement of right atrial (RA) and right ventricular (RV) pressures in bioprosthetic valve tricuspid stenosis shows the pressure gradient (the difference between the RA and RV pressures), and absence of the usual inspiratory decrease in RA pressure. The large "a" wave is evident in the right atrial pressure tracing at the end of diastole

Tricuspid valve disease

Stenosis

Tricuspid stenosis is usually due to rheumatic heart disease, prosthetic valve stenosis, or carcinoid syndrome. If the gradient is greater than 4 mmHg or the valve area is less than 2 cm², then the patient has severe tricuspid stenosis (Figure 12.8). The diastolic murmur of tricuspid stenosis increases with inspiration; the neck veins show a large "a" wave and slow Y descent. Surgical therapy is usually required.

Regurgitation

Tricuspid regurgitation is usually functional and due to pressure or volume overload of the right ventricle, most often secondary to mitral

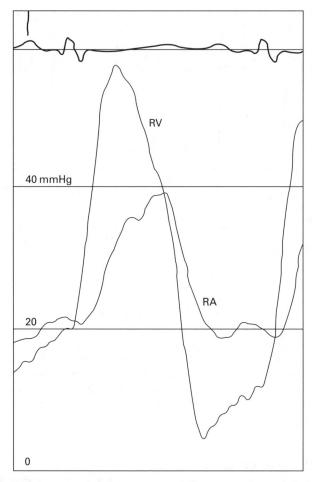

Figure 12.9 Pressure measurements in combined tricuspid regurgitation and stenosis. Hemodynamic measurements of right atrial (RA) and right ventricular (RV) pressures in a patient with carcinoid syndrome shows an enormous "v" wave in the RA trace during ventricular systole. During systole the right atrial pressure is "ventricularized", while during diastole a significant pressure gradient exists between the two chambers

valve disease. In patients with rheumatic mitral stenosis, 20% have significant tricuspid regurgitation. Of these, 80% have functional tricuspid regurgitation and 20% have organic tricuspid regurgitation. The most sensitive physical signs are prominent "v" waves in the jugular pulse and a pulsatile liver (Figure 12.9). The holosystolic murmur may be soft, uncharacteristic, or completely absent in as many as 50% of patients with tricuspid regurgitation, so that the bedside diagnosis is made by placing the "eyes on the neck veins, and a hand on the liver". The primary therapy is directed at the associated

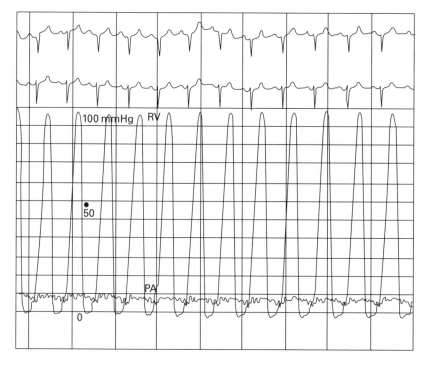

Figure 12.10 Hemodynamic measurements in pulmonary valve stenosis. Simultaneous measurement of right ventricular (RV) and pulmonary artery (PA) pressures in a patient with congenital pulmonary valve stenosis reveals a pressure gradient exceeding 100 mmHg and characteristically low pulmonary artery pressures

conditions such as mitral stenosis or right ventricular failure. Thus, mechanical therapy for mitral stenosis, or diuretic therapy for right heart failure are most commonly used. Patients with severe or organic tricuspid regurgitation occasionally require surgical therapy with valvuloplasty.

Pulmonary valve stenosis

Pulmonary valve stenosis is almost always congenital in etiology. By convention, the severity of pulmonary valve stenosis is classified according to the peak to peak systolic gradient measured between the right ventricle and the pulmonary artery at cardiac catheterization (Figure 12.10). Patients with pressure gradients above 80 mmHg are considered to have severe pulmonary valve stenosis and should be treated with balloon valvuloplasty. Patients with pressure gradients between 40 and 80 mmHg have moderate pulmonary stenosis and should be sponsored for balloon valvuloplasty if they are symptomatic. Those with gradients less than 40 mmHg have mild pulmonary valve stenosis and are unlikely to have progressive disease.

Infective endocarditis

The cardiac valves are among the structures included in the endocardial surface of the heart. Infection of the endocardial surface of the heart by microbial organisms is commonly but not always associated with pre-existing valvular heart disease. Infective endocarditis has an incidence of two to six cases per 100 000 persons per year, and it carries a 10–30% risk of mortality when treated with antibiotics and a 100% mortality if untreated.

Clinical classifications

Three practical classifications of infective endocarditis exist. Infective endocarditis may be classified according to clinical presentation, type of patient (host substrate), or specific etiology. According to the first classification scheme, when infective endocarditis presents as an acute fulminant infection it is termed "acute bacterial endocarditis" and a highly virulent organism such as *Staphylococcus aureus* is usually responsible. When infective endocarditis presents with an insidious clinical course, it is called "subacute bacterial endocarditis" and less virulent organisms such as *Streptococcus viridans* are implicated, although the more destructive organism *Enterococcus* may also present in this manner. In a more practical classification, the clinician can prescribe empiric antibiotics before the etiology is identified, and infective endocarditis can be categorized according to the underlying substrate as either native valve endocarditis, prosthetic valve endocarditis, or intravenous drug abuse-related endocarditis. Of these, native valve endocarditis accounts for approximately 60–80% of cases. Again, different microorganisms and clinical courses are associated with each category. Ultimately, infective endocarditis is described by etiology.

Acute bacterial endocarditis is a rapidly progressive illness characterized by high fever and rigors. It carries a high incidence of complications and has the potential to result in sudden cardiac decompensation. Acute bacterial endocarditis involves highly invasive, virulent organisms and requires a small innoculum to cause infection. It is most commonly associated with *Staphylococcus aureus*, but also occurs with fungi, Gram negative rods, and polymicrobial infection. Risk factors for acute bacterial endocarditis include intravenous drug abuse, the presence of prosthetic valves, and the immunocompromised state. Unfortunately, this process may also afflict individuals without underlying valvular pathology.

Subacute bacterial endocarditis is more common than acute bacterial endocarditis, and usually presents over a period of weeks to months with an indolent, slowly progressive course. Because organisms responsible for subacute presentations are less virulent than those that cause acute presentations, a larger innoculum is required to produce an infection. The most common etiologic agents are α hemolytic streptococci, namely *Streptococcus viridans*, *Streptococcus bovis*, and *Streptococcus (Enterococcus) faecalis*. Subacute bacterial endocarditis occurs most often on damaged native valves.

Experimental studies and clinical observations suggest that pre-existing damage to an endocardial surface such as valvular endocardium is a necessary event for the development of infective endocarditis. The most common cause of endothelial injury is turbulent blood flow resulting from hemodynamic abnormalities such as underlying valvular stenosis or regurgitation. These abnormalities can lead to high velocity jets that mechanically injure the endothelial surface. Other causes of endothelial injury include iatrogenic damage such as indwelling intravenous catheters or prosthetic valves, immune complex deposition as in systemic lupus erythematosus, and intravenous injection of foreign substances with illicit drugs. About 70–75% of patients with endocarditis have evidence of underlying structural or hemodynamic abnormalities by clinical or laboratory examination.

Once the endocardial surface of a valve is injured, platelets adhere to the exposed subendocardium and form a sterile thrombus composed of fibrin termed as "vegetation". This process is referred to as non-bacterial thrombotic endocarditis or "marantic" endocarditis. Non-bacterial thrombotic endocarditis makes the endocardium more hospitable to microbes in two ways. First, the fibrin–platelet deposits provide a surface for adherence by bacteria. Second, the fibrin covers adherent organisms and protects them from host defenses by inhibiting chemotaxis and migration of phagocytes.

When non-bacterial thrombotic endocarditis is present, the exposure of microorganisms to the injured surface can lead to infective endocarditis. Three factors determine the ability of an organism to induce infective endocarditis: access to the bloodstream, survival of the organism in the circulation, and adherence of the bacteria to the endocardium. Bacteria are introduced into the bloodstream whenever a mucosal or skin surface harboring an organism is traumatized, such as following dental procedures or during non-sterile intravenous drug use. However, although transient bacteremia is a relatively common event, only those microorganisms that are both suited for survival in the circulation and able to adhere to the vegetation will cause an infection. For example, Gram positive organisms account for approximately 90% of cases of endocarditis, in large part because of their resistance to destruction in the circulation by complement. Moreover, the ability of certain streptococcal species to produce dextran (a cell wall component that adheres to thrombus) correlates with the ability to incite endocarditis. Likewise, certain staphylococcal species are able to promote adherence via binding to fibronectin.

When organisms penetrate into the previously sterile vegetations on the injured endocardial surface, they are protected from phagocytic activity by overlying fibrin. The organisms multiply and cause further enlargement of the infected vegetation. The presence of an infected vegetation provides a source for continuous bacteremia and can lead to several complications. These complications may occur as a result of mechanical cardiac injury, systemic or pulmonary emboli, or immunologically mediated injury such as antigen–antibody deposition. Local extension of the infection within the heart can result in valvular destruction and congestive heart failure, abscess formation, or erosion into the cardiac conduction system. Portions of a vegetation may embolize to anywhere in the body to produce infection or infarction. Activation of the immune system may lead to immune complex deposition resulting in glomerulonephritis, arthritis, or vasculitis.

Clinical manifestations and evaluation

The underlying etiology and host substrate determine the type of presentation, tempo, and manifestations of infective endocarditis. The most common presenting symptoms include fever and other non-specific constitutional symptoms such as fatigue, anorexia, weakness, myalgias, chills, and night sweats. The diagnosis of infective endocarditis requires a high degree of suspicion on the part of the clinician. A history of valvular heart disease, recent critical illness, chronic dialysis, a recent invasive procedure, or intravenous drug use are risk factors for infective endocarditis.

Systemic inflammatory response produced by the infection is responsible for the fever and splenomegaly that may be present on examination. The infection also produces a number of laboratory findings, including an elevated white cell count with a left shift, an "anemia of chronic disease", or an elevated erythrocyte sedimentation rate.

Physical examination may identify the murmur of the underlying valvular pathology that predisposed the patient to infective endocarditis. On the other hand, auscultation may also reveal a new murmur of valvular insufficiency due to valve destruction from the infective endocarditis process. Because infective endocarditis may affect any of the cardiac valves, heart murmurs in this condition may be referable to any valve. Right sided valvular lesions, although rare in most types of endocarditis, are particularly common in endocarditis in intravenous drug users. Serial examinations in acute endocarditis may reveal changing murmurs of worsening regurgitation. Physical examination may also reveal evidence of congestive heart failure, septic emboli, or stroke. Evidence of symptomatic emboli to the central nervous system is seen in up to 33% of patients with infective endocarditis, and may produce a transient ischemic attack, hemiparesis, hemiplegia, headache, seizures, encephalitis, meningitis, brain abscess, or visual changes. Injury to the kidneys attributable to either immunologically mediated damage or emboli may be identified via hematuria or flank pain. Lung infarction (pulmonary embolus) or infection (pneumonia) is particularly common with right sided lesions and endocarditis associated with intravenous drug use. Infarction and seeding of the vasa vasora or arterial wall will produce a "mycotic aneurysm", which weakens the vessel wall and may ultimately result in rupture and hemorrhage. Mycotic aneurysms may be found in the aorta, viscera, or periphery, but are particularly dangerous in cerebral vessels as rupture may result in a fatal intracranial hemorrhage.

Other cutaneous, oral mucosal, and ocular findings of infective endocarditis, which are associated with septic emboli or immune complex mediated vasculitis in the extremities, should be sought. Petechiae may appear as tiny, circular, red-brown discolorations found on mucosal surfaces and skin. Splinter hemorrhages, which are much more often the result of external trauma, are longitudinal hemorrhages under the nails that result from subungual microemboli in infective endocarditis. Painless, slightly nodular discolorations found on the palms and soles are called Janeway's lesions. Tender, pea sized, erythematous nodules found primarily in the pulp space of the fingers and toes are termed Osler's nodes. Emboli to the retina produce Roth spots, which are microinfarctions that appear as white dots with a hemorrhagic surround.

The diagnosis and appropriate treatment of endocarditis depends on the identification of the responsible microorganism by blood culture. Ideally, blood cultures should be drawn at three distinct times from separate sites to both avoid confusion between contaminants and the responsible organism and optimize the yield. Treatment can then be tailored to the specific microorganism according to its antibiotic sensitivities. A specific etiologic agent will be identified by culture approximately 95% of the time. Recent exposure to antibiotics, fastidious organisms (i.e. difficult to grow in culture), or rare organisms (i.e. yeast, Gram negative organisms) may result in negative cultures or so-called "culture negative endocarditis".

Table 12.4 Empiric therapy for infective endocarditis

Host substrate	Antibiotics
Native valve endocarditis	
Acute presentation	Gentamicin, oxacillin or vancomycin
Subacute presentation	Gentamicin, ampicillin
Prosthetic valve endocarditis	
Early (<60 days postoperative)	Gentamicin, vancomycin
Late (≥60 days postoperative)	Gentamicin, vancomycin, cephalosporin
Intravenous drug use endocarditis	Gentamicin, oxacillin, cephalosporin

When patients present with the clinical syndrome of infective endocarditis, three sets of blood cultures should be obtained. Empiric therapy should be started, however, before the results of blood cultures are available. "Cephalosporin" refers to a third generation cephalosporin such as ceftriaxone.

The electrocardiogram is useful in acute endocarditis in identification of invasion of the conduction system by infection or abscess formation, which may appear as a heart block or arrhythmia. Doppler echocardiography is diagnostically useful if the vegetations are visualized. The size of the vegetations relates roughly to the risk for embolization. Echocardiography is extremely helpful in the determination of individual valve involvement, valvular competence, and the identification of complications such as abscess formation. Transesophageal echocardiography is the most sensitive method of imaging for these purposes.

Treatment

Treatment of endocarditis entails high dose, intravenous antibiotic therapy for 4–6 weeks (Table 12.4). Although it is critical to start empiric antibiotics while waiting for the culture results, the final antibiotic regimen should be tailored to the identification and sensitivities of the causative organism. Persistent infection in the face of appropriate antibiotic treatment should prompt a search for metastatic sites of infection. Surgical intervention[1] is indicated for the following:

- valve dysfunction and persistent infection after 7–10 days of appropriate antibiotic therapy as indicated by the presence of fever, leukocytosis, and bacteremia if non-cardiac causes of infection are excluded
- acute aortic or mitral regurgitation with heart failure
- recurrent embolic events
- evidence of annular or aortic abscess, or sinus or aortic true or false aneurysm
- fungal infection.

Surgical intervention is considered for infection with Gram negative organisms (or organisms with a poor response to antibiotics) and for prosthetic valve endocarditis. Surgical correction consists of valve replacement and debridement.

The most important aspect of therapy is prevention of infective endocarditis, namely the administration of antibiotics before and immediately following procedures that result in bacteremia in susceptible individuals.[8,9]

Case studies

Case 12.1

An 83-year-old woman presents with persistent anorexia, refractory congestive heart failure, and a new heart murmur 2 weeks after completing a course of antibiotics for prosthetic valve endocarditis. The patient had a lifelong history of a heart murmur caused by mild aortic stenosis. She had an episode of unexplained *Staphylococcus aureus* bacteremia 10 years before admission and was treated with antibiotics for 6 weeks for possible endocarditis, although no definite evidence was identified. She was otherwise well until 6 months before admission, when she developed congestive heart failure requiring urgent admission to a hospital in another city. Evaluation showed evidence of pulmonary edema and a murmur consistent with aortic stenosis. Doppler echocardiographic examination showed a sclerocalcific aortic valve with reduced leaflet motion, peak instantaneous aortic gradient of 80 mmHg, and reduced left ventricular ejection fraction of 25%.

Cardiac catheterization showed the following (expressed as values at rest [normal]). Pressures (mmHg): mean right atrial 9 (0–8), right ventricular (systolic/end-diastolic) 45/10 (15–30/0–8), pulmonary arterial (systolic/diastolic) 45/28 (15–30/4–12), mean pulmonary artery wedge 27 (4–12), systemic arterial (systolic/diastolic) 126/72 (110–140/60–90), left ventricular (systolic/end-diastolic) 198/35 (110–140/5–13). Mean aortic valve gradient (mmHg): 66 (0). Cardiac output (l/min): 4·5. Cardiac index (l/min per m²): 2·5 (2·5–4·2). Arteriovenous oxygen difference (mmHg): 45 (30–50). Oxygen consumption index (ml/min/m²): 101 (100–125). Aortic valve area (cm²): 0·7 (>4·0).

Coronary arteriography showed a 50% lesion in the mid-portion of the left anterior descending artery and no other significant coronary artery disease.

Aortic balloon valvuloplasty was carried out as a bridge to surgical aortic valve replacement. The following parameters before (and after) valvuloplasty were recorded. Pressures (mmHg): systemic arterial (systolic/diastolic) 125/70 (130/80), left ventricular (systolic/end-diastolic) 201/36 (161/34). Mean aortic valve gradient (mmHg): 67 (28). Cardiac output (l/min): 4·5 (4·4). Aortic valve area (cm^2): 0·9 (>4·0).

Symptoms of congestive heart failure improved in response to valvuloplasty, and she was treated with digoxin 0·25 mg/day orally, furosemide 120 mg/day orally, enalapril 5 mg/day orally, and potassium chloride 24 mEq/day orally. The patient was discharged from the hospital but noted gradually worsening congestive heart failure 3 months later associated with evidence of aortic valve restenosis by Doppler echocardiogram, showing a peak instantaneous gradient of 55 mmHg and ejection fraction of 25%.

Aortic valve replacement with a Carpentier–Edwards pericardial valve and single coronary artery bypass grafting with a saphenous vein graft to the left anterior descending artery was successfully carried out 3 months before admission. After discharge from the hospital, the patient felt well with class I congestive heart failure. Two weeks after discharge, however, she suddenly developed fever, chills, and anorexia. Blood cultures were obtained and within 18 hours showed growth of group B β-hemolytic streptococci. The patient was treated initially with penicillin G 20 million units/day and gentamicin 80 mg every 8 hours intravenously. Gentamicin was discontinued after the organism was found to be sensitive to penicillin. The patient became afebrile within 24 hours of institution of antibiotic therapy and developed no complications of endocarditis, such as systemic embolization, congestive heart failure, aortic insufficiency, persistent sepsis, or heart block. She was discharge to home to complete a 6 week course of antibiotics.

After completion of antibiotics, the patient initially felt well and was able to resume normal activities such as light housework and shopping with assistance. During the week before admission, however, she noted persistent anorexia, new symptoms of paroxysmal nocturnal dyspnea, and temperature ranging from 99° to 100·4°F (37·2–37·9°C). On examination, a new murmur of aortic insufficiency was detected.

Past medical history. Other active medical problems included upper gastrointestinal hemorrhage during warfarin therapy administered for atrial fibrillation, complicated by acute blood loss and profound anemia to hematocrit 15·1%, which was attributed to a prepyloric gastric ulcer and documented by upper endoscopy. This was successfully treated with blood transfusion and amoxicillin for *Helicobacter pylori*. Medications on admission included digoxin 0·25 mg/day orally, furosemide 60 mg/day orally, potassium chloride 24 mEq/day, and omeprazole 20 mg/day orally.

Examination. Physical examination: the patient appeared acutely ill. No abnormalities of skin, nail beds, or oral mucosa. Temperature: 99·6°F (37·6°C). Pulse: 66 beats/min, irregular. Blood pressure: 150/60 mmHg in right arm. Jugular venous pulse: 10 cm. Cardiac impulse: displaced laterally to anterior axillary line. First heart sound: soft. Second heart sound: split normally on inspiration. No added sounds. Grade 3/6 diastolic decrescendo murmur heard at left sternal border. Grade 3/6 mid-systolic murmur in aortic area. Chest examination: reduced air entry, rales in the lower half of the lungs bilaterally. Abdominal examination: soft abdomen, no tenderness, and no masses. Normal liver span. Mild foot edema. Femoral, popliteal, posterior tibial, and dorsalis pedis pulses: all normal volume and equal. Carotid pulses: normal, no bruits. Optic fundi: normal.

Investigations. Electrocardiogram: atrial fibrillation with slow ventricular response of 61 beats/min, axis 0°, ST-TW changes consistent with digoxin effect or inferolateral ischemia. Chest *x* ray: moderate cardiomegaly and interstitial pulmonary edema, without pleural effusion or infiltrate. Doppler echocardiography: aortic perivalvular leak, and a poorly defined mass at the level of the aortic valve sewing ring adjacent to the left sinus of Valsalva.

Questions

1. What is the underlying cause of this patient's current problem?
2. What treatment is required for this patient?
3. When you admit any patient to hospital with infective endocarditis, which consultants should be called immediately?
4. What are the indications for valve surgery in patients with infective endocarditis?
5. What are the best empiric antibiotic regimens for infective endocarditis that should be started before the results of blood cultures are obtained?

Answers

Answer to question 1   This patient presents with congestive heart failure, fever, and a new perivalvular leak after treatment with antibiotics for prosthetic valve endocarditis. She has relapsed prosthetic valve endocarditis associated with an abscess in the sewing ring of the aortic prosthesis.

Answer to question 2   For immediate control of infection the patient should be admitted to hospital and treated again with penicillin G 20 million units/day and gentamicin 80 mg every 8 hours intravenously after blood cultures are obtained. For treatment of congestive heart failure and monitoring of potential cardiovascular complications, the patient requires intravenous furosemide 60–120 mg/day, enalapril 5–10 mg/day orally, and continuous electrocardiographic monitoring. For cure of endocarditis, the patient requires repeat aortic valve replacement and debridement of the sewing ring abscess.

Answer to question 3 The treatment of endocarditis requires a team approach with immediate consultations and coordinated care from a cardiologist, a cardiac surgeon, and an infectious disease specialist.

Answer to question 4 Surgical intervention[1] is indicated for the following: valve dysfunction and persistent infection after 7–10 days of appropriate antibiotic therapy, as indicated by the presence of fever, leukocytosis, and bacteremia if non-cardiac causes of infection are excluded; acute aortic or mitral regurgitation with heart failure; recurrent embolic events; evidence of annular or aortic abscess, or sinus or aortic true or false aneurysm; and fungal infection. It is considered for infection with Gram negative organisms (or organisms with a poor response to antibiotics) and for prosthetic valve endocarditis. Surgical correction consists of valve replacement and debridement.

Answer to question 5 For patients with a subacute presentation affecting native valves, streptococcal and enterococcal etiologies are the most likely etiologies and should be treated with ampicillin and gentamicin. For patients with early postoperative endocarditis (<90 days) affecting prosthetic valves, *S. aureus* and *S. epidermidis* species are most common and should be covered with vancomycin and gentamicin. For patients with late postoperative endocarditis (>90 days) affecting prosthetic valves, streptococcal, staphylococcal, and Gram negative species have been reported and should be treated with vancomycin, gentamicin, and a third generation cephalosporin. For endocarditis associated with intravenous drug abuse, vancomycin, gentamicin, and a third generation cephalosporin should be used for Gram negative etiologies.

Thus, empiric antibiotic regimens recommended for the various clinical classifications of endocarditis are based on the statistical likelihood of specific etiologies causing endocarditis for each patient group. In the case shown here, with early postoperative endocarditis, the etiology was identified as a streptococcal species (a rare cause of endocarditis); this would have been covered by empiric use of vancomycin and gentamicin, but it is more adequately treated with the specific regimen of penicillin after identification of the organism and its sensitivities are known.

Progress

After 4 days of treatment for congestive heart failure and infection, the patient underwent repeat aortic valve replacement. She was cardioverted to normal sinus rhythm and had no recurrence of congestive heart failure during her stay in hospital. Repeat Doppler echocardiogram showed normal aortic valve prosthesis and improved ejection fraction of 45%. She received a total of 6 weeks of intravenous penicillin and lifetime prophylaxis at times of risk.

Case 12.2

An 80-year-old woman presents with a 2 month history of congestive heart failure and a single episode of near fainting while walking up stairs 1 week before admission. The patient has a 10 year history of a heart murmur caused by mild aortic stenosis, as documented by Doppler echocardiography showing a 16–25 mmHg peak instantaneous gradient. She underwent regular follow up office visits every 4 months and repeat Doppler echocardiography every 12 months. Two months before admission, she noted mild dyspnea while walking up stairs. Because the patient also had a head cold at the time, she thought the shortness of breath was related to the coincidental viral syndrome and did not report this to her physician, although the mild dyspnea persisted after the symptoms of coryza spontaneously disappeared. She did become alarmed, however, when she almost passed out while walking upstairs carrying a bundle of laundry. She presented to her physician who found no significant change on physical examination but found that the peak instantaneous gradient on Doppler measurement had increased to 64 mmHg from 25 mmHg 1 year before. She was referred for cardiac catheterization. The patient had a history of gastroesophageal reflux treated with antacids but no other cardiovascular or significant medical history.

Examination. Physical examination: the patient appeared well. Temperature: 98°F (36·7°C). Pulse: 75 beats/min, low volume. Blood pressure: 170/90 mmHg in right arm. Jugular venous pulse: 5 cm. Cardiac impulse: slightly prominent at mid-clavicular line. First heart sound: normal. Second heart sound: soft and single. No added sounds. Grade 1/6 diastolic decrescendo murmur heard at left sternal border. Grade 3/6 coarse mid-systolic murmur at left sternal border radiating to carotids. Chest examination: normal air entry, no rales, or rhonchi heard. Abdominal examination: soft abdomen, no tenderness, and no masses. Normal liver span. No peripheral edema. Femoral, popliteal, posterior tibial, and dorsalis pedis pulses: all normal volume and equal. Carotid pulses: delayed upstroke, no bruits. Optic fundi: normal.

Investigations. Laboratory investigations: hemoglobin 13·0 g/dl (130 g/l), hematocrit 36%, white blood cell count $7·7 \times 10^3/\mu l$, platelets $234 \times 10^3/\mu l$, International Normalized Ratio 1·0, partial thromboplastin time 30·1 seconds. Potassium 4·0 mEq/l (4·0 mmol/l), creatinine 0·7 mEq/l (62 mmol/l).

Electrocardiogram: normal sinus rhythm of rate 68 beats/min, PR 0·20, axis −22°, left ventricular hypertrophy with repolarization changes consistent with strain or ischemia. Echocardiography: normal left ventricular function with estimated ejection fraction 70%, mild concentric left ventricular hypertrophy, calcified and thickened aortic valve leaflets with diminished motion, and peak instantaneous gradient 64 mmHg.

Cardiac catheterization showed the following (expressed as values at rest [normal]). Pressures (mmHg): mean right atrial 4 (0–8), right ventricular (systolic/end-diastolic) 36/8 (15–30/0–8), pulmonary arterial (systolic/diastolic) 36/18 (15–30/4–12), systemic artery (systolic/diastolic) 205/70 (110–140/60–90), left ventricle (systolic/end-diastolic) 255/15 (110–140/5–13). Mean aortic valve gradient (mmHg): 55 (0). Cardiac output (l/min): 4·8. Cardiac index (l/min per m^2): 3·1 (2·5–4·2). Arteriovenous oxygen difference (mmHg): 36 (30–50). Oxygen consumption index (ml/min per m^2): 111 (100–125). Aortic valve area (cm^2): 0·6 (>4·0).

Coronary arteriography showed significant two vessel coronary artery disease with a 70% stenosis at the origin of the first diagonal branch, and an 80% stenosis of the posterior descending artery. No left ventriculogram was performed, because of the presence of severe aortic stenosis. After cardiac catheterization, the patient developed lightheadedness associated with a heart rate of 30 beats/min and blood pressure 50 mmHg systolic during compression of the femoral artery after the cardiac catheterization sheaths were removed.

Questions

1. What is the patient's presenting problem for which she was referred for cardiac catheterization?
2. What is the etiology of the patient's acute problem after cardiac catheterization, why is this especially serious in a patient with aortic stenosis, and how should it be treated?
3. In general, what are indications for valve surgery in patients with aortic stenosis?
4. Should this patient be treated with balloon aortic valvuloplasty?
5. What is the lowest ejection fraction acceptable for patients undergoing aortic valve replacement for aortic stenosis?

Answers

Answer to question 1   The patient has critical aortic stenosis, as defined by the presence of symptoms of congestive heart failure, presyncope, and an aortic valve area ≤0·7 cm^2.

Answer to question 2   The patient is experiencing a vagal reaction attributed to the discomfort of femoral compression. This is a critical situation in a patient with aortic stenosis because the maintenance of cardiac output and blood pressure in aortic stenosis depends on adequate preload. The peripheral vasodilatation that accompanies a vagal reaction abruptly decreases preload, and the underfilled and hypertrophied left ventricle is unable to maintain the pressure needed to generate a gradient across the stenotic aortic valve. Blood pressure and cardiac output fall precipitously. This hemodynamic situation is difficult to reverse, but a quick response with 1·0 mg atropine and intravenous fluids in this case resulted in heart rate of 76 beats/min and a systolic blood pressure of 110 mmHg. She was then immediately referred for aortic valve replacement and saphenous vein bypass grafting to the diagonal branch and posterior descending artery. She had an uneventful postoperative course and was discharged to home 8 days after surgery.

Because patients with aortic stenosis frequently suffer from shifts in volume after cardiac catheterization from several etiologies, such as osmotic diuresis from contrast agents and attempts at volume repletion, they are at increased risk for hemodynamic complications after the procedure. It has therefore been the policy in several institutions to schedule cardiac catheterization on the same day as valve surgery for patients with critical aortic stenosis. There is no advantage in waiting any longer than this in patients who have documented severe aortic stenosis.

Answer to question 3   Aortic valve replacement is indicated for persons with symptomatic severe aortic stenosis, or patients with severe aortic stenosis undergoing coronary artery surgery or surgery of the aorta or other valves.[1] Patients with valve area ≤ 0.7 cm^2 by Doppler echocardiography or by hemodynamic measurement should be considered for valve replacement if they have symptoms of angina, syncope, or congestive heart failure. The postoperative survival statistics showing 70% survival or more after 15 years significantly exceed the natural history of symptomatic aortic stenosis, with median survivals of 5, 3, and 2 years after the onset of angina, syncope, or congestive heart failure in aortic stenosis, respectively.

Answer to question 4   Initial enthusiasm for aortic valvuloplasty has been replaced by marked skepticism when it was revealed that the hemodynamic improvements in aortic valvuloplasty are modest, almost always temporary, and associated with survival that is not different from the natural history of severe, symptomatic aortic stenosis.[14,17] Thus, the procedure is not recommended as definitive therapy for patients with aortic stenosis but only for patients who are potential surgical candidates. Aortic valvuloplasty may be considered as a "bridge" to valve replacement in patients who are hemodynamically unstable or have a reversible contraindication to valve surgery such as sepsis or prerenal azotemia, or for patients who require major non-cardiac surgery on an emergency basis such as internal fixation of hip fracture.

Answer to question 5 No lower limit for ejection fraction has been defined as a contraindication to aortic valve replacement for severe aortic stenosis. Unlike balloon aortic valvuloplasty, which produces such a mild hemodynamic benefit that no significant improvement in ejection fraction is detectable, aortic valve replacement results in a predictable increase in ejection fraction for patients with reduced left ventricular function. If, however, left ventricular function is so poor that the mean aortic valve gradient is below 30 mmHg, then aortic valve replacement should not be considered because the operative mortality is prohibitive.[16]

Case 12.3

A 67-year-old general surgeon was admitted with a long history of mitral regurgitation and general fatigue. The patient was first told of a heart murmur when he was 12 years old. He remained well, however, until 3 years before admission when he noted progressively worsening fatigue on exertion and occasional palpitations. His past history included *S. viridans* endocarditis in 1953, gastroesophageal reflux, and prostatism.

Examination. Physical examination: the patient appeared normal. No abnormalities of skin, nail beds, or oral mucosa. Temperature: 98·6°F (37°C). Pulse: 100 beats/min, frequent premature beats. Blood pressure: 110/75 mmHg in right arm. Jugular venous pulse: 12 cm. Cardiac impulse: displaced laterally to anterior axillary line. First heart sound: soft. Second heart sound: split normally on inspiration. No added sounds. Grade 3/6 holosystolic murmur at cardiac apex with a mid-systolic click. Chest examination: normal air entry, no rales or rhonchi. Abdominal examination: soft abdomen, no tenderness, and no masses. Normal liver span. Mild foot edema. Femoral, popliteal, posterior tibial, and dorsalic pedis pulses: all normal volume and equal. Carotid pulses: normal, no bruits. Optic fundi: normal.

Investigations. Laboratory investigations: hemoglobin 16 g/dl (16 g/l), hematocrit 47%, white blood cell count 6·5 × 10³/µl, platelets 179 × 10³/µl, International Normalized Ratio 1·0, partial thromboplastin time 26·7 seconds, potassium 4·4 mEq/l (4·4 mmol/l), creatinine 1·1 mEq/l (97 mmol/l).

Electrocardiogram: normal sinus rhythm, at a rate of 100 beats/min, PR 0·21, axis 20°; otherwise within normal limits. Rest Doppler echocardiography: normal left ventricular size, vigorous contractile function, and mild concentric left ventricular hypertrophy. There was moderate myxomatous thickening and redundancy of the mitral valve with holosystolic bulging of both leaflets and more prominent posterior leaflet prolapse associated with at least moderately severe regurgitation. Exercise echocardiography: limited exercise capacity. The patient was able to exercise for 5 min on a standard Bruce protocol and stopped because of fatigue. There was no evidence of ischemia or left ventricular decompensation.

Cardiac catheterization showed the following (expressed as values at rest [normal]). Pressures (mmHg): mean right atrial 13 (0–8), right ventricular (systolic/end-diastolic) 42/16 (15–30/0–8), pulmonary arterial (systolic/diastolic) 42/20 (15–30/4–12), pulmonary artery wedge (mean, v) 26, 34 (4–12), systemic arterial (systolic/diastolic) 126/72 (110–140/60–90), left ventricular (systolic/end-diastolic) 126/25 (110–140/5–13). Cardiac output (l/min): 4·0. Cardiac index (l/min per m²): 2·1 (2·5–4·2). Arteriovenous oxygen difference (mmHg): 60 (30–50). Oxygen consumption index (ml/min per m²): 125 (100–125). Left ventricular end-diastolic volume index (ml/m²): 113 (50–90). Left ventricular end-systolic volume index (ml/m²): 39 (15–30). Left ventricular stroke volume index (ml/m²): 74 (35–75). Left ventricular ejection fraction (%): 65 (50–80).

Coronary arteriography showed no evidence of coronary artery disease. The patient underwent mitral valve repair and Duran ring annuloplasty. The anterior leaflet was myxomatous and regurgitant at the posteromedial commissure. The anterior leaflet was brought to the level of the posterior leaflet with three sutures placed near the posteromedial commissure. There was a cleft in the anterior leaflet at the anterolateral commissure, which was closed with two sutures. Because the annulus continued to appear to be eccentric, a Duran ring was sutured to the annulus, which corrected the deformity of the valve. Intraoperative assessment showed no evidence of residual mitral regurgitation. Postoperative Doppler echocardiography showed evidence of trace mitral regurgitation and well preserved left ventricular function. After discharge from the hospital, the patient gradually showed improvement in exercise tolerance and returned to working on a full-time basis.

Questions

1. What medical therapy could have been used in this patient with mitral regurgitation?

2. What anatomic features made this patient an ideal candidate for mitral valve repair versus mitral valve replacement? What features may have made this patient less suitable for repair?
3. What is the effect of mitral valve repair on left ventricular ejection fraction? What is the effect of mitral valve replacement?

Answers

Answer to question 1   By reducing the resistance to forward flow, vasodilator therapy may reduce the degree of regurgitation in patients with mitral regurgitation. Because sodium retention is almost always seen with vasodilators, diuretic therapy is often required as well. For patients with impaired left ventricular function, digoxin therapy is indicated. Anticoagulation with warfarin sodium is indicated if atrial fibrillation is present. Antibiotic prophylaxis is important in patients with mitral regurgitation.

Answer to question 2   The patient had myxomatous degeneration of the mitral valve, predominantly affecting the posterior leaflet. This is an ideal anatomic substrate for surgical repair. The patient had a history of endocarditis, however. Many patients with a history of endocarditis often have extensive valve destruction, thus reducing the likelihood of successful repair. This patient had a cleft in the anterior leaflet of the mitral valve that may have been a residual defect from prior endocarditis. Because the cleft was small, it was easily repaired with sutures.

Answer to question 3   A study from the Mayo Clinic[20] reported that ejection fractions decreased by an average of 10% for patients undergoing surgery for mitral regurgitation, from 62 ± 10% to 52 ± 13%. The type of surgery had a small effect on the change in ejection fraction: mean ejection fraction decreased from 63 ± 9% to 54 ± 11% in 195 patients undergoing valve repair, and from 60 ± 12% to 49 ± 15% in 214 patients undergoing valve replacement. The slight improvement in ejection after mitral valve repair is attributed to better maintenance of mitral architecture, including integrity of papillary muscles, chordae, leaflets, and annulus, than that achieved with valve replacement.

References

1   Bonow R, Carabello BA, de Leon AC, *et al*. ACC/AHA guidelines for the management of patients with valvular heart disease: a report of the American College of Cardiology/American Heart Association Task Force on Practice Guidelines (Committee on Management of Patients with Valvular Heart Disease). *J Am Coll Cardiol* 1998;**32**:1486–588.

2   Wood P. *Chronic rheumatic heart disease in diseases of the heart and circulation.* Philadelphia: J B Lippincott, 1968.

3   Rowe JC, Bland EF, Sprague HB, White PD. The course of mitral stenosis without surgery: ten- and twenty-year perspectives. *Ann Intern Med* 1960;**52**:741.

4   Ellis LB, Singh JB, Morales DD, Harken DE. Fifteen to twenty-year study of one thousand patients undergoing closed mitral valvuloplasty. *Circulation* 1973; **48**:357–64.

5   Lock JE, Khalilullah M, Shirivastrava S, Bahl V, Keane JF. Percutaneous catheter commisurotomy in rheumatic mitral stenosis. *N Engl J Med* 1985;**313**:1515–18.

6   Dalen JE. Mitral stenosis. In: Dalen JE, Alpert JS, eds. *Valvular heart disease.* Boston: Little, Brown and Co, 1981:41–98.

7   Carabello BA, Crawford FA. Valvular heart disease. Review article. *N Engl J Med* 1997;**337**:32–41.

8   Dajani AS, Taubert KA, Wilson W, *et al.* Prevention of bacterial endocarditis. Recommendations by the American Heart Association. *JAMA* 1997;**277**:1794–801.

9   Durack DT. Prevention of infective endocarditis. *N Engl J Med* 1995;**332**:38–44.

10 Palacios IF, Block PC, Wilkins GT, Weyman AE. Follow-up of patients undergoing percutaneous mitral balloon valvotomy. Analysis of factors determining restenosis. *Circulation* 1989;**79**:573–9.

11 Bittl JA. Mitral balloon dilatation. Long-term results. *J Card Surg* 1994;**9(suppl)**: 213–17.

12 Turi ZG, Reyes VP, Raju BS, *et al.* Percutaneous versus surgical closed commisurotomy for mitral stenosis. *Circulation* 1991;**83**:1170–85.

13 Reyes VP, Baju BS, Wynne J, *et al.* Percutaneous balloon valvuloplasty compared with open surgical commissurotomy for mitral stenosis. *N Engl J Med* 1994; **331**:961–7.

14 O'Keefe JH, Vlietstra RE, Bailey KR, Holmes DR. Natural history of candidates for balloon aortic valvuloplasty. *Mayo Clin Proc* 1987;**62**:986–91.

15 Vekshtein VI, Alexander RW, Yeung AC, *et al.* Coronary atherosclerosis is associated with left ventricular dysfunction and dilatation in aortic stenosis. *Circulation* 1990;**82**:2068–76.

16 Carabello BA, Green LH, Grossman W, Cohn LH, Koster JK, Collins J. Hemodynamic determinants of prognosis of aortic valve replacement in critical aortic stenosis and advanced congestive heart failure. *Circulation* 1980;**62**:42–8.

17 Otto CM, Mickel MC, Kennedy JW, *et al.* Three-year outcome after balloon valvuloplasty: insights into prognosis after valvular aortic stenosis. *Circulation* 1994;**89**:642–50.

18 Marks AR, Choong CY, Sanfilippo AJ, Ferre M, Weyman AE. Identification of high-risk and low-risk subgroups with mitral valve prolapse. *N Engl J Med* 1989; **320**:1031–6.

19 Ross J. Afterload mismatch in aortic and mitral valve disease: implications for surgical therapy. *J Am Coll Cardiol* 1985;**5**:811–26.

20 Enriquez-Sarano M, Schaff HV, Orszulak TA, Tajik AJ, Bailey KR, Frye RL. Valve repair improves the outcome of surgery for mitral regurgitation. A multivariate analysis. *Circulation* 1995;**91**:1022–8.

21 Bland EF, Wheeler EO. Severe aortic regurgitation in young people. *N Engl J Med* 1957;**256**:667–71.

22 Shores J, Berger KR, Murphy EA, Pyeritz RE. Progression of aortic dilatation and the benefit of long-term β-adrenergic blockade in Marfan's syndrome. *N Engl J Med* 1994;**330**:1335–41.

13: Pericardial disease, disease of the aorta, and heart tumors

JOHN A OSBORNE, LEONARD S LILLY

Pericardial disease

The pericardium is a supportive tissue that surrounds the heart. It consists of a tough fibrous outer coat (the parietal pericardium) and a thin, inner serosal lining (the visceral pericardium). Between these two layers, the normal pericardium contains up to 50 ml plasma ultrafiltrate, which allows cardiac contraction and relaxation to occur in a minimum friction environment. The most common affliction of the pericardium is acute inflammation, known as pericarditis.

Acute pericarditis

Etiology

Many medical and surgical conditions can result in pericardial inflammation (Box 13.1). The most common form is "idiopathic" pericarditis, which occurs in otherwise healthy individuals. Serologic studies have documented that such cases are frequently associated with an acute viral infection, particularly caused by echovirus and coxsackie virus group B. Because of the essentially identical presentation and course of "idiopathic" and documented viral pericarditis, they are considered the same clinical syndrome. Other viruses that have been implicated in acute pericarditis are adenovirus, varicella, and Ebstein–Barr virus. In patients with AIDS, additional viral causes include cytomegalovirus and herpes simplex.

Tuberculosis is now an uncommon cause of pericarditis in industrialized societies. However, its incidence is increased among immunocompromised individuals, including those with AIDS. Tuberculous infection may spread directly to the pericardium from the lungs and mediastinal lymph nodes, or indirectly via hematogenous dissemination.

Other types of bacterial pericarditis are uncommon and usually occur in immunocompromised individuals or those with pre-existing medical illnesses. Bacterial pericarditis can develop via extension from infection in the mediastinum (for example, infection following

Box 13.1 Causes of acute pericarditis

Idiopathic
Infectious
    Viral (especially echovirus, coxsackie virus group B)
    Bacterial (including tuberculosis)
Non-infectious
    Uremia
    Following acute myocardial infarction or cardiac surgery
    Neoplastic
    Following radiation therapy
    Connective tissue diseases
    Trauma
    Medication related (Box 13.2)

thoracic surgery or penetrating chest trauma), contiguous spread from endocarditis or pneumonia, or by way of hematogenous dissemination during bacteremia of any cause. The most commonly implicated bacteria are staphylococci, streptococci, and Gram negative bacilli. Rarely, fungi, protozoa, or rickettsial organisms have been identified as causes of pericarditis.

Uremic pericarditis is an important complication of chronic renal failure. The mechanism by which uremia results in pericardial inflammation is not known, and there is no direct correlation between the concentration of nitrogen metabolites and this form of pericarditis, which may even occur during the first several months of dialysis therapy.

Pericarditis following myocardial infarction may occur in two forms. The first occurs within the first few days of acute myocardial infarction (AMI) and is due to extension of myocardial inflammation to the adjacent pericardium. Clinically, this form of pericarditis is detected in a minority of patients following AMI. The second form of post-AMI pericarditis occurs rarely 2 weeks to several months following AMI, and is known as Dressler's syndrome. The cause of this complication is not known but it may be of autoimmune origin related to antigens released from necrotic myocardial cells. A similar syndrome may occur several weeks following cardiac surgery when the pericardium has been opened (termed "post-pericardiotomy" pericarditis).

Neoplastic invasion of the pericardium occurs most commonly from cancers of the lungs or breast, or with lymphoma. Tumor extends to the pericardium by direct invasion from neighboring tissues or via hematogenous spread. Primary malignancy of the pericardium, such as mesothelioma, is very rare.

Radiation-induced pericarditis sometimes occurs following therapeutic irradiation of the mediastinum. The frequency of this complication is related to the volume of the pericardium exposed and is especially likely to occur when a dose greater than 4000 rads has been delivered. Pericardial injury may occur soon after radiation therapy or, commonly, often several months later. It is usually necessary to perform cytologic examination of the pericardial fluid to distinguish between radiation-induced and recurrent neoplastic pericarditis.

Several medications can cause pericardial inflammation and pericardial effusion (Box 13.2). In some cases (for example, procainamide, hydralazine, isoniazid, methyldopa, and diphenylhydantoin) pericarditis is due to the induction of a lupus-like syndrome. In other cases (for example, minoxidil and anthracycline antitumor agents) pericardial effusions develop via an unknown mechanism.

Box 13.2 Medication-related pericarditis or pericardial effusion

Drug-induced lupus
    Procainamide
    Hydralazine
    Isoniazid
    Methyldopa
    Diphenylhydantoin
Not associated with drug-induced lupus
    Minoxidil
    Anthracycline antitumor drugs

Pathophysiology

The acute inflammation of pericarditis is accompanied by local vasodilatation, increased vascular permeability with leaking of protein into the pericardial space, and leukocyte exudation, initially by neutrophils and later by mononuclear cells. On gross pathologic examination, the pericardium has a shaggy appearance. In bacterial pericarditis the pericardial effusion is grossly purulent, whereas grossly hemorrhagic fluid is often present with neoplastic or tuberculous disease.

Portions of the visceral and parietal pericardium may become thickened and fused, and this process occasionally leads to dense scar formation with impaired cardiac filling, resulting in constrictive pericarditis.

Clinical features

The most common symptoms of acute pericarditis are chest pain and fever (Box 13.3). The pain may be intense, and is generally localized to the retrosternal area and left precordium. It may radiate to the neck, back, and ridge of the left trapezius muscle. The pain may mimic that of myocardial infarction, but is usually sharp or "stabbing". Unlike AMI, the pain of pericarditis is typically pleuritic (aggravated by inspiration or coughing) and is positional. It may be worse when lying supine, whereas sitting and leaning forward may reduce the discomfort.

Box 13.3 Clinical features of acute pericarditis

Chest pain: pleuritic and positional
Fever
Pericardial friction rub
Electrocardiographic abnormalities: diffuse ST-segment elevation, PR depression

---

Physical examination A pericardial friction rub is the most common physical finding in acute pericarditis. It is a scratchy sound produced by the movement of the inflamed pericardial layers against one another, and is best heard using the diaphragm of the stethoscope while the patient leans forward. In its full form, a pericardial friction rub consists of three components corresponding to the major phases of cardiac movement: ventricular contraction, ventricular relaxation, and atrial contraction. The absence of a friction rub does not exclude the diagnosis of acute pericarditis because it can be transient. Sometimes only one or two of the components of the rub are heard and can be confused with a heart murmur.

The electrocardiogram is abnormal in more than 90% of patients with acute pericarditis, and electrocardiographic features often help to distinguish this syndrome from other forms of cardiac disease. The most common abnormality is diffuse ST-segment elevation (Figure 13.1), which is related to epicardial inflammation. This finding is usually present in most of the electrocardiographic leads with the notable exception of aVR and V_1. Distinguishing the ST-segment elevation of pericarditis from that of AMI is of extreme clinical importance (Table 13.1). In pericarditis the direction of the ST segment is concave upward, whereas in AMI it is usually convex upward. Unlike the diffuse ST-segment elevation that is characteristic of acute pericarditis, in AMI the ST elevation is localized to the region of myocardial injury, with reciprocal ST depression in the opposite leads. The evolution of the ST- and T-wave abnormalities is also different. Within hours of an AMI ST-segment elevation is accompanied by T-wave inversion and Q-wave development; in pericarditis, however, T-wave inversion does not occur until days, or weeks, after the ST segment has returned to

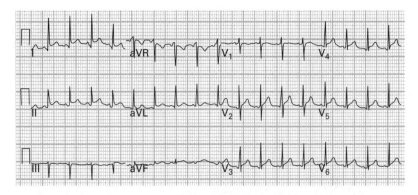

Figure 13.1 Electrocardiogram in acute pericarditis. There is diffuse elevation of the ST segments, with ST-segment depression only in lead aVR. There is depression of the PR segment, best visualized in lead II

Table 13.1 Electrocardiographic features of pericarditis versus acute myocardial infarction

Entity	Shape of ST elevation	ECG leads affected	Timing of ST-T evolution	PR segment
Pericarditis	Concave upward	Diffuse	Days to weeks	Often depressed
Acute myocardial infarction	Convex upward	Localized to infarcting region; reciprocal ST depression in opposite leads	Hours	Normal

its baseline, and Q waves never develop. In 80% of patients with acute pericarditis, depression of the PR segment is evident and is thought to reflect abnormalities of atrial repolarization; PR depression does not occur in AMI.

Chest radiography may be diagnostically useful in acute pericarditis, but only if a larger pericardial effusion is present. If more than 250 ml of fluid has developed, then the cardiac silhouette becomes symmetrically enlarged. Often, pleural effusions are also present due to inflammation of the adjacent pleural surfaces.

Echocardiography is a much more sensitive tool for the detection of pericardial effusion; as little as 15 ml can be identified within the pericardial space by this technique (Figure 13.2). Small pericardial effusions collect posterior to the left ventricle because of the effects of gravity. As effusions become larger, they wrap circumferentially

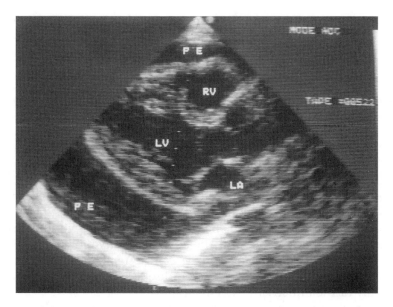

Figure 13.2 Two-dimensional echocardiogram, parasternal long-axis view, demonstrating a pericardial effusion (PE) posterior to the left ventricle (LV). LA, left atrium; RV right ventricle

around the heart. When more than 250 ml has accumulated, the effusion appears anterior to the heart as well.

Treatment

Idiopathic or acute viral pericarditis is usually a self-limited condition that spontaneously improves in 1–3 weeks. Reduced physical activity is recommended in order to alleviate pain by reducing the interaction of the inflamed pericardial layers. Anti-inflammatory drugs are generally effective at reducing pericardial pain. Aspirin is a commonly used analgesic in this situation, although large doses (4–6 g/day) may be required for symptomatic relief. Other non-steroidal anti-inflammatory drugs, such as ibuprofen or indomethacin, are also effective. Corticosteroids are useful for severe or recurrent pericardial pain, but should not be used in uncomplicated cases. Patients treated with steroids have a high relapse rate of pericarditis, making it difficult to taper this therapy without a resurgence of pain. This may lead to a prolonged course of steroid therapy, with its attendant long-term side effects. Recent studies have shown that oral colchicine, an antigout drug, may be useful in reducing the symptoms of pericarditis.

Other forms of pericarditis necessitate other specific treatments. Tuberculous pericarditis requires prolonged multidrug, antituberculous therapy. Purulent pericarditis mandates rapid aggressive therapy, almost always with catheter drainage of the pericardium and intensive antibiotic regimens. Pericarditis in the setting of uremia usually resolves following intensive dialysis. The forms of pericarditis that follow myocardial infarction are treated in a similar manner as acute viral pericarditis, including rest and aspirin. In this setting, non-steroidal anti-inflammatory drugs other than aspirin should generally be avoided; they have been associated with impaired healing of infarcted tissue. During the acute stages of myocardial infarction, anticoagulant therapy is relatively contraindicated if pericarditis is present because it may lead to intrapericardial hemorrhage.

Neoplastic involvement of the pericardium is usually indicative of widely metastatic cancer, and therapy is palliative; drainage of the pericardial fluid causing tamponade can be temporarily life saving. Pericarditis due to connective tissue diseases generally responds to therapy of the underlying systemic illness.

In rare situations pericarditis recurs repetitively and requires institution of steroid therapy or surgical removal of the pericardium.

Complications of pericarditis

There are two serious complications of pericarditis: cardiac tamponade and chronic constrictive pericarditis. Although systolic contractile function is usually normal, diastolic filling of the right and left ventricles is impaired in each of these complications (Figure 13.3). In the case of cardiac tamponade, impaired diastolic filling is due to the accumulation of pericardial fluid that surrounds the cardiac chambers and subjects them to high external pressure. In constrictive pericarditis, a rigid scarred pericardium surrounds the heart and limits ventricular filling. Impaired filling of the ventricle leads to signs of left and right sided heart failure, including pulmonary congestion and jugular venous distension. Reduced filling of the ventricles (for example, lower preload) also decreases their forward stroke volumes so that cardiac output falls, manifested by a decline in systemic blood pressure.

Cardiac tamponade

Cardiac tamponade can result from most causes of pericarditis as well as from acute bleeding into the pericardium caused by chest trauma or perforation of a cardiac chamber during cardiac catheterization or pacemaker placement. Whether a pericardial effusion results in cardiac

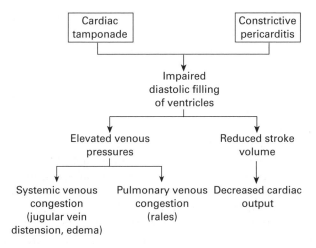

Figure 13.3 Pathophysiology of cardiac tamponade and constrictive pericarditis

tamponade depends on the volume of pericardial fluid and the rate at which it accumulates. Because the pericardium is a stiff, relatively non-distensible structure, the sudden introduction of as little as 50–100 ml of fluid into the pericardial space can dramatically increase intrapericardial pressure and result in tamponade physiology. Such is often the case following penetrating chest trauma, with hemorrhage into the pericardial space. In many cases of acute pericarditis however, the rate of fluid accumulation is relatively slow, so that the pericardium gradually stretches and may accommodate greater amounts of fluid (up to 1–2 l) before pressure rises sufficiently to compromise cardiac chamber filling.

Cardiac tamponade should be suspected in any patient with known pericarditis or chest trauma who develops signs and symptoms of systemic vascular congestion and decreased cardiac output. The main physical findings include sinus tachycardia, jugular venous distension, hypotension, and soft heart sounds (due to the insulating effect of the pericardial effusion between the heart and the chest wall). Dyspnea and tachypnea are frequently present, reflecting pulmonary congestion and decreased oxygen delivery to the peripheral tissues.

An important physical sign in cardiac tamponade is known as pulsus paradoxus. It is an exaggeration of a normal decline in blood pressure following inspiration. It refers to an abnormal decline in systolic blood pressure of more than 10 mmHg during inspiration, which can be measured at the bedside using a standard blood pressure cuff. Pulsus paradoxus is thought to develop in cardiac tamponade because the high pressure pericardial effusion forces the two ventricles to share a common reduced space. Normal inspiratory augmentation of right ventricular filling in tamponade therefore results in the proportional decline in left ventricular filling, followed by falls in stroke volume and systolic blood pressure. Pulsus paradoxus strongly suggests the presence of cardiac tamponade in appropriate clinical situations, but may also occur in other conditions in which respiration is exaggerated, such as severe asthma and chronic obstructive lung disease.

Electrocardiographic features of cardiac tamponade include sinus tachycardia, reduced limb lead voltage (due to the insulating effect of the surrounding pericardial fluid), and sometimes electrical alternans. The latter may be seen when huge pericardial effusions are present and is due to beat to beat alterations in the electrical axis of the heart as it swings within the large volume. The most useful non-invasive test in the diagnosis of cardiac tamponade is echocardiography. The key finding relates directly to the elevated pressure within the pericardial sac that transiently equals, or exceeds, that in the cardiac chambers during diastole. As a result, early diastolic "collapse" of the right ventricle is an echocardiographic hallmark of this condition.

Treatment of cardiac tamponade requires removal of the high pressure pericardial fluid. This is most safely accomplished under fluoroscopy in the cardiac catheterization laboratory. A catheter is introduced into the pericardial space, usually from a subxiphoid approach in order to avoid trauma to the coronary arteries. Another catheter is passed intravenously into the right heart chambers, and simultaneous measurements of intracardiac and pericardial pressures are recorded. In cardiac tamponade, the pericardial pressure is elevated and equal to the diastolic pressures within each of the cardiac chambers; all of the latter are elevated to the same degree because of the compressive force of the surrounding effusion. Recordings of the right atrial pressure are also abnormal (Figure 13.4): there is loss of the normal rapid Y descent because compression of the right ventricle prevents rapid early diastolic filling of that chamber.

Following removal of a sufficient amount of pericardial fluid the pericardial pressure returns to normal (approximately 0 mmHg) and diastolic pressures within the heart chambers separate to their normal values. The obtained pericardial fluid sample may identify the underlying pericardial pathology, and most importantly should be stained and cultured for bacteria, fungi, and acid fast bacilli, as well as undergo cytologic examination for malignancy. Cytologic examination of pericardial fluid is diagnostic of tumor in 85% of malignant effusions.

If cardiac tamponade recurs, then repeat pericardiocentesis can be performed or a draining catheter may be left in the pericardial space for several days. In some cases, a more definitive procedure is necessary to prevent recurrent tamponade, including surgical removal of part, or all, of the pericardium.

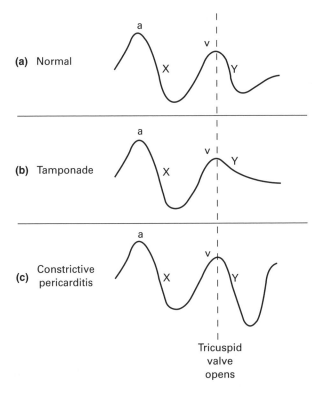

Figure 13.4 Right atrial pressure tracings in cardiac tamponade and constrictive pericarditis. **(a)** Normal right atrial pressure tracing. In early diastole the tricuspid valve opens and the Y descent is inscribed as blood quickly flows from the right atrium to the right ventricle. **(b)** In cardiac tamponade, the high pressure external to the cardiac chambers prevents normal right ventricular filling and the Y descent is blunted. **(c)** In constrictive pericarditis, very early diastolic flow is normal so that the Y descent is present, and because the "a" and "v" waves are higher than normal the Y descent appears unusually prominent. Reproduced with permission from Lilly (1993)

Constrictive pericarditis

Constrictive pericarditis (or "pericardial constriction") is the other serious potential complication of acute pericarditis, and it generally presents in a more chronic and insidious manner than does cardiac tamponade. Although tuberculosis was formerly the major source of pericardial constriction, it is an uncommon cause in the current era (Table 13.2). Most often, constrictive pericarditis follows known or occult "idiopathic" pericarditis. Other risk factors for this complication are previous mediastinal radiation therapy and cardiac operations during which the pericardium had been entered and has

413

Table 13.2 Causes of constrictive pericarditis	
Cause	%
Idiopathic	42
After radiotherapy	31
After cardiac surgery	11
Postinfective	6
Connective tissue disorders	4
Neoplastic	3

Modified from Cameron *et al.* (1987) with permission

presumably become inflamed. In the presence of constrictive pericarditis diastolic filling of the ventricles is reduced because chronic scarring of the pericardium prevents the cardiac chambers from expanding normally. Thus, there is a secondary elevation in pulmonary and systemic venous pressures (see Figure 13.3).

The symptoms and signs of constrictive pericarditis reflect the elevation in pulmonary and systemic venous pressures, with the gradual development of bilateral (especially right sided) congestive heart failure. Therefore, common physical findings in a patient with chronic constrictive pericarditis include jugular venous distension, hepatomegaly, ascites, and peripheral edema. On cardiac examination, an early diastolic "knock" may follow the second heart sound along the left sternal border in patients with severe calcific constriction. It reflects the sudden cessation of ventricular diastolic filling imposed by the rigid pericardial sac.

Unlike cardiac tamponade, constrictive pericarditis does not usually cause pulsus paradoxus. In constrictive pericarditis, negative intrathoracic pressure generated during inspiration is not transmitted through the rigid pericardial shell, and therefore inspiratory augmentation of right ventricular filling does not occur. Instead, in the presence of severe pericardial constriction, when inspiration draws blood toward the thorax it "accumulates" in the systemic veins, causing the jugular veins to become more distended. This inspiratory augmentation of jugular venous distension is known as Kussmaul's sign.

The chest radiograph in constrictive pericarditis shows calcification of the pericardium in up to 50% of patients with this condition, which is usually best visualized on the lateral projection (Figure 13.5). The electrocardiogram often shows non-specific ST and T wave abnormalities. Less commonly, atrial arrhythmias such as atrial fibrillation occur.

Echocardiographic features of constrictive pericarditis are subtle because the pericardium is often not well imaged. The pericardium

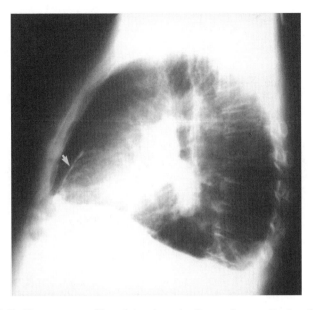

Figure 13.5 Chest *x* ray film, lateral projection, of a patient with chronic constrictive pericarditis. Calcification of the pericardium is present (arrow)

appears thickened, the ventricular cavities are small and contract vigorously, and ventricular filling terminates abruptly in early diastole as the chambers reach the limits imposed on them by the rigid pericardial shell. Cardiac Doppler flow patterns are abnormal in constrictive pericarditis, showing reversed hepatic vein flow in late systole and in mid-diastole. Magnetic resonance imaging or computed tomography are superior to transthoracic echocardiography in the assessment of pericardial thickness.

The diagnosis of constrictive pericarditis may be confirmed by cardiac catheterization. There is elevation, and equalization, of diastolic pressures in each of the cardiac chambers. However, unlike cardiac tamponade, the ventricular pressure tracings show an early diastolic "dip and plateau" configuration (Figure 13.6). This pattern reflects the sudden cessation of filling in early diastole as further expansion of the ventricles is prevented by the surrounding rigid pericardium. Also, unlike cardiac tamponade, there is a prominent Y descent of the right atrial pressure tracing (see Figure 13.4); as the tricuspid valve opens in early diastole, the right atrium quickly empties its contents into the right ventricle during the brief period before filling is abruptly terminated.

Treatment of constrictive pericarditis requires surgical removal of the rigid pericardium. Symptoms and signs of constriction may not

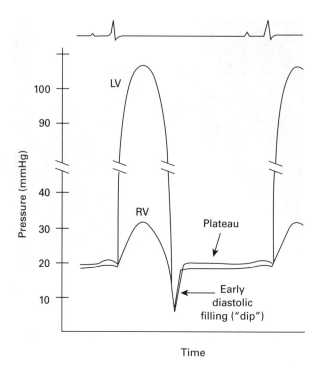

Figure 13.6 Right and left ventricular pressure tracings in constrictive pericarditis. There is elevation and equalization in diastolic pressures. After rapid filling in early diastole, there is sudden cessation of further filling ("dip and plateau"). LV, left ventricular; RV, right ventricular

resolve immediately following surgery because of associated stiffness of the neighboring epicardium, but eventual symptomatic improvement is expected in nearly all patients who survive surgery.

Case studies

Case 13.1

A 44-year-old accountant presents to the emergency department because of severe chest pain that began 12 hours ago and has increased progressively in intensity. The pain is sharp, most pronounced over the left precordium, and radiates toward the neck and left shoulder. It intensifies when he breathes in and is eased somewhat when he leans forward. There is no associated nausea or diaphoresis. He has had no cough, hemoptysis, or chills. He takes no medications.

His past medical history is unremarkable. There is no history of exertional chest pain, or gallbladder or peptic ulcer disease. There is no history of hypertension, diabetes, cigarette smoking, or family history of premature coronary disease. One month before admission he had an upper respiratory infection that did not require antibiotic therapy.

Examination. Physical examination: the patient prefers to lean forward to reduce his chest pain. Temperature: 100·6°F (38·1°C). Weight: 180 lb (81·5 kg). Pulse: 102 beats/min, regular, normal sinus rhythm. Blood pressure: 130/80 mmHg. Respiratory rate: 18/min. Jugular venous pulse: 5 cm. Cardiac impulse: normal. First heart sound: normal. Second heart sound: splits normally on inspiration. At the apex and left sternal edge a two-component friction rub is present, which is loudest when the patient leans forward. Chest examination: normal air entry, no rales or rhonchi. Abdominal examination: soft abdomen, no tenderness. Normal liver span. No other obvious abnormalities. No peripheral edema. Femoral, popliteal, and foot pulses: normal. Carotid pulses: normal, without bruits.

Investigations. Chest *x* ray: cardiac silhouette size at top limits of normal and clear lung fields. Electrocardiogram: sinus tachycardia, diffuse elevation of the ST segments in each of the precordial leads and most of the limb leads. Complete blood count: white blood cell count 10 300/mm^3 with normal differential, hematocrit 42%. Chemistries: normal electrolytes, blood urea nitrogen, creatinine, and liver functions. Creatine kinase: 110 (110 U/l [normal 10–70] or 1·8 µkat/l [Normal = 0·42–1·5]), no MB fraction detected. Echocardiogram: normal left and right ventricular size and contractile function. Normal size atria, no valvular disease, moderate size posterior pericardial effusion (approximately 100 ml) without evidence of cardiac chamber compression.

Hospital course. The patient was admitted for observation and control of chest pain with oral ibuprofen and intravenous morphine. He slept comfortably, but on the second hospital day appears dyspneic and tachypneic (respiratory rate 26/min). The heart rate is 130 beats/min and regular. The blood pressure is 102/60 mmHg with 14 mm pulsus paradoxus (decline in systemic systolic pressure during inspiration). The heart sounds and pericardial friction rub are softer as compared with the examination the previous day. Emergent echocardiography shows a marked increase in the volume of pericardial effusion, now encircling the heart (<250 ml), with early diastolic collapse of the right ventricular cavity. In the cardiac catheterization laboratory, the following pressures are recorded (mmHg): pericardium 18, right atrium (18), right ventricle 34/18, pulmonary artery 34/16, pulmonary capillary wedge (18), aorta (during expiration) 98/64. (The figures in brackets indicate mean pressures). Emergency pericardiocentesis is performed, with removal of 22 cm^3 of straw colored pericardial effusion. There is a rapid rise in systemic blood pressure to 132/80 mmHg, the pericardial pressure falls to 0 mmHg, and the right atrial mean pressure falls to 5 mmHg. Subsequent Gram's stain, acid fast bacilli smear, cultures, and cytology of the pericardial fluid are negative.

Questions

1. What is the differential diagnosis of the patient's presenting chest pain?
2. What features of the electrocardiogram can help distinguish pericarditis from acute myocardial infarction (AMI) and from the early repolarization variant seen in some healthy young individuals?
3. What is the differential diagnosis of the etiology of pericarditis in this case?
4. What do the hemodynamic data obtained in the cardiac catheterization laboratory indicate? What features of this case differentiate cardiac tamponade from constrictive pericarditis and restrictive cardiomyopathy?

Answers

Answer to question 1 The pain is sharp, pleuritic, and positional, which is typical of acute pericarditis. The discomfort of AMI is usually described as a "pressure" and is neither positional nor pleuritic, although the pattern of radiation may be similar to that of pericardial disease; often there is a history of exertional angina. The pain of aortic dissection is an intense tearing or "ripping" pain that often migrates along the path of the dissection lesion. Pulmonary causes of chest pain include acute pneumonia, pneumothorax, and pulmonary embolism. Pneumonia is associated with fever, cough, and sputum production, with evidence of consolidation by auscultation and percussion. Pneumothorax causes sudden sharp pleuritic unilateral chest pain with decreased breath sounds and hyperresonance of the affected side. The pain of pulmonary embolism is pleuritic but not usually positional; a pleural friction rub may correspond to the respiratory cycle (as opposed to the pericardial friction rub, which relates to the cardiac cycle).

Gastrointestinal causes of severe pain include esophageal spasm and acute cholecystitis. The former is accompanied by difficult swallowing during pain, and the latter is usually associated with right upper quadrant tenderness, nausea, vomiting, and a history of fatty food intolerance.

Answer to question 2 The electrocardiogram of acute pericarditis demonstrates diffuse ST-segment elevation in most of the electrocardiographic leads. The ST-segment elevation usually appears in a concave upward direction and PR-segment depression is often present. In contrast, the electrocardiogram of AMI shows localized ST-segment elevation in the leads overlying the affected segment with reciprocal ST-segment depression in the opposite leads. In AMI, the ST-segment elevation more often appears in a convex upward configuration, and PR-segment depression does not occur.

The electrocardiogram in individuals with "normal" early repolarization can appear quite similar to that of acute pericarditis. However, in acute pericarditis the height of ST elevation is usually greater than 25% of the height of the T wave, whereas in early repolarization it is less than 25% and PR-segment depression does not occur.

Answer to question 3 In this otherwise healthy man who had sustained an upper respiratory tract infection 3 weeks before presentation, the probable etiology is viral pericarditis. There was no clinical or laboratory evidence of chronic renal failure, AMI, or connective tissue disease. He was not taking any drugs that result in pericarditis. There was no history of mediastinal radiation therapy or known neoplastic disease.

Analysis of the pericardial fluid did not show evidence of malignancy. Gram's stain and acid fast stain of the pericardial fluid were negative. However, the sensitivity of diagnosis of tuberculosis by this technique is low. When tuberculous pericarditis is strongly suspected a PPD (the intracutaneous tuberculin skin test when the antigen is tuberculin purified protein derivative) should be placed and consideration given to pericardial biopsy, which improves the sensitivity of diagnosis. Recent small studies have shown that a high concentration of adenosine deaminase in the pericardial fluid should suggest the diagnosis of tuberculous pericarditis in the appropriate clinical setting.

Answer to question 4 The hemodynamic data show an elevation in pericardial pressure as well as elevation, and equalization, of the diastolic pressures within each of the cardiac chambers. This is consistent with cardiac tamponade due to the pressure exerted on the cardiac chambers by surrounding pericardial fluid. In constrictive pericarditis the pericardial pressure would not be obtainable (the pericardial space is obliterated by scar formation and often calcification) but the diastolic chamber pressures would be elevated and equal because of the hemodynamic effect of the constricting pericardial shell. In addition, in pericardial constriction the configuration of diastolic right and left ventricular filling would show a "dip and plateau" pattern caused by abrupt early cessation of diastolic filling.

The hemodynamics of restrictive cardiomyopathy are often quite similar to those of constrictive pericarditis. However, in the former condition systolic left ventricular dysfunction is often present as well, with pulmonary hypertension and elevation in right ventricular systolic, as well as diastolic pressure. To differentiate between these entities additional studies are often needed, including computed tomography or magnetic resonance imaging (the pericardium is thickened in constrictive pericarditis but not in restrictive cardiomyopathy) or myocardial biopsy (abnormal in restrictive cardiomyopathy but normal in constrictive pericarditis).

Diseases of the aorta

Normal aortic anatomy

The aorta is the largest of the arterial conductance vessels and serves a variety of functions beyond the simple transmission of blood to the peripheral circulation. It also assists in the pumping of blood by the heart, as well as in the modulation of blood pressure by feedback control of the systemic vascular resistance. The specialized anatomy of the aorta facilitates these multiple functions. The normal aortic wall consists of three layers (the intima, media, and adventitia) and a neurogenic plexus. The intima is comprised of a single layer of endothelial cells. The intima is surrounded by the media, a thick layer of spirally arranged intertwining sheets of tough, resilient elastic tissue, with a small amount of smooth muscle and collagen between the elastic layers. The large amount of elastic tissue gives the aorta tremendous tensile strength and elasticity, so that in systole the rapid ejection of blood from the left ventricle creates a pressure wave that produces radial expansion of the aorta and energy transfer to the aortic wall. During diastole the aorta recoils, converting the potential energy imparted during systole to kinetic energy and thereby propels blood into the peripheral vessels. The outermost layer of the aorta is the adventitia, which is chiefly made up of collagen and houses the vasa vasorum and lymphatics. The vasa vasorum is a network of small blood vessels encompassing the aorta that supplies a capillary network to the adventitia and media of the thoracic aorta. Finally, pressure responsive afferent receptors lie within the wall of the ascending aorta and the aortic arch, and are responsible for sending impulses via the vagus nerve to modulate heart rate and systemic resistance.

Pathogenesis of aortic diseases

The diseases that affect the aorta do so by degenerative processes that weaken the arterial wall. These disorders may be either acquired or congenital. Regardless of the cause, once dilatation at the site of weakness is initiated wall tension increases according to the Laplace relationship (i.e. wall stress = [pressure × radius]/wall thickness) and further expansion occurs, which can lead to intramural or extramural rupture of the aorta. The most common contributors are atherosclerosis, hypertension, and loss of distensibility with advanced age. Less common factors that contribute to aortic disease include congenital defects such as bicuspid aortic valve and aortic coarctation, autoimmune mediated diseases, syphilis, and trauma (Box 13.4). In Marfan's syndrome there is degeneration of the aortic media due to loss of the normal elastic and fibromuscular elements, which is caused by an inherited defect in the collagen binding protein fibrillin.

Box 13.4 Examples of predisposing factors in aortic disease

Atherosclerosis
Hypertension
Advanced age
Cystic medial necrosis (idiopathic, Marfan's syndrome), Ehlers–Danlos syndrome, infectious aortitis (syphilis, mycotic aneurysms), vasculitis, trauma

---

Aortic aneurysms

Aortic aneurysms are abnormal localized dilatations of the vessel, in distinction to "ectasia", which is diffuse enlargement of the aorta that may occur with aging. It is also important to distinguish true aneurysms from pseudoaneurysms. A pseudoaneurysm is a contained aortic rupture in which the wall of the pseudoaneurysm is comprised of a mass of connective tissue surrounding extravasated blood. The dilated wall of a true aneurysm contains all of the layers of the aorta, namely the intima, media, and adventitia.

True aneurysms develop morphologically as either fusiform or saccular. A fusiform aneurysm is cylindrical and affects the entire circumference of the aorta. In contrast, the less common saccular aneurysm is an outpouching of only a portion of the circumference.

The saccular outpouchings are frequently connected to the body of the aorta by a small neck, which as a result of its limited communication to the aorta may protect the thin wall of the aneurysm from rupture by reducing the force of intra-aortic pressure. In contrast, the entire circumference of the fusiform aneurysm is exposed to the pulsatile distending force during cardiac systole.

The most common factor leading to aortic aneurysm formation is atherosclerosis. Other etiologies and contributors include hypertension, connective tissue and inflammatory conditions (for example syphilitic aortitis), trauma, and cystic medial degeneration (see Box 13.4). The lesions of atherosclerosis initially affect the intima; however, as the disease progresses and extracellular lipid accumulates, the supporting medial layer thins and dilates. Atherosclerotic aneurysms can develop at any location along the aorta, but more than 75% appear in the abdominal aorta and that condition is discussed in detail below. The thoracic aorta is less commonly affected by atherosclerosis, and within that segment the descending aorta is involved more often than the ascending portion. When the aortic arch and descending portions of the thoracic aorta contain atherosclerotic aneurysms, there is often extensive involvement of the abdominal aorta as well.

Aneurysms of the ascending aorta are less commonly atherosclerotic in origin and more often are due to cystic degeneration of the medial layer as a result of hypertension, aging, or connective tissue disorders such as Marfan's syndrome.

Although thoracic aortic aneurysms are often asymptomatic, they may produce a localized deep aching sensation that is not related to physical activity. In addition, their presence may be signaled by compression of neighboring structures. Pressure against the esophagus and trachea result in dysphagia and respiratory complaints (cough, hemoptysis, dyspnea), respectively. Tension on the recurrent laryngeal nerve causes hoarseness. Aneurysms of the ascending aorta may result in dilatation of the aortic valve annulus with valvular regurgitation.

Thoracic aneurysms may rupture without warning into the mediastinum, bronchi, or pleural space. Alternatively, an aneurysm may leak slowly into the vessel wall, resulting in localized pain as a harbinger of rupture.

Abdominal aortic aneurysms

Clinical features

Abdominal aneurysms are typically atherosclerotic and arise most frequently distal to the renal arteries. They are usually asymptomatic and discovered incidentally on routine physical examination or by abdominal radiography or ultrasound examinations. Unfortunately, the physical examination is neither sensitive nor specific for the detection of an abdominal aneurysm, and when detected its size tends to be overestimated by palpation. When symptoms are present, they include a sense of abdominal fullness or pain located in the hypogastrium or the lower back. The pain is usually steady with a gnawing quality, and may last for hours or days at a time. Expansion or impending rupture may be heralded by the sudden development of pain that is constant and severe, sometimes with radiation to the groin. Acute rupture of an abdominal aortic aneurysm is typically accompanied by hemorrhagic shock, manifested by hypotension, vasoconstriction, mental obtundation, and oliguria. Rupture into the abdominal cavity may cause sudden abdominal distension, whereas rupture into a gastrointestinal viscus (for example, the duodenum) presents as massive gastrointestinal hemorrhage. Another potential complication is peripheral embolization of mural thrombus that forms within the aneurysm.

Diagnosis

As indicated above, physical examination is not reliable in the diagnosis and sizing of abdominal aortic aneurysms. An epigastric bruit may be heard but is non-specific. A lateral abdominal radiograph is inexpensive and reliably detects the outline of the aneurysm if the wall is calcified (Figure 13.7). However, visible calcification is not the case in a quarter of patients with abdominal aortic aneurysms. In contrast, cross-sectional ultrasonography is very sensitive, yields an accurate size measurement, and is easily performed. Ultrasonography is therefore the procedure of choice for screening for this condition.

Computed tomography and magnetic resonance imaging can provide even greater detail than ultrasonography, and provide better intraluminal characterization of the aneurysm and its relationship to surrounding structures, such as the renal arteries and the spine. Abdominal aortic angiography is not always accurate in sizing an abdominal aneurysm because the full width may be masked by the presence of non-opacified mural thrombus.

Natural history

There is a crucial relationship between the size of an aortic aneurysm and risk for spontaneous rupture. Fifty percent of abdominal aortic aneurysms that are more than 6 cm in diameter rupture within 1 year, as compared with 15–20% of aneurysms that have a smaller diameter. The average aneurysm expansion rate is 0·4–0·5 cm/year. Larger aneurysms expand slightly more rapidly. At

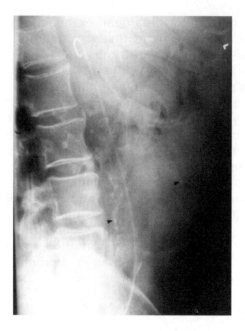

Figure 13.7 Lateral abdominal x ray film demonstrating the calcified wall of an abdominal aortic aneurysm (arrows). Courtesy of Dr Mark Creager

least 30% of deaths in patients with aortic aneurysms are attributed to acute aortic rupture, whereas nearly half are due to associated cardiovascular disease, especially coronary atherosclerosis.

Surgical management

Because of the increased risk for spontaneous rupture and death, elective surgery is advised for all abdominal aortic aneurysms that are 6 cm or more in diameter. Mortality for emergency aneurysmectomy for a ruptured abdominal aneurysm is 35–60%, even at experienced centers, with the limiting factor being the timeliness of the diagnosis and the speed of surgical repair. In contrast, elective resection of abdominal aortic aneurysms has an operative mortality of only 2–5%. In patients with aneurysms of 4–6 cm in diameter, close clinical and radiologic follow up is advised, with surgery indicated if there is evidence of rapid expansion such as acute onset of associated pain.

Surgical correction consists of resection of the aneurysm and insertion of a synthetic graft. Clinical studies are in progress to evaluate the use of intravascular stenting to obviate the need for surgical repair in high risk patients.

Aortic dissection

Dissection of the aorta is a life-threatening disorder in which a blood-filled channel separates the layers of the aortic media, dividing the intima from the adventitia. This process may involve the entire length of the aorta or isolated portions of it.

Pathophysiology

A prerequisite for aortic dissection is degeneration of collagen and elastic tissue often with cystic changes, most frequently due to cystic medial necrosis or chronic hypertension. Cystic medial degeneration is also seen in hereditary defects of connective tissue, including Marfan's syndrome and Ehlers–Danlos syndrome. Other conditions that predispose to dissection include coarctation of the aorta, bicuspid aortic valve, and Noonan's and Turner's syndromes. There is also an increased frequency of aortic dissection during pregnancy, usually occurring in the last trimester.

It is not known whether the causal event in aortic dissection is a tear within the intima with secondary dissection into the medial layers, or alternatively primary hemorrhage within a diseased media followed by disruption of the subjacent intima and subsequent propagation of the dissection as high pressure flow is forced through the intimal tear (Figure 13.8). Longitudinally, the dissection may extend for only several centimeters or may involve the entire course of the aorta. The process of dissection is exacerbated by hemodynamic forces generated by the pulse wave of each cardiac cycle (dP/dt) and the level of blood pressure.

Untreated dissections lead to rupture through the adventitia anywhere along the aorta, including into the pericardium or left pleural space. Extension into the aortic root can disrupt the aortic valve annulus and produce aortic regurgitation. Propagation of the dissection may occlude aortic branch vessels resulting in stroke (carotid occlusion), myocardial infarction (coronary occlusion), asymmetric arm pulses (subclavian artery occlusion), or compromise of the renal or splanchnic beds.

Classification

More than 95% of aortic dissections arise in one of two locations. The first is in the ascending aorta within several centimeters of the aortic valve; this is the most common site but it is underreported because dissection there is often quickly lethal. The second location is in the descending aorta, just distal to the origin of the left subclavian artery at the site of the ligamentum arteriosum. There are two

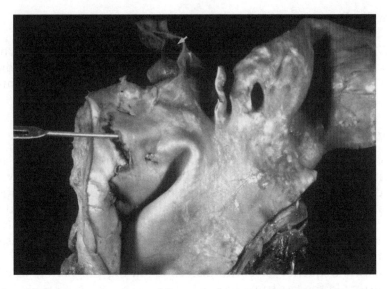

Figure 13.8 Autopsy specimen of the aorta from a patient who had sustained a proximal (type A) dissection. A metal probe is inserted into the origin of the dissection in the proximal aorta. There is extension of the dissecting hematoma into the brachiocephalic artery (arrow). Courtesy of Dr Gail Winters

classifications schemes used to describe the location and extent of aortic dissections: The DeBakey classification and the Stanford (or Daily) classification.

The DeBakey classification divides aortic dissections into three types.

- Type 1: the intimal tear originates in the ascending aorta and extends beyond the ascending aorta and the aortic arch into the distal aorta.
- Type 2: dissection is confined to the ascending aorta.
- Type 3: dissection originates in the descending aorta and propagates distally: type 3a, limited to the thoracic aorta; type 3b, extension of the dissection below the diaphragm.

The Stanford classification system is more commonly used and simply divides dissections according to whether the ascending aorta is involved (Figure 13.9).

- Type A: all ascending aortic dissections and those descending aortic dissections that extend retrograde to involve the arch and ascending aorta (corresponds to DeBakey types 1 and 2).
- Type B: descending aortic dissections without proximal extension (corresponds to DeBakey type 3).

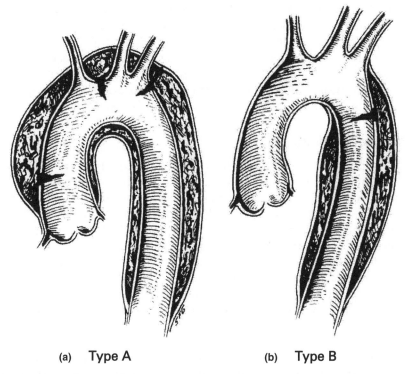

(a) **Type A**　　　　　　　　　(b) **Type B**

Figure 13.9 Stanford system for classification of aortic dissections. **(a)** Type A (proximal) aortic dissection with an intimal tear in the ascending aorta. The dissection involves the aortic arch and extends distally. **(b)** Type B (distal) aortic dissection. The intimal flap is located in the descending aorta (below the level of the ligamentum arteriosum) and does not extend proximally. Reproduced with permission from Izzo *et al.* (1993)

The distinction of whether dissection involves the proximal aorta in these classification systems is critically important because involvement at that site often portends a worse outcome and need for surgical repair. Approximately two-thirds of aortic dissections are of Stanford type A and one-third are of type B.

Clinical features

Men are twice as likely as women to develop an aortic dissection, and the peak incidence is in the sixth and seventh decades of life. The most common presenting symptom is severe pain, which is most intense at its onset and may cause the patient to writhe in agony. It is described as of tearing, ripping, or stabbing quality. Pain in the anterior chest is more common in proximal dissections, whereas pain in the interscapular region is more typical of distal aortic involvement.

Of patients with dissection of the descending aorta, 90% report back pain. Pain in the neck, throat, jaw, or teeth often accompanies dissections that involve the aortic arch. Often, the pain of aortic dissection migrates as a reflection of propagation of the dissection along the length of the aorta. Less common modes of presentation include congestive heart failure, acute cerebral vascular accident, syncope, or paraplegia (see below). Most patients have a history of hypertension.

Physical findings

Most patients with aortic dissection are hypertensive on presentation. If shock is present, aortic rupture or accompanying cardiac tamponade (due to retrograde dissection into the pericardial sac) may be the cause. If the dissection occludes the origin of a subclavian artery, then a difference in systolic blood pressure is recorded between the two arms (15% of patients).

Aortic valve regurgitation occurs in one-third of acute aortic dissections. On cardiac auscultation a diastolic murmur with a musical quality is heard best along the right sternal border. There are three mechanisms by which acute aortic insufficiency develops in this situation.

- The dissection may cause dilatation of the aortic root, widening the valve annulus so that aortic leaflets are unable to coapt properly during diastole.
- In an asymmetric dissection, pressure from the dissecting hematoma may depress one leaflet below the line of closure of the others.
- Annular support of the leaflets or the leaflets themselves may become torn by the dissection so as to render the valve incompetent.

Neurologic manifestations are common in aortic dissection and may present as acute cerebrovascular accidents (due to occlusion of flow into a carotid artery), ischemic peripheral neuropathy, or ischemic paraparesis. Horner's syndrome may occur due to compression of the superior cervical sympathetic ganglion, or vocal cord paralysis and hoarseness due to pressure against the left recurrent laryngeal nerve.

Differential diagnosis

When aortic dissection presents with chest pain and hemodynamic compromise it is not uncommon to wrongly suspect myocardial ischemia as the cause. The danger of this misdiagnosis is that the therapeutic management of myocardial ischemia often involves anticoagulation and treatment with thrombolytic agents to dissolve

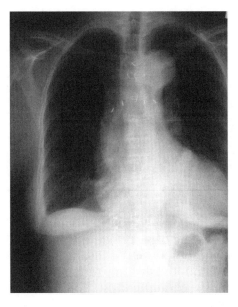

Figure 13.10 Chest *x* ray film from a patient with an acute type A aortic dissection. The superior mediastinum is enlarged

intracoronary blood clots. This strategy can rapidly be fatal if the correct diagnosis is aortic dissection. Other diagnoses that mimic the presentation of aortic dissection include thoracic non-dissecting aneurysms, esophageal spasm, musculoskeletal pains, pericarditis, and acute aortic insufficiency without dissection.

Investigations

Anemia is a common finding in patients with aortic dissection, as is leukocytosis. Thrombocytopenia can also occur due to low grade intravascular coagulation, with a rise in the prothrombin time accompanied by a fall in circulating fibrinogen levels. The bilirubin level may also rise due to hemolysis of blood trapped in the false lumen. The electrocardiogram often shows signs of left ventricular hypertrophy secondary to a history of hypertension and, usually, the absence of acute ischemic changes. If ischemic changes are seen, then they may implicate retrograde dissection into a coronary artery.

A suggestive chest radiographic finding is the presence of an abnormally wide superior mediastinum, representing aortic enlargement (Figure 13.10). However, the lack of mediastinal enlargement does not exclude the diagnosis. A much less common finding on the plain radiograph is the "calcium sign". This sign is

Table 13.3 Comparison of diagnostic studies in aortic dissection

Diagnostic study	Sensitivity (%)	Specificity (%)	Accuracy (%)	Positive predictive value (%)	Negative predictive value (%)
Transthoracic echocardiography	59	83	70	81	62
Transesophageal echocardiography	98	77	90	88	95
Computed tomography	94	87	91	92	90
Magnetic resonance imaging	98	98	98	98	98

pathognomonic of aortic dissection and is identified as a separation of the intimal calcification from the adventitial border of greater than 1 cm. Many other non-invasive imaging modalities are available to aid in the diagnosis of aortic dissection, each providing certain advantages and limitations.

Echocardiography is often helpful in the diagnosis of this condition. Transthoracic two-dimensional echocardiograms may show a widened aortic root accompanied by an intimal "flap". Echocardiography is also a sensitive means to detect accompanying pericardial effusion and/or evidence of aortic insufficiency. Unfortunately, the sensitivity of transthoracic echocardiography for detecting proximal aortic dissections is under 60% (Table 13.3), and it is only rarely of benefit in determining the length of aortic involvement by the dissection.

Conversely, transesophageal echocardiography has become the echocardiographic standard in diagnosis of aortic dissection. It permits high resolution visualization of the aortic root and descending aorta; only a localized region of the ascending aorta and arch evades visualization by this technique. The sensitivity of transesophageal echocardiography for the diagnosis of aortic dissection is nearly 98% (see Table 13.3). It can be performed quickly at the bedside, and does not utilize ionizing radiation. Its drawback is that it is a semi-invasive procedure and can be uncomfortable.

Computed tomography with intravenous contrast is also sensitive for the diagnosis of proximal and distal aortic dissections (Figure 13.11). The disadvantage is the need for intravenous contrast and ionizing radiation. Magnetic resonance imaging can accurately identify the presence and extent of aortic dissections (see Table 13.3). The chief disadvantages are the long imaging times required to obtain the study and the inability to monitor closely the critically ill patient while within the protected magnet area.

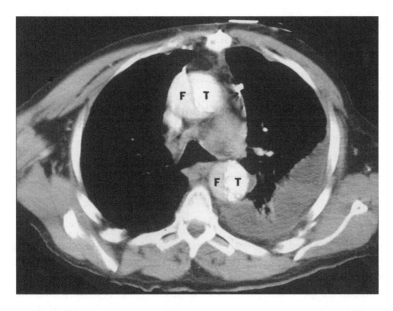

Figure 13.11 Computed tomography of the chest in a patient with aortic dissection. The dissection is visible as a flap separating the true lumen (T), which is enhanced with intravenous contrast from the false lumen (F)

The role of catheterization and angiography has lessened with the advent of the above non-invasive imaging techniques. Despite its invasive nature, cost, and exposure to intravenous contrast agents, angiography is sometimes required to define the full extent of the dissection, to outline the relationship of the dissection to the major aortic branches, and to localize precisely the site of the intimal tear.

Given the wealth of imaging modalities available, local expertise should dictate which of these is performed.

Management

Initial medical management of aortic dissection includes elimination of pain with analgesics; reduction in systolic blood pressure to 100–120 mmHg (mean blood pressure 60–75 mmHg); and reduction in the force of left ventricular contraction (dP/dt). Frequently used agents in this regard include intravenous β-blockers (for example metoprolol or esmolol) and sodium nitroprusside. Overall in-hospital mortality is 27%.

In type A dissection, mortality is 58% in patients not receiving surgery (usually because of advanced age and comorbidity) and 26%

Table 13.4 Surgical versus medical therapy in aortic dissection

Indication	Details
Surgical therapy	Acute dissection of the ascending aorta
	Acute distal dissection complicated by: vital organ compromise, rupture or impending rupture, retrograde extension into the ascending aorta, dissection in Marfan's syndrome
Medical therapy	Uncomplicated distal aortic dissection
	Stable chronic dissection (uncomplicated by aortic valve insufficiency)

in those managed surgically. Thus, early and aggressive surgical intervention is necessary to improve survival (Table 13.4). Surgical correction involves excision of the intimal tear, obliteration of the false channel by oversewing the aortic edges, restoration of aortic valve competence, and sometimes replacement of a portion of the aorta with a synthetic graft.

It has been shown clearly that surgical results are superior to those with medical therapy in acute proximal aortic dissection. Conversely, surgery does not improve outcome as compared with medical therapy in uncomplicated cases of acute distal aortic dissection. Medically treated patients with type B dissection have a mortality of 11% and in those patients treated surgically the mortality is 31%. Once a patient with a distal aortic dissection is stabilized on intravenous β-blocker/antihypertensive therapy, oral agents can be substituted and the patient followed for changes in clinical symptoms.

Case studies

Case 13.2

A 69-year-old man presented to the emergency department with 1 hour of severe upper back pain. The pain was intrascapular and had a "ripping" quality that radiated to his neck and anterior chest. The intensity of pain was not affected by his position (standing or lying down) or by inspiration. The discomfort was accompanied by sweating and light-headedness, but he denied shortness of breath, nausea, or vomiting.

He had a history of hypertension for 20 years that had been treated with diuretics and β-blockers. He had a 45 pack-year smoking history.

There was also a long history of coronary artery disease. He had sustained an inferior wall myocardial infarction 9 years ago and has continued to experience chronic stable angina with good exercise tolerance.

Examination. Physical Examination: the patient was pale and writhing with pain. Temperature: 97·9°F (36·6°C). Weight: 167 lb (75·7 kg). Pulse: 110 beats/min, regular, normal sinus rhythm. Blood pressure: 180/90 mmHg in the left arm and 140/80 mmHg in the right arm, confirmed by repeated measurements. Respiratory rate: 20/min. Jugular venous pulse: 8 cm. Cardiac impulse: normal. First heart sound: normal. Second heart sound: splits normally on inspiration. Loud fourth heart sound at the apex. Grade 2/4 early diastolic murmur at the right upper sternal border. Chest examination: normal air entry, no rales or rhonchi. Abdominal examination: soft abdomen, no tenderness. Normal liver span. No other obvious abnormalities. A bruit was present at the umbilicus, which radiated toward the femoral arteries. No peripheral edema. Femoral, popliteal, and foot pulses were equally diminished. Carotid pulses: decreased, with a bruit over the right carotid. Neurologic examination: normal.

Investigations. Chest x ray: markedly widened superior mediastinum and mild cardiomegaly. There was blunting of the left costophrenic angle without evidence of pulmonary edema. Electrocardiogram: sinus tachycardia at 112 beats/min with left ventricular hypertrophy and secondary repolarization abnormalities in the lateral leads. There was evidence of an old inferior myocardial infarction with Q waves in leads II, III, and aVF. Compared with an electrocardiogram obtained 1 year earlier, there was no change except that the heart rate was faster. Hematologic studies: notable for a hematocrit of 35·5%, a white blood cell count of 16 300/mm³, and a platelet count of 167 000/mm³. Coagulation studies: normal. Blood chemistries: normal electrolytes, blood urea nitrogen, creatinine, and liver function tests. Creatine kinase: within normal limits. Magnetic resonance imaging: Figure 13.12. Subsequent aortic angiography: Figure 13.13.

Questions

1. What is the differential diagnosis of this patient's back and chest pain?
2. What do the imaging studies demonstrate?
3. What other diagnostic procedures could be performed to achieve a rapid diagnosis? Which is the best test to perform?
4. How should the patient be managed initially?
5. What is the role of medical versus surgical treatment in this case?

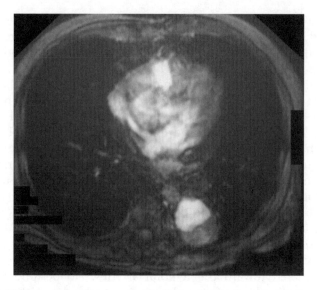

Figure 13.12 Magnetic resonance image from patient presented in Case 13.2

Answers

Answer to question 1 This hypertensive man presents with the acute onset of back pain described as having a "tearing" quality with radiation anteriorly, accompanied by diaphoresis and light-headedness. His physical examination is notable for hypertension but with unequal pulses in his arms and a number of vascular bruits on examination with diminished peripheral pulses. The superior mediastinum is widened on the chest *x* ray film.

The most common diagnosis to consider in patients with a history of coronary artery disease and acute chest pain is myocardial ischemia or infarction. The lack of acute changes on the electrocardiogram during pain rule against these diagnoses. Other clues, however, point squarely to the diagnosis of aortic dissection: the quality and location of the pain, the presence of unequal pulses in the upper extremities (especially with concomitant hypertension), and the widened mediastinum on chest *x* ray. The presence of carotid bruits (which may indicate underlying atherosclerotic disease or extension of the dissection into the carotid arteries), abdominal bruits, and decreased peripheral pulses can be observed in aortic dissection, but are not specific findings in a patient with known atherosclerosis. The described diastolic murmur represents aortic insufficiency, which may be due to retrograde dissection into the aortic root and distortion of the aortic valve annulus, or due to primary aortic valvular disease.

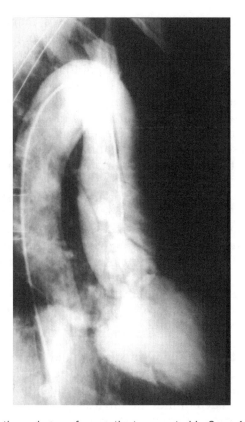

Figure 13.13 Aortic angiogram from patient presented in Case 13.2

Other causes of chest pain and/or mediastinal widening need to be considered within the differential diagnosis. A thoracic atherosclerotic (non-dissecting) aneurysm may cause chest or back pain and increased aortic size within the mediastinum, but the pain is usually more chronic and "gnawing" in quality. Pericarditis (see above) results in pleuritic, positional "sharp" chest pain, and is usually accompanied by a pericardial friction rub and diffuse ST-segment elevation. Mediastinal enlargement in pericarditis is usually confined to the cardiac silhouette, when a large effusion is present. Recall that pericardial involvement can complicate aortic dissection if the latter progresses retrograde into the pericardial sac; hemopericardium with cardiac tamponade generally follow with a high mortality rate.

Esophageal disorders that can result in severe chest discomfort (esophageal spasm or rupture) are accompanied by dysphagia, nausea and/or emesis, but not the hemodynamic or chest x ray findings observed in this case.

Answer to question 2 Figure 13.12 shows a magnetic resonance angiogram of the thoracic cavity. In this angiogram, rapid blood flow is recorded as lighter shading while slower flow is indicated in darker tones. The heart is anterior in this photo (blurred due to motion artifact), and the descending aorta is located posteriorly. Within the aorta a partition is visualized, which is the intimal "flap" of the dissection. On one side of the flap normal blood flow is present and is the lighter of the two zones. This represents the "true lumen" of the aorta. The "false lumen" is the channel created by the dissection process within the media of the aorta and is the darker of the two zones.

This patient subsequently underwent contrast aortography (Figure 13.13). The thoracic angiogram shows the catheter in the "true" aortic lumen. In this study the entire length of the dissection is visualized from its origin just above the aortic valve to its distal aspect within the descending aorta. Also note the opacification of the left ventricle, which indicates aortic regurgitation through an incompetent aortic valve. These studies show this to be a proximal (type A) dissection with involvement of the ascending aorta as well as the arch and descending aorta.

Answer to question 3 The ideal study would be one that is readily available, quickly performed, sensitive for the diagnosis of dissection anywhere along the aorta, able to identify the site of intimal disruption (which determines the surgical approach), and can identify concomitant aortic regurgitation or pericardial effusion. Historically the "gold standard" for the diagnosis of aortic dissection has therefore been invasive catheterization and angiography. However, the newer non-invasive modalities are highly sensitive and often eliminate the need for angiography. These include magnetic resonance imaging, transesophageal echocardiography, and computed tomography.

Although the positive and negative predictive values favor magnetic resonance imaging over the other non-invasive imaging studies (see Table 13.3), the use of magnetic resonance imaging in this setting may be limited by the long image acquisition time. In addition, for critically ill patients magnetic resonance imaging is not practical because it is impossible to attach intravenous infusion pumps with metallic components or mechanical ventilators to the patient within the magnetic imaging field. The advantage of transesophageal echocardiography is that it is usually readily available; it is portable, accurate, and quick to perform and interpret; and it is less costly than magnetic resonance imaging. It can be used to detect aortic regurgitation and to assess ventricular function. Computed tomography is also sensitive and accurate, but suffers the disadvantages of its lack of portability and the inability to assess aortic regurgitation. Thus there are clear trade-offs with any of these non-invasive techniques; therefore, at each medical center the best diagnostic test for aortic dissection is the one that can be performed most rapidly and with the greatest local expertise.

Answer to question 4 Once the diagnosis of a proximal aortic dissection is confirmed, the immediate management strategy is to call for surgical consultation followed by emergent repair. Medical management (antihypertensive and vasodilator therapy, as described below) should not delay surgical intervention. Ideally, surgical evaluation should proceed in parallel with the diagnostic strategy if the initial differential diagnosis includes aortic dissection.

For patients with a distal (type B) aortic dissection, the goal is to lower intra-aortic pressure and the force of ventricular contraction (dP/dt) in order to prevent further extension of the dissection. This is initially accomplished by the administration of intravenous β-blockers (typically metoprolol or the short-acting agent esmolol), as well as antihypertensive/vasodilator therapy using agents such as intravenous nitroprusside. Once stabilized, oral β-blockers and other antihypertensive agents can be substituted.

Answer to question 5 Proximal (type A) aortic dissections should be repaired surgically to improve survival, whereas distal (type B) aortic dissections are treated medically with control of blood pressure as outlined above. However, there are exceptions to this rule. Type B aortic dissections complicated by compromise of blood flow to vital organs, impending aortic rupture, or retrograde extension into the ascending aorta should prompt surgical repair. In addition, aortic dissections in all patients with Marfan's syndrome should be surgically repaired because of the high incidence of redissection if treated only with medications.

The patient in this case underwent successful surgical repair of the ascending aorta and replacement of the aortic valve, followed by aggressive long-term antihypertensive therapy.

Heart tumors

Tumors of the heart are uncommon but can cause significant morbidity, often in young individuals. Tumors may be primary, but are more often metastatic from extracardiac sites. Cardiac neoplasms may be asymptomatic. Alternatively, they may result in a constellation of findings due to their ability to act as space occupying lesions and interfere with normal intracardiac blood flow, cause pulmonary or systemic embolism, invade and destroy myocardial

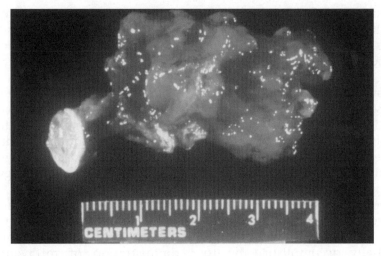

Figure 13.14 Gross pathologic specimen of a resected left atrial myxoma. The tumor consists of a stalk with large gelatinous, shiny lobules

tissue, and cause constitutional symptoms that mimic systemic illnesses.

Primary benign tumors of the heart

Approximately 75% of the primary tumors of the heart are benign and 25% are malignant. Cardiac myxomas are the most common primary tumors, and are usually pathologically benign and curable in general. Myxomas, such as the one presented in the case history below, appear as large gelatinous, shiny, lobular masses, often several centimeters in diameter (Figure 13.14). Microscopically, they consist of scattered stellate cells in a mucinous matrix. They may arise from the endothelium of any cardiac chamber. However, 75% of myxomas appear in the left atrium, approximately 20% in right atrium, and the remainder in the ventricles or on the surface of the cardiac valves. Atrial myxomas are most often pedunculated and 85% of the time arise from the fossa ovalis in the mid-atrial septum. Myxomas appear as solitary lesions 95% of the time, and in the remainder multiple tumors are present. Up to 10% of myxomas occur in a hereditary manner.

The clinical relevance of cardiac myxomas is due to three features of the tumor. First, these are generally large, mobile, space occupying lesions that can obstruct the inflow of blood to or outflow from the cardiac chamber in which they appear. Second, friable tumor fragments or superimposed thrombi embolize to the systemic circulation in 30–70% of patients with left atrial myxoma. In a similar manner, pulmonary embolism may result from emboli derived from a right atrial myxoma. Finally, constitutional symptoms such as fever, chills, sweats, fatigue, and myalgias occur and may be related to necrosis of portions of the myxoma or tumor secretory products.

Left atrial myxomas may transiently obstruct blood flow across the mitral valve during diastole. Symptoms are intermittent and may relate to changes in body position due to the movement of the tumor within the chamber. In such patients, episodic dyspnea, light-headedness and syncope often occur. The physical examination of a patient with left atrial myxoma may demonstrate the stigmata of peripheral systemic emboli and an abnormal cardiac examination. In early diastole, a low-pitched "tumor plop" may be heard, as the mobile tumor strikes the mitral valve or heart chamber wall. If partial obstruction of transmitral flow ensues, then a diastolic murmur mimicking mitral stenosis can be heard. In some cases, chronic repetitive traumatic injury of the mitral valve by the myxoma may result in leaflet damage and the murmur of mitral regurgitation.

Patients with right atrial myxoma may also manifest positional dyspnea and syncope because of intermittent obstruction of the tricuspid valve. In addition, symptoms typical of pulmonary emboli may result if there is dislodgement of tumor fragments. Signs of right sided heart failure may also appear, including jugular venous distension, hepatomegaly, and peripheral edema. A tall "a" wave may be present in the jugular venous pulse if right atrial contraction causes the tumor to partially obstruct blood flow across the tricuspid valve.

Laboratory studies in patients with myxomas reveal anemia, leukocytosis, and an elevated erythrocyte sedimentation rate. The chest x ray film usually demonstrates a normal cardiac silhouette; rarely, calcification within a myxoma may be visualized on the plain film. The electrocardiogram may demonstrate left or right atrial enlargement, reflecting obstructed blood flow in the chamber that contains the tumor. The most useful imaging modality is two-dimensional echocardiography because myxomas are usually readily identified using this technique (Figure 13.15). Although less convenient to perform, computed tomography and magnetic resonance imaging have sensitivities of detection similar to that of echocardiography.

The curative treatment of an intracardiac myxoma is surgical excision. Rarely, the tumor recurs (most often in the familial forms of myxoma), so that yearly echocardiography is recommended for 5 years following excision of the tumor.

Cardiac myxomas have been reported as part of a syndrome including lentigines, blue nevi, and various endocrine abnormalities

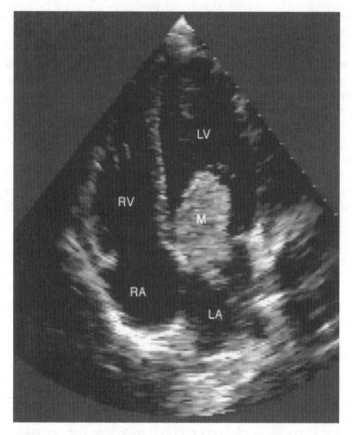

Figure 13.15 Echocardiogram, apical four chamber view, demonstrating a mass (M) extending between the left atrium (LA) and left ventricle (LV). RA, right atrium; RV, right ventricle

(Cushing's disease, acromegaly, testicular tumors, and myxoid fibroadenomas of the breast).

Other benign tumors of the heart are often asymptomatic, but they too may obstruct intracardiac blood flow or result in arrhythmias and/or conduction disturbances. Fibroelastomas are sometimes found as an incidental finding on echocardiography. They arise as small masses on the cardiac valves or adjacent endothelium. They are seldom symptomatic, but occasionally interfere with valvular function. Rhabdomyomas are the most common cardiac tumors in children. They generally occur within the ventricles, are often multiple, and depending on their size and location they may mimic valvular stenosis, restrictive or hypertrophic cardiomyopathy, or result in congestive heart failure. Cardiac lipomas are often an incidental finding at autopsy. Sometimes they become quite large and obstruct intracardiac flow or cause arrhythmias.

Primary malignant tumors of the heart

Primary cardiac malignant tumors are usually a form of sarcoma and appear more commonly in the right side of the heart. Symptoms arise from intracavitary growth as well as invasion of the myocardium, conduction system, and pericardium. Depending on the size and rate of progression, malignant cardiac tumors can result in sudden congestive heart failure, syncope, arrhythmias, and conduction disturbances. Myocardial invasion can result in electrocardiographic abnormalities that mimic acute myocardial infarction. Erosion into the pericardium results in large hemorrhagic effusions. In most cases, death occurs within weeks to months following initial presentation of malignant cardiac tumors. Cures are uncommon, even with surgical and radiation therapy. Rarely, cardiac transplantation has been performed successfully. Of the modalities available to image suspected malignant cardiac tumors, magnetic resonance stands out because it provides superb anatomic detail that can delineate the extent of tumor invasion and the relationship to normal cardiac structures.

Metastatic tumors to the heart

Metastatic tumors to the heart are much more common than primary cardiac tumors. They are found in 10% of patients who die from extracardiac malignancies, but they are rarely symptomatic during life. Cardiac metastases are most commonly found in patients with cancer of the lung, breast, melanoma, leukemia, and lymphoma. Metastases arising from Kaposi's sarcoma have been found in patients with AIDS. Metastatic cardiac tumors may invade the heart via the blood stream, the lymphatic system, or by direct invasion from the primary neoplastic site. Grossly, they may appear as small nodules or as a diffuse infiltration into the myocardium and/or pericardium.

When symptomatic, clinical findings are similar to those of primary cardiac malignant tumors. Most commonly, symptoms are attributable to pericardial metastasis with large malignant hemorrhagic effusions, which often result in cardiac tamponade. Infiltrating tumor can also encase the heart and result in physiology resembling that of constrictive pericarditis.

The prognosis of an individual with metastatic cardiac tumor is poor, and therapy is generally palliative. In rare cases, cardiac invasion may respond to radiation or chemotherapy. Acute deterioration due to cardiac tamponade is treated by pericardiocentesis or, if recurrent, by surgical creation of a pericardial window for continued drainage.

Occasionally, certain carcinomas of extracardiac origin may extend into the inferior vena cava and enter the right heart chambers via that route. Such lesions are often readily visualized by echocardiography or other imaging modalities. Examples of such tumors include renal cell and hepatocellular carcinoma.

Case studies

Case 13.3

A 22-year-old male college student and football player has been in previously good health. Over the months before admission he noted intermittent low grade fever, fatigue, and decreased appetite. Over the 2 weeks before admission he experienced repeated episodes of severe light-headedness and sudden dyspnea with rapid changes in position, such as jumping to catch the football. The coach dismissed him from the football team because of his poor performance. His mother, however, was not satisfied that a cause had been found for his symptoms, and brought him to the hospital for evaluation. His past medical history is unremarkable. He is a non-smoker, non-drinker, and denies use of illicit drugs.

Examination. Physical examination: the patient appeared tired. No peripheral stigmata of embolic phenomena. Temperature: 99°F (37·2°C). Weight: 200 lb (90·6 kg). Pulse: 64 beats/min, regular, normal sinus rhythm. Blood pressure: 120/80 mmHg. Jugular venous pulse: 5 cm. Cardiac impulse: normal. First heart sound: normal. Second heart sound: splits normally on inspiration. In the left lateral decubitus position, at the apex, an intermittent early diastolic low frequency sound was heard, which was followed by a brief diastolic murmur. Chest examination: normal air entry, no rales or rhonchi. Abdominal examination: soft abdomen, no tenderness. Normal liver span. No other obvious abnormalities. No peripheral edema. Femoral, popliteal, and foot pulses were equally diminished. Carotid pulses: normal, no bruits.

Investigations. Hematocrit: 44%. White blood cell count: 8 300/mm^3. Erythrocyte sedimentation rate: 34. Electrocardiogram: sinus rhythm with normal intervals and axis; a normal tracing. Echocardiography: 5 cm × 5 cm mobile mass within the left atrium (see Figure 13.15). It appears pedunculated and attached to the mid-portion of the atrial septum. During diastole, the mass prolapses into the mitral valve orifice with partial obstruction of left ventricular inflow.

Questions

1. What is the differential diagnosis of the echocardiographic lesion?
2. Is this likely to be a benign or malignant lesion?
3. What complications may arise from this process?
4. What therapy is indicated?

Answers

Answer to question 1 This young man presents with recent onset of constitutional symptoms, positional light-headedness, and a large mass within the left atrium that appears pedunculated. The differential diagnosis of this lesion includes a large thrombus, an intracardiac tumor or possibly infective endocarditis. Any of these conditions may present with the described constitutional symptoms. There is no apparent clinical reason for this individual to have an intracardiac thrombus. Notably, the left atrium is not significantly enlarged, and he does not have mitral valve disease or atrial fibrillation. The pedunculated mass appears to be attached to the interatrial septum, which is the most typical position for a left atrial myxoma. Conversely, thrombus within the left atrium is most commonly observed in the region of the atrial appendage. Blood cultures had been obtained but were negative, ruling against endocarditis.

Answer to question 2 Of the heart tumors, the location, pedunculated attachment, and origin at the mid-intra-atrial septum in this case are most consistent with a cardiac myxoma, as described below. Myxomas are usually pathologically benign and are surgically curable.

Answer to question 3 The clinical presentation of left atrial myxoma includes constitutional symptoms (fever, chills, sweats, fatigue, myalgias), systemic emboli including stroke, and obstruction in intracardiac blood flow. In this young man's case, sudden changes in position resulted in syncope due to obstruction of diastolic blood flow across the mitral valve into the left ventricle.

Answer to question 4 The presence of a left atrial myxoma with evidence of obstructed blood flow or embolization is a medical emergency, and prompt surgical excision should follow.

Further reading

Diseases of the pericardium

Cameron J, Oesterle SN, Baldwin JC, Hancock EW. The etiology spectrum of constrictive pericarditis. *Am Heart J* 1987;**113**:354–60.

Fowler NO. *The pericardium in health and disease.* New York: Futura Publishing Co, 1985.

Klein AL, Cohen GI. Doppler echocardiographic assessment of constrictive pericarditis, cardiac amyloidosis, and cardiac tamponade. *Cleve Clin J Med* 1992;**59**:278–90.

Lilly LS, ed. *Pathophysiology of heart disease.* Philadelphia: Lea & Febiger, 2002.

Oh JK, Hatle LK, Seward JB, et al. Diagnostic role of Doppler echocardiography in constrictive pericarditis. *J Am Coll Cardiol* 1994;**23**:154–62.

Shabetai R, ed. Diseases of the pericardium. *Cardiol Clin* 1990;**8**:579–716.

Singh S, Wann LS, Schuchard GH, et al. Right ventricular and right atrial collapse in patients with cardiac tamponade: a combined echocardiographic and hemodynamic study. *Circulation* 1984;**70**:966.

Soulen RL, Stark DD, Higgins CB. Magnetic resonance imaging of constrictive pericardial disease. *Am J Cardiol* 1985;**55**:480.

Spodick DH. Macrophysiology, microphysiology, and anatomy of the pericardium: a synopsis. *Am Heart J* 1992;**124**:1046–51.

Diseases of the aorta

Belkin M, Donaldson MC, Whittemore AD. Abdominal aortic aneurysms. *Curr Opin Cardiol* 1994;**9**:581–90.

Cigarroa JE, Isselbacher EM, DeSanctis RW, Eagle KA. Diagnostic imaging in the evaluation of suspected aortic dissection: old standards and new directions. *N Engl J Med* 1993;**328**:35–43.

Ernst CB. Abdominal aortic aneurysm. *N Engl J Med* 1993;**328**:1167–72.

Hagan PG, Nienaber CA, Isselbacher EM, et al. The International Registry of Acute Aortic Dissection (IRAD). *JAMA* 2000;**283**:897–903.

Izzo JL, Black HR, ed. *Hypertension primer: the essentials of high blood pressure.* Dallas: American Heart Association, 1993.

Kouchokos NT, Daigenis D. Surgery of the thoracic aorta. *N Engl J Med* 1997;**336**:1876–87.

Nienaber CA, von Kodolitsch Y, Nicolas V, et al. Definitive diagnosis of thoracic aortic dissection: the emerging role of noninvasive imaging modalities. *N Engl J Med* 1993;**328**:1–9.

Heart tumors

Reynen K. Cardiac myxomas. *N Engl J Med* 1995;**333**:1610–17.

Fyke FE III, Seward JB, Edwards WD, et al. Primary cardiac tumors: experience with 30 consecutive patients since the introduction of two-dimensional echocardiography. *J Am Coll Cardiol* 1985;**5**:1465–73.

Reeder, GS, Khandheria BK, Seward JB, et al. Transesophageal echocardiography and cardiac masses. *Mayo Clin Proc* 1991;**66**:1101–9.

Salcedo EE, Cohen GI, White, RD, Davison MB. Cardiac tumors: diagnosis and management. *Curr Probl Cardiol* 1992;**17**:73–137.

14: Pulmonary embolism and pulmonary hypertension

SAMUEL Z GOLDHABER

Pulmonary embolism and deep venous thrombosis (DVT) result in hundreds of thousands of hospitalizations, and attempts at prompt diagnosis and appropriate treatment of this illness cost billions of dollars annually. The incidence of pulmonary embolism and DVT increases steadily with age. For patients with pulmonary embolism, the most dangerous period precedes ascertainment of the correct diagnosis. The latter is quite difficult despite the availability of traditional tests such as lung scanning, right heart catheterization, and pulmonary angiography, as well as plasma D-dimer enzyme linked immunosorbent assay (a blood screening test), leg ultrasonography with color Doppler imaging (to detect venous thrombosis), chest computed tomography scanning, and echocardiography.

Contemporary diagnosis of pulmonary embolism emphasizes a strategy that integrates clinical findings with a variety of diagnostic modalities.[1–4]

The optimal approach to treatment (primary therapy with thrombolysis or embolectomy versus secondary prevention with anticoagulation alone) is somewhat controversial. Risk stratification has emerged as the key concept in planning the treatment of patients with pulmonary embolism. Because pulmonary embolism is difficult to diagnose, expensive to treat, and occasionally lethal despite therapy, utilization of primary preventive measures is extraordinarily important.[5] Fortunately, a variety of effective mechanical measures and pharmacologic agents can be employed. Primary prophylaxis is cost effective. For every 1 000 000 patients undergoing operation who receive primary prophylaxis against DVT and pulmonary embolism, approximately US$60 000 000 can be saved in direct healthcare costs.

Pathophysiology

The most spectacular advance in the molecular medicine of venous thrombosis is the discovery of a specific genetic mutation, termed factor V Leiden, which predisposes to pulmonary embolism and DVT. This mutation results from a single nucleotide substitution of adenine for guanine 1691, which replaces the amino acid arginine with glutamine at position 506. This change eliminates the protein C cleavage site in factor V. Consequently, resistance to activated protein C (aPC) is the phenotypic expression of this genetic mutation.

Normally, one can add a specified amount of aPC to plasma and observe prolongation in the activated partial thromboplastin time. However, patients with "aPC resistance" have an inadequate prolongation in partial thromboplastin time. In contrast to classic coagulation protein deficiencies, which are rare (such as antithrombin III, protein C, and protein S), aPC resistance occurs frequently among patients with venous thrombosis.

The allelic frequency of the factor V Leiden mutation is about 3% in healthy American male physicians. In the Physicians' Health Study, the prevalence of the factor V mutation was three times higher among men who developed venous thrombosis.[6]

The ramifications of testing for factor V Leiden are far reaching. For example, in a case–control study of premenopausal women who developed DVT, the risk for thrombosis among users of oral contraceptives was increased fourfold. However, the risk for thrombosis among carriers of the factor V Leiden mutation was eightfold as compared with non-carriers. When the risks associated with oral contraceptive use and factor V Leiden were combined, the rate of thrombosis increased more than 30-fold.

A careful family history is the most rapid and cost effective method to identify a genetic predisposition to venous thrombosis.

Conditions that increase venous stasis or cause endothelial damage are likely to predispose to venous thrombosis, especially among patients who already have subclinical hypercoagulable states. These conditions include surgery, immobilization, trauma, obesity, increasing age, oral contraceptives, pregnancy, cancer (particularly occult adenocarcinoma), stroke, spinal cord injury, and indwelling central venous catheters. Of course, patients who have had a prior pulmonary embolism or DVT are particularly susceptible to recurrences, even many years after the initial event.

Most pulmonary emboli result from thrombi that originate in the pelvic or deep veins of the leg, and occasionally thrombi in the axillary or subclavian veins embolize to the pulmonary arteries. Almost half of patients with proximal leg DVT have asymptomatic pulmonary emboli. When venous thrombi become dislodged from their sites of formation, they flow through the venous system to the pulmonary arterial circulation. Although extremely large emboli may lodge at the bifurcation of the pulmonary artery, forming a "saddle embolus", more commonly a second, third, or fourth order pulmonary vessel is affected.

Pulmonary embolism can have the following pathophysiologic effects:

- increased pulmonary vascular resistance due to vascular obstruction, neurohumoral agents, or pulmonary artery baroreceptors
- impaired gas exchange due to increased alveolar dead space from vascular obstruction and hypoxemia from alveolar hypoventilation, low ventilation/perfusion units, and right to left shunting, as well as impaired carbon monoxide transfer due to loss of gas exchange surface
- alveolar hyperventilation due to reflex stimulation of irritant receptors
- increased airway resistance due to bronchoconstriction
- decreased pulmonary compliance due to lung edema, lung hemorrhage, and loss of surfactant.

Right heart failure

The hemodynamic response to pulmonary embolism depends on the size of the embolus, coexistent cardiopulmonary disease, and neurohumoral activation. Pulmonary artery obstruction and circulating neurohumoral substances reduce the pulmonary vascular bed and cause an increase in right ventricular afterload. As right ventricular and pulmonary artery pressures rise, the right ventricle dilates, becomes hypokinetic, and ultimately fails. Progressive right heart failure leads to reduced forward cardiac output and is usually the cause of death from acute pulmonary embolism.

Sudden increases in right ventricular pressure adversely affect left ventricular function because of the anatomic juxtaposition of the two ventricles and "ventricular interdependence". Moderate right ventricular hypertension can displace the interventricular septum toward the left ventricle, resulting in decreased left ventricular diastolic filling and end-diastolic volume (Figure 14.1).[7] The subsequent reduction in coronary artery perfusion pressure to the overloaded right ventricle may cause progressive right ventricular ischemia and failure. Ultimately, right ventricular infarction, circulatory arrest, and death may ensue.

Diagnosis

The differential diagnosis of pulmonary embolism is broad and covers a spectrum from life-threatening disease such as acute myocardial infarction to innocuous anxiety states (Box 14.1). Some patients have concomitant pulmonary embolism and other illnesses. Thus, for example, if pneumonia or heart failure do not respond to appropriate therapy, then the possibility of coexisting pulmonary embolism should be considered.

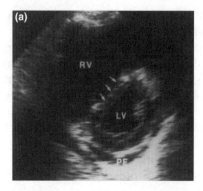 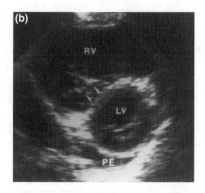

Figure 14.1 Parasternal short axis views of the right ventricle (RV) and left ventricle (LV) in **(a)** diastole and **(b)** systole. There is diastolic and systolic bowing of the interventricular septum (arrows) into the left ventricle compatible with right ventricular volume and pressure overloads, respectively. The right ventricle is appreciably dilated and markedly hypokinetic, with little change in apparent right ventricular area from diastole to systole. PE, small pericardial effusion. Reprinted with permission from Come[7]

Box 14.1 Differential diagnosis of pulmonary embolism

Myocardial infarction
Pneumonia
Congestive heart failure
Cardiomyopathy
Primary pulmonary hypertension
Asthma
Pericarditis
Intrathoracic cancer
Rib fracture
Pneumothorax
Costochondritis
"Musculoskeletal pain"
Anxiety; hyperventilation syndrome

Paradoxic embolism may present with a sudden, devastating stroke and concomitant pulmonary embolism. Such patients often have a patent foramen ovale evident on echocardiography. Among patients suspected of paradoxic embolism, occult leg vein thrombosis is frequently present and often is confined to the calves.

Non-thrombotic pulmonary embolism is less common than thrombotic pulmonary embolism. Fat embolism syndrome is most often observed after blunt trauma complicated by long bone fractures. Among cancer patients, tumor embolism is more difficult to diagnose clinically than thrombotic pulmonary embolism because presenting

Table 14.1 Primary pulmonary hypertension versus recurrent pulmonary embolism

Variable	PPH	Recurrent pulmonary embolism
Similarities		
Symptoms	Fatigue, dyspnea on exertion (most common); chest pain; syncope, hemoptysis, cyanosis (also common)	
Clinical course	Progressive dyspnea, right heart failure	
Hemodynamics	Elevated right heart pressures, normal pulmonary capillary wedge pressure	
Histology	Thrombotic lesions usually present	
Treatment	Includes anticoagulation	
Differences		
Age (years)	20–40	>50
Female:male ratio	4:1	1:1
Clinical course	Continued deterioration	Deterioration, with intermittent stabilization
Perfusion lung scan	No segmental perfusion defects	Segmental or larger perfusion defects
Pulmonary artery systolic pressure (mmHg)	>60	<60
Pulmonary angiogram	"Pruning"	Intraluminal filling defects
Confounding problems with angiogram	Thrombi may occur on or distal to PPH lesions	"Pruning" can also suggest pulmonary embolism
Diagnostic modalities	Lung biopsy	Pulmonary angioscopy; chest computed tomography or pulmonary angiography
Therapy	Anticoagulation; high dose nifedipine or diltiazem; long-term continuous intravenous prostacyclin; bosentan	Anticoagulation; inferior vena cava interruption; thromboendarterectomy

PPH, primary pulmonary hypertension

symptoms and signs are similar in both conditions. Air embolus can occur during placement or removal of a central venous catheter.[8] Intravenous drug abusers may inadvertently inject a variety of substances that contaminate their drug supply, such as hair, talc, and cotton. These patients are also susceptible to septic pulmonary embolus, which may be accompanied by endocarditis of the tricuspid or pulmonic valves.

Distinguishing between pulmonary embolism and primary pulmonary hypertension requires special consideration (Table 14.1). Primary pulmonary hypertension is a disease of unclear etiology in which the pulmonary vasculature undergoes extensive remodeling, leading to elevations in pulmonary artery pressure and pulmonary vascular resistance. The sustained increases in right ventricular afterload result initially in right ventricular hypertrophy and subsequently in right heart dilatation and depressed cardiac function.

Both primary pulmonary hypertension and thrombotic pulmonary embolism are treated with anticoagulants. However, the prognosis with primary pulmonary hypertension is usually more ominous.

In considering the diagnosis of thrombotic pulmonary embolism, clinical clues remain of paramount importance. Unexplained dyspnea, light-headedness, and chest pain are three of the most common presenting symptoms of hemodynamically important pulmonary embolism. Whereas dyspnea, syncope, or cyanosis portends a major life-threatening pulmonary embolism, pleuritic chest pain often signifies that the embolism is small and located in the distal pulmonary arterial system, near the pleural lining.

Pulmonary embolism should be suspected in hypotensive patients in the following circumstances[9]:

- there is evidence of or there are predisposing factors for venous thrombosis, and
- there is clinical evidence of acute cor pulmonale (acute right ventricular failure) such as distended neck veins, a third heart sound (S_3) gallop, or a parasternal lift due to right ventricular pressure overload, tachycardia, or tachypnea, and especially if
- there is electrocardiographic evidence of acute cor pulmonale manifested by a new S_1-Q_3-T_3 pattern, new incomplete right bundle branch block, or right ventricular ischemia.

Patients with massive pulmonary embolism present with systemic arterial hypotension and usually have anatomically widespread thromboembolism. Primary therapy with thrombolysis or embolectomy offers the greatest chance of survival.[10] A moderate to large pulmonary embolus may be associated with right ventricular hypokinesis seen on echocardiography despite normal systemic arterial pressure. There is increasing evidence that such patients may benefit from primary therapy with thrombolysis or embolectomy (in addition to secondary prevention with anticoagulation) in order to avert recurrent embolism. Small to moderate pulmonary emboli are usually found in the presence of both normal right heart function and normal systemic arterial pressure. These patients have a good prognosis with secondary prevention measures, such as either adequate anticoagulation or an inferior vena cava filter. Pulmonary infarction is often accompanied by severe pleuritic chest pain and, rarely, by a small amount of hemoptysis. Despite the discomfort usually experienced, the associated pulmonary embolus is almost always anatomically small and hemodynamically inconsequential.

Venous thrombosis as a surrogate for pulmonary embolism

The presence of confirmed DVT is usually an adequate surrogate for pulmonary embolism. Therefore, symptoms and signs of DVT should also be sought when investigating the possibility of pulmonary embolism. DVT may be described as an intermittent "pulling" sensation at the insertion of the lower calf muscle into the posterior portion of the lower leg. An insidious feeling of calf cramping may subsequently become more pronounced, and warmth, swelling, or erythema may ensue. Eventually, the discomfort and abnormal physical findings may extend proximally into the popliteal fossa or thigh. Occasionally, a cord may be palpable, or prominent venous collaterals may appear. However, Homans' sign, defined as increased resistance or pain during dorsiflexion of the foot, is unreliable and non-specific.

In patients with prior DVT, the sudden onset of diffuse leg swelling usually indicates venous insufficiency and not recurrent venous thrombosis. Other clues to venous insufficiency include brownish pigmentation (and rarely ulceration) of the medial malleolus, or pain, cramping, or calf mottling and discoloration when standing.

Laboratory and imaging tests

Classic chest radiograph findings include focal oligemia (Westermark's sign), indicating massive central embolic occlusion, or a peripheral wedge shaped density above the diaphragm (Hampton's hump), indicating pulmonary infarction. Enlargement of a central pulmonary artery, especially with progressive expansion on serial radiographs, is a cardinal sign of pulmonary hypertension on plain chest radiography.

Enlargement of the right descending pulmonary artery (Palla's sign) to greater than 16 mm diameter also suggests pulmonary arterial hypertension. Chest radiography can also help identify patients with other diseases, such as lobar pneumonia or pneumothorax, which can mimic pulmonary embolism. However, patients with these illnesses can also have concomitant pulmonary embolism.

The electrocardiogram is useful not only to help exclude acute myocardial infarction but also because patients with a large pulmonary embolism may have electrocardiographic manifestations of right heart strain (Box 14.2).[9] The differential diagnosis of new right heart strain includes acute pulmonary embolism, acute asthma, or exacerbation of chronic bronchitis in patients with chronic obstructive pulmonary disease.

Box 14.2 Electrocardiographic findings in pulmonary embolism[9]

Incomplete or complete right bundle branch block
S in leads I and aVL >1·5 mm
Transition zone shift to V_5
QS in leads III and aVF, but not in lead II
QRS axis >90° or indeterminate axis
Low limb lead voltage
T-wave inversion in leads III and aVF or in leads V_1–V_4

Unfortunately, the time honored screening test of abnormal room air arterial blood gases is not useful in triaging patients suspected of having pulmonary embolism.[11] Although arterial blood gases are inexpensive and readily available, extensive analyses of the large Prospective Investigation of Pulmonary Embolism Diagnosis (PIOPED) database[12] indicate that even sophisticated calculations of the alveolar–arterial oxygen difference do not accurately separate patients with pulmonary embolism from those without pulmonary embolism. Therefore, arterial blood gases should not be obtained as a screening test in patients with suspected pulmonary embolism.

The most promising blood test for pulmonary embolism is an abnormally elevated level of enzyme linked immunosorbent assay (ELISA) determined plasma D-dimer (>500 ng/ml), which has a more than 90% sensitivity for identifying patients with pulmonary embolism proven by lung scan or by angiogram.[13,14] This test relies on the principle that most patients with pulmonary embolism have ongoing endogenous fibrinolysis that is not effective enough to prevent pulmonary embolism but that does break down some of the fibrin clot to D-dimers (Figures 14.2 and 14.3[15]). These D-dimers can be assayed by monoclonal antibodies that are commercially available. Although elevated plasma concentrations of D-dimers are sensitive for the presence of pulmonary embolism, they are not specific. Levels are elevated in patients for at least 1 week postoperatively and are also increased in patients with myocardial infarction, sepsis, or almost any other systemic illness. Therefore, the plasma D-dimer ELISA is best utilized when suspected pulmonary embolism patients have no coexisting acute systemic illness. The usual D-dimer measurement obtained in hospital laboratories employs a latex agglutination assay to detect disseminated intravascular coagulation. Unlike the ELISA, the latex agglutination assay is simply not sensitive enough for reliable pulmonary embolism screening.[14] Therefore, use of an ELISA based assay is necessary to "rule out pulmonary embolism".

Ventilation/perfusion lung scanning is the principal diagnostic imaging test for suspected acute pulmonary embolism (Table 14.2). Small particulate aggregates of albumin or microspheres labeled

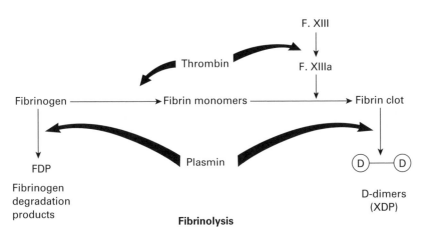

Blood activation

Fibrinolysis

Figure 14.2 Plasma D-dimer is generated exclusively from plasmin breakdown of fibrin clot. The D-dimers can be measured using commercially available enzyme linked immunosorbent assay (ELISA) kits. Plasma D-dimer ELISA is an excellent screening test for pulmonary embolism. Elevated levels are sensitive and normal levels have a high negative predictive value for pulmonary embolism at angiograph

with a γ emitting radionuclide (usually technetium) are injected intravenously and are trapped in the pulmonary capillary bed. A perfusion scan defect suggests decreased blood flow, possibly due to pulmonary embolism. Ventilation scans, obtained with radiolabeled inhaled gases such as xenon or krypton, may improve the specificity of the perfusion scan. Abnormal ventilation scans indicate non-ventilated lung, thereby providing possible explanations for perfusion defects other than acute pulmonary embolism. The ventilation/ perfusion scan is most useful if it is normal or if it demonstrates a pattern that is suggestive of a high probability of pulmonary embolism. The diagnosis of pulmonary embolism is very unlikely (<5% chance) in patients with normal and near normal scans; in contrast, it is about 90% certain in patients with high probability scans. A high probability scan for pulmonary embolism is defined as having two or more segmental perfusion defects in the presence of normal ventilation. Unfortunately, fewer than half of patients with angiographically confirmed pulmonary embolism have a high probability scan. Intermediate probability scans or low probability scans with high clinical suspicion do not exclude pulmonary embolism.[15] In PIOPED, 40% of patients with high clinical suspicion

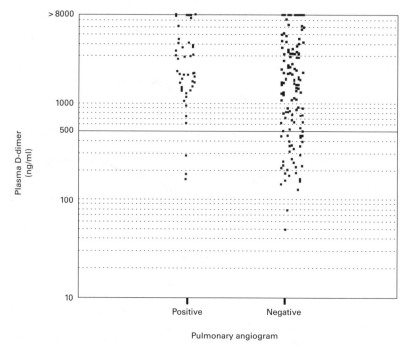

Figure 14.3 Distribution of plasma D-dimer levels, sorted according to angiographic findings, among 173 patients with suspected acute pulmonary embolism. Reprinted with permission from Goldhaber *et al.*[15]

for pulmonary embolism and "low probability" scans did, in fact, have pulmonary embolism at angiography (Table 14.2).

Ultrasonography of the leg veins is usually accurate in diagnosing proximal leg DVT in symptomatic outpatients but it is an insensitive screening test for DVT in asymptomatic inpatients.[16] Overall, about one-third of pulmonary embolism patients have no venographic evidence of leg DVT. Therefore, if clinical suspicion of pulmonary embolism is high, then the diagnosis of pulmonary embolism should be pursued even in the absence of DVT.

Bedside echocardiography is particularly useful among clinically unstable patients who seem "too ill" to undergo lung scanning or pulmonary angiography. If transthoracic echocardiographic images are technically inadequate, then transesophageal echocardiography should be considered. Although it is unusual for echocardiography to demonstrate a thrombus in the main pulmonary artery or at its proximal bifurcation, a constellation of indirect findings will often suggest pulmonary embolism (Box 14.3). However, patients can also have a normal echocardiogram despite anatomically extensive

Table 14.2 PIOPED: pulmonary embolism status

Ventilation/perfusion lung scan category	Clinical probability (%)			
	80–100	20–70	0–19	0–100
High	28/29 (96)	70/80 (88)	5/9 (56)	103/118 (87)
Intermediate	27/41 (66)	66/236 (28)	11/68 (16)	104/345 (30)
Low	6/16 (40)	30/191 (16)	4/90 (4)	40/296 (14)
Very low	0/5 (0)	4/62 (6)	1/61 (2)	5/128 (4)
Total	61/90 (68)	170/569 (30)	21/228 (9)	252/887 (28)

Values are presented as number of patients with pulmonary embolism/total number of patients in the respective probability category (%). Adapted with permission from the PIOPED Investigators[15]

pulmonary embolism. Echocardiography for suspected pulmonary embolism can also help to exclude other life-threatening conditions, such as ventricular septal rupture, aortic dissection, and pericardial tamponade. The distinction is important because patients with these alternative, grave illnesses require urgent therapy that differs radically from that for pulmonary embolism.

Box 14.3 Echocardiographic findings in pulmonary embolism

Right ventricular dilatation
Right ventricular hypokinesis (especially the right ventricular free wall)
Bowing of the interventricular septum into the left ventricle
Extrinsic compression of an intrinsically normal left ventricle
Tricuspid regurgitation
Pulmonary artery dilatation
Decreased inspiratory collapse of inferior vena cava

Right heart catheterization and pulmonary angiography

Before undertaking diagnostic pulmonary angiography, accurate and high quality recordings of right heart pressures and waveforms should be obtained. A carefully performed right heart catheterization may provide important clues to alternative diagnoses such as cardiac tamponade and left ventricular failure. Patients with dyspnea and pulmonary hypertension might have intracardiac shunting, which can be defined most precisely by an oxygen saturation run. If the pressure tracing "dampens" or "wedges" in the proximal pulmonary artery without balloon expansion, then anatomically massive pulmonary embolism should be suspected before injection of contrast agent. Even when the angiographic diagnosis is in fact pulmonary embolism, a carefully performed right heart catheterization can provide clues about the age of the thrombus, based on the degree of elevation of the pulmonary artery systolic pressure. In general, if the pulmonary artery systolic pressure exceeds approximately 50 mmHg, then the differential diagnosis should include chronic pulmonary embolism and acute pulmonary embolism superimposed on chronic pulmonary embolism.

Pulmonary angiography can almost always be accomplished safely if:

- selective angiography is performed, with the perfusion lung scan serving as a road map to the angiographer
- soft, flexible catheters with side holes are employed, rather than stiff catheters with end holes
- a low osmolar contrast agent is utilized to minimize the transient hypotension, heat, and coughing sensation that often occurs with conventional radiocontrast agents.

Among patients undergoing pulmonary angiography, an intraluminal filling defect seen in more than one projection is the most reliable feature to diagnose pulmonary embolism. Standard contrast pulmonary angiography can detect emboli accurately in peripheral vessels as small as 1–2 mm. Secondary signs of pulmonary embolism reflect decreased perfusion and consist of abrupt occlusion ("cut-off") of vessels, oligemia or avascularity of a segment, a prolonged arterial phase with slow filling and emptying of veins, and tortuous tapering peripheral vessels.

Pulmonary angiography may also help diagnose chronic pulmonary embolism. Arteries may appear "pouched", and thrombus appears organized with a concave edge. Band-like defects called webs may be present, in addition to intimal irregularities and abrupt narrowing or occlusion of lobar vessels.

With increasing frequency, chest computed tomography scanning with contrast is replacing classical contrast pulmonary angiography, which is now being reserved for patients who have equivocal chest computed tomography scans or who require therapeutic procedures such as catheter embolectomy in the interventional laboratory.

Overall diagnostic strategy

An integrated diagnostic approach is advocated, which combines clinical assessment, lung scanning, and evaluation for DVT. This strategy narrows the number of patients who require pulmonary angiography. Often, a definitive diagnosis can be obtained by combining clinical likelihood, plasma D-dimer ELISA, leg ultrasonography, lung scan, and

Pulmonary embolus diagnosis strategy

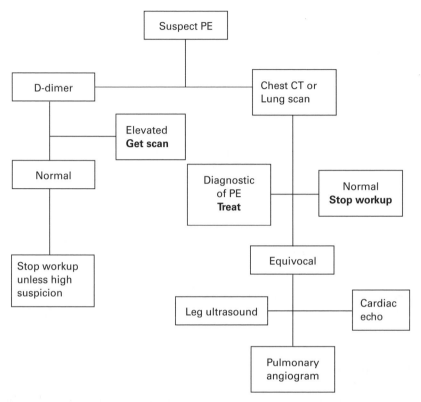

Figure 14.4 Proposed diagnostic strategy for suspected pulmonary embolism (PE) that integrates the clinical likelihood of pulmonary embolism with the results of the plasma D-dimer enzyme linked immunosorbent assay, lung scan, echocardiogram, and leg ultrasound to help decide whether to perform pulmonary angiography. CT, computed tomography

chest computed tomography scan results. When the plasma D-dimer ELISA is elevated in the presence of a normal leg ultrasound, normal echocardiogram, and non-diagnostic lung scan and chest computed tomography scan, the clinical setting may warrant pulmonary angiography (Figure 14.4). Ordinarily, pulmonary angiography is unnecessary for patients with high probability lung scans, even if thrombolysis is planned. This strategy is analogous to the widely accepted practice of empirically administering thrombolysis to patients with chest pain and ST-segment elevation on electrocardiogram who have suspected (but not definitely proven) acute myocardial infarction, rather than proceeding with diagnostic coronary angiography.

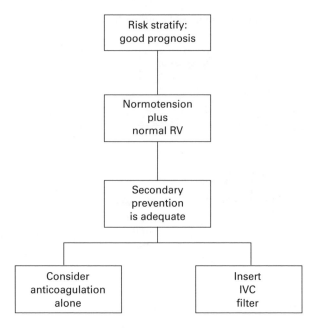

Figure 14.5 Risk stratification: pulmonary embolism patients with good prognosis have good outcomes with secondary prevention alone

Management

We consider patients with pulmonary embolism to be hemodynamically unstable if they have right ventricular hypokinesis, usually documented on echocardiogram, even in the presence of a normal systemic arterial pressure.[15–17] Such patients may initially appear deceptively stable based on the clinical evaluation alone. We use echocardiographic assessment of right ventricular function to help risk stratify pulmonary embolism patients into good prognosis (Figure 14.5) or ominous prognosis (Figure 14.6) groups. Pulmonary embolism patients with good prognosis do well clinically with anticoagulation alone or filter placement (secondary prevention). Pulmonary embolism patients with ominous prognosis may have better outcomes if primary therapy is utilized (i.e. thrombolysis or embolectomy) in addition to anticoagulation.

Despite adequate heparin anticoagulation, patients with right ventricular hypokinesis are at high risk for recurrent pulmonary embolism and clinical deterioration, even if they are normotensive initially.[1] Therefore, they are potential candidates for primary therapy with thrombolysis or mechanical intervention. If patients are candidates for thrombolysis, then we administer thrombolysis in

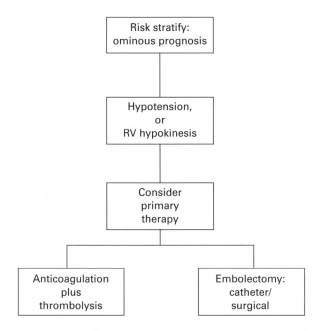

Figure 14.6 Risk stratification: pulmonary embolism patients with ominous prognosis may have improved outcomes if primary therapy (thrombolysis or embolectomy) is utilized in addition to anticoagulation

preference to embolectomy, which is reserved for those few instances in which thrombolysis fails or for situations in which thrombolysis is contraindicated. Dobutamine – a β-adrenergic agonist with positive inotropic and pulmonary vasodilating effects – should be utilized to treat right heart failure and cardiogenic shock. In general, volume loading is ill advised because increased right ventricular dilatation can lead to even further reductions in left ventricular forward output.

Anticoagulation

Unfractionated heparin is administered immediately, as soon as pulmonary embolism is suspected clinically. Initiate heparin with a bolus of 5000–10 000 units followed by a continuous intravenous infusion of approximately 1250 units/hour while the diagnostic work up is pursued. The partial thromboplastin time should then be adjusted to a target of at least twice the control value. In established pulmonary embolism, failure to use heparin in adequate doses can prolong the duration of hospital stay, predispose to recurrent pulmonary embolism, and increase the costs of medical care. Low molecular weight heparin is evolving as a contemporary alternative to unfractionated heparin for management of acute pulmonary embolism.

Bleeding and thrombocytopenia are the major side effects of short-term unfractionated heparin administration. When unfractionated heparin is administered chronically (the usual case when pulmonary embolism is being treated during pregnancy), heparin associated osteopenia may develop. Oral anticoagulation with warfarin can be started as soon as the partial thromboplastin time is within the therapeutic range. Patients should receive at least 5 days of heparin while an adequate level of oral anticoagulation is established. The prothrombin time, utilized to adjust the dose of oral anticoagulation, should be reported according to the well standardized International Normalized Ratio (INR) but not according to the prothrombin time ratio or the prothrombin time expressed in seconds. The target INR range is 2·0–3·0. However, for patients with pulmonary embolism and antiphospholipid antibodies, more intensive anticoagulation, with a target INR range of 3·0–4·0, will result in fewer recurrent embolic events.

After discontinuation of anticoagulation, the risk for recurrent pulmonary embolism is surprisingly high. Patients with underlying cancer that is not cured or massive obesity should probably be anticoagulated indefinitely. For other patients, I anticoagulate the first episode of isolated calf vein thrombosis for 3 months, and proximal DVT or pulmonary embolism for 6 months.

Inferior vena cava filter

An inferior vena caval filter does not directly treat an established pulmonary embolism[16] but it does provide secondary prevention of recurrent pulmonary embolism. Accepted indications for filter insertion include established venous thrombosis with active, clinically important bleeding that prohibits the use of heparin; and recurrent pulmonary embolism despite adequate anticoagulation. An inferior vena cava filter may also be used adjunctively to prevent recurrent pulmonary embolism among hemodynamically compromised pulmonary embolism patients who cannot be treated with thrombolytic therapy. Whenever possible, anticoagulation should also be utilized to prevent further thrombosis.

Thombolysis

Thrombolysis (Box 14.4)[10,17] and mechanical catheter interventions[18] debulk clot and provide primary treatment of pulmonary embolism. Over the past decade, the administration of thrombolysis to pulmonary embolism patients has been streamlined so that it is safer, less expensive, and less time consuming (Table 14.3).

Box 14.4 US Food and Drug Administration approved thrombolytic regimens for pulmonary embolism

Streptokinase (approved in 1977): 250 000 IU as a loading dose over 30 min, followed by 100 000 U/hour for 24 hours
Urokinase (approved in 1978): 2000 IU/lb as a loading dose over 10 min, followed by 2000 IU/lb per hour for 12–24 hours
Recombinant tissue-type plasminogen activator (approved in 1990): 100 mg as a continuous peripheral intravenous infusion administered over 2 hours

---

Contraindications to thrombolysis include intracranial disease, recent surgery, or trauma. There is about a 1% risk for intracranial hemorrhage. Careful patient screening for potential contraindications is the best way to minimize bleeding risk.

Embolectomy

There has been a resurgence of interest in aggressive interventional management of pulmonary embolism, often undertaken in the cardiac catheterization laboratory.[18,19] The Greenfield embolectomy device is probably the most frequently used catheter based method of extracting

Table 14.3 Old and new concepts in pulmonary embolism thrombolysis

Variable	Concept	
	Old	New
Diagnosis	Mandatory pulmonary angiogram	High probability lung scan, suggestive echocardiogram (if hypotensive), or chest computed tomography scan with contrast
Indications	Systemic arterial hypotension	Hypotension or normotension with accompanying right ventricular hypokinesis
Time window	5 days or less	14 days or less
Agents	Streptokinase or urokinase	rt-PA
Dosing regimens	24 h streptokinase or 12–24 h urokinase	100 mg/2 h rt-PA
Route	Via pulmonary artery catheter	Via peripheral vein
Coagulation tests	"DIC screens" every 4–6 h during infusion	PTT at conclusion of thrombolysis

DIC, disseminated intravascular coagulation; PTT, partial thromboplastin time; rt-PA, recombinant tissue-type plasminogen activator pulmonary arterial thrombus. It consists of a 10 F steerable catheter with a suction cup attached at the tip. Because of the cup's large size, a surgical venotomy is utilized, usually in the right internal jugular vein. A steerable handle controls progression of the catheter through the right cardiac chambers and the pulmonary arterial branches. If catheter based strategies fail, then emergent surgical embolectomy with cardiopulmonary bypass can be undertaken.[20] A non-randomized comparison of recombinant tissue-type plasminogen activator thrombolysis versus surgical embolectomy indicated that both approaches can be lifesaving in the majority of patients with massive pulmonary embolism. It is best to refer patients for embolectomy before the development of overt cardiogenic shock.

Pulmonary thromboendarterectomy

Patients with chronic pulmonary hypertension due to prior pulmonary embolism may be virtually bedridden with breathlessness because of high pulmonary arterial pressures. They should be considered for pulmonary thromboendarterectomy which, if successful, can reduce and at times even cure pulmonary hypertension. The operation involves a median sternotomy, institution of cardiopulmonary bypass, and deep hypothermia with circulatory arrest periods. Incisions are made in both pulmonary arteries. The surgeon performing thromboendarterectomy creates an endarterectomy plane and then dissects endothelialized thrombus from as many involved pulmonary vessels as possible. At selected centers, pulmonary thromboendarterectomy can be performed with good results and at an acceptable risk among patients debilitated from chronic pulmonary hypertension due to pulmonary embolism.

Primary prevention

Primary prophylaxis is of paramount importance because pulmonary embolism is both difficult to recognize and expensive to treat. Fortunately, mechanical and pharmacologic prophylaxis modalities are widely available and usually effective (Table 14.4).

Case studies

Case 14.1

A 21-year-old woman, who was 8 weeks pregnant and nulliparous, was hospitalized with suspicion of pulmonary embolism. She had

Table 14.4 Primary prevention of pulmonary embolism

Condition	Strategy
Total hip or knee replacement; hip or pelvis fracture	Warfarin (target INR 2·0–2·5) for 4–6 weeks Low molecular weight heparin for 5–14 days (for example enoxaparin 40 mg/daysubcutaneously or dalteparin 5000 units/day) IPC ± warfarin
Gynecologic cancer surgery	Coumadin (target INR 2·0–2·5) ± IPC Unfractionated heparin 5000 U every 8 h ± IPC or enoxaparin 40 mg/day or dalteparin 5000 units/day
Urologic surgery	Warfarin (target INR 2·0–2·5) ± IPC
Thoracic surgery	IPC plus unfractionated heparin 5000 U every 8 h
High risk general surgery (for example prior VTE, current cancer, or obesity)	IPC or graded compression stockings plus unfractionated heparin 5000 U every 8 h or enoxaparin 40 mg/day or dalteparin 5000 units/day
General, gynecologic, or urologic surgery (without prior VTE) for non-cancerous conditions	Graded compression stockings plus unfractionated heparin 5000 U every 12 h or enoxaparin 40 mg/day or dalteparin 2500 units/day IPC alone
Neurosurgery, eye surgery, or other surgery when prophylactic anticoagulation is contraindicated	Graded compression stockings ± IPC
Medical conditions	Graded compression stockings ± heparin 5000 U every 8–12 h or enoxaparin 40 mg/day IPC alone

INR, International Normalized Ratio; IPC, intermittent pneumatic compression; VTE, venous thromboembolism

complained of pleuritic chest and back discomfort for 1 week. Her primary care provider estimated the overall likelihood of pulmonary embolism to be 50%. She was previously healthy. A "cold" (viral syndrome) was going around the family.

Examination. Physical examination: the patient appeared tearful and anxious. No abnormalities of skin, nail beds, or oral mucosa. Pulse: 88 beats/min. Blood pressure: 105/65 mmHg in right arm. Respiratory rate: 24/min. Jugular venous pulse: 8 cm. Cardiac impulse: normal. First heart sound: normal. Second heart sound: split normally on inspiration. No added sounds or murmurs. Chest examination: normal air entry, no rales or rhonchi. Abdominal examination: soft abdomen, no tenderness, and no masses. Normal liver span. No peripheral edema. Femoral, popliteal, posterior tibial, and dorsalis pedis pulses: all normal volume and equal. Carotid pulses: normal, no bruits. Optic fundi: normal.

Investigations. Chest *x* ray and electrocardiogram: normal. Ventilation/perfusion lung scan: intermediate probability for pulmonary embolism. Leg ultrasound: negative for DVT. Echocardiogram: normal, including normal right ventricular function. D-dimer: a plasma D-dimer enzyme linked immunosorbent assay (ELISA) was 2003 ng/ml (normal <500 ng/ml).

Questions

1. Based on the lung scan result and the primary care provider's clinical impression, what is the PIOPED estimate of her likelihood of having a pulmonary embolism?
2. What is the differential diagnosis?
3. How does the elevated plasma D-dimer ELISA affect your estimate of the likelihood of pulmonary embolism?
4. How does the normal echocardiogram affect your estimate of the likelihood of pulmonary embolism?
5. What is the "down side" of empiric treatment for pulmonary embolism?
6. What are the possible advantages and disadvantages of pulmonary angiography?
7. What do you think was actually done in this case, and what was the outcome?

Answers

Answer to question 1 With an intermediate clinical suspicion and intermediate probability lung scan, the PIOPED estimate of her likelihood of pulmonary embolism is 28% (see Table 14.2).

Answer to question 2 The differential diagnosis includes acute viral illness, muscoloskeletal pain, pericarditis, and pulmonary embolism.

Answer to question 3 The presence of a markedly elevated plasma D-dimer level means that the D-dimer cannot be used in this case to exclude pulmonary embolism. If the clinical suspicion is sufficiently high, then the work up for pulmonary embolism should continue or, alternatively, the patient should be treated empirically for pulmonary embolism.

Answer to question 4 The normal echocardiogram does not exclude pulmonary embolism, but it does indicate that if pulmonary embolism is present then the prognosis will be favorable with secondary prevention alone (i.e. anticoagulation). There will be no need to consider thrombolytic therapy or embolectomy.

Answer to question 5 The "down side" of empiric treatment spans a range of medical, psychologic, and social considerations. Medically, if she does not really have pulmonary embolism, then she would be exposed unnecessarily to heparin. Although in her age group bleeding is exceedingly rare, prolonged exposure to heparin places her at risk for developing heparin associated osteopenia or thrombocytopenia. She and society would also incur the expense and inconvenience of full dose heparin during pregnancy, followed by warfarin postpartum. She would be instructed to avoid all forms of estrogen and progesterone contraceptives, as well as postmenopausal hormone replacement therapy. Finally, she would be labeled as having suffered a pulmonary embolism, without solid evidence to support this contention. Because of the inherited nature of some pulmonary emboli, she would always be concerned about whether her children would be at risk for venous thrombosis.

Answer to question 6 If chest computed tomography scan or classic pulmonary angiography were normal, then she could be discharged within several hours of completing the procedure. The fetal exposure to radiation during pulmonary angiography is well below the recommended maximum for pregnancy.

Answer to question 7 After considerable discussion, the patient and her primary care provider agreed to proceed with cardiac catheterization and pulmonary angiography. Appropriate lead shielding of the abdomen was employed, and fluoroscopy time was kept to a minimum. Right heart pressures were entirely normal (right atrial 5 mmHg, pulmonary artery 25/9 mmHg), but angiography demonstrated a large right lower lobar pulmonary embolism (Figure 14.7). Therefore, she was maintained on continuous intravenous heparin for her entire pregnancy and was anticoagulated with warfarin postpartum. Her delivery was entirely unremarkable and she was discharged home uneventfully.

Case 14.2

A 53-year-old man presented with gradually worsening dyspnea on exertion. He complained of fatigue and inability to work and pursue leisure activities without marked shortness of breath.

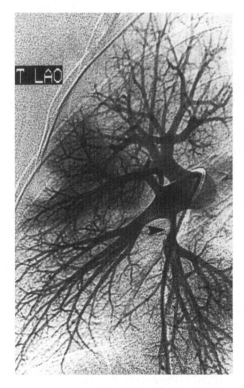

Figure 14.7 Pulmonary angiography with digital subtraction (left anterior oblique projection) demonstrates a large, acute embolus in the right lower lobar pulmonary artery (arrowhead)

At age 25 years he had suffered bilateral DVT of the legs but did not receive a prolonged course of anticoagulation because of a duodenal ulcer 3 years previously. At age 36 years he presented with syncope accompanied by tachycardia and diaphoresis. His electrocardiogram at that time was notable for atrial fibrillation and inverted T waves in leads V_1–V_3. Five years later he complained of exertional dyspnea. A lung scan demonstrated a high probability of pulmonary embolism. At that time his mean pulmonary arterial pressure was 32 mmHg, and a pulmonary angiogram was positive for pulmonary embolism. He was placed on warfarin. During the ensuing 12 years of anticoagulation, his dyspnea worsened to the point where he could not pursue the active lifestyle that he desired.

Examination. Physical examination: the patient appeared normal. No abnormalities of skin, nail beds, or oral mucosa. Pulse: 94 beats/min, normal character, irregularly irregular. Blood pressure: 120/80 mmHg in right arm. Jugular venous pulse: 10 cm. Cardiac impulse: normal. First heart sound: normal: Second heart sound: split normally on inspiration. Gallop rhythm and grade 2/6 holosystolic murmur heard at left lower sternal border, which increased with inspiration. Chest examination: normal air entry, no rales or rhonchi. Abdominal examination: soft abdomen, no tenderness, and no masses. Normal liver span. No peripheral edema. Femoral, popliteal, posterior tibial, and dorsalis pedis pulses: all normal volume and equal. Carotid pulses: normal, no bruits. Optic fundi: normal.

Investigations. Electrocardiogram: atrial fibrillation at a rate of 94/min; QRS axis of 116°; right axis deviation; right ventricular hypertrophy; left posterior fascicular block; diffuse ST and T wave abnormalities. Echocardiogram: very enlarged and moderately hypertrophied right ventricle with moderately reduced systolic function; the left ventricle was relatively small with marked septal flattening and abnormal septal motion but preserved systolic function.

Questions

1. What is the pathophysiology of this patient's condition?
2. What risks are associated with various management strategies?
3. What further diagnostic tests might be considered?
4. What do you think was actually done in this case, and what was the outcome?

Answers

Answer to question 1 This patient has chronic thromboembolic pulmonary hypertension. Pulmonary hypertensive changes develop in the small muscular arteries and arterioles. The lesions include medial hypertrophy, concentric and eccentric intimal fibrosis, thrombotic lesions, and plexogenic lesions.

Dyspnea is associated with an increase in dead space ventilation, resulting in high minute ventilation demands and an inability of cardiac output to meet metabolic demands.

Findings on physical examination are influenced by the degree of pulmonary hypertension and right ventricular dysfunction that is present. This patient has evidence of tricuspid regurgitation and right heart failure on physical examination. This was corroborated by his electrocardiogram and echocardiogram.

Answer to question 2 If treated medically he would continue to receive warfarin and would be placed on round the clock oxygen. His dyspnea and right ventricular failure would, nevertheless, inexorably worsen. With pulmonary thromboendarterectomy he would have an operative mortality of about 10%. If he survived the operation, then he could expect substantial functional improvement.

Answer to question 3 If his functional disability were uncertain, then exercise testing could be done. Also, pulmonary function tests could be obtained. In this patient's case, these ancillary tests were not felt to be necessary in order to decide on a course of action.

Answer to question 4 Right heart catheterization and pulmonary angiography were repeated, as part of a preoperative evaluation for planned pulmonary thromboendarterectomy. Catheterization demonstrated a right atrial pressure of 10 mmHg, right ventricular pressure 55/10 mmHg, and pulmonary arterial pressure 55/28 mmHg, with a mean pulmonary arterial pressure of 35 mmHg. Pulmonary angiography (Figure 14.8a) revealed total occlusion of his left lower lobe pulmonary arteries.

He underwent pulmonary thromboendarterectomy. The surgeon endarterectomized multiple large thrombi that were chronic and laminated (Figure 14.8b). The patient has subsequently done well and is no longer incapacitated in any way. He runs a factory and hunts and fishes in his leisure time.

Case 14.3

A 67-year-old Hispanic man presented to the emergency department with a chief complaint of 6 days of shortness of breath. Hypertension was well controlled on verapamil SR 240 mg/day; he underwent surgery many years ago to correct an undescended testicle. He had no family history of venous thrombosis. He was a retired farmer and had quit smoking cigarettes 40 years ago.

Examination. Physical examination: the patient appeared to have mild respiratory distress. No abnormalities of skin, nail beds, or oral mucosa. Pulse: 100 beats/min, normal character. Blood pressure: 140/80 mmHg in right arm. Jugular venous pulse: 15 cm. Cardiac impulse: normal. First heart sound: normal: Second heart sound: single. No added sounds. Grade 1/6 holosystolic murmur at left lower sternal border. Chest examination: normal air entry, no rales or rhonchi. Abdominal examination: soft abdomen, no tenderness, and no masses. Normal liver span. No peripheral edema. Lower extremities appeared normal. Femoral, popliteal, posterior tibial, and dorsalis pedis pulses: all normal volume and equal. Carotid pulses: normal, no bruits. Optic fundi: normal.

Investigations. Electrocardiogram: emergency department (Figure 14.9a) and prior comparison electrocardiogram (Figure 14.9b) are provided.

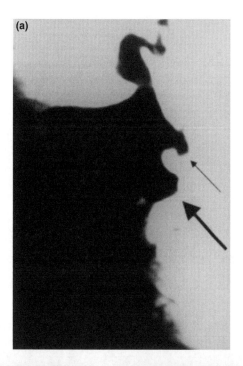

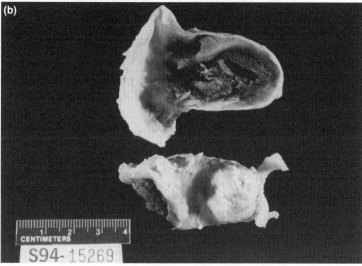

Figure 14.8 Pulmonary angiogram. **(a)** Left pulmonary arteriogram of a 53-year-old man (Case 14.2) with chronic pulmonary embolism causing total occlusion of left lower lobar pulmonary arteries (thin and thick arrows). **(b)** This patient underwent pulmonary thromboendarterectomy and large and extensive thrombi were surgically removed. The endarterectomy specimen contained laminated thrombus adherent to the endothelial wall

(a)

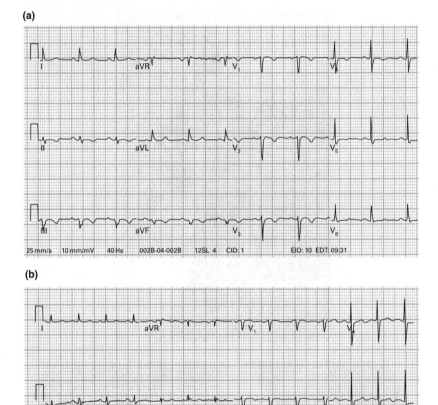

(b)

Figure 14.9 Electrocardiograms for the patient presented in Case 14.3. **(a)** Emergency department and **(b)** prior comparison electrocardiograms

Chest *x* ray: normal. Lung scan: emergency department (Figure 14.10) perfusion scan is provided. Ventilation scan: normal. Echocardiogram: emergency department echocardiogram (Figure 14.11) is provided; pulmonary arterial systolic pressure estimated at 50 mmHg.

Questions

1. Interpret the electrocardiograms (see Figure 14.9).
2. Interpret the lung scan (see Figure 14.10). What is the PIOPED estimate of the likelihood of pulmonary embolism?

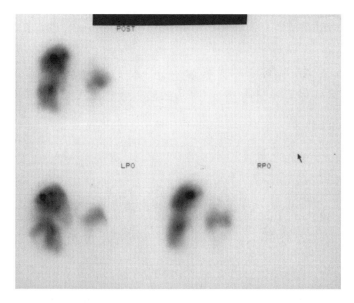

Figure 14.10 Emergency department perfusion lung scan for the patient presented in Case 14.3. Three views are shown. LPO, left posterior oblique; Post, posterior; RPO, right posterior oblique

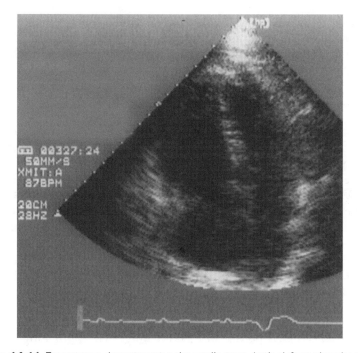

Figure 14.11 Emergency department echocardiogram (apical four chamber view) for the patient presented in Case 14.3

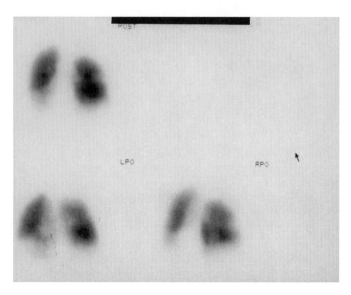

Figure 14.12 Perfusion lung scan 1 week after admission of the patient presented in Case 14.3. LPO, left posterior oblique; Post, posterior; RPO, right posterior oblique

3. Interpret the echocardiogram (see Figure 14.11).
4. How does the echocardiogram impact on the treatment plan?
5. What do you think was actually done in this case, and what was the outcome?

Answer

Answer to question 1 The emergency department electrocardiogram demonstrates a normal sinus rhythm at a rate of 63 beats/min. The QRS axis is –30°. The QRS interval is widened, indicating a mild intraventricular conduction defect. There are T-wave inversions in leads V_1–V_4. Without a prior electrocardiogram the significance of the T-wave inversions is uncertain. The prior comparison tracing is available, however, and we observe that the T-wave inversions were not present previously. Thus, the emergency department tracing suggests new right ventricular strain (see Box 14.2). Of note, in the emergency department the patient was not tachycardic and his axis had shifted leftward as compared with the prior electrocardiogram.

Answer to question 2 The lung scan (see Figure 14.10) shows markedly decreased perfusion of both lungs. The right lung is more affected than the left lung. In the presence of a normal chest *x* ray and ventilation scan, the lung scan reveals a high probability for

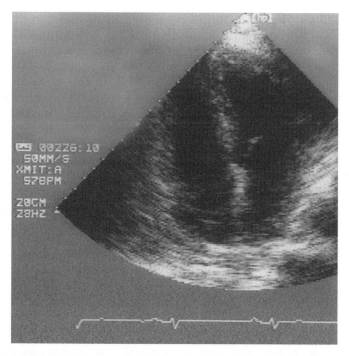

Figure 14.13 Echocardiogram (apical four chamber view) 1 week after admission of the patient presented in Case 14.3

pulmonary embolism. Because of the combination of high clinical suspicion and a high probability scan, the PIOPED estimate of pulmonary embolism at angiography is 96% (see Table 14.2).

Answer to question 3 The echocardiogram (see Figure 14.11), apical four chamber view, shows the left ventricle in the upper right, the right ventricle in the upper left, the left atrium in the lower right, and the right atrium in the lower left. The right ventricle and right atrium are dilated as compared with the left ventricle and left atrium. The right ventricular free wall was hypokinetic and, overall, there was moderate right ventricular hypokinesis.

Answer to question 4 The echocardiogram demonstrates right heart failure and risk stratifies this patient as having a pulmonary embolism with an ominous prognosis, despite his normal heart rate and blood pressure (see Figure 14.6). Even if he is treated with appropriate doses of heparin, he is at risk for recurrent pulmonary embolism.[15-17] The echocardiogram raises the consideration of primary therapy of the pulmonary embolism, either with thrombolysis or embolectomy.

Answer to question 5 Pulmonary embolism was suspected in the emergency department, and therefore he was heparinized before obtaining the lung scan and echocardiogram. The patient had no contraindications to thrombolysis. His blood pressure had been well controlled on verapamil SR 240 mg/day. With the hope of rapidly reversing his right heart failure, he received the US Food and Drug Administration approved dosing regimen of tissue-type plasminogen activator (tPA; i.e. 100 mg as a continuous infusion over 2 hours; see Box 14.4). During the 2 hour infusion of tPA, heparin was suspended. Heparin was then restarted, without a bolus, after the tPA infusion.

He experienced dramatic clinical improvement with rapid resolution of his dyspnea. One week later, just before hospital discharge, the lung scan and the echocardiogram were repeated. Both imaging tests were almost completely normal.

References

1 Goldhaber SZ. Pulmonary embolism. *N Engl J Med* 1998;339:93–104.
2 Goldhaber SZ, Ridker PM, eds. *Thrombosis and thromboembolism.* New York: Marcel Dekker, 2002.
3 Goldhaber SZ. Echocardiography in the management of pulmonary embolism. *Ann Intern Med* 2002;136:691–700.
4 Gelfand EV, Piazza G, Goldhaber SZ. Venous thromboembolism guidebook. *Crit Pathways Cardiol* 2002;1:26–43.
5 Goldhaber S. *Prevention of venous thromboembolism.* New York: Marcel Dekker, 1993.
6 Ridker P, Hennekens C, Lindpaintner K, Stampfer M, Eisenberg P, Miletich J. Mutation in the gene coding for coagulation factor V and risks of future myocardial infarction, stroke, and venous thrombosis in apparently healthy men. *N Engl J Med* 1995;332:912–17.
7 Come PC. Echocardiographic evaluation of pulmonary embolism and its response to therapeutic interventions. *Chest* 1992;101(suppl):151S–162S.
8 Muth CM, Shank ES. Gas embolism. *N Engl J Med* 2000;342:476–82.
9 Sreeram N, Cherlex E, Smeets J, Gorgels A, Wellens H. Value of the 12-lead electrocardiogram at hospital admission in the diagnosis of pulmonary embolism. *Am J Cardiol* 1994;73:298–303.
10 Jerjes-Sanchez C, Ramirez-Rivera A, Garcia ML, *et al.* Streptokinase and heparin versus heparin alone in massive pulmonary embolism: a randomized controlled trial. *J Thromb Thrombolysis* 1995;2:227–9.
11 Stein P, Goldhaber S, Henry J, Miller A. Arterial blood gas analysis in the assessment of suspected acute pulmonary embolism. *Chest* 1996;109:78–81.
12 PIOPED Investigators. Value of the ventilation/perfusion scan in acute pulmonary embolism. Results of the Prospective Investigation of Pulmonary Embolism Diagnosis (PIOPED). *JAMA* 1990;263:2753–9.
13 Bounameaux H, de Moerloose P, Perrier A, Reber G. Plasma measurement of D-dimer as diagnostic aid in suspected venous thromboembolism: an overview. *Thromb Haemost* 1994;71:1–6.
14 de Moerloose P, Minazio P, Reber G, Perrier A, Bounameaux H. D-dimer determination to exclude pulmonary embolism: a two-step approach using latex as a screening tool. *Thromb Haemost* 1994;72:89–91.
15 Goldhaber SZ, Simons GR, Elliott CG, *et al.* Quantitative plasma D-dimer levels among patients undergoing pulmonary angiography for suspected pulmonary embolism. *JAMA* 1993;270:2819–22.

16 Ginsberg JS. Management of venous thromboembolism. Review. *N Engl J Med* 1996;**335**:1816–28.

17 Goldhaber S, Haire W, Feldstein M, *et al*. Alteplase versus heparin in acute pulmonary embolism: randomized trial assessing right ventricular function and perfusion. *Lancet* 1993;**341**:507–11.

18 Greenfield LJ, Proctor MC, Williams DM, Wakefield TW. Long-term experience with transvenous catheter pulmonary embolectomy. *J Vasc Surg* 1993;**18**:450–7.

19 Koning R, Cribier A, Gerber L, *et al*. A new treatment for severe pulmonary embolism: percutaneous rheolytic thrombectomy. *Circulation* 1997;**96**:2498–500.

20 Aklog L, Williams CS, Byrne JG, Goldhaber SZ. Acute pulmonary embolectomy: a contemporary approach. *Circulation* 2002;**105**:1416–19.

15: Non-cardiac surgery in patients with heart disease

THOMAS H LEE

Management of the patient with cardiac disease through non-cardiac surgical procedures is a common and difficult challenge for internists, cardiologists, surgeons, and anesthesiologists. The goal of the initial evaluation is often described as a request for "clearance" of the patient for the procedure, but this terminology is inappropriate and even risky from a medicolegal perspective, because the term "clearance" implies a guarantee that the procedure will not have complications. Every procedure, even in patients without any apparent risk factors, carries some chance of complications. Hence, the true objectives include the following:

- to assess the patient's risk for cardiac complications
- to determine whether specialized cardiac testing may be appropriate to refine this risk assessment
- to identify risk reduction strategies
- to manage the patient postoperatively in order to reduce risk and detect complications.

An important principle in the management of patients with cardiac disease through non-cardiac surgery is that the strategy should minimize the patient's overall risk for poor outcomes.[1] Therefore, clinicians cannot restrict their assessment to the risk associated with the procedure itself; they must also consider the risk associated with alternative strategies. For example, evaluation of the patient with coronary artery disease and an abnormal stress perfusion imaging scan who is about to undergo vascular surgery must include an estimate of the risk of the procedure with, and without, coronary revascularization. It should also include an estimate of the mortality with coronary angiography and revascularization, the risk for stroke and non-fatal myocardial infarction with various strategies, and the possibility that the test has provided a false positive result (Table 15.1).[2]

There are rarely "right" or "wrong" answers to the questions that arise in the care of the patient with heart disease who is undergoing non-cardiac surgery, because even the most carefully considered strategy will be associated with some finite rate of complications. Instead, clinicians should seek to keep that complication rate to a

Table 15.1 Probability of various outcomes for patients undergoing vascular surgery with positive dipyridamole thallium scans

Factor	Baseline (%)	Range (%)
Mortality		
Coronary angiography	0·3	0·1–0·5
Coronary angioplasty	1·8	1·0–2·5
Coronary bypass surgery:		
Elective	3·6	2·0–5·0
Emergency	6·1	3·4–8·5
Vascular surgery in presence of:		
Trivial coronary disease	1·5	0·8–3·3
Operable coronary disease	4·5	2·3–10
Inoperable coronary disease	9·0	4·6–20
Non-fatal myocardial infarction		
Coronary angiography	0·15	0·07–0·25
Coronary angioplasty	6·0	3·0–10·0
Coronary bypass surgery	5·8	3·0–10·0
Vascular surgery in presence of:		
Trivial coronary disease	2·0	0·5–4·0
Operable coronary disease	6·0	3·3–10·0
Inoperable coronary disease	9·0	5·0–15·0
Non-fatal stroke		
Coronary angiography	0·15	0·07–0·25
Coronary angioplasty	0·15	0·05–0·30
Coronary bypass surgery	1·5	1·0–3·0
Vascular surgery	0·5	0·1–1·7
Costs (in US$1000s)		
Coronary angiography	6	4·0–9·0
Coronary angioplasty	15	8·0–20·0
Coronary bypass surgery	32	23·0–45·0
Vascular surgery	24	17·5–31·0
Risk reduction by PTCA or CABG		
Death	66	50–80
Non-fatal myocardial infarction	50	35–70
Diagnostic testing		
Pretest probability of coronary artery disease	60	30–90
Sensitivity of dipyridamole thallium	80	NA
Specificity of dipyridamole thallium	78	NA
Post-test probability	85	61–97
Vascular surgery patients:		
Trivial disease	41	32–66
Operable disease	55	30–64
Inoperable	4	3–5
Operable patients treated with PTCA	50	30–70

This table shows estimates of various outcomes and costs that were considered in a decision analysis examining various strategies for patients undergoing vascular surgery who had abnormal dipyridamole thallium scintigraphy tests. For references used to derive these estimates, see the original article.[2] CABG, coronary artery bypass grafting; NA, not applicable; PTCA, percutaneous transluminal coronary angioplasty minimum through careful clinical evaluation, judicious use of tests, and close postoperative follow up. Recent guidelines can assist in these choices.[3]

Risk assessment

Because of demographic trends and technical advances, an increasing number of elderly patients are now considered candidates for major non-cardiac surgical procedures. In addition to their advanced age, these patients have high rates of chronic health problems. Furthermore, they are more likely to have one of the major predictors of increased perioperative cardiovascular risk (myocardial infarction, heart failure, and death), including the following[3]: unstable angina or a myocardial infarction within 1 month, decompensated heart failure, significant arrhythmias (high grade atrioventricular block, symptomatic ventricular arrhythmias, underlying heart disease, and supraventricular arrhythmias with poor rate control), and severe valvular heart disease (especially aortic stenosis). Although patients undergoing these procedures are older and sicker and one might suspect that the complication rates ought to be rising for non-cardiac surgery, the rates of adverse outcomes have actually decreased over the past 20 years. Perioperative myocardial infarction occurs after elective procedures in only about 1% of cases, and cardiac deaths occur in only about 0·5% of general surgical patients.

This risk varies widely for different types of procedures (Table 15.2).[3] In general, abdominal aortic aneurysm and other major vascular surgery carry the highest risk for cardiac complications, whereas major elective orthopedic surgery carries a low risk for such events. The clinician who is caring for a patient with heart disease should not assume that similar strategies should be used for different types of operations. For example, a more aggressive strategy, perhaps leading to coronary angiography and revascularization, might be appropriate for patients with stable angina undergoing abdominal aortic aneurysm repair. However, if these same patients were undergoing a cataract operation or even a total hip replacement, then a more conservative approach should be used, with emphasis on careful monitoring of hemodynamic status during and after surgery.

The preoperative evaluation is therefore undergoing constant change and has evolved into a search for a "needle in a haystack" (i.e. the high risk patient amid a population with a very low overall risk). In this search, the clinician must rely on a limited database to identify higher risk candidates who may warrant special management strategies. These clinical data usually include a history, physical

Table 15.2 Risk for cardiac death or non-fatal myocardial infarction with non-cardiac surgical procedures

Degree of risk	Procedures
High (often >5%)	Emergency major operations (especially in the elderly)
	Major vascular surgery (especially of the aorta)
	Peripheral vascular surgery
	Procedures with anticipated major blood loss and/or fluid shifts
Intermediate (usually <5%)	Intraperitoneal and intrathoracic surgery
	Carotid endarterectomy
	Head and neck surgery
	Prostate surgery
	Orthopedic surgery
Low (preoperative cardiac testing usually not required)	Endoscopic procedures
	Cataract surgery
	Breast surgery
	Superficial procedure (Mohs' surgery)

Data from the American College of Cardiology/American Heart Association[3]

examination, chest radiography, electrocardiogram, and a serum chemistry evaluation of renal function. More specialized (and costly) testing technologies should be reserved for specific subsets of this patient population. Importantly, stress testing and other non-invasive tests used to detect myocardial ischemia should not be used routinely for perioperative risk stratification.[4]

Coronary artery disease

Recent acute myocardial infarction

The most important cause of cardiac complications after non-cardiac surgery is coronary artery disease, and recent acute myocardial infarction has traditionally been recognized as the worst prognostic factor. Pooled data from the 1960s and 1970s indicated that recurrent myocardial infarction or cardiac death occurred in about 30% of patients who underwent non-cardiac surgery within 3–6 months. Complication rates were about 5% if more than 6 months had elapsed since acute myocardial infarction. More recent data indicate that the risk for complications after recent myocardial infarction has fallen, and that the risk is fairly stable at about 2% 3 months after the infarction.[5] Undoubtedly, patient selection plays an important role in the achievement of such low complication rates, and one should not assume that all postinfarction patients can undergo non-cardiac procedures with low risk. However, improved surgical and anesthesia techniques, wider use of hemodynamic monitoring, and the impact of coronary revascularization procedures have all contributed to this improvement.

Many patients with acute myocardial infarction, or needing revascularization, undergo percutaneous coronary interventions and intracoronary stent placement. Because some data suggest a high stent thrombosis rate for elective surgery performed within 2 weeks of stent placement, recent guidelines suggest delaying elective surgery for 2–4 weeks.[3] In addition patients at risk for myocardial ischemia undergoing non-cardiac or vascular surgery appear to benefit from perioperative β-blocker therapy, which reduces early and late cardiovascular morbidity and mortality.[6,7] It is recommended that, in the absence of major contraindications, prophylactic β-blockade should be used in intermediate and high risk patients who are not already taking β-blockers, and especially in patients for whom coronary revascularization is not a serious consideration.[3] When possible the β-blocker dose should be adjusted to achieve a resting heart rate of 50–60 beats/min and this is most easily accomplished in the weeks before elective procedures.

The data relating to non-cardiac surgery following myocardial infarction have led to recommendations that purely elective surgery be delayed until 6 months after the acute event.[8] When emergency surgery is necessary, patients who have had more recent infarctions should undergo hemodynamic monitoring with a pulmonary artery catheter and arterial line. Fluctuations in left heart filling pressures or blood pressure should be treated promptly. When surgery is semielective, but prolonged delay may carry its own risks, such as in a patient with a potentially resectable malignancy, surgery can be undertaken at 4–6 weeks after infarction if the patient is judged to be at low risk on the basis of performance on a stress test. Higher risk patients should be considered for coronary angiography and revascularization with either bypass graft surgery or percutaneous coronary angioplasty before their non-cardiac operations, provided the combined morbidity and mortality of the investigations, revascularization, and the non-cardiac surgery are thought to be acceptable as compared with the risk associated with non-cardiac surgery alone.

Unstable angina

Patients with unstable angina are rarely considered for elective non-cardiac surgery, and patients with recent episodes of unstable angina can be considered comparable to patients who have had recent myocardial infarctions. Elective surgery should generally be postponed until the patient's functional status has improved and ischemic symptoms are stabilized. Non-invasive and invasive testing should be considered for preoperative risk stratification. If the operation cannot be delayed, then the patient should undergo the procedure with hemodynamic monitoring to reduce volume shifts that may induce ischemia. Patients with unstable cardiac ischemic syndromes who must undergo higher risk procedures, such as major vascular operations, may benefit from use of an intra-aortic balloon pump. An alternative strategy that is often used in patients who require vascular operations such as carotid endarterectomy is simultaneous performance of the non-cardiac operation and coronary artery bypass graft surgery.

Stable angina

Patients with stable angina who have ischemic chest pain only with strenuous physical exertion have a low overall risk for complications. However, physicians can be misled by casual histories of the frequency of angina. This is because patients often reduce their activity levels to avoid cardiac or non-cardiac symptoms, particularly if they have non-cardiac conditions that limit their mobility. Some clinicians therefore have a low threshold for performing coronary angiography and revascularization procedures for operative patients with angina or histories of myocardial infarction.

In apparent support of this approach are non-randomized data demonstrating that patients with New York Heart Association functional class I or II anginal symptoms have higher mortality rates with non-cardiac surgery if they have not undergone previous coronary artery bypass graft surgery.[9] However, the operative mortality risk associated with elective coronary artery bypass graft surgery would counterbalance potential benefits of this strategy in patients with mild stable angina (see Table 15.1). Thus, instead of routine angiography, evaluation of patients with stable angina should focus on assessment of the threshold at which ischemia is induced, which is usually readily accomplished by stress testing if the clinician is concerned after taking a careful angina history. Low risk patients are those with either no ischemia during stress testing or ischemia induced at a high level of exercise (>7 METs), and high risk patients are those whose angina or ischemia is induced at a low level of activity (<4 METs, equivalent to light house work or walking one to two blocks on level ground).[3]

Functional status   Regardless of whether a patient has known or suspected coronary disease, a major determinant of surgical risk is functional status. In general, patients who are in functional class I or early class II (which implies that they can do exercise equivalent to carrying two grocery bags up a flight of stairs) can achieve a heart rate and blood pressure equivalent to what would be expected with general anesthesia and surgery. If such an activity level can be achieved, then the risk for perioperative infarction is probably no higher than 1–4%, with a risk for perioperative cardiac death below 2%.

Congestive heart failure

Patients with a history of congestive heart failure are at increased risk for perioperative volume overload and other major cardiovascular complications (Table 15.3).[10] Pulmonary edema occurs in about 16% of patients who have signs or symptoms of congestive heart failure at the time of surgery, with an even higher risk among patients who have jugular venous distension or an third heart sound (S_3) gallop (Table 15.3). Patients who have a history of heart failure but who are not in failure at the time of surgery have about a 6% risk for pulmonary edema – a finding that suggests that appropriate treatment of the manifestations of heart failure may reduce complication rates. New onset of pulmonary edema or heart failure is rare in patients with no history of heart failure, and when it occurs it is related to a postoperative myocardial infarction in about 30% of cases.

One important reason for the increased risk for complications is the volume shifts associated with surgery; hence, procedures associated with larger volume shifts, such as major vascular procedures, have been found to carry an increased risk for complications. The risk associated with these shifts is exacerbated by the effects of anesthetic agents, which include impairment in cardiac contractility and vasodilatation. Finally, diuretic therapy can lead to a mild hypovolemic state in many patients that has no hemodynamic consequences under normal conditions but can contribute to hypotension when vasodilator agents are administered. Therefore, diuretic therapy should usually be withheld before surgery in patients whose examination reveals an orthostatic fall in blood pressure.

The management of patients who are at high risk for postoperative pulmonary edema may be improved by perioperative hemodynamic monitoring with a pulmonary artery catheter.[11] For patients with severe heart failure and low blood pressures, intra-arterial blood pressure monitoring may also help guide treatment.

Valvular heart disease

Aortic stenosis

Patients with preoperative valvular heart disease have about a 20% risk for new, or worse, heart failure developing during the perioperative period. In the preoperative evaluation of patients with heart murmurs, the most important lesion to detect is severe aortic

Table 15.3 Correlation between preoperative clinical findings and postoperative heart failure

Characteristic	n (total = 1001)	Pulmonary edema (%)	Worsened heart failure or pulmonary edema (%)
No prior history of heart failure	853	2	4
History of heart failure but not evident on preoperative examination or chest radiography	87	6	16
Left heart failure on preoperative examination or chest radiography	66	16*	26*
Jugular venous distension	23	30*	35*
S_3 gallop	17	35*	47*
History of pulmonary edema	22	23*	32*
Preoperative NYHA functional class for CHF:			
I	935	3	5
II	15	7	7
III	34	6	8
IV	17	25	31

*$P<0.01$ (comparison of patients with findings with those without). CHF, congestive heart failure; NYHA, New York Heart Association. Table adapted with permission from Goldman et al.[10]

stenosis. This lesion is increasing in prevalence as the population ages, and carries risks for perioperative mortality as high as 13%.[5] The narrowing of the aortic valve restricts the ability of the cardiac output to rise in response to vasodilatation or volume loss, thus placing the patient at high risk for shock. In addition, the left ventricular hypertrophy that is induced by high pressures within this chamber leads to a decrease in ventricular compliance and impaired diastolic filling. Therefore, these patients may become unstable, with the development of hypovolemia, tachycardia, or atrial fibrillation.

Echocardiography with Doppler analysis allows a reliable non-invasive diagnosis of aortic stenosis. In the vast majority of patients with advanced symptoms, such as chest pain, syncope, or evidence of heart failure, aortic valve replacement should be strongly considered before non-cardiac surgery. If, on careful questioning, a patient with non-invasive evidence of aortic stenosis does not have any of these symptoms despite a reasonable activity level, then the patient may undergo most operations without valve replacement, but should have invasive hemodynamic monitoring initiated before surgery and for 24–48 hours postoperatively. Occasionally, a patient may have evidence of severe aortic stenosis but be asymptomatic because non-cardiac conditions greatly limit the patient's activity level; if the cardiac stress of the planned general surgical procedure clearly exceeds the stress of the activities that the patients can perform, then aortic valve replacement may be indicated even in the absence of cardiac symptoms. Finally, in patients with severe aortic stenosis who are not candidates for aortic valve surgery or who refuse surgery, non-cardiac surgery can be performed with a mortality of approximately 10%. Rarely, aortic balloon valvuloplasty is performed in an attempt to reduce the risk associated with non-cardiac surgery.

Mitral stenosis

In patients with mitral stenosis, tachycardia associated with the stresses of surgery can lead to a precipitous fall in cardiac output and development of pulmonary edema caused by a decrease in emptying time for the left atrium. Fluid shifts that might be well tolerated by a patient without mitral stenosis can cause major changes in cardiac output, because high filling pressures are needed to force blood across the stenotic valve. Hence, blood loss or venodilatation can decrease left ventricular filling and compromise output. However, vigorous volume replacement can lead to pulmonary edema. Patients with moderate or severe mitral stenosis may therefore benefit from invasive hemodynamic monitoring if significant fluid shifts are expected with surgery. Perioperative heart rate control and avoidance of excess volume shifts is the key to safe non-cardiac surgery in the patient with mitral stenosis.

Patients with mitral stenosis are also at increased risk for development of supraventricular tachyarrhythmias. If a supraventricular tachycardia develops, then the cardiac output may fall even in patients with only mild or moderate severity of mitral stenosis. The consequences can be hypotension and pulmonary edema. In the past, many clinicians prescribed digitalis for patients with mitral stenosis and normal sinus rhythm in an attempt to prevent a rapid ventricular response if atrial fibrillation or another supraventricular tachycardia occurred. The ability of "on board" digitalis to slow the initial ventricular response to a tachyarrhythmia at a time of heightened sympathetic activity is questionable; furthermore, intravenous calcium channel blockers (verapamil and diltiazem) or β-blockers (esmolol) are now available to control heart rate. Adenosine can be used to terminate supraventricular arrhythmias.

Aortic and mitral regurgitation

In chronic aortic and mitral regurgitation the left ventricle is subjected to high volume loads that can cause a loss of contractility. These patients are at increased risk for volume overload during the perioperative period, but they are not as sensitive to small shifts in hemodynamic status or changes in heart rate as are patients with aortic stenosis or mitral stenosis. Therefore, patients with regurgitant lesions can often be managed without hemodynamic monitoring during the perioperative period if they are not in congestive heart failure at the time of the preoperative evaluation. The clinician should be aware that even minor reductions in left ventricular systolic function (left ventricular ejection fraction) in patients with mitral regurgitation may be an indicator of impaired ventricular function and contractile reserve because the low impedance left atrium is "reducing the afterload" of the ventricle.

Antibiotics and anticoagulants

Patients with any of these valvular abnormalities or with prosthetic valves should receive appropriate antibiotic prophylaxis before procedures that are associated with bacteremia. In addition, patients with prosthetic valves may require other special management strategies. Patients who have been anticoagulated because of a non-bioprosthetic valve may encounter thromboembolic complications when anticoagulation is discontinued around the time of surgery. This risk appears to be higher with caged-disk prostheses used in the mitral valve position than in the aortic valve position. When warfarin is stopped it takes about 4 days for the International Normalized Ratio (INR) to reach 1·5, when surgery can be performed safely.[12] After warfarin is restarted about 3 days are required for the INR to reach 2·0. Therefore, the temporary discontinuation of warfarin exposes the patient to the risk for thromboembolism equivalent to 1 day without anticoagulation before and after surgery. If necessary, intravenous heparin therapy can be used to bridge this gap.

A reasonable strategy that balances the risk for such events against the risk for perioperative bleeding is to stop oral anticoagulants in patients with prosthetic valves in the aortic position 2–3 days before surgery, and to perform the operation when the prothrombin time has fallen to within 1–2 seconds of the control value. Once hemostasis is achieved postoperatively (usually at 12–24 hours) intravenous heparin is initiated and continued until therapeutic anticoagulation with oral warfarin is achieved. For patients with mechanical prostheses in the mitral position, a similar approach can be used except that intravenous heparin should be initiated preoperatively as soon as warfarin is discontinued, and continued until about 6 hours before surgery. This approach, which reflects the higher embolic risk in such patients, may necessitate admission about 2–3 days before surgery.

Hypertrophic cardiomyopathy

Patients with hypertrophic cardiomyopathy are at increased risk for hemodynamic instability with non-cardiac surgery. The cause of pulmonary edema in these patients is left ventricular stiffness, which leads to impaired diastolic filling and, in some patients, a dynamic obstructive outflow gradient. Any perturbation that reduces left ventricular volume (reduced blood volume, increased venous capacitance, decreased systemic vascular resistance) will increase the outflow obstruction. Drugs that increase myocardial contractility, such as β-adrenergic agonists (for example, dobutamine), should be avoided in these patients, whereas β-blockers and calcium channel blocking agents may be useful in optimizing hemodynamics by both slowing the heart rate and improving ventricular relaxation. Because increased left ventricular filling pressures and adequate left ventricular volume are critical for maintenance of cardiac output, volume depletion, drug-induced venodilatation, and new atrial fibrillation are hazardous for these patients. Adverse cardiac events in these patients at the time of non-cardiac surgerey are related to major surgery of long duration.[3] In these patients, spinal anesthesia must be used only with extreme caution.[13] If major fluid shifts are expected, then a pulmonary artery catheter should be considered. Hypotension occurring during or after surgery should be promptly treated with volume expansion.

Arrhythmias

Arrhythmias and conduction abnormalities occur commonly during the perioperative period, regardless of whether patients have underlying heart disease and regardless of the type of anesthesia. Among 5013 patients undergoing surgery, Vanik and Davis[14] found a 16% incidence of arrhythmias among patients with no known heart disease. Clinically significant arrhythmias occurred in only about 0·7% of patients without cardiac histories, but in patients with a prior history of heart disease with or without arrhythmias, 174 (32%) of 551 patients had perioperative arrhythmias, including 14 (3%) who had clinically significant arrhythmias.

Patients with five or more ventricular premature contractions (VPCs) per minute at any time are at increased risk for perioperative

Table 15.4 Multifactorial Index of Cardiac Risk in non-cardiac surgery

Aspect of assessment	Finding	Points
History	Myocardial infarction within 6 months	10
	Age over 70 years	5
Physical examination	S_3 or jugular venous distension	11
	Important aortic stenosis	3
Electrocardiogram	Rhythm other than sinus or sinus plus APBs on last preoperative electrocardiogram	7
	More than five premature ventricular beats/min at any time preoperatively	7
	Poor general medical status*	3
	Intraperitoneal, intrathoracic, or aortic surgery	3
	Emergency operation	4
Total		53

*Electrolyte abnormalities (potassium <3·0 mEq/l [3·0 mmol/l] or HCO_3 <20 mEq/l [<20 mmol/l]); renal insufficiency (blood urea nitrogen >50 mg/dl [>17·9 mmol/l] or creatinine >3·0 mg/dl [>265 μmol/l]); abnormal blood gases (partial O_2 tension <60 mmHg or partial CO_2 tension >50 mmHg); abnormal liver status (elevated serum aspartate transaminase or signs on physical examination of chronic liver disease); or any condition that has caused the patient to be chronically bedridden. APB, atrial premature beat; S_3, third heart sound. Adapted with permission from Goldman et al.[15]

cardiac complications (Tables 15.4 and 15.5).[15–19] However, the clinical importance of VPCs (and of supraventricular arrhythmias) appears to be as a marker for underlying myocardial dysfunction. In general, in patients without evidence of structural heart disease, the presence of complex VPCs is not associated with increased cardiac mortality or morbidity.[20]

The patient with ventricular arrhythmias and myocardial dysfunction is at higher risk for perioperative congestive heart failure and cardiac death, but this risk is mainly a reflection of the myocardial dysfunction. Prophylactic antiarrhythmic therapy will not correct the underlying dysfunction. Therefore, such therapy should be reserved for patients with serious arrhythmias, such as those with histories of hemodynamically significant ventricular arrhythmias or sudden death. A general principle is that addition of new drugs just before a patient goes into the operating room is not advisable; if arrhythmias worsen or become hemodynamically significant, then the anesthesiologist can respond quickly.

Similarly, prophylactic placement of a temporary pacemaker is rarely indicated for asymptomatic conduction abnormalities such as preoperative sinus bradycardia or chronic bifascicular heart block

Table 15.5 Major complication rates in studies that analyzed the multifactorial risk index

		Study (patients)			
Class	Definition (points)	Goldman et al.[15] (unselected non-cardiac surgery patients >40 years old)	Zeldin[17] (unselected non-cardiac surgery patients >40 years old)	Detsky et al.[18] (preoperative medical consultations)	Jeffrey et al.[19] (abdominal aortic aneurysm surgery)
I	0–5	5/537 (1%)	4/590 (1%)	8/134 (6%)	4/56 (7%)
II	6–12	21/316 (7%)	13/453 (3%)	6/85 (7%)	4/35 (11%)
III	13–25	18/130 (14%)	11/74 (15%)	9/45 (20%)	3/8 (38%)
IV	≥26	14/18 (78%)	7/23 (30%)	4/4 (100%)	0
All patients		58/1001 (6%)	35/1140 (3%)	27/268 (10%)	11/99 (11%)

Complication rates by multifactorial risk index. Adapted with permission from Goldman[16]

(i.e. left bundle branch block or complete right bundle branch block with anterior or posterior fascicular block). Pacemakers should generally be reserved for patients who meet criteria for permanent pacemaker implantation. If the planned surgery is elective, then a permanent pacemaker can be placed beforehand. If the procedure is emergent or is likely to induce a transient bacteremia, a temporary pacemaker may be inserted preoperatively, and a permanent pacemaker can be placed subsequently.

Some cardiologists recommend that an exception to this policy be made for patients with preoperative left bundle branch block who undergo perioperative placement of a pulmonary artery catheter. This procedure is associated with the development of a new right bundle branch block in about 5% of cases.[21] Although a new right bundle branch block may be well tolerated by most patients, in the presence of a left bundle branch block it can occasionally lead to development of complete heart block. Hence, a method for ventricular pacing should be available before right heart catheterization in patients with a left bundle branch block.

Pacemakers and implantable cardioverter–defibrillators

Radiofrequency current, which flows between the device and an indifferent electrode on the patient's skin, is used with electrocautery during surgery. If the cautery device is close to the pacemaker or if the current path flows along the axis of the pacemaker or implantable cardioverter–defibrillator (ICD) lead, then the pacemaker or ICD may reset, or be inhibited or stimulated. The use of bipolar pacer leads has reduced, but not eliminated, the likelihood of this happening. The following recommendations are made if surgical procedures are contemplated.[3]

- The device should be interrogated to determine the patient's natural rhythm, and the battery strength and pacemaker settings.
- During surgery rate responsive programs should be deactivated.
- ICD devices should be programmed off during surgery.
- Pacing thresholds should be evaluated if the patient is pacer dependent.
- If cardioversion is required then the paddles should be placed as far from the device as possible and oriented in the direction most likely to be perpendicular to the device leads, which is usually an anteroposterior paddle position.

Other risk factors

The risk for perioperative cardiac death is about 10 times higher for patients older than 70 years than for younger patients, even after adjustment for their higher prevalence of cardiac disease and other conditions.[9] Risk assessment of elderly patients is therefore particularly important, but it may be complicated by the high prevalence of comorbid medical conditions among the elderly and hindered by inability of many elderly patients to undergo treadmill exercise testing. Because the risk for cardiac complications is highest in patients who cannot exercise, alternative tests for evaluating the inducibility of ischemia are particularly useful in this population (see below).

The type and timing of the surgery are also important predictors of perioperative cardiovascular risk (see Table 15.1). Major intra-abdominal, intrathoracic, or aortic procedures are associated with higher risks than are other types of operations,[9] presumably because of factors including the prevalence of coronary artery disease in patients who require these procedures; hemodynamic and electrolyte shifts associated with the surgery; and the degree of respiratory compromise and postoperative pain associated with these procedures. The risk associated with any operation increases fourfold if it is performed emergently instead of electively, probably because of general medical problems that cannot be corrected before emergency operations. Abnormalities such as hypoxia, carbon dioxide retention, acidosis, hypokalemia, elevated liver function enzyme levels, and evidence of renal failure are all associated with increased risk.

Cardiac Risk Index

Perhaps the best known system for integrating clinical data in order to estimate the risk for cardiac complications with non-cardiac surgery is the Cardiac Risk Index, which was developed by Goldman *et al.* in the 1970s on the basis of prospectively collected data on 1001 patients (see Table 15.3).[9] In the Cardiac Risk Index, points are assigned to each factor that can be used to place patients into approximate risk classes (see Table 15.4). In the original series of patients, more than half of all patients were placed into risk class I, and the risk for life-threatening or fatal cardiac complications in such patients was less than 1%. In risk classes II and III, the rate of complications was higher, but only 2% of patients died perioperatively. Only 18 patients were in risk class IV, but 56% of them died from cardiac causes.

In prospective testing at other institutions in varying patient populations the Cardiac Risk Index stratified patients reliably into risk groups, but recent data indicate that lower mortality rates can be achieved in high risk patients through patient selection and hemodynamic monitoring.[16] Furthermore, the Cardiac Risk Index may not fully reflect the impact on risk of factors such as the precise type of surgery performed, prior histories of class III or IV angina, remote myocardial, and pulmonary edema. Modifications to adjust for such factors have been proposed, and updated versions of the Cardiac Risk Index can be expected in the years ahead. However, improvements in risk stratification based upon routine clinical data are likely to be incremental at best.

Data from 4315 patients aged 50 years or older at Brigham and Women's Hospital[22] indicate that the Cardiac Risk Index continued to stratify patients according to their risk for complications; however, more than 90% of patients undergoing elective procedures fall into low risk classes (classes I and II). As a result, even though the Cardiac Risk Index remains valid, most patients who suffer major complications are in low risk classes. In that study, six independent predictors of complications were identified and included in a Revised Cardiac Risk Index. These predictors are as follows: high risk surgery, history of ischemic heart disease, history of congestive heart failure, history of cerebrovascular disease, preoperative treatment with insulin, and preoperative serum creatinine greater than 2·0 mg/dl (>177 mmol/l). Receiver operating characteristic curve analysis in the validation cohort indicated that the diagnostic performance of this Revised Cardiac Risk Index was superior to that of other published risk prediction indices. New types of data to improve the clinical evaluation, such as the information available from non-invasive tests, are likely to have greater impact on preoperative risk assessment than a more refined risk index.

Another useful approach was described by Ashton *et al.*,[23] based on data collected from a Veterans Affairs Medical Center population of 1487 men undergoing major non-emergent non-cardiac operations (Table 15.6). This population had a relatively high overall rate of

Table 15.6 Incidence of perioperative infarction, cardiac mortality, and all-cause mortality in a Veterans Affairs Medical Center population

Strata (description)	Estimated prevalence of coronary disease	AMI	Cardiac deaths	Overall deaths
High risk (patients with coronary artery disease: history of MI or ECG evidence of MI, typical angina pectoris, angiographically documented significant coronary artery disease, or history of coronary bypass surgery)	Nearly 100%	4·1%	2·3%	4·1%
Intermediate risk (patients without evident coronary artery disease but with atherosclerotic disease elsewhere: history of stroke, previous or planned vascular surgery, carotid bruit, transient ischemic attack, claudication, or atypical chest pain)	30–70%	0·8%	0·4%	3·5%
Low risk (patients without evidence of atherosclerotic disease but who are either older than 75 years or who have a high atherogenic risk factor profile: based on age, sex, smoking, blood pressure, glucose tolerance, and cholesterol, patients who have a ≥15% likelihood of a cardiac event within 6 years)	5–30%	0	0·4%	3·1%
Negligible risk (patients without evidence of atherosclerosis and with low atherogenic risk factor profiles)	Almost 0%	Not known	0	1·2%

ECG, electrocardiographic; MI, myocardial infarction. Adapted from Ashton et al.[23]

perioperative myocardial infarction, and so the rates cited (Table 15.6) may not be accurate in other populations. However, those data demonstrate the low rate of major complications even in patients in intermediate and high risk categories.

Specialized testing

Patients with evidence of ischemia during preoperative non-invasive testing have higher rates of cardiac complications with non-cardiac surgery, but clinicians should not assume that all patients require non-invasive testing, or that all patients with abnormal test results should undergo coronary angiography and revascularization. These tests should be performed when the information might change management. Hence, they are not likely to be useful for patients who are at such low risk for complications that an abnormal exercise test is not likely to alter management, such as a patient with atypical chest pain who is undergoing cataract surgery. Similarly, non-invasive testing is not likely to alter the management of very high risk patients, such as those with ischemic pain at low levels of exertion or rest. These patients usually warrant aggressive management of their coronary artery disease before any elective non-cardiac procedures. Eagle et al.[24] recommended that testing technologies be reserved for routine use in patients with intermediate probabilities of complications, such as patients with one or two clinical predictors of adverse outcomes.

The recent guidelines[3] stratify intermediate risk patients (those with mild angina, prior myocardial infarction, compensated or prior heart failure, diabetes mellitus, or renal insufficiency) into those who have moderate or excellent functional capacity and those who do not (i.e. <4 METs). In intermediate risk patients with moderate or excellent functional capacity, only those undergoing a high risk surgical procedure require non-invasive testing. Patients with stable angina usually do well with most major non-cardiac operations if angina is their only risk factor, but the clinician must determine whether patients with apparently stable angina are active enough so that they routinely increase cardiovascular work to a level comparable to that of surgery. If the patient's activity level is uncertain, then a test aimed at provoking ischemia may provide important information. Patients with poor functional capacity (<4 METs) all undergo non-invasive testing, and if this suggests significant myocardium at risk (reversible ischemia) then empiric β-blockade or coronary angiography is recommended. If the patient undergoes coronary angiography, then subsequent care is dictated by angiography findings and treatment results, and can include cancellation or delay of surgery, coronary revascularization preceding non-cardiac surgery, or intensified medical care.

Many patients cannot undergo adequate treadmill exercise testing because of poor conditioning or non-cardiac disorders, but various non-invasive tests are now available to assist in the evaluation of these patients. These tests use pharmacologic agents including dipyridamole, adenosine, and dobutamine to provoke ischemia. Methods for detecting ischemia include various radionuclides and echocardiography. An alternative to these tests is ambulatory ischemia monitoring, which uses ST-segment patterns to detect electrocardiographic ischemia.[25] Data demonstrating the superiority of any one testing technology over the others are not impressive; hence, clinicians should develop an understanding of the testing technologies that are most readily available at their institutions.

Even if patients have an abnormal test result, coronary angiography and revascularization is not always clearly the best strategy. A decision analysis was conducted in order to explore whether preoperative coronary angiography and revascularization versus proceeding directly to surgery improved short-term outcomes.[2] This decision analysis focused on patients who were undergoing elective vascular surgery who had either no angina or mild angina, and a positive dipyridamole thallium scan result. The researchers used published data (see Table 15.1) to compare the expected outcomes of three major strategies:

- proceeding directly to surgery
- coronary angiography, followed by coronary revascularization for patients with high risk coronary anatomy; in this strategy vascular surgery would be canceled in patients with severe inoperable coronary artery disease
- Coronary angiography, followed by coronary revascularization for high risk coronary anatomy before vascular surgery; in this strategy vascular surgery would be undertaken in patients with inoperable coronary disease.

Among the factors considered in the analysis were the mortality of performing vascular surgery in the presence of trivial coronary diseases (estimate 1·5%), operable coronary disease (estimate 4·5%), and inoperable coronary disease (estimate 9%). Other key factors included the mortality associated with coronary angiography and revascularization, and the sensitivity and specificity of non-invasive testing.

The researchers concluded that the best strategy was proceeding to vascular surgery with close monitoring of cardiac status, which had an expected mortality similar to that with the second strategy using coronary angiography.[2] The reason that proceeding directly to vascular surgery was a competitive strategy in the analysis was that the risk associated with operating on patients with severe coronary disease in this population was offset by the risks associated with coronary angiography and revascularization. The costs expected with the first strategy were more than one-third lower than those expected with the two strategies using coronary angiography. The attractiveness of this "conservative" strategy has been enhanced by more recent studies showing marked reduction in risk for complications in this population if they are treated with perioperative β-blockade.[6,7]

The researchers who performed the analysis did not conclude that coronary angiography was not useful before vascular surgery.[2] Rather, they recommended that coronary angiography be reserved for patients with a very high expected operative mortality due to vascular surgery in whom it could be anticipated that the mortality of coronary revascularization would be reasonably low. In short, that analysis emphasizes the importance of considering the risks associated with overall management of the patient, and not just the risk of the operation. Some implications of this approach include the following.

- Coronary angiography is probably quite appropriate in patients who have "high risk" thallium scans, showing a large amount of myocardium in jeopardy or accumulation of thallium in pulmonary fields.
- Coronary angiography may not be beneficial for patients who have a high risk for morbidity or mortality if they undergo revascularization.
- In procedures associated with a lower risk for cardiac complications than vascular procedures, the threshold for proceeding to coronary angiography after an abnormal non-invasive test result should be even higher. This is because the potential benefit for that patient from revascularization before surgery is lower than in vascular surgery patients, but the risks from coronary angiography and revascularization remain the same.

Postoperative medical management

Most perioperative myocardial infarctions occur within 48 hours of surgery, but complications such as congestive heart failure and hypertension frequently occur 3–5 days after surgery, when extravascular fluid returns to the intravascular space thus increasing cardiac preload and work. Therefore, the care of the surgical patient does not end when the patient returns to the surgical floor; consultants and other physicians should continue to follow the patient carefully during this high risk period.

Because of anesthesia and postoperative pain management, only about half of postoperative infarctions are accompanied by a complaint of chest pain. Nevertheless, most postoperative myocardial infarctions are associated with symptoms or signs such as decreased blood pressure, congestive heart failure, arrhythmias, or a change in mental status. The occurrence of any such unusual events should precipitate consideration of an underlying cardiovascular problem.

Definitive diagnosis of postoperative infarctions is difficult, however. Electrocardiogram interpretation is often complicated by the high prevalence of ST-segment or T-wave changes of doubtful significance in postoperative patients. Similarly, cardiac enzyme levels may be difficult to interpret because the trauma of surgery can be expected to lead to abnormalities in creatine kinase (CK), lactate dehydrogenase (LDH), and LDH isoenzyme levels. CK-MB is also now recognized to exist in small amounts in non-cardiac tissues; hence, even in the absence of cardiac complications, surgery frequently produces a rise in CK-MB that is easily detectable with CK-MB mass assays. Newer assays, such as those for cardiac troponins I and T, may provide improved specificity and more accurate diagnosis.

Congestive heart failure is often caused by postoperative surgical problems that increase myocardial demands, but some patients develop mild heart failure about 12–36 hours postoperatively, when mobilization of intraoperative fluid begins. Diuretic therapy is usually sufficient to manage these volume shifts, but all patients with postoperative heart failure should be evaluated carefully to determine whether a perioperative myocardial infarction may have occurred.

Postoperative arrhythmias

New onset of supraventricular tachyarrhythmias or development or worsening of ventricular arrhythmias during the postoperative period often reflects increased sympathetic tone in response to surgery, but arrhythmias may also indicate underlying ischemia. In general, new postoperative supraventricular tachyarrhythmias do not require cardioversion because they usually resolve either with continuation or resumption of the patient's chronic cardiac medications, or with treatment with β-blockers or calcium channel blockers. Electrical cardioversion can be used if cardiac output is compromised or evidence of ischemia develops.

Case studies

Case 15.1

A 73-year-old white male with coronary artery disease was found to have an abdominal aortic aneurysm during a preoperative evaluation for adenocarcinoma of his left lung.

The patient had a remote history of prior myocardial infarction and had undergone coronary artery bypass graft surgery 12 years before admission. For several years he was asymptomatic from a cardiovascular perspective, but over the past 3 years he had developed a stable angina syndrome with exertion, consisting of discomfort in his upper chest, neck, and shoulders, occasionally spreading to his left arm. This complaint usually occurred after walking distances of 150 yards or more.

He had no history of syncope, presyncope, or symptoms of congestive heart failure.

He was a former heavy smoker, and frequently had respiratory infections characterized by a productive cough. The evaluation of one such episode led to detection of a 2 cm nodule in his left lung. The patient was scheduled for a lobectomy.

During his preoperative evaluation, he was found to have a pulsatile abdominal mass. Ultrasound and angiographic evaluation led to diagnosis of an infrarenal aortic aneurysm measuring 6 cm on frontal views and 7 cm in the anteroposterior views. This aneurysm extended into the common iliac arteries bilaterally.

Examination. Physical examination: the patient appeared normal. No abnormalities of skin, nail beds, or oral mucosa. Pulse: 76 beats/min, normal character. Blood pressure: 130/80 mmHg in right arm. Jugular venous pulse: 8 cm. Cardiac impulse: normal. First heart sound: normal. Second heart sound: split normally on inspiration. Fourth heart sound (S_4) gallop and grade 2/6 ejection systolic murmur. Chest examination: normal air entry, no rales or rhonchi. Abdominal examination: soft abdomen, no tenderness. Pulsatile abdominal mass. Normal liver span. No peripheral edema. Femoral, popliteal, posterior tibial, and dorsalis pedis pulses: all diminished bilaterally. Carotid pulses: normal, no bruits. Optic fundi: normal.

Investigations. Electrocardiogram: sinus rhythm with the ventricular rate at 68 beats/min, PR interval 188 ms, QRS duration of 124 ms. There was left ventricular hypertrophy with QRS widening and repolarization abnormality. There was a prior inferior myocardial infarction. The patient underwent a dipyridamole thallium scintigraphy scan, which showed an apical and septal reversible perfusion defect consistent with ischemia. An echocardiogram showed an end-diastolic diameter of 5·1 cm (normal 3·5–6·0 cm) and end-systolic diameter of 3·3 cm (normal 2·1–4·0 cm). The overall left ventricular size was normal and the ejection fraction was estimated to be 65%. There was 2+ mitral regurgitation.

Questions

1. How does the presence of potentially curable lung cancer influence the patient's management?
2. What was this patient's risk for complications with abdominal aortic aneurysm repair as assessed from his clinical data?
3. Should this patient have to undergo coronary angiography prior to surgery?
4. What management strategies might reduce this patient's risk of complications?

Answers

Answer to question 1 The patient's lung cancer made all of the decisions more complex in this case. The lesion was potentially curable, but a long delay in resection would decrease the chances that the patient's tumor would metastasize. Even if the tumor were resected immediately, however, the patient's chances of surgical cure were less than 50%. This uncertain prognosis called into question the appropriateness of recommendations that his asymptomatic aortic aneurysm be resected, and made coronary revascularization of even less certain benefit. The decision to proceed with abdominal aortic aneurysm repair before lung cancer resection was based in part on concern that hypertensive episodes associated with surgery and postoperative pain might cause rupture of a fairly large aneurysm.

Answer to question 2 According to the Cardiac Risk Index, this patient had 5 points for age over 70 years and 3 points for needing aortic surgery (see Table 15.4). The total of 8 points placed the patient in Cardiac Risk Index class II, which was associated with a major complication rate of 11% in one series of patients undergoing abdominal aortic aneurysms (see Table 15.5.)

Answer to question 3 Whether the patient has coronary artery disease is not in question. The issue is whether the patient should undergo coronary revascularization before abdominal aortic aneurysm repair and lung cancer resection. Although randomized trials to test this strategy have not been performed, many clinicians would recommend coronary angiography followed by angioplasty or bypass surgery before (or simultaneously with) repair of an abdominal aortic aneurysm, because of the high risk of major hemodynamic shifts during this procedure. However, in this case, the patient would have been confronting the serial risks of three major procedures. Therefore, after discussion with the patient, the decision was made to proceed directly to abdominal aortic aneurysm repair.

Answer to question 4 Hemodynamic monitoring with a pulmonary artery catheter and a radial arterial line can be used to minimize hemodynamic shifts. Hypovolemia due to blood loss can be rapidly detected and treated using such monitoring, and hypertension can be reduced with intravenous vasodilator therapy.

Case 15.2

A 67-year-old white male with severe congestive heart failure due to ischemic heart disease is diagnosed with lung cancer.

The patient had recently presented with pneumonia in his left lower lobe. After treatment with antibiotics, his symptoms and the infiltrate on chest radiography resolved, but he was found to have a 3 cm nodule. Bronchoscopy revealed this nodule to be a squamous cell carcinoma. A staging evaluation revealed no metastases, and the patient was considered potentially curable with surgical therapy.

The patient had a major anterolateral myocardial infarction 7 years before admission, and had undergone bypass surgery because of recurrent ischemia. Since then, he had had occasional chest pressure that was variably associated with exercise. He slept on three pillows and had occasional leg edema. He had no syncope or presyncope. He was treated with anticoagulants because echocardiographic evaluations had revealed poor left ventricular function and thrombus. His regimen included warfarin 5 mg/day, captopril 18·5 mg orally three times daily, furosemide 160 mg orally twice daily, digoxin 0·25 mg/day orally, and potassium supplementation. He also used a steroid inhaler and an atropine inhaler for treatment of occasional wheezing that was considered to represent reactive airway disease.

Examination. Physical examination: the patient appeared normal. Pulse: 88 beats/min, normal character. Blood pressure: 100/60 mmHg in right arm. Jugular venous pulse: 10 cm. Cardiac impulse: normal. First heart sound: normal. Second heart sound: split normally on inspiration. No added sounds. Grade 3/6 apical holosystolic murmur. Chest examination: bilateral basal rales. Abdominal examination: soft abdomen, no tenderness and no masses. Normal liver span. No peripheral edema. Femoral, popliteal, posterior tibial, and dorsalis pedis pulses: all normal volume and equal. Carotid pulses: normal, no bruits. Optic fundi: normal.

Investigations. Electrocardiogram: normal sinus rhythm with frequent premature supraventricular complexes, left anterior hemiblock, left ventricular hypertrophy, evidence of a lateral infarction. Echocardiogram: left atrium 4·4 cm (normal 1·9–4·0 cm), left ventricular end-diastolic diameter 8·2 cm (normal 3·5–6·0 cm), end-systolic diameter 7·5 cm (normal 2·1–4·0 cm). His left atrium was moderately dilated and there were multiple regional wall motion abnormalities. He had 3+/4+ mitral regurgitation. The estimated ejection fraction was 30%. He also had 3+ tricuspid regurgitation. He underwent a dipyridamole thallium test, which showed a marked increase in left ventricular volume, and marked decrease in uptake in the apex and the apical two-thirds of the anterior wall, consistent with a transmural myocardial infarction in the left anterior descending coronary artery region. There was also moderate to marked decrease in uptake in the inferior wall, consistent with a mixed transmural/non-transmural myocardial infarction. There was moderate decreased uptake in the septum, consistent with a non-transmural myocardial infarction. The lateral wall was well perfused, suggesting that his left circumflex was his only patent coronary artery. No ischemia was detected.

Questions

1. What was this patient's risk for cardiovascular complications with surgery?
2. Should he undergo coronary angiography and coronary revascularization before chest surgery?
3. What would you have recommended if the dipyridamole thallium scan had shown a considerable amount of myocardium in jeopardy?
4. What measures might reduce the patient's risk for complications?

Answers

Answer to question 1   This patient had 14 points according to the Cardiac Risk Index (11 points for the third heart sound [S_3] gallop and jugular venous distension; 3 points for thoracic surgery), which placed him at high risk for complications (see Tables 15.4 and 15.6). This classification reflects the high probability of complications in patients with severe left ventricular dysfunction.

Answer to question 2   Despite the patient's high risk, there is no evidence that the risk could be reduced through coronary revascularization. The dipyridamole thallium scan did not show evidence of myocardium in jeopardy. Hence, the physicians concluded that the risk associated with coronary revascularization was not warranted.

Answer to question 3   Neither the patient nor his physicians were enthusiastic about the prospect of performing coronary artery bypass graft surgery upon a patient with moderate sized lung cancer. However, the high risk associated with the operation would have been even higher if the patient showed evidence of a large amount of myocardium in jeopardy. Therefore, before the dipyridamole thallium scan, the patient and his physicians agreed on a detailed plan. According to this plan, if the non-invasive study suggested that much of his remaining myocardium was in jeopardy, then they would perform coronary angiography and, if feasible, angioplasty. Elective bypass surgery would not have been considered if the patient's coronary anatomy did not lend itself to angioplasty, but emergency bypass surgery would have been performed if the angioplasty had been complicated by acute closure. There are no data from prospective trials that support or undermine this plan; for this reason, the physicians considered discussion of potential strategies before performance of the non-invasive test for ischemia to be particularly important.

Answer to question 4 Hemodynamic monitoring with a pulmonary artery catheter and a radial arterial line can be used to minimize hemodynamic shifts. Hypovolemia due to blood loss can be rapidly detected and treated using such monitoring, and hypertension can be reduced with intravenous vasodilator therapy.

Case 15.3

A 76-year-old female with lumbar spinal stenosis was considered for surgery because of intractable pain. The patient had a long history of exertional dyspnea and leg edema. She also had about one episode per week of an epigastric and substernal chest burning that was not associated with exertion. Prior echocardiographic studies had shown a markedly hypertrophied left ventricle with a normal ejection fraction. She had been treated for pulmonary congestion due to presumed diastolic dysfunction with verapamil 240 mg/day orally, furosemide 180 mg/day orally, and potassium 20 mEq orally three times daily. Other medical problems included diabetes, for which she took daily insulin, and restrictive lung disease that was believed to be due to obesity.

Examination. Physical examination: the patient was obese and in a wheelchair, unable to stand. Respiratory rate: 18/min. Pulse: 70 beats/min, normal character. Blood pressure: 130/80 mmHg in right arm. Jugular venous pulse: not visible. Cardiac impulse: normal. First heart sound: normal. Second heart sound: split normally on inspiration. Grade 2/6 murmur at the left sternal border that did not change with handgrip or Valsalva. Chest examination: bilateral basal rales. Abdominal examination: soft abdomen, no tenderness and no masses. Normal liver span. Moderate edema of lower extremities.

Investigations. Electrocardiogram: sinus rhythm, left ventricular hypertrophy with non-specific ST-T-wave abnormalities. An echocardiographic study showed mild dynamic obstruction in the left ventricular outflow track, and abnormal, diffuse upper septal thickening. Right heart structures were normal in size and function. There was mild tricuspid regurgitation consistent with a right heart systolic pressure of 35–40 mmHg.

Questions

1. Should this patient undergo a non-invasive test for ischemia, such as a dipyridamole thallium scintigraphy?
2. Should this patient receive general or spinal/epidural anesthesia?
3. What might be the consequences of postoperative tachyarrhythmias in this patient?

Answers

Answer to question 1 Even if a non-invasive test for ischemia suggested that the patient had myocardium in jeopardy as the cause of her chest discomfort, the basic management plan would not have been altered. Major elective orthopedic surgery is associated with a low cardiovascular complication rate, and even if the patient had known coronary disease the physicians would have been unlikely to recommend coronary angiography and coronary revascularization, or to have suggested hemodynamic monitoring for this low risk procedure. Had the patient been scheduled for a higher risk procedure, such as major vascular surgery, then the physicians would have considered a non-invasive test for ischemia because the patient's poor functional status made her history of chest pain unreliable.

Answer to question 2 In general, the risks for major complications associated with spinal, epidural, and general anesthesia are similar. However, spinal and epidural anesthesia are relatively contraindicated in patients with hypertrophic cardiomyopathies because venodilatation can rapidly reduce venous return to the heart. Because this patient's hypertrophied left ventricle is especially dependent on high filling pressures, this reduction in venous return could lead to abrupt severe falls in cardiac output.

Answer to question 3 Although this patient's dynamic outflow obstruction was not severe, she was at risk for hypotension due to reduced cardiac output if she developed a tachycardia because of an arrhythmia or sinus tachycardia resulting from pain or blood loss. Patients with hypertrophic cardiomyopathy require longer filling times for their left ventricle in order to achieve a normal volume. Faster heart rates decrease the amount of time between each systole during which the ventricle can fill. If this patient developed atrial fibrillation, then she would also have lost her "atrial kick" – the augmentation in left ventricular filling that occurs with each atrial contraction. Therefore, tachyarrhythmias were an especially serious potential problem for her.

References

1 Mangano DT, Goldman L. Preoperative assessment of patients with known or suspected coronary disease. *N Engl J Med* 1995;**333**:1750–6.

2 Mason JJ, Owens DK, Harris RA, Cooke JP, Hlatky MA. The role of coronary angiography and coronary revascularization before noncardiac vascular surgery. *JAMA* 1995;**273**:1919–24.

3 ACC/AHA Guideline Update for Perioperative Cardiovascular Evaluation for Noncardiac Surgery. ACC/AHA Guideline Update for Perioperative Cardiovascular Evaluation for Noncardiac Surgery: Executive Summary. *Circulation* 2002;**105**: 1257–67.

4 Lee TH. Reducing cardiac risk in noncardiac surgery [editorial]. *N Engl J Med* 1999;**341**:1838–40.

5 Rao T, El-Etr A. Myocardial infarction following anesthesia in patients with recent myocardial infarction. *Anesth Analg* 1981;**60**:271–2.

6 Mangano DT, Layug EL, Wallace A, Tateo I, for the Multicenter Study of Perioperative Ischemia Research Group. Effect of atenolol on mortality and cardiovascular morbidity after noncardiac surgery. *N Engl J Med* 1996;**335**: 1713–20.

7 Poldermans D, Boersma E, Bax JJ, *et al.* The effect of bisoprolol on perioperative mortality and myocardial infarction in high-risk patients undergoing vascular surgery. *N Engl J Med* 1999;**341**:1789–94.

8 Weitz H, Goldman L. Noncardiac surgery in the patient with heart disease. *Med Clin North Am* 1987;**71**:413–32.

9 Foster E, Davis K, Carpenter J, *et al.* Risk of noncardiac operation in patients with defined coronary disease: the Coronary Artery Surgery Study (CASS) Registry experience. *Ann Thorac Surg* 1986;**41**:42–50.

10 Goldman L, Caldera D, Southwick F, *et al.* Cardiac risk factors and complications in non-cardiac surgery. *Medicine* 1978;**57**:357–70.

11 Katz J, Cronan L, Barash P, *et al.* Pulmonary artery flow guided catheters in the perioperative period. *JAMA* 1977;**237**:2832–4.

12 Kearon C, Hirsh J. Management of anticoagulation before and after elective surgery. *N Engl J Med* 1997;**336**:1506–11.

13 Thompson R, Liberthson R, Lowenstein E. Perioperative anesthetic risk of noncardiac surgery in hypertrophic obstructive cardiomyopathy. *JAMA* 1985;**254**:2419–21.

14 Vanik P, Davis H. Cardiac arrhythmias during halothane anesthesia. *Anesth Analg* 1968;**47**:299–307.

15 Goldman L, Caldera DL, Nussbaum SR, *et al.* Multifactorial index of cardiac risk in noncardiac surgical procedures. *N Engl J Med* 1977;**297**:845–50.

16 Goldman L. Multifactorial index of cardiac risk in noncardiac surgery: ten-year status report. *J Cardiothorac Anesth* 1987;**1**:237–44.

17 Zeldin R. Assessing cardiac risk in patients who undergo noncardiac surgical procedures. *Can J Surg* 1984;**27**:402–4.

18 Detsky A, Abrams H, Forbath N, Scott J, Hilliard J. Cardiac assessment for patients undergoing noncardiac surgery. A multifactorial clinical risk index. *Arch Intern Med* 1986;**146**:2131–4.

19 Jeffrey C, Kunsman J, Cullen D, Brewster D. A prospective evaluation of cardiac risk index. *Anesthesiology* 1983;**58**:462–4.

20 Kennedy H, Whitlock J, Sprague M, *et al.* Long term follow up of asymptomatic healthy subjects with frequent and complex ventricular ectopy. *N Engl J Med* 1985; **312**:193–7.

21 Sprung C, Pozen R, Rozanski J, *et al.* Advanced ventricular arrhythmias during bedside pulmonary artery catheterization. *Am J Med* 1982;**72**:203–8.

22 Lee TH, Marcantonio ER, Mangione CM, *et al.* Derivation and prospective validation of a simple index for prediction of cardiac risk of major noncardiac surgery. *Circulation* 1999;**100**:1043–9.

23 Ashton C, Petersen N, Wray N, *et al*. The incidence of perioperative myocardial infarction in men undergoing noncardiac surgery. *Ann Intern Med* 1993;**118**: 504–10.
24 Eagle K, Coley C, Newell J, *et al*. Combining clinical and thallium data optimizes preoperative assessment of cardiac risk before major vascular surgery. *Ann Intern Med* 1989;**110**:859–66.
25 Raby K, Goldman L, Creager M, *et al*. Correlation between preoperative ischemia and major cardiac events after peripheral vascular surgery. *N Engl J Med* 1989; **321**:1296–300.

16: Heart disease in pregnancy

JOHN D RUTHERFORD

During a normal pregnancy there are major changes in blood volume, total body water and sodium, and cardiovascular hemodynamics, in part because of increases in steroid hormones, including estrogens. Cardiac output (the product of stroke volume and heart rate) increases by 40–50%, reaches a peak in mid-pregnancy, and is either maintained or declines slightly at term. There is an inverse relationship between this increase in cardiac output and a significant fall in peripheral arterial resistance (and mean arterial blood pressure), with diastolic blood pressure falling more than systolic blood pressure and pulse pressure increasing. In addition, red blood cell mass increases progressively during pregnancy by 30–40%, with a greater increase in plasma volume resulting in the "physiological anemia of pregnancy". Total body water and exchangeable body sodium increase with activation of the renin–angiotensin system and lowering of the osmotic thresholds for thirst stimulation and vasopressin release. This results in a fall in plasma sodium and osmolality, and clinical edema is found in up to 80% of healthy pregnant women.

Because resting cardiac output is increased the maximal cardiac output induced by exercise is achieved at a lower level of work, and as pregnancy advances there is a gradual increase in resting oxygen consumption. Serial echocardiography shows that the cardiac adaptation to normal pregnancy is a gradual increase in all cardiac dimensions that is more pronounced on the right side of the heart, and that mild, transient tricuspid and mitral regurgitation are normal findings.[1]

Because of the changes in hemodynamics associated with pregnancy, particularly the major increase in cardiac output and the fall in systemic vascular resistance, certain cardiac conditions will be well tolerated and others poorly tolerated (Table 16.1).

Peripartum cardiomyopathy

Peripartum cardiomyopathy is a rare and poorly understood condition that is defined clinically as the development of cardiac failure in the last month of pregnancy, or within 5 months of delivery, in the absence of either recognizable heart disease before the last month of pregnancy or an identifiable cause for the heart failure.[2] Echocardiographic demonstration of left ventricular systolic

Table 16.1 Prognosis of cardiac conditions

Well versus poorly tolerated	Cardiac condition
Well tolerated	Asymptomatic patients – those NYHA functional class I Valvular regurgitation: mild and moderate mitral and aortic regurgitation Left to right shunt (without pulmonary hypertension): ASD, VSD, PDA
Poorly tolerated	Breathless at rest – NYHA functional class IV Valvular stenoses: moderate to severe mitral and aortic stenosis Right to left shunt: Eisenmenger's syndrome Pulmonary hypertension: moderate to severe Marfan's syndrome Myocardial infarction

ASD, atrial septal defect; NYHA, New York Heart Association; PDA, patent ductus arteriosus; VSD, ventricular septal defect

dysfunction is an important component of the diagnosis. Among a large series of patients with cardiomyopathy, the women with peripartum cardiomyopathy appeared to have a better survival (94% at 5 years) than did patients with other etiologies.[3]

After the diagnosis is made some patients' cardiac function can rapidly revert to normal, whereas others have persistent evidence of cardiac dysfunction beyond 6–12 months of diagnosis. The persistence of cardiac dysfunction beyond 6–12 months often indicates a long-term problem and almost always supports an absolute contraindication to a repeat pregnancy. Even in patients who appear to have "recovered" from peripartum cardiomyopathy, and who have normal resting ventricular function, there may be impaired contractile reserve. Finally, a few patients may rapidly deteriorate, fail medical therapy, and require cardiac transplantation.

Valvular heart disease

In pregnant patients who are asymptomatic or who have mild cardiac symptoms, the lesions of mild or moderate mitral or aortic valve regurgitation are usually well tolerated. The reduced peripheral vascular resistance (or afterload) of pregnancy tends to diminish the degree of regurgitation and, provided the patient maintains sinus rhythm, the increased hemodynamic load of pregnancy is usually well tolerated. For patients with overt cardiac symptomatology, or major degrees of aortic or mitral regurgitation, the hemodynamic changes of pregnancy may impose an excessive load and lead to hemodynamic compromise. In marked contrast, mitral and aortic valve stenosis are generally poorly tolerated during pregnancy. The severity of the fixed stenosis is accentuated by the increase in cardiac output of pregnancy, and in patients with mitral stenosis the increase in heart rate during pregnancy shortens diastole and increases left atrial pressure.

Mitral stenosis

Mitral stenosis is the commonest and most important rheumatic cardiac lesion seen in pregnancy. The dominant symptom is breathlessness, and the onset of atrial fibrillation may be associated with marked decompensation and should be considered a medical emergency. In patients with mitral stenosis both diuretics and β-blockers can safely be used during pregnancy. New onset arrhythmias, such as atrial fibrillation or supraventricular tachycardia, should be treated promptly. The use of β-blockers, or perhaps digitalis, may be appropriate for controlling the ventricular response; however, acute pulmonary edema may ensue rapidly if the ventricular rate is not controlled and sinus rhythm regained. Therefore, for rapid atrial fibrillation associated with symptoms, prompt cardioversion is recommended.

If a patient in sinus rhythm, with mitral stenosis, becomes pregnant and has symptoms during the first trimester of pregnancy, despite diuretic therapy, then it is doubtful that the patient and/or fetus will tolerate the lesion hemodynamically throughout pregnancy, labor, delivery, and the puerperium. In such patients, with symptomatology of greater than New York Heart Association functional class II, consideration should be given to either surgical intervention or mitral balloon valvuloplasty in appropriate candidates. Generally, pregnancy does not influence the maternal surgical results, but there is a fetal mortality of approximately 10%, and surgery early in pregnancy may be associated with abortion and later in pregnancy with premature labor.

With severe mitral valve stenosis, there is a pregnancy-related mortality of up to 5%. Labor, delivery, and especially the immediate postpartum period appear to be the times of greatest risk. In patients with severe symptoms, a rise in pulmonary capillary wedge pressure of approximately 10 mmHg may be anticipated immediately postpartum. Clark *et al.*[4] recommended that such patients should have oxygen administration in labor in the recumbent position; a pulmonary artery wedge catheter should be placed to monitor hemodynamics during early labor induction, and reduction in pulmonary capillary wedge pressures to approximately 14 mmHg is a desired goal. They recommend epidural anesthesia during the active phase of labor, careful monitoring during the puerperium, and use of cesarean section for obstetric indications alone.

Valve replacements

Both valve surgery during pregnancy and pregnancy in patients who have had a valve replacement are hazardous to the mother and to the fetus.[5] Mechanical prosthetic valves carry a risk for thromboembolic events, patients require lifelong anticoagulation, and associated pregnancy carries an estimated maternal mortality of up to 4%. Biologic prostheses may structurally deteriorate, especially during the second and third decades of life, although some suggest that these valves may be the preferred replacement in women who are anticipating having a child in an attempt to avoid the deleterious effects of anticoagulation.

Anticoagulation

Pregnant patients with rheumatic mitral valve disease (and associated paroxysmal or chronic atrial fibrillation), with heart valve replacements, and with a history of recurrent pulmonary thromboembolism may require anticoagulants during pregnancy. Warfarin crosses the placenta, is teratogenic, and its use during the first trimester of pregnancy carries a significant risk to the fetus. Exposure in the weeks 6–9 of gestation may produce the fetal warfarin syndrome, and spontaneous abortions, stillbirths, and neonatal deaths may occur. In a review of anticoagulant use in pregnant women with prosthetic heart valves,[6] use of oral anticoagulation throughout pregnancy was associated with warfarin embryopathy in 6·4% of live births, which was eliminated with substitution of heparin at or before 6 weeks of gestation. When heparin was used between weeks 6 and 12, in place of continued warfarin therapy, the risk for valve thrombosis increased from 4% to 9%. The estimated risk for maternal hemorrhage in a woman taking anticoagulants is 2·5%, with the majority of episodes occurring at the time of delivery.

Unfractionated heparin is often used during pregnancy and its complications include hemorrhage, thrombocytopenia, and symptomless bone loss (osteopenia). Low molecular weight heparins and heparinoids are increasingly being used during pregnancy. They do not appear to cross the placenta, are less likely to cause heparin-induced thrombocytopenia, may result in a lower risk for heparin-induced osteopenia, and have the potential for once daily administration.

Because of the current uncertainty of adequate protection of patients with the use of full dose heparin, the optimal management of women with mechanical heart valves may involve the use of warfarin throughout pregnancy except for two time periods, namely between 6 and 12 weeks gestation (in order to eliminate the risk for warfarin embryopathy) and after 36 weeks of gestation (in order to minimize the risk for maternal hemorrhage at the time of labor and delivery).[6] During these periods, adjusted dose unfractionated heparin should be used to maintain a therapeutic mid-interval activated partial thromboplastin time of 2·0–2·5 times control.

Planned pregnancy in patients on long-term anticoagulants

In women of childbearing age who require long-term anticoagulants, the risks for anticoagulant therapy during pregnancy must be explained before conception. If pregnancy is desired, then a reasonable approach is to perform frequent pregnancy tests and to substitute heparin for warfarin when pregnancy is achieved. This assumes that warfarin is safe during the first 4–6 weeks of gestation,[7] and after 12 weeks warfarin therapy is reinstituted.

Coronary artery disease

With increasing age and duration of fertility of mothers, and with more than half of the total births occurring in women aged 30–44 years, coronary artery disease during pregnancy is likely to be encountered with increasing frequency. In pregnancy, coronary artery disease presenting as angina has been associated with smoking alone, vasospastic angina, pre-eclampsia, homozygous familial hypercholesterolemia, and diabetes mellitus.

Acute myocardial infarction presenting during pregnancy is very rare (incidence 0·1%) but is potentially lethal for both the mother and the fetus.[8] Usually, women who have a myocardial infarction before the age of 40 years have either insulin requiring diabetes mellitus, a strong family history of premature coronary artery disease, and/or hypertension and hyperlipidemia. Cocaine abuse should also be considered and spontaneous coronary artery dissection is a rare entity, usually reported in women. The latter condition occurs one-third of the time during pregnancy or the puerperium, and presents with sudden death or an unstable coronary syndrome. The left anterior descending coronary artery is usually involved, and if the patient survives the initial event long-term survival is possible.[9]

It is important to realize that, during the peripartum period (whether or not acute myocardial infarction has occurred), total creatine phosphokinase and creatine kinase-MB increase markedly during normal vaginal deliveries. They reach a peak of two to four times baseline levels 24 hours postpartum.[10] Evolving electrocardiographic changes, coupled with echocardiographic evidence of regional wall motion abnormalities, are essential in making a diagnosis of acute myocardial infarction during this period. Thrombolytic agents used during pregnancy for venous thrombosis, pulmonary embolism, and thrombosed prosthetic heart valves are associated with a maternal mortality of 1–2%, a fetal mortality of 6%, and hemorrhagic complications in 8%. Such risks may outweigh any potential benefits. Successful percutaneous transluminal coronary angioplasty has been performed during pregnancy.

Any management plan of a patient with an acute coronary syndrome requires close consultation between the cardiologist, the obstetric service, and the anesthesiology service in order to coordinate and plan an elective labor or provide optimal management of an unexpected premature labor. In addition, the team needs to develop a strategy to provide a greater chance of prompt and effective rescue of the fetus in the event of sudden maternal demise. Because the course of events can change dramatically and rapidly, it is important that the goals of therapy and the alternatives be explained simply and clearly to the patient and her relatives.

Intracardiac shunts

The most common left to right cardiac shunts encountered in women of childbearing age are atrial or ventricular septal defects. In the absence of significant cardiac symptomatology or pulmonary hypertension, the outcome of pregnancy is usually normal and uncomplicated because the normal, major fall in systemic vascular resistance during pregnancy tends to diminish the magnitude of the left to right shunting. However, serious and fatal maternal and fetal problems can occur during pregnancy in patients with shunts associated with cardiac arrhythmias, right heart failure, or pulmonary hypertension.

Pulmonary hypertension

Pulmonary hypertension is associated with substantially increased maternal mortality. Maternal mortality approaches 50% in

Eisenmenger's syndrome, and 30% in primary and pulmonary hypertension. Most deaths occur within the month after delivery, and neonatal survival is over 85%. The predictive risk factors for maternal mortality are late diagnosis and late admission to hospital.[11]

In patients with primary pulmonary hypertension both pregnancy termination and tubal ligation may be indicated. If a patient elects to continue with pregnancy, bed rest should be enforced and consideration should be given to full dose anticoagulation. In addition to adequate oxygenation with careful hemodynamic monitoring, inhaled nitric oxide therapy and treatment with pulmonary vasodilators (nifedipine and prostacyclin) may be associated with improved hemodynamics and successful completion of pregnancy.

In patients with Eisenmenger's syndrome (patients with large intracardiac defects that allow free communication between the systemic and pulmonary circulations, and who have predominantly right to left shunting secondary to fixed and markedly elevated pulmonary vascular resistance), high maternal and fetal mortality rates are observed. With pregnancy, and the usual maternal hemodynamic alterations (increased cardiac output and a major full and systemic vascular resistance), patients with Eisenmenger's syndrome have more right to left shunting, experience deeper cyanosis, and have a reduced systemic arterial oxygen saturation and a rise in hematocrit. This is among the few cardiac conditions for which sterilization may be recommended because pregnancy is poorly tolerated and the maternal mortality is high.[11,12] If termination of pregnancy is not feasible, or is declined, then supportive measures must include avoidance of operative procedures and hypotension, hypovolemia, and thromboembolic phenomena. Gleicher *et al.*[12] recommended hospitalization and prolonged bed rest, anticoagulation of patients from mid-pregnancy, non-induced labor, administration of high concentrations of oxygen during labor, epidural anesthesia, and non-induced vaginal delivery with elective low forceps to shorten the second stage of labor.

Marfan's syndrome

Marfan's syndrome is an autosomal dominant connective tissue disorder. It has substantial cardiovascular manifestations as a consequence of mutations in fibrillin, a glycoprotein associated with elastin, resulting in defective connective tissue. The cardiovascular manifestations of the disease typically involve the supporting tissues of the aorta and the cardiac valves. The natural history of the untreated disease is that life expectancy is reduced by 30–50%, mainly because of aortic root dilatation resulting in dissection, aortic rupture, or regurgitation of the aortic or mitral valves. The increased cardiovascular stresses of pregnancy increase the risk for aneurysmal dissection, and this risk increases with maternal age.

In a major, prospective evaluation of the outcome of pregnancy in Marfan's syndrome patients, it was found that most patients with mild cardiovascular involvement can safely undergo pregnancy.[13] Lower risk women with Marfan's syndrome were those with minor cardiovascular involvement and an aortic root diameter of less than 40 mm. In contrast, patients at higher risk (those with aortic root dilatation, aortic regurgitation, or a history of dissection) appeared to be at increased risk for dissection during pregnancy.[14] In adolescent and adult patients with classic Marfan's syndrome and mild to moderate dilatation of the aortic root, β-blocker therapy slowed the rate of aortic dilatation and reduced the development of aortic complications.[15] Although there is no similar information in pregnant women with Marfan's syndrome, β-blockers are given to all such patients, even during pregnancy, because it is felt that the maternal advantages of β-blockers far outweigh their potential adverse affects on the fetus.

It is recommended that all women with Marfan's syndrome have preconceptional assessment of echocardiographic and clinical status, and genetic counseling regarding the risk for cardiovascular complications during pregnancy and the risk for inheritance. During pregnancy, echocardiographic surveillance should continue and transthoracic echocardiograms should be performed every 6–10 weeks (the interval being determined by initial echocardiographic findings). It should be stressed that, even in patients with a normal aortic root and no evidence of valvular dysfunction, the presence of Marfan's syndrome alone can predispose a patient to a poor outcome with morbid or fatal events. Patients with moderate or greater aortic regurgitation or an aortic root diameter exceeding 40 mm should be advised that their cardiovascular risk during pregnancy is likely to be greatly increased.

In most patients with Marfan's syndrome a vaginal delivery with adequate analgesia is recommended, provided the progress of labor is satisfactory and the second stage of labor is not prolonged. Cesarean section is usually reserved for standard obstetric indications.

Cardiac arrhythmias

The common arrhythmias that occur during pregnancy include premature atrial ventricular beats, re-entrant supraventricular tachyarrhythmias, and occasional tachyarrhythmias associated with Wolff–Parkinson–White syndrome.[16] If patients have asymptomatic or mildly symptomatic ventricular or supraventricular premature beats in the presence of normal cardiac function, then treatment is not usually necessary. A history of caffeine use, alcohol use, or other precipitants of arrhythmias should be sought (for example, sympathomimetic amine inhalers for asthma). Vagal maneuvers are always taught to the patient and should be attempted initially in all patients with such arrhythmias. If vagal maneuvers are not effective, then patients may be treated with digitalis, β-blocking agents, adenosine, or intravenous verapamil. Adenosine has been used to treat maternal supraventricular arrhythmias, without any adverse effects attributable to adenosine in the fetus or newborn reported.

Ventricular tachycardia has been reported in pregnant patients with and without detectable structural heart disease. Therapy with lidocaine is used acutely, and subsequent recurrence may be prevented with β-blocking drugs, procainamide, or quinidine.

Cardiopulmonary resuscitation

If a cardiac arrest occurs in a pregnant woman, then standard resuscitative measures and procedures should take place. If ventricular fibrillation is present then the patient should be defibrillated according to protocol. Closed chest compressions and supportive ventilation should be conducted in accordance with usual protocols. Airway control is extremely important and, in order to reduce the effects of the gravid uterus on cardiac output and venous return, a pillow or wedge should be placed under the right abdominal flank and hip to displace the uterus to the left side of the abdomen.[17] If cardiopulmonary resuscitation is required for the mother before the onset of fetal viability (approximately week 24 of gestation), then the main objective is to resuscitate the mother. After this stage of pregnancy, consideration has to be given to delivery of the fetus, which is usually expedited by emergency cesarean section within 5–15 min if cardiopulmonary resuscitation is unsuccessful. Because of these considerations, careful coordination is required between cardiology, obstetric, and anesthesiology services in patients at risk for ventricular fibrillation (for example, acute myocardial infarction) who should be cared for in facilities that are capable of delivering this type of complicated, emergency care involving the mother and child.

Antibiotic prophylaxis

The American Heart Association Committee on Prevention of Bacterial Endocarditis does not recommend prophylaxis for cesarean section or in the absence of infection for urethral catheterization, uncomplicated vaginal delivery, therapeutic abortion, dilatation and curettage, sterilization procedures, or insertion or removal of intrauterine devices.[18] However, prophylaxis is recommended for certain cardiac conditions (mitral valve prolapse with valvular regurgitation, prosthetic cardiac valves) if urinary tract infection is present.

Case studies

Case 16.1

A 28-year-old woman presents to the emergency room in the fourth month of her first pregnancy with a 24 hour history of rapid heart beat and increasing shortness of breath. She is known to have rheumatic heart disease. At the age of 21 years she had an echocardiogram, which revealed moderate mitral stenosis and mild aortic regurgitation.

Examination. Physical examination: the patient was acutely breathless. Pulse: 150 beats/min, irregularly irregular. Blood pressure: 110/80 mmHg in right arm. Jugular venous pulse: "v" waves to the angle of the jaw. Cardiac impulse: parasternal lift. First heart sound: variable. Second heart sound: accentuated. Grade 3/6 holosystolic murmur at the left sternal edge. Chest examination: extensive rales. Abdominal examination: soft abdomen, no tenderness, and no masses. Pulsatile liver. No peripheral edema. No evidence of swollen legs or deep calf thrombosis.

Investigations. Electrocardiogram: atrial fibrillation 150 beats/min; no evidence of right or left ventricular hypertrophy. Swan–Ganz catheter pressures (mmHg): pulmonary capillary wedge 25, pulmonary arterial 55/30, right atrial "v" waves to 20.

In summary, this 28-year-old woman is 4 months pregnant and presents with new onset atrial fibrillation, pulmonary edema, a holosystolic murmur at the left sternal edge associated with "v" waves to the angle of the jaw, and a pulsatile liver.

Questions

1. What is the differential diagnosis, what diagnostic test should be performed, and what treatment should be administered acutely?
2. What is the likelihood this patient will complete pregnancy without further cardiac complications taking medical therapy? Should consideration be given to cardiac surgery or to percutaneous mitral balloon valvuloplasty in order to relieve the mitral stenosis?

Answers

Answer to question 1   The patient was known to have moderate mitral stenosis 7 years ago and now presents in the fourth month of her first pregnancy with uncontrolled or rapid atrial fibrillation, and acute pulmonary edema. With the increase in cardiac output associated with pregnancy in the presence of mitral stenosis, the onset of atrial fibrillation has shortened the diastolic filling period of the heart, and left atrial pressure has risen to approximately 25 mmHg, exceeding the colloid osmotic pressure and resulting in pulmonary edema. The pulmonary artery pressure is moderately elevated and the patient has the classic findings of tricuspid regurgitation ("v" waves, holosystolic murmur in the tricuspid area, which may increase with inspiration, and a pulsatile liver). The tricuspid regurgitation is probably secondary to dilatation of the right ventricle and the tricuspid annulus, in association with an elevated right ventricular systolic pressure due to pulmonary hypertension of 55 mmHg or greater, secondary to mitral valve disease (in this instance mitral stenosis).

Acute onset of breathlessness in pregnancy raises the possibility of peripartum cardiomyopathy; this patient presents in the fourth month of her first pregnancy and has known heart disease. Patients with peripartum cardiomyopathy present in the last month of pregnancy or within 5 months of delivery, and they do not have recognizable heart disease before the last month of pregnancy or an identifiable cause for the heart failure. This patient has known rheumatic heart disease. New onset of atrial fibrillation is associated with valvular heart disease, and especially mitral stenosis, but one should also consider concurrent infection (urinary or respiratory) as a possible precipitant, hyperthyroidism, or cardiomyopathy (see above). Pregnancy is considered to cause a hypercoagulable state, and pulmonary embolism may be associated with acute breathlessness in pregnancy. This patient has no evidence of deep venous thrombosis and there is no recent history of immobilization. The constellation of signs and symptoms suggests that mitral valve disease is more likely, but if indicated an ultrafast computed tomography or a ventilation/perfusion scan could be performed to explore the diagnosis of pulmonary embolism.

A two-dimensional echocardiogram was ordered and this confirmed the presence of moderate to severe mitral stenosis with a mobile, non-thickened, non-calcified valve, and moderate to severe tricuspid regurgitation with peak pulmonary pressures of approximately 55 mmHg and a dilated right ventricle. No mitral regurgitation was seen. No overt thrombus was seen in the left atrium.

The development of acute pulmonary edema in a patient with mitral stenosis and new onset atrial fibrillation is a medical emergency, especially during pregnancy. The most important acute treatment is to try to restore the patient to sinus rhythm. Restoration of sinus rhythm (usually by cardioversion) is the optimal treatment for this patient, but if there is a reason this cannot be attempted, rate control of the heart is very important.

Electrical cardioversion was attempted acutely in this patient but failed. She was treated with oxygen, furosemide, verapamil (to slow her ventricular rate), and procainamide as an antiarrhythmic. Eight hours later she reverted to normal sinus rhythm. She was stabilized on a medical regimen of digoxin 0·125 mg/day, verapamil 160 mg/day, procainamide 1250 mg four times daily, and full dose subcutaneous heparin in order to maintain a therapeutic mid-interval activated partial thromboplastin time of 2·0–2·5 times control.

Answer to question 2   The patient presents with a number of features that suggest that her cardiac condition will be poorly tolerated during pregnancy. She presents with breathlessness at rest (i.e. New York Heart Association functional class IV), relatively early in pregnancy (4 months), and has mitral valve stenosis (moderately severe to severe) associated with secondary pulmonary hypertension and tricuspid regurgitation. The increased cardiac output associated with pregnancy and the fixed mitral valvular stenosis puts her at risk for recurrent pulmonary edema, especially if she does not maintain normal sinus rhythm.

The relatively young age of the patient and the features of her mitral valve noted at the time of echocardiography, including the lack of valvular rigidity, calcification, or thickening, and the lack of overt thrombus, make her a candidate for balloon mitral valvotomy. The fact that she presented with atrial fibrillation would increase her risk for having a clot in the left atrium or appendage. She has been treated with anticoagulants for a few days; however, if there were concerns immediately before a contemplated balloon valvuloplasty then a transesophageal echocardiogram might be performed in order to exclude overt cardiac thrombus. Usually, a history of chronic atrial fibrillation in the absence of long-term therapeutic anticoagulation would be a relative contraindication to the procedure. The percutaneous technique involves advancing a balloon from the right atrium through the interatrial septum, and inflating it within the mitral valve orifice. Complications include cerebral emboli (1%), cardiac perforation (1%), severe mitral regurgitation requiring mitral valve surgery (2%), and a small residual atrial septal defect.

This particular patient was considered a good candidate for this procedure but was concerned about the potential complications and refused to consider it. She was evaluated by a cardiac surgeon, who offered the opinion that she would need mitral valve surgery (repair or replacement) as well as tricuspid valve surgery (annuloplasty), at a risk of 5% maternal mortality and 5–10% fetal mortality (associated with cardiopulmonary bypass). The patient decided she wished to continue medical therapy including rest, medications (digoxin 0·125 mg/day, verapamil 160 mg/day, procainamide 1250 mg four times daily, and full dose subcutaneous heparin), and frequent outpatient surveillance. On this regimen she remained stable and delivered a normal male infant at term without complications. She was not given antibiotic prophylaxis at the time of delivery.

When her child was 10 months old she discussed the issue of family planning and indicated that she wished to consider having another child within the next 18 months. It was decided that because her echocardiographic evaluation suggested "moderate to severe" rather than "critical" mitral stenosis, she should undergo elective cardiac catheterization to evaluate further her valvular heart disease and provide additional information on which to base advice. At that time her medications included digoxin 0·125 mg/day, verapamil 160 mg/day, furosemide 40 mg/day, and warfarin to achieve an International Normalized Ratio of 2·0–3·0. Her chest *x* ray taken before elective cardiac catheterization is shown in Figure 16.1.

Cardiac catheterization hemodynamics. Pressures (mmHg): left ventricular 112/12, wedge 25/22 (mean 19), pulmonary arterial 31/8 (mean 23), right ventricular 31/8, right atrial 11/7 (6). Mean mitral valve gradient: 9 mmHg. Mitral valve area: 1·8 cm^2 (normal 4–6 cm^2 and severe mitral stenosis <1·3 cm^2).

Comment. It is interesting to note in the non-pregnant state that her echocardiogram and cardiac catheterization hemodynamics are concordant and show that she has moderate mitral stenosis. Her right atrial and right ventricular pressures are near normal. These hemodynamics are measured with the patient mildly sedated at rest and do not reflect changes associated with physical activity or at times of hemodynamic stress. In contrast, when she presented 10 months previously in the fourth month of pregnancy with new onset atrial fibrillation, she had moderate pulmonary hypertension (pulmonary arterial pressure 50/30 mmHg), she had clinical features of tricuspid regurgitation ("v" waves in jugular venous pressure, tricuspid holosystolic murmur at left sternal edge, and pulsatile liver), and her right atrial pressure was 20 mmHg. This illustrates the consequences of the hemodynamic stresses associated with pregnancy combined with mitral stenosis. With the increased cardiac output of pregnancy her mitral stenosis became hemodynamically more important, and the onset of atrial fibrillation decompensated her into acute pulmonary edema. Secondary to her mitral stenosis and pregnancy, she developed moderate pulmonary hypertension,

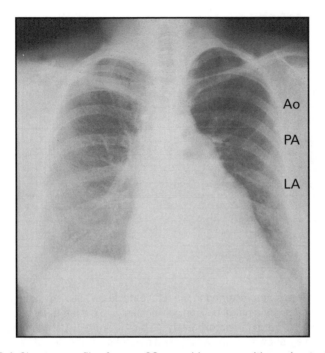

Figure 16.1 Chest *x* ray film from a 28-year-old woman with moderate to severe mitral stenosis in the non-pregnant state at a time when she was in normal sinus rhythm and had no clinical evidence of tricuspid regurgitation. Her overall heart size is at the upper limits of normal and the contours of the left heart border show her aorta (Ao), pulmonary artery (PA), and left atrium or left atrial appendage (LA), and her pulmonary vascularity is near normal

dilatation of the right ventricle, and functional tricuspid regurgitation, which disappeared in the non-pregnant state. Obviously, there was concern that she would be at risk for these same events during a subsequent pregnancy, but the patient was not inclined to have attempted mitral balloon valvuloplasty with its possible complications while she felt well. Six months later she developed symptomatic rapid atrial fibrillation in the non-pregnant state associated with marked breathlessness. She agreed to proceed with percutaneous mitral balloon valvuloplasty.

Hemodynamics before (and immediately after) mitral valvuloplasty. Pressures (mmHg): right atrial 7, right ventricular 36/8, pulmonary arterial 36/21 (24/12), left atrial 18 (7), left ventricular 92/7 (95/7), aorta 92/64 (95/67). Cardiac index: 2·9 l/min per m² (2·9 l/min per m²). Mitral valve gradient 9 mmHg (< 2·0 mmHg). Mitral valve area: 1·6 cm² (>3·0 cm²). Left ventricular angiogram: no mitral regurgitation.

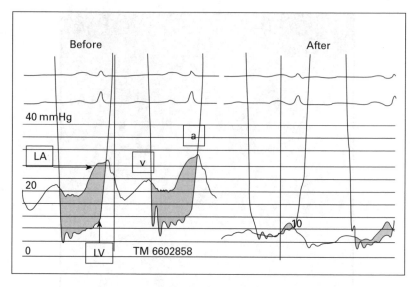

Figure 16.2 Pressures recorded in the left ventricle (LV) and left atrium (LA) before and after percutaneous mitral balloon valvuloplasty. In the left atrial trace before the procedure, an "a" wave of approximately 30 mmHg and a "v" wave of approximately 23 mmHg are shown, with a LV end-diastolic pressure of approximately 10–12 mmHg. The mean gradient across the mitral valve was 9 mmHg and is represented by the shading between the direct LA pressure trace and the LV trace. After the procedure, the LA "a" wave approximates the LV end-diastolic pressure at about 9 mmHg. The LV angiogram after the procedure showed no mitral regurgitation, and the absence of large "v" waves in the LA trace is consistent with this. Note that the gradient across the mitral valve has disappeared

The patient had an uncomplicated mitral balloon valvuloplasty, which relieved her mitral stenosis (Figure 16.2). She subsequently had a further uneventful, successful, normal pregnancy within the next 2 years.

Case 16.2

A 27-year-old woman was referred by an obstetrician for a cardiac evaluation after her first office visit at week 13 of her first pregnancy. Ultrasonography revealed subsequently that she was having twins. Over the preceding month she had noted moderate shortness of breath during normal physical activity. She commented that she had similar symptoms 6 years previously before she had had an atrial septal defect repaired in another city. She remembered that she was told before the cardiac surgery that she had "a 2:1 left to right shunt" and that her pulmonary artery pressure was 70 mmHg.

Examination. Physical examination: the patient was pink without evidence of cyanosis. There was no evidence of clubbing of the extremities. Pulse: 70 beats/min, normal character. Blood pressure: 90/55 mmHg in right arm. Jugular venous pulse: normal. Cardiac impulse: prominent parasternal lift, and palpable pulmonary component of second heart sound. First heart sound: normal. Second heart sound: loud. Pulmonary click heard. No murmurs. Chest examination: normal air entry, no rales or rhonchi. Abdominal examination: soft abdomen, no tenderness, and no masses. Normal liver span. No peripheral edema. Femoral, popliteal, posterior tibial, and dorsalis pedis pulses: all normal volume and equal. Carotid pulses: normal, no bruits.

Investigations. Electrocardiogram (Figure 16.3): normal sinus rhythm with a mean frontal plane axis of approximately 110°, R/S ratio in V_1 >1, and ST-segment depression and T-wave inversions in the right precordial leads consistent with right ventricular hypertrophy. Two-dimensional echocardiogram: markedly dilated right atrium, right ventricle, and pulmonary artery, with paradoxic motion of the interventricular septum, suggesting that right ventricular pressure might exceed left ventricular pressure. Left ventricular systolic function was preserved and there were no abnormalities of the mitral or aortic valves. There was mild tricuspid regurgitation and the right ventricular systolic pressure was estimated to be 100 mmHg. Color Doppler and a bubble study suggested a residual defect at the site of the atrial septal defect repair, with bidirectional shunting across the atrium.

Questions

1. What is the risk to the mother and fetus of this pregnancy? What would you recommend to the patient?

Answers

Answer to question 1 The patient has clinical evidence of severe pulmonary hypertension, presumably secondary to an atrial septal defect that was repaired 6 years previously. Echocardiography now shows evidence of a residual shunt and severe pulmonary hypertension, with paradoxic motion of the interventricular septum and an estimated right ventricular pressure of 100 mmHg while her systolic blood pressure is approximately 90 mmHg. The patient probably has Eisenmenger's syndrome; maternal mortality approaches 50%, and fetal (or neonatal) mortality is around 10–15%. There is no

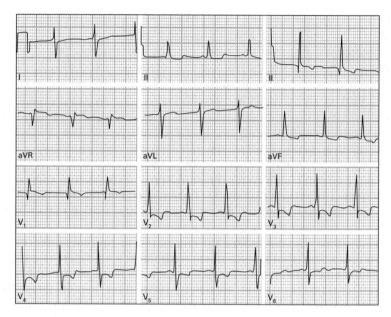

Figure 16.3 This is a 12-lead electrocardiogram (from left to right and top to bottom the leads displayed are I, II, III; aVR, aVL, aVF, V_1 to V_3, V_4 to V_6). The presence of right axis deviation of about +110 (or more), the R/S ratio in V_1 of >1, the R wave in V_1 7 mm or more, the qR pattern in V_1, and the ST-T segment changes in V_2–V_3 changes consistent with strain all suggest right ventricular hypertrophy

medical therapy (for example, pulmonary vasodilators) to offer in this situation to treat the pulmonary hypertension, which is markedly elevated and "fixed". Indeed, administering vasodilators may be dangerous because they will shunt directly into the systemic circulation and may cause hypotension. A less likely possibility is that she has two conditions, namely an atrial septal defect and primary pulmonary hypertension. Although this is unlikely, the maternal mortality with primary pulmonary hypertension of this severity approaches an unacceptable 30%. Because of the unacceptably high maternal mortality, Eisenmenger's syndrome is one of the few cardiac conditions for which termination of pregnancy is recommended. The patient was advised to consider terminating the pregnancy and to have a tubal ligation. She elected to seek a second opinion from the medical center who performed her cardiac surgery 6 years previously. Those physicians decided to perform a cardiac catheterization to examine her cardiac hemodynamics, and this was performed within 2 weeks.

Cardiac catheterization at 14–15 weeks of pregnancy. Oxygen saturations (%): arterial 94, wedge 88, right pulmonary arterial 79, right ventricular 81, low right atrial 77, superior vena cava 67, inferior vena cava 76. Left to right shunt: 1·5–1·0. Pressures (mmHg): wedge 10, right pulmonary arterial 80/38 (mean 52). Pulmonary vascular resistance: 499 dynes·s/cm^5 (normal range 20–130 dynes·s/cm^5). Breathing 100% oxygen: mean right pulmonary arterial pressure 35 mmHg, pulmonary vascular resistance 486 dynes·s/cm^5.

Comment. The saturations show a "step-up" at right atrial level, indicating a left to right shunt. The pulmonary pressures and vascular resistances are markedly elevated, and after administration of 100% oxygen there is a fall in mean pulmonary arterial pressure but the pulmonary vascular resistance is unchanged ("fixed") and is approximately five times normal.

The patient accepted the advice offered at the time of her initial cardiac evaluation during pregnancy and from the physicians who gave the second opinion, and the pregnancy was terminated and a tubal ligation was performed. After seeking multiple opinions as to whether the benefits of repairing the atrial septal defect a second time in the presence of severe, fixed pulmonary hypertension outweighed the risks associated with surgery, the patient decided to continue medical therapy (anticoagulation with warfarin). She is alive and well at follow up 16 years later.

References

1   Campos O, Andrade JL, Bocanegra J, *et al.* Physiologic multivalvular regurgitation during pregnancy: a longitudinal Doppler echocardiographic study. *Int J Cardiol* 1993;40:265–72.
2   Pearson GD, Veille JC, Rahimtoola S, *et al.* Peripartum cardiomyopathy: National Heart, Lung, and Blood Institute and Office of Rare Diseases (National Institutes of Health) workshop recommendations and review. *JAMA* 2000;283:1183–8.
3   Felker GM, Thompson RE, Hare JM, *et al.* Underlying causes and long-term survival in patients with initially unexplained cardiomyopathy. *N Engl J Med* 2000; 342:1077–84.
4   Clark SL, Phelan JP, Greenspoon J, *et al.* Labor and delivery in the presence of mitral stenosis: central hemodynamic observations. *Am J Obstet Gynecol* 1985;152:984–8.
5   Sadler L, McCowan L, White H, Stewart A, Bracken M, North R. Pregnancy outcomes and cardiac complications in women with mechanical, bioprosthetic and homograft valves. *Br J Obstet Gynaecol* 2000;107:245–53.
6   Chan WS, Anand S, Ginsberg JS. Anticoagulation of pregnant women with mechanical heart valves: a systematic review of the literature. *Arch Intern Med* 2000;160:191–6.
7   Ginsberg JS, Hirsh J. Use of antithrombotic agents during pregnancy. *Chest* 1998;114(suppl):524S–30S.
8   Hands M, Johnson MD, Saltzman DH, Rutherford J. The cardiac, obstetric, and anesthetic management of pregnancy complicated by myocardial infarction. *J Clin Anesth* 1990;2:258–68.
9   Madu EC, Kosinski DJ, Wilson WR, Burket MW, Fraker TD, Ansel GM. Two-vessel coronary artery dissection in the peripartum period. Case report and literature review. *Angiology* 1994;45:809–16.
10 Abramov Y, Abramov D, Abrahamov A, Durst R, Schenker J. Elevation of serum creatine phosphokinase and its MB isoenzyme during normal labor and early puerperium. *Acta Obstet Gynecol Scand* 1996;75:255–60.

11 Weiss BM, Zemp L, Seifert B, Hess OM. Outcome of pulmonary vascular disease in pregnancy: a systematic overview from 1978 through 1996. *J Am Coll Cardiol* 1998;**31**:1650–7.

12 Gleicher N, Midwall J, Hochberger D, *et al*. Eisenmenger's syndrome and pregnancy. *Obstet Gynecol Surv* 1979;**34**:721–41.

13 Rossiter JP, Repke JT, Morales AJ, Murphy EA, Pyeritz RE. A prospective longitudinal evaluation of pregnancy in the Marfan syndrome. *Am J Obstet Gynecol* 1995;**173**:1599–606.

14 Elkayam U, Ostrzega E, Shotan A, Mehra A. Cardiovascular problems in pregnant women with the Marfan syndrome. *Ann Intern Med* 1995;**123**:117–22.

15 Shores J, Berger KR, Murphy EA, Pyeritz RE. Progression of aortic dilatation and the benefit of long-term β-adrenergic blockade in Marfan's syndrome. *N Engl J Med* 1994;**330**:1335–41.

16 Page RL. Treatment of arrhythmias during pregnancy. *Am Heart J* 1995;**130**:871–6.

17 Anonymous. Guidelines for cardiopulmonary resuscitation and emergency cardiac care. Emergency Cardiac Care Committee and Subcommittees, American Heart Association. Part IV. Special resuscitation situations. *JAMA* 1992;**268**:2242–50.

18 Dajani AS, Taubert KA, Wilson W, *et al*. Prevention of bacterial endocarditis. Recommendations by the American Heart Association. *JAMA* 1997;**277**:1794–801.

17: Cardiovascular pharmacology

CARLOS M SOTOLONGO, JAMES D MARSH

Discussion of pharmacologic agents in this chapter is descriptive, not prescriptive. Only selected drugs are discussed. One must be familiar with the package insert regarding exact indications, contraindications, and dosages before actual drug administration.

Case 17.1

A 55-year-old male automobile assembly line worker, Mr Bostock, presents with central chest discomfort that occurs with exertion, most commonly when he is working around his home on weekends. Over the past few months this has occurred several times a week. It is a squeezing sensation in the middle of his chest that is provoked by exertion such as painting the ceiling or mowing the lawn, and it is relieved by resting for a few minutes. The discomfort does not radiate. It is not positional and does not occur at rest. It is sometimes associated with sweating but is not associated with shortness of breath. Once or twice he has had the discomfort initially when he starts his shift on the assembly line, but with continued moderate activity the discomfort does not recur.

The patient is a former 15 pack-year smoker, having stopped 5 years ago. He does not have a history of cough or wheezing. He has been told he has borderline hypertension but has not required medication. He is unaware of his serum cholesterol level. His father had a myocardial infarction at age 60 years.

Examination. Physical examination: the patient was muscular. No abnormalities of skin, nail beds, or oral mucosa. Pulse: 85 beats/min, normal character. Blood pressure: 145/90 mmHg in right arm. Jugular venous pulse: normal. Cardiac impulse: normal. First heart sound: normal. Second heart sound: split normally on inspiration. Fourth heart sound heard. No murmurs. Chest examination: normal air entry, no rales or rhonchi. Abdominal examination: soft abdomen, no tenderness, and no masses. Normal liver span. No peripheral edema. Femoral, popliteal, posterior tibial, and dorsalis pedis pulses: all normal volume and equal. Carotid pulses: normal, no bruits. Optic fundi: normal.

Investigations. Routine laboratory tests, including fasting lipid panel: entirely normal. Resting 12-lead electrocardiogram: minor non-specific ST-T wave abnormalities, no evidence of left ventricular hypertrophy.

Questions

1. What is the most likely diagnosis?
2. Is further testing needed at this time? If so, what test?
3. How would you manage this man with pharmacotherapy?
4. What are the pharmacologic properties of aspirin, metoprolol, and nitrates that modify angina pectoris? Why are these drugs appropriate in this setting?

Answers

Answer to question 1

The symptoms are typical of angina pectoris. The character of the discomfort and the description that it is always effort related and is relieved by resting make this the most likely diagnosis. The pattern is relatively stable, the discomfort has never occurred at rest, and it has been occurring for several weeks. The evaluation and management can probably be done safely on an outpatient basis.

Answer to question 2

The patient's physician has diagnosed angina on the basis of his history. Now there is a need to determine whether significant myocardial ischemia is induced by increased metabolic demand of the heart during a "stress" test. Therefore, a symptom limited, treadmill exercise, perfusion imaging nuclear scan is ordered. Mr Bostock exercises for 6 min achieving a workload of 7 METs, and stops because of chest tightness. The electrocardiogram shows 1 mm ST-segment depression in leads V_3–V_6, and nuclear perfusion images show a moderate sized anterolateral defect at peak exertion that reperfuses on delayed images.

Answer to question 3

After discussion, the patient and his physician decide to initiate medical therapy and the therapy he is started on includes the following: aspirin 81 mg/day (antiplatelet), metoprolol 50 mg twice daily (β-blocker), isosorbide dinitrate 20 mg three times daily (nitrate), and sublingual nitroglycerin as needed for discomfort and to take prophylactically before activities that are likely to induce angina.

Answer to question 4

Aspirin

Mode of action Aspirin (acetylsalicylic acid) is a non-steroidal anti-inflammatory drug that inhibits platelet function. Aspirin acetylates cyclo-oxygenase in platelets, blocking formation of thromboxane A_2 from arachidonic acid. Thus, aspirin abolishes the potent vasoconstricting and platelet aggregating effect of thromboxane A_2. Because the acetylation of cyclo-oxygenase is essentially irreversible, the platelets present at the time at which aspirin is administered are affected for their lifetime (8–10 days).

Pharmacokinetics Aspirin is rapidly absorbed in the stomach and small intestine. Peak plasma levels occur within 15–20 min. The antiplatelet effect is manifest within 1 hour. For the antiplatelet effect, one dose per day or every other day is needed. The clinical antiplatelet effect persists for about 5 days after the last dose.

Side effects Gastrointestinal side effects are most common and are dependent on dose, dosing interval, and duration of treatment. They include dyspepsia, nausea and vomiting. Gastrointestinal effects may be reduced with enteric coated aspirin. There is a 3% incidence of gastrointestinal bleeding, usually from multiple discrete ulcers or hemorrhagic gastritis.

Indications for Mr Bostock The indication in this case is primary prevention of cardiovascular events: aspirin use is likely to reduce the risk for myocardial infarction in men over the age of 50 years. Studies of dosage and platelet function suggest that, for prevention of myocardial infarction, low doses of aspirin are adequate (100 mg/day or less).[1,2]

Other indications *Secondary prevention.* In patients with acute coronary syndromes (acute non-ST-segment elevation myocardial infarction, unstable angina), aspirin decreases rates of non-fatal reinfarction and cardiovascular death.[3] It has a similar effect in patients with chronic stable angina and after myocardial infarction. Aspirin is used to prevent vessel closure after percutaneous transluminal coronary angioplasty (combined initially with clopidogrel) and to prevent graft closure after coronary artery bypass graft surgery. At the time of acute ST-segment elevation myocardial infarction aspirin use, either in conjunction with fibrinolytic therapy or alone, reduces cardiac mortality.[4]

Atrial fibrillation. For non-valvular atrial fibrillation aspirin is effective in preventing cerebral and systemic emboli. In patients in atrial fibrillation at low risk for cerebral emboli, its efficacy in preventing stroke is similar to that of warfarin.[3]

β-Adrenergic receptor blockers

β-Blocking drugs are widely used for several indications in patients with cardiovascular disease. The endogenous neurotransmitter and hormone norepinephrine (noradrenaline) and the hormone epinephrine (adrenaline) bind to β_1- and β_2-adrenergic receptors in myocardium and in vascular smooth muscle. In myocardium, the adrenergic agonists norepinephrine and epinephrine produce positive inotropic and chronotropic effects, enhance conduction, and in vascular tissue they produce vasodilation via β-adrenergic pathways (and vasoconstriction via α-adrenergic pathways). β-Adrenergic agonists modulate the renal production of renin, and via the renin–angiotensin–aldosterone system they modulate blood pressure (see Chapter 4). β-Adrenergic blockers (antagonists) partly or completely block the agonist effects.

In the human heart there is a mixture of β_1- and β_2-adrenergic receptors, typically expressed at a ratio of about 65%/35%, respectively. There is a large number of β-adrenergic blocking drugs clinically available, with some or little selectivity for β_1- and β_2-receptors; pure antagonism for the receptor or partial agonism; different degrees of lipophilicity; and highly varying pharmacokinetics, with half-lives varying from 8 min to 30 hours.

β-Adrenergic blockers are commonly used to treat angina pectoris. The drug decreases heart rate, contractility, and blood pressure, thereby decreasing three major determinants of myocardial oxygen consumption and improving the myocardial oxygen supply/demand ratio. By blocking the effects of catecholamines on the myocardium and conduction system, β-adrenergic blockers decrease the excitability of tissue, and the prevalence of atrial and ventricular arrhythmias. When β-adrenergic blockers are administered in the hours following myocardial infarction, the short-term mortality of the patient is improved, probably because of both effects cited above. When administered to survivors of myocardial infarction for the 1–3 years after the infarct, β-adrenergic blockers decrease mortality during this period of time as well. The mechanism is less certain, but may be due to prevention of ischemic events and/or arrhythmias (Table 17.1).

Table 17.1 β-Adrenergic blocking drugs

Drug	β₁ selective?	Typical intravenous dose	Typical oral dose	Indications
Propranolol	No	1–3 mg	40 mg three times daily	Angina, arrhythmias, hypertension
Metoprolol	Yes	5–15 mg (divided doses)	50 mg twice daily	Angina, myocardial infarction, hypertension, arrhythmias
Atenolol	Yes	5–10 mg (divided doses)	50 mg/day	Angina, hypertension, myocardial infarction, arrhythmias

Dosing See Table 17.1.

Adverse effects There are many potential adverse effects from β-adrenergic blockers because they interrupt one arm of the autonomic nervous system, which innervates many organs in the body. Bronchospasm due to β-adrenergic blockers is a common problem. The presence of bronchospastic pulmonary disease is thus a contraindication to their use. (Drugs with relative β_1-receptor selectivity, if used in a low dose, may produce little aggravation of bronchospasm, but β_1/β_2 selectivity of all drugs is only relative and not absolute; in high doses β_1-receptor selectivity is lost. Because there are other pharmacologic options available to reduce heart rate and blood pressure, we do not recommend use of β-blockers in any patient with known or induced bronchospasm.)

Other common adverse effects of β-adrenergic blockers can be predicted from the withdrawal of sympathetic tone, and can include excess bradycardia, hypotension, and high degree heart block. Many patients with advanced heart failure have high sympathetic tone, which may aggravate their heart failure by producing downregulation of β-adrenergic receptors. However, it has emerged that several β-blockers (carvedilol,[5] bisoprolol, extended release metoprolol) improve mortality and quality of life, and reduce hospitalization in patients with mild to moderate (New York Heart Association functional class II or III) heart failure.[6] Initiation of this therapy requires individualized drug dosing and very careful clinical monitoring.

Indications for Mr Bostock Metoprolol is a good choice for management of angina because he does not have a history of bronchospastic pulmonary disease. The antihypertensive effect may also be of benefit.

Table 17.2 Nitrate drugs

Drug	Onset	Duration	Dosing intervals
Nitroglycerin	0·5–5 min	10–30 min	As needed
Sublingual nitroglycerin aerosol	0·5–5 min	10–30 min	As needed
Isosorbide dinitrate	30–45 min	2–8 h	Three times daily
Nitropaste 2%	20–60 min	3–8 h	Three times daily
Nitropatch	30–60 min	8–14 h	Every day
Isosorbide mononitrate	30 min	8–14 h	Every day

Nitrates

Organic nitrates and nitrites are used to treat several cardiovascular disorders, including myocardial ischemia, congestive heart failure, and hypertensive crisis. There are many preparations of nitrates with similar pharmacodynamics but distinct pharmacokinetic properties (Table 17.2).

Mode of action Organic nitrates interact with intracellular sulfhydral groups (for example, thiols found on cysteine) to form unstable intermediates, known as S-nitrosothiols, which spontaneously generate nitric oxide. Nitric oxide is thought to be identical to the endogenous compound endothelial derived relaxing factor. Nitric oxide/endothelial derived relaxing factor activates guanylate cyclase in vascular smooth muscle, which leads to an increase in intracellular cyclic guanosine monophosphate, which is responsible for the observed clinical response of vasodilatation via sequestration of intracellular calcium and/or dephosphorylation of myosin light chains. At low concentrations (<50 micrograms/min), nitroglycerin infusion is primarily a venodilator and by increasing venous capacitance it decreases preload. At higher concentrations arterial dilatation occurs.

The pathogenesis of chronic stable angina and unstable angina differ significantly but both respond to nitroglycerin. Chronic stable angina is usually brought on by "supply and demand" mismatch, that is, an increase in oxygen demand with a fixed coronary blood flow (see Chapter 7). The end result is an increase in left ventricular end-diastolic pressure and wall tension, as well as a sympathetic response characterized by increased systolic blood pressure (afterload) and heart rate. These hemodynamic events lead to increased myocardial oxygen demand and angina. Nitrates produce vasodilatation of venous system with resultant decreases in left ventricular end-diastolic pressure, left ventricular volume, and wall tension. Nitrates also vasodilate the coronary arteries, increasing coronary blood flow and decreasing angina.[7] Patients with coronary artery disease also have abnormal endothelial function characterized by paradoxic coronary vasoconstriction in response to various substances, probably because of decreased endogenous endothelial derived relaxing factor production. Nitrates do not require normal endothelium to produce relaxation of vascular smooth muscle. Also, there is strong evidence to support an antiplatelet effect of nitroglycerin.

Indications for Mr Bostock Administration of a long-acting nitrate preparation should favorably alter hemodynamics and decrease the frequency and severity of angina for Mr Bostock, and allow him to perform more physical activity and delay the onset of angina. The use of sublingual nitroglycerin acutely and prophylactically will also help.

Other indications *Acute coronary syndromes (unstable angina and non-ST-segment elevation acute myocardial infarction).* The pathogenesis of these syndromes is most commonly a rupture of an atherosclerotic plaque with exposure of proaggregatory substances (for example, collagen), which initiates intracoronary platelet aggregation and thrombus formation. In patients with unstable angina a significant decrease in progression to myocardial infarction has been shown in patients who receive heparin, aspirin, and β-blockers, but not with nitroglycerin. Intravenous nitroglycerin is used at low doses (<50 micrograms/min) because symptoms are improved.[8] With all doses of continuously infused nitroglycerin, at least partial pharmacologic tolerance to the drug develops within 24 hours. When intravenous nitroglycerin is being weaned off, longer-acting nitrates should be administered to avoid "rebound ischemia". In acute anterior myocardial infarction, early initiation of intravenous nitroglycerin tends to improve mortality, infarct size, and left ventricular remodeling.

Congestive heart failure. Patients with the most severe heart failure tend to derive the most clinical benefit from nitrates. In this setting, nitrates decrease preload by venodilatation and decrease afterload by arterial dilatation, thereby improving cardiac output. Long-acting nitrates are often administered in combination with hydralazine (a direct acting arteriolar dilator) for patients with class III–IV congestive heart failure. This combination improves both symptoms and survival. Nitrates and hydralazine are the standard of care in heart failure patients who are unable to tolerate converting enzyme inhibitors.

Adverse effects Adverse effects are predominantly manifest in the cardiovascular system, and include headache, hypotension, syncope, gastrointestinal upset, contact dermatitis, methemoglobinemia (rare), and tachyphylaxis. Metabolism occurs in the liver by the glutathione–organic nitrate reductase system. Tachyphylaxis in response to the hemodynamic effects of nitroglycerin occur with prolonged use and is improved by lower doses of nitrates or by an 8–10 hour nitrate-free period every day. Tachyphylaxis is thought, in part, to be secondary to depletion of sulfhydral groups; this nitrate-free period permits repletion of these compounds.

Case 17.1 (continued)

Mr Bostock returns to see his physician in 1 week. He has had no further angina, but finds that he routinely gets a headache 30 min after taking the isosorbide dinitrate. Headaches have not decreased in severity over the week and he finds them intolerable, despite taking acetaminophen for headache relief. His physician continues all his medications, except that she stops the isosorbide dinitrate and starts diltiazem (long acting) 180 mg/day (calcium channel blocker).

Questions

5. Why are headaches occurring?
6. How do calcium channel antagonists work; is there a difference among the three subclasses of calcium channel antagonists?

Answers

Answer to question 5

Headaches are common with nitrates. The headaches are due to cerebral venous and arteriolar dilatation, and are usually dose related. For some patients, headaches improve over several days; for others they are intractable, even with a low dose of nitrates.

Answer to question 6

Calcium channel blockers

Mechanism of action Calcium channel blockers decrease myocardial ischemia by producing dilatation of coronary arteries as well as peripheral arteriolar dilatation, lowering afterload and thus reducing myocardial oxygen demand. To varying degrees, all calcium channel blockers have a negative inotropic effect, which would tend to

Table 17.3 Calcium channel blockers

Drug	Subclass	Indication	Typical total dose (24 h)	Sinus rate	Atrio-ventricular conduction
Nifedipine	Dihydropyridine	Chronic angina, hypertension	20–120 mg	↑	↑
Diltiazem	Benzothiazipine	Angina, hypertension, atrial fibrillation	90–360 mg	↓	↓
Verapamil	Phenylalkylamine	Angina, hypertension, atrial fibrillation	60–180 mg	↓	↓

decrease myocardial ischemia as well. Some subclasses of calcium channel blockers also lower heart rate. There are important differences in the pharmacodynamics of the three major subclasses of calcium channel blockers: dihydropyridines (represented by nifedipine), benzothiazipines (represented by diltiazem), and phenylalkylamines (represented by verapamil). All are effective arteriolar dilators and effective antihypertensive drugs. Verapamil, diltiazem, and to a less degree nifedipine, and some other dihydropyridines, have a negative inotropic effect on the myocardium, which may become clinically significant when the ejection fraction is under 40–45% (Table 17.3). Drugs from all three classes are effective antianginal agents and effective antihypertensive drugs. In angina patients they all reduce symptoms and improve exercise performance. Drugs from all three classes are available in short-acting (about 6 hours) and long-acting (12–24 hours) formulations.

Indications for patient For Mr Bostock, a drug from any of the three subclasses of calcium channel blockers would probably be effective for angina, would improve exercise performance, and would be well tolerated.

Case 17.1 (continued)

Mr Bostock does well for 3 years, rarely having angina. In fact, on his own he discontinued taking all of his medications. On getting up from bed one morning he developed severe chest pain, associated with diaphoresis, dyspnea, and a sense of doom. He was taken to the nearest emergency room within 1 hour of the onset of the chest discomfort. Electrocardiograms and subsequent cardiac enzymes confirmed the clinical suspicion of an ST-segment elevation inferior myocardial infarction. It was decided to treat him with antithrombotic therapy and a thrombolytic drug.

As the drugs were being prepared he started vomiting; his heart rate decreased to 30 beats/min. A junctional bradycardia was noted on the monitor. Atropine (0·5 mg intravenously) was administered and sinus rhythm at 95 beats/min was restored. He was given an aspirin and the thrombolytic drug. The chest pain worsened; he was given a small dose of intravenous morphine, intravenous nitroglycerin was instituted, and metoprolol 5 mg intravenous (repeated once) was administered. The chest pain improved, and 1 hour after the thrombolytic drug was administered, the chest pain suddenly resolved. However, repeated runs of ventricular tachycardia were noted on the monitor. The rate was about 150 beat/min. Mr Bostock became near syncopal during the ventricular tachycardia, which lasted about 30 seconds. Accordingly, lidocaine (100 mg bolus, followed by continuous infusion at 2 mg/min) was instituted. He was rebolused with 50 mg lidocaine intravenous 30 min after the first bolus. The ventricular tachycardia did not recur, and Mr Bostock clinically stabilized.

Questions

7. Why use antithrombotic therapy in an acute myocardial infarction? How does heparin help in this setting? How does aspirin help?
8. What is the mechanism of action of atropine?
9. What actions of intravenous nitroglycerin are of particular help in the setting of acute myocardial infarction?
10. What are the mechanisms of action of streptokinase and of tissue plasminogen activator?
11. What is the mechanism of action of lidocaine?

Answers

Answer to question 7

Aspirin (an antiplatelet agent) was administered to decrease the contribution of platelet aggregation to the thrombus formation in the coronary artery that was producing the infarction.

Answer to question 8

Atropine blocks the effect of the neurotransmitter acetylcholine at muscarinic cholinergic receptors. Both the gastrointestinal tract and the heart (particularly the conduction system) are rich in vagal efferent fibers for which acetylcholine is the neurotransmitter. The effect on the heart produced by stimulation of the vagus nerve (and blocked by atropine) includes decreased automaticity of the sinoatrial node and atrioventricular node, and slowing of conduction in the atrioventricular node. In acute myocardial infarction, especially that involving the inferoposterior wall, there is often intense vagal stimulation. This commonly produces vagally mediated reflux bradycardia and high degree atrioventricular block, as well as intense gastrointestinal symptoms, including vomiting. Administration of atropine intravenously (0·5–1·0 mg) blocks the muscarinic cholinergic receptors, abolishes the effect of the parasympathetic stimulation, and thus ameliorates the bradycardia, atrioventricular block, and gastrointestinal symptoms that are often seen in this clinical setting.

Answer to question 9

Intravenous nitroglycerin favorably alters the myocardial oxygen supply/demand relationship in myocardial ischemia and infarction (see mechanisms of action of nitrates, above). In addition to thrombus formation in myocardial infarction, there is a variable degree of coronary vasoconstriction produced in part by vasoactive substances released from platelets in the coronary thrombus. Nitroglycerin, in the doses that are usually given intravenously, has a direct coronary vasodilator effect, improving oxygen delivery. Second, nitroglycerin, by producing venodilatation, reduces preload, left ventricular size, wall stress, and myocardial oxygen consumption. Finally, intravenous nitroglycerin produces systemic arteriolar dilatation, leading to decreased afterload and decreased myocardial oxygen consumption.[8]

Answer to question 10

Thrombolytic agents

After a thrombus is formed, fibrinolysis is achieved by converting plasminogen into plasmin, which has protease activity capable of breaking down the fibrin component of a thrombus. The conversion of plasminogen to plasmin is mediated by several factors, including factor XIIa and tissue plasminogen activator (t-PA), which is synthesized and released by endothelial cells. These agents have been shown to lower mortality of patients with ST-segment elevation acute myocardial infarction when administered within 12 hours of the onset of symptoms.[9] There are numerous pharmacologic activators of plasminogen used clinically, including t-PA, streptokinase, retaplase, and tenecteplase.

Tissue plasminogen activator   The human protein t-PA is produced using recombinant DNA technology (rt-PA). t-PA binds to fibrin in formed thrombus with high affinity, and once bound the complex activates local plasminogen. Because of its binding to fibrin, there is relatively little systemic fibrinolysis. Typically, a total dose of 100 mg is administered intravenously over 90 min: a 15 mg bolus, followed by 50 mg over an hour, and 35 mg over the last 30 min. Advantages over streptokinase include lower incidences of allergic reactions, hypotension, and bleeding complications. It can be used repeatedly without concern for anaphylactic reactions. Disadvantages include a slightly higher incidence of hemorrhagic stroke, primarily in patients over 75 years of age; also, t-PA is very expensive.

Streptokinase   The thrombolytic agent streptokinase is a bacterial protein produced by group C β-hemolytic streptococcal cultures. By binding directly to plasminogen, the complex becomes enzymatically active and converts plasminogen into plasmin. Streptokinase is not highly fibrin selective and induces a greater degree of systemic thrombolytic effect than does t-PA. The dosage for acute myocardial infarction is 1·5 million units administered over 60 min. Advantages include its efficacy profile being generally similar to rt-PA; it is relatively inexpensive.

Adverse effects. Allergic reaction, and hypotension during infusion are relatively common. Because it is a bacterial protein and has antigenic properties, it cannot be readministered for 6 months. Bleeding is a common side effect that can be minimized by avoiding cannulation of non-compressible vessels, arterial punctures, or intramuscular injections.

Adjuvant agents for thrombolysis   Thrombolytic therapy is aimed at dissolution of the thrombus but it does not remedy the underlying cause. In treatment following myocardial infarction there is a paradoxic prothrombotic state, because the underlying stimulus responsible for the original thrombus (i.e. plaque rupture) is still present. Hence, adjuvant antithrombotic treatment is critical.[8,10] Aspirin at doses of at least 160 mg decreases mortality by 23% in acute myocardial infarction and 42% in conjunction with thrombolytics. In addition, heparin therapy decreases mortality and reocclusion following t-PA administration. This efficacy of heparin is less clear cut with streptokinase. Heparin is initiated during infusion of thrombolytic agent and continued for 24–72 hours.

Indications for thrombolytics

- Chest pain consistent with acute myocardial infarction.
- ST-segment elevation of at least 0·1 mV in two contiguous leads or new onset of bundle branch block.
- Time of onset of symptoms: most beneficial if symptoms are less than a few hours from onset at the time of administration, but benefits are seen up to 12 hours after the onset of symptoms.

Contraindications Contraindications to thrombolytic therapy are many. Among the considerations are excluding from therapy any patient with a significant chance of more than trivial bleeding.

Answer to question 11

Lidocaine is a class 1B antiarrhythmic agent. Like other class I agents, it blocks sodium channels. However, unlike some other class I agents, it promotes repolarization. This protects against QT prolongation and associated proarrhythmic effects.

Electrophysiologic properties

Lidocaine is particularly efficacious in the ischemic myocardium. It decrease automaticity, action potential duration, and effective refractory period of Purkinje fibers and ventricular muscle, with little or no effect on atria, atrioventricular node, or accessory pathways.

Hemodynamic effects

This drug is usually well tolerated at therapeutic dose. It may produce a modest decrease in ventricular contractility in those patients with severely depressed systolic function.

Pharmacokinetics

Lidocaine is available only in intravenous form. It is metabolized rapidly by the liver into various less active agents. The elimination half-life is 1–2 hours.

Adverse effects

Cardiovascular It rarely causes bradyarrhythmias but needs to be used cautiously in patients with underlying heart block.

Non-cardiovascular Most common adverse effects are due to central nervous system excitability or depression. Lidocaine may result in drowsiness, confusion, nervousness, or seizures. Particularly vulnerable are older patients with underlying hepatic disease or decrease in hepatic blood flow, such as patients in heart failure.

Dosage The usual loading dose is 1–2 mg/kg, followed by 1–2 mg/min continuous infusion. Because of the short half-life of the drug for optimal dosing, after an initial intravenous bolus patients should be rebolused (using half the initial dose) 20–40 min later. In older patients, or those with heart failure, a continuous infusion overnight of 2 mg/min or more will invariably lead to central nervous system toxicity. Therapeutic plasma levels are 2–5 micrograms/ml.

Drug interactions Drugs that decrease hepatic blood flow, such as β-blockers, may lead to decreased lidocaine metabolism and increased toxicity. Cimetidine also decreases its metabolism.

Indications Because it has little or no effect on atrial refractory period, it is not useful in supraventricular tachyarrhythmias and may actually accelerate accessory pathway conduction in patients with Wolff–Parkinson–White syndrome. Its greatest efficacy is in ventricular tachyarrhythmias, particularly in the setting of an acute ischemic syndrome. In acute myocardial infarction, lidocaine reduces the rate of ventricular fibrillation, but has no effect on mortality.

Case 17.1 (continued)

Four days following acute myocardial infarction, Mr Bostock had an episode of near syncope. Monomorphic, sustained ventricular tachycardia (a 90 second episode) was noted on the cardiac monitor. Evaluation by echocardiography demonstrated moderately depressed left ventricular function. A symptom limited exercise test was negative for ischemia and for arrhythmias. His physician decided on an empiric trial of quinidine to suppress the ventricular arrhythmia, and quinidine gluconate (324 mg every 8 hours) was started. Forty-eight hours later, near syncope occurred again. The cardiac monitor showed polymorphic ventricular tachycardia (torsades de pointes) at a rate of 170 beat/min, lasting for 60 seconds. Quinidine was discontinued. This arrhythmia did not recur. Mr Bostock's physician considered alternative approaches, including electrophysiologic testing or empiric therapy with flecainide, sotalol, or amiodarone. After discussing the options with Mr Bostock, amiodarone was started. A loading program of 1200 mg/day for 7 days was administered, followed by maintenance therapy at 200 mg/day.

Questions

12. What is the mechanism of action of quinidine and of procainamide? Why did torsades de pointes occur?
13. What are the mechanisms of action of flecainide, sotalol, and amiodarone?

Answers

Answer to question 12

Quinidine

Quinidine inhibits sodium channels as well as the repolarizing potassium channels, which results in prolonging the action potential duration and the effective refractory period.

Hemodynamics   Quinidine has little, if any, negative inotropic effect and seldom worsens heart failure when given orally. It is rarely used parenterally.

Pharmacokinetics   After oral administration, bioavailability is 90%. It is metabolized in the liver to hydroxyquinidine, which also possesses antiarrhythmic effects. It is eliminated largely by the hepatic route; however, 20–30% is excreted in the urine. Steady state plasma levels are reached within 24 hours and elimination half-life is 6–8 hours.

Dosing   Quinidine is available orally as quinidine sulfate, quinidine gluconate, and quinidine sulfate extended release, which are administered every 6, 8, and 12 hours, respectively. The usual starting dose is 1·2–1·4 g/daily. Because of its adverse effects profile and idiosyncratic reactions, quinidine therapy usually should not be initiated on an outpatient basis (Table 17.4).

Adverse effects   *Cardiovascular.* Proarrhythmic adverse effects include increased frequency of ventricular premature depolarizations, ventricular tachycardia, and torsades de pointes. Although usually manifest in the first few days after initiating drug treatment, torsades de pointes can occur at any time. The incidence of torsades de pointes is 1–8% and occurs as an idiosyncratic reaction to quinidine, and is not dose dependent. In patients with sick sinus syndrome quinidine may lead to bradycardia; in patients with atrial fibrillation or flutter the ventricular response can be increased.

Table 17.4 Antiarrhythmic drugs

Drug	Class	Typical dose	Adverse effects
Quinidine gluconate	1A	324 mg three times daily	Diarrhea, tinnitus, torsade de pointes
Procainamide (sustained release)	1A	750 mg three times daily	Gastrointestinal effects; systemic lupus erythematosus-like syndrome
Flecainide	1C	100 mg twice daily	Heart block, proarrhythmia, central nervous system symptoms
Sotalol	III	80–160 mg twice daily	Proarrhythmia, β-blocking effects
Amiodarone	I, II, III, IV	200–800 mg/day (maintenance dose)	See Table 17.6

Non-cardiac. Non-cardiac effects are the most common adverse effects and include diarrhea (reported in up to one-third of patients), nausea, flu-like symptoms, tinnitus, headaches, light-headedness, loss of hearing, and elevated liver enzymes. Thrombocytopenia is secondary to quinidine–platelet immunogen complex. These adverse effects account for the most common reasons to discontinue quinidine therapy.

Drug interactions Most pronounced is an increase in serum digoxin level, which may lead to bradycardia and predispose the patient to torsades de pointes. The therapeutic effects of warfarin are also enhanced. Cimetidine can decrease hepatic metabolism of quinidine.

Indications Quinidine is used for supraventricular and ventricular tachyarrhythmias. In the past it has been used for maintaining sinus rhythm chronically in such patients or in those with paroxysmal atrial fibrillation. Although its efficacy is as good as other type 1 antiarrhythmics, a meta-analysis of several trials showed a threefold increase in mortality when compared with placebo.[11] Quinidine is also effective in treating other types of supraventricular tachyarrhythmias such as Wolff–Parkinson–White syndrome. However, with radiofrequency ablations of these re-entrant tachycardias, its use is becoming less frequent. Finally, it is not as efficacious as amiodarone or sotalol in treating patients with aborted sudden cardiac death.

Procainamide

Procainamide is a class 1A antiarrhythmic agent with electrophysiologic properties similar to those of quinidine. However, the QT interval is not prolonged to the same extent and QRS is usually unchanged. It suppresses automaticity at therapeutic levels and decreases conduction velocity in the atria, ventricles, His–Purkinje system, and accessory pathways.

Hemodynamic effects α-Adrenergic blockade mediated peripheral vasodilatation may lead to hypotension when procainamide is given as an intravenous bolus. At therapeutic doses, the negative inotropic effect is negligible.

Phamacokinetics Bioavailability following absorption is 75–90%. It undergoes hepatic acetylation to form a second biologically active antiarrhythmic, namely N-acetyl procainamide, which may represent a half of total drug in the plasma. Both are excreted in the urine.

Adverse effects *Cardiovascular.* Heart block may be seen in some patients and caution is needed when used in patients with marked disturbances in conduction. Proarrhythmic effects are dose related. Torsades de pointes occurs less frequently than with quinidine. Procainamide may also produce a paradoxic increase in ventricular response in patients with atrial fibrillation or flutter who are not on rate controlling drugs.
Non-cardiac. Non-cardiac adverse effects are more common than adverse cardiac effects. A positive antinuclear antibody ANA titer is seen in 50–60% of patients, with a significant amount of these patients progressing to develop a systemic lupus erythematosus-like syndrome. Patients who are "slow acetylators" and have higher levels of plasma procainamide are at increased risk for this syndrome. Drug discontinuation is required. Other adverse effects include bone marrow suppression, which is usually seen during the first 3 months of therapy.

Indications Indications for use are similar to those of quinidine, with similar efficacy in treating supraventricular and ventricular tachyarrhythmias. Indications include conversion of atrial fibrillation or flutter to sinus rhythm, and maintaining sinus rhythm chronically. It is also efficacious in patients with atrioventricular node re-entrant tachycardia and Wolff–Parkinson–White syndrome. It is used to suppress or prevent recurrence of life-threatening ventricular arrhythmias either by itself or in conjunction with amiodarone. If it is difficult to decide whether a "wide complex" tachycardia is ventricular tachycardia or supraventricular tachyarrhythmia with

Table 17.5 Electrocardiographic effects of antiarrhythmic drugs

Drug	Class	Effect on electrocardiogram intervals			Heart rate	Left ventricular function
		PR	QRS	QT		
Digoxin		↑		↓	↓	↑
Procainamide	1a	↑	↑	↑	→	↓
Quinidine	1a	↑↓	↑	↑	↑	→
Lidocaine	1b			↓	→	→
Flecainide	1c	↑	↑		→	↓
Propranolol	2	↑			↓	↓
Amiodarone	3	↑		↑	↓	→
Sotalol	3	↑		↑	↓	↓
Verapamil	4	↑			↓	↓
Diltiazem	4	↑			↓	↓

aberration, then procainamide is an appropriate antiarrhythmic to consider using.

Dosage The usual loading dose is 1 g given orally or slowly intravenously, followed either by 2–4 mg/min infusions or 2–6 g/day orally. Procainamide (slow release) is given at 6 hour intervals. When plasma levels are obtained, one must check both procainamide and N-acetyl procainamide levels.

Drug interactions Cimetidine will prolong the half-life. There is no interaction with digoxin or warfarin.

Answer to question 13

Flecainide

Mode of action Flecainide is a potent inhibitor of the sodium channel and produces a dose-related decrease in conduction throughout the myocardium; it exhibits its greatest effect on the His–Purkinje system.[12]

Hemodynamics Flecainide has a negative inotropic effect that is almost exclusively seen in patients with depressed ventricular function (Table 17.5).

Pharmacokinetics Bioavailability after oral administration is nearly 95%. There is no first pass effect and steady state is reached within 3–4 days. Half-life is 13–19 hours. It is excreted renally.

Adverse effects Flecainide, like all antiarrhythmic agents, can be proarrhythmic or worsen baseline arrhythmias. Adverse proarrhythmic events are strongly correlated with the presence of structural heart disease. Exacerbation of heart failure is also correlated with severity of underlying ventricular dysfunction and functional class. In patients with pacemakers, the pacing threshold may be increased and needs to be followed closely.

Dosage Usual starting dose is 50–100 mg twice daily and can increase by 50 mg every 4 days. Dosage should not exceed 150–200 mg twice daily.

Drug interactions Digoxin serum concentrations are increased by less than 20%. Propanolol coadministration will result in higher flecainide plasma levels.

Indications *Supraventricular tachyarrhythmia.* Flecainide has good efficacy and safety for patients with paroxysmal supraventricular tachycardia and paroxysmal atrial fibrillation, particularly in patients with no structural heart disease.

Ventricular tachyarrhythmias. Flecainide is very efficacious in suppressing ventricular premature depolarizations and non-sustained ventricular tachyarrhythmias; however, the clinical importance of this is questionable. In addition, when used following myocardial infarction to suppress ventricular premature depolarizations and non-sustained ventricular tachycardia, there is a twofold increase in mortality when compared with placebo. This is believed to be secondary to a proarrhythmic effect and worsening heart failure. Flecainide is approved for treatment of life-threatening ventricular tachycardia.

Sotalol

Sotalol is a non-selective β-adrenergic blocking agent that also possesses antiarrhythmic properties.[13] It is classified as a class III antiarrhythmic drug based on its ability to inhibit the potassium channel and thus prolong the action potential and increase the refractory period. QT prolongation is dose dependent.

Hemodynamics Unlike other β-adrenergic blockers, which exhibit negative inotropic effects, sotalol may actually improve ventricular contractility by increasing the action potential duration and allowing more time for calcium influx. The net result is little change in ventricular function. However, sotalol can worsen heart failure in patients with underlying ventricular dysfunction.

Pharmacokinetics After oral administration, absorption and bioavailability are nearly 100%. It does not undergo a first pass effect. It is excreted unchanged by the kidneys. Elimination half-life is 7–18 hours and steady state is reached within 3 days.

Dosing Dosing needs to be adjusted for creatinine clearance. In patients with normal renal function, dosing begins at 40–80 mg twice daily and can be increased to 160 mg twice daily.

Adverse effects Discontinuation of sotalol secondary to adverse effects is approximately 15%.

Cardiovascular. Sotalol at high doses may contribute to worsening heart failure in patients with baseline ventricular dysfunction. It can cause sinus bradycardia and atrioventricular blocks. As with any antiarrhythmic drug, sotalol may be proarrhythmic. The incidence of torsades de pointes is 3–4%. It is usually seen within the first week and it is clearly dose dependent. Sotalol should be used cautiously with QT intervals greater than 500 ms, and once QT interval exceeds 550 ms one needs to consider strongly a decrease in dose or discontinuation of drug.

Non-cardiovascular. Other adverse effects include fatigue, dizziness, nausea, vomiting, rash, and bronchospasm.

Indications Sotalol is very effective in supraventricular and ventricular tachyarrhythmias. In patients with atrial fibrillation who have undergone electrical cardioversion, sotalol is as effective as and better tolerated than quinidine in maintaining sinus rhythm. Because of its β-adrenergic blocking actions, patients who developed atrial fibrillation were less symptomatic secondary to better heart rate control. Sotalol is as effective as amiodarone in treatment of hemodynamically significant ventricular tachycardia and survivors of sudden cardiac death. It needs to be used cautiously during the first few weeks following myocardial infarction because there may be an increase in mortality during this period.

Amiodarone

Amiodarone is also classified as a class III antiarrhythmic drug.[14] However, it is unique because it possesses mechanisms of action from all four antiarrhythmic drug categories.

Mode of action Amiodarone prolongs the action potential and refractoriness of all cardiac tissue, thus increasing the QT interval. It reduces automaticity by decreasing resting membrane potential. It slows conduction through both the atrioventricular node and accessory pathways, such as those seen in Wolff–Parkinson–White syndrome, via its antisympathetic activity and possibly by its calcium channel blocking effects.

Hemodynamics Even though amiodarone possesses mild negative inotropic effects, it is usually well tolerated hemodynamically, even in patients with severely depressed left ventricular systolic function. This is in part due to its peripheral vasodilatory effect.

Pharmacokinetics Amiodarone bioavailability after oral dosing varies between 20% and 80%. It undergoes a large first pass effect by the liver, resulting in a biologically active compound. It is almost exclusively hepatically cleared and has a large volume of distribution. The half-life varies between 20 and 180 days. As a result, a large loading dose is required before adipose tissue is saturated and plasma levels are within the "therapeutic" range (i.e. 1–2·5 mg/l). Below this level patients tend not to respond clinically and above 2·5 mg/l there is a disproportionate increase in toxicity/therapeutic ratio.

Dosing Generally amiodarone is administered by an oral loading dose of 1200–1600 mg/day for 1 week. The usual maintenance dose is 200–800 mg/day.

Adverse effects (Table 17.6) Between 10% and 25% of patients are unable to tolerate the adverse effects of amiodarone. Although most of the adverse effects are benign and reversible, there is a significant incidence of morbidity and mortality.[15] Most adverse effects are dose and duration dependent.

Recommended monitoring See Table 17.7.

Drug interactions Amiodarone increases digoxin and warfarin effects, and the dosages of these drugs need to be decreased. Concomitant use with quinidine or procainamide increases QT interval and incidence of torsades de pointes. β-Blockers and calcium channel blockers may exacerbate bradyarrhythmias.

Indications Amiodarone appears to reduce the risk for cardiac arrest or sudden death in myocardial infarct survivors with left ventricular dysfunction and in patients with clinical heart failure.[15,16] In patients with atrial fibrillation, who have no structural heart disease and have failed to respond to or cannot tolerate flecainide, propafenone or sotalol, low-dose amiodarone (i.e. 200–400 mg/day) is effective at maintaining sinus with a relatively low risk of toxicity. In patients

Table 17.6 Adverse effects of amiodarone

System	Effects
Cardiovascular	Sinus bradycardia. Low incidence of proarrhythmic effects
Pulmonary	Amiodarone pulmonary toxicity (5–10% incidence): non-productive cough, dyspnea, fever, pulmonary infiltrates on chest x ray, >15% decrease in diffusing capacity for carbon monoxide or lung volume. Usually slowly reversible; may benefit from steroids
Thyroid	Hyperthyroidism; hypothyroidism
Dermatologic	Photosensitivity. Blue-gray discoloration of skin
Ocular	Microdeposits on cornea; usually not a clinical problem; reversible
Gastrointestinal	Nausea, constipation, anorexia, cholestasis, hepatitis. If transaminase levels are increased more than threefold over normal, then a decrease in dose or drug discontinuation is usually necessary

Table 17.7 Recommended monitoring during amiodarone therapy

Investigation	Timing
Complete blood count	Baseline, every 6 months
Liver enzymes	Baseline, every 6 months
Thyroid studies	Baseline, every 6 months
Chest x ray	Baseline, every 6 months
Pulmonary function test	Baseline, with symptoms
Ophthalmologic	Baseline, every 6 months

with atrial fibrillation and structural heart disease (heart failure, significant left ventricular hypertrophy, and patients with coronary artery disease who have failed sotalol), amiodarone is used to maintain sinus rhythm in those with paroxysmal or persistent atrial fibrillation.

Case 17.1 (continued)

Mr Bostock did well over the subsequent year. His medical regimen was stabilized and included aspirin 81 mg/day, atenolol 50 mg/day, enalapril 10 mg/day, and amiodarone 200 mg/day. He remained symptom free. His serum cholesterol level rose despite attention to his diet. His fasting lipid profile was as follows: total cholesterol

225 mg/dl (8·7 mmol/l), low-density lipoprotein (LDL)-cholesterol 165 mg/dl (6·4 mmol/l), high-density lipoprotein (HDL)-cholesterol 30 mg/dl (0·8 mmol/l), and fasting triglycerides 180 mg/dl (2·0 mmol/l), with a cholesterol/HDL ratio of 7·5.

Mr Bostock initially was started on nicotinic acid, but this was stopped because of severe headaches. His physician considered prescribing gemfibrozil, but he was instead treated with lovastatin 10 mg/day, which was subsequently increased to 20 mg/day. Two months later, the total cholesterol was 190 mg/dl (4·9 mmol/l), LDL-cholesterol 135 mg/dl (3·49 mmol/l), and HDL-cholesterol 40 mg/dl (1·0 mmol/l), with a cholesterol/HDL ratio of 4·7. For secondary prevention of coronary heart disease events, the goal of therapy is to achieve an LDL below 100 mg/dl (<2·6 mmol/l) and a cholesterol/HDL ratio below 5·0. Therefore, therapy had not achieved the LDL target and the options were to increase the dose of the 3-hydroxy-3-methylglutaryl coenzyme A reductase inhibitor (statin) or add a second drug. Probably, an increase in dose of the statin with monitoring of liver function tests would be the first step.

Questions

14. What is the mechanism of action of nicotinic acid, of fibric acid compounds, and of drugs such as lovastatin?
15. How do cholesterol lowering medications interact with the other medications that Mr Bostock was taking?

Answers

Answer to question 14

There are several cholesterol and triglyceride lowering compounds that one might consider for a patient such as Mr Bostock. The properties of representative compounds are outlined in Table 17.8. Among the considerations in choosing a lipid lowering drug are the lipid profile (predominantly high LDL and low HDL in this case), tolerability, and cost, as well as potential for interaction with other drugs.

Answer to question 15

In general, lipid lowering drugs have more important drug interactions than many other classes of cardiovascular drugs. These are

Table 17.8 Lipid lowering drugs

Lipid lowering drug	Nicotinic acid (niacin)	Fibric acid compounds (gemfibrozil, clofibrate)	Statins (for example simvastatin, lovastatin, atorvastatin)
Description	Naturally occurring vitamin	Multiple mechanisms of action	HMG-CoA reductase inhibitors
Pharmacokinetics	Well absorbed in gastrointestinal tract; high first pass effect; 90% renal excretion	Well absorbed in gastrointestinal tract; both hepatic and renal excretion	30–40% absorbed orally; hydrolyzed by liver to active drug; hepatically excreted
Adverse effects	Flushing, itching (blocked by NSAIDs), peptic ulcer disease, nausea, gout, hyperglycemia	Well tolerated generally; gastrointestinal symptoms	Well tolerated generally; gastrointestinal symptoms; headache. Myositis (rare). Elevation in liver function tests
Dosage	250 mg/day; titrate slowly up to 1000 mg twice daily	Gemfibrozil 600 mg twice daily, clofibrate 1 g twice daily	10–80 mg/day; dose at bedtime
Drug interactions	When used with HMG-CoA reductase inhibitors, can lead to myositis	When used with HMG-CoA reductase inhibitors, can lead to myositis; potentiates effect of warfarin	Rhabdomyolysis can occur with concomitant therapy with ciclosporin, fibric acid compounds, or nicotinic acid
Monitoring	Liver function tests (AST, ALT), uric acid, glucose		Liver function tests (AST, ALT); creatine kinase every 2–3 months for first year then every 6 months
Efficacy	Reduces LDL 20–35%, reduces TGs 10–20%, increases HDL 10–20%	Most effective in lowering TGs (30–60%), reduces LDL 10%, increases HDL 5–10%	Reduces LDL 20–30%, reduces TGs 10–20%, increases HDL 5–10%

ALT, alanine aminotransferase; AST, aspartate aminotransferase; HDL, high-density lipoprotein; HMG-CoA, 3-hydroxy-3-methylglutaryl coenzyme A; LDL, low-density lipoprotein; NSAID, non-steroidal anti-inflammatory drug; TG, triglyceride

outlined in Table 17.8. There are no major drug interactions between lovastatin and the other drugs that are part of Mr Bostock's regimen.

Case 17.2

Ms Adair is a 40-year-old woman, employed as a nurse, who is an alcoholic. She sees her physician because of ankle edema that has been progressive over 2 months.

Examination. Physical examination: the patient appeared normal. Pulse: 80 beats/min, normal character. Blood pressure: 110/75 mmHg in right arm. Jugular venous pulse: normal. Cardiac impulse: normal. First heart sound: normal. Second heart sound: split normally on inspiration. Fourth heart sound heard. Chest examination: normal air entry, basilar rales. Abdominal examination: soft abdomen, no tenderness and no masses. Normal liver span. Mild lower extremity edema.

Investigations. Chest *x* ray: mild cardiomegaly. Electrocardiogram: non-specific ST-T abnormalities.

Her physician counsels her regarding stopping drinking, and starts her on hydrochlorothiazide 25 mg/day. The ankle edema improves. She returns 1 year later in florid heart failure. On her own she stopped alcohol consumption entirely 1 month previously.

Examination. Physical examination: the patient appeared breathless and had moderate edema of her lower extremities from the thighs distally. Pulse: 105 beats/min, normal character. Blood pressure: 130/85 mmHg in right arm. Jugular venous pulse: 10 cm. Cardiac impulse: normal. First heart sound: normal. Second heart sound: split normally on inspiration. Quadruple gallop heard: S_3, S_4. Chest examination: rales heard through two-thirds of chest. Abdominal examination: soft abdomen, no tenderness, and no masses. Enlarged liver.

Hydrochlorothiazide is discontinued; furosemide 40 mg/day, enalapril 10 mg/day, and digoxin 0·25 mg/day are started, along with a potassium supplement. An echocardiogram reveals global hypokinesis of the left ventricle with an ejection fraction of about 30%. There is mild impairment in right ventricular function.

Questions

1. What is the mechanism of action of these diuretics?
2. What is the mechanism of action of enalapril?
3. What is the mechanism of action of digoxin?

Answers

Answer to question 1

Hydrochlorothiazide is one of several thiazide diuretics that are available for clinical use. As a group, they inhibit sodium, chloride, and water reabsorption in the distal convoluted tubules, probably mediated via luminal receptors. The diuretic and natriuretic effect of hydrochlorothiazide is less than that induced by loop diuretics

Table 17.9 Diuretics

Drug	Hydrochlorothiazide	Furosemide (oral)	Furosemide (intravenous)
Pharmacokinetics	Variable gastrointestinal tract absorption; onset of diuretic effect 1 h; duration of diuretic effect 6–12 h	60–70% gastrointestinal absorption; onset of diuretic effect: 1 h; duration of effect 4–6 h	Onset of vasodilator effect 1–2 min; onset of diuretic effect 5–10 min; duration of effect 3–4 h
Adverse effects	Hypokalemia, hypomagnesemia, hyponatremia; hyperuricemia, hyperglycemia, volume depletion; orthostatic hypotension	Hypokalemia, hypomagnesemia, hyponatremia; hyperuricemia, hyperglycemia; volume depletion; orthostatic hypotension	Hypokalemia, hypomagnesemia, hyponatremia; hyperuricemia, hyperglycemia; volume depletion; orthostatic hypotension; ototoxicity (dose dependent)
Dosage	25–100 mg/day orally; sometimes used in fixed dose combination with other diuretics and antihypertensives	10–80 mg orally once or twice daily	10–160 mg intravenously up to every 4 h
Drug interactions	Probenecid, non-steroidal anti-inflammatory drugs	Non-steroidal anti-inflammatory drugs	Non-steroidal anti-inflammatory drugs
Monitoring	K$^+$, Mg^{2+}, glucose, uric acid	K$^+$, Na$^+$, Mg^{2+}, glucose, uric acid	
Indications	Hypertension, mild to moderate congestive heart failure	Hypertension, congestive heart failure	Congestive heart failure, pulmonary edema

because 90% of sodium reabsorption occurs before reaching the distal tubules. (Diuretic properties are summarized in Table 17.9.)

Furosemide is the loop active diuretic used most commonly. Loop diuretics are the most potent diuretics used. Their mode of action is through inhibition of active sodium–chloride transport in the ascending limb of the loop of Henle in the nephron. This inhibition leads to excretion of salt and water. When used intravenously, furosemide also produces vasodilatation.

Answer to question 2

Angiotensin-converting enzyme inhibitors

The renin–angiotensin–aldosterone system (RAAS) plays a vital role in maintaining homeostasis, particularly with regard to blood pressure regulation and fluid and electrolyte balance.[17] Renin is secreted by the kidney and converts angiotensinogen to angiotensin I, which is converted to the physiologically active angiotensin II by angiotensin-converting enzymes (ACEs), located in the highest concentration in pulmonary capillary endothelium. Angiotensin II has multiple effects, including potentiation of sympathetic activity, renal sodium retention, stimulation of thirst, and antagonism of vasodilator agents such as bradykinin. The end result is systemic vasoconstriction and elevation in blood pressure. Angiotensin II is also a growth factor that produces a hypertrophic response and remodeling in the heart. In heart failure patients, there is an enhancement of neurohormonal activation (including of the RAAS).

The mechanism of action of ACE inhibitors is inhibition of ACEs, which are found in endothelium and also in cardiac muscle. Several ACE inhibitors are clinically used that have similar modes of action and side effect profiles, but differ in their pharmacodynamics. With the exception of captopril and lisinopril, most ACE inhibitors are prodrugs and are transformed to their active form by de-esterification of the prodrug in the liver. Prodrug activation is decreased in patients with liver disease or those with abnormal liver blood flow (for example, heart failure). Most of the drug elimination is via the kidneys with little hepatic excretion.

Hemodynamics By virtue of decreasing circulatory concentration of angiotensin II and catecholamines, and increasing the concentration of powerful vasodilators such as bradykinin and prostaglandins, ACE inhibitors cause a decrease in heart rate, left ventricular and right ventricular end-diastolic pressures, right atrial pressure, and blood pressure, which result in an increased cardiac output and a decrease in myocardial oxygen demand.

Adverse effects As a group, ACE inhibitors are very well tolerated with few and mild side effects. Discontinuation of the drug secondary to side effects occurs in 5% of patients. The adverse effects that may occur are as follows.

Cough. Cough is common, occurring in 5–20% of patients. It is the most common reason for discontinuation of the drug. It is usually a non-productive cough that can develop at any time but it is rare after 6 months of therapy. It does not respond to antitussive agents. The mechanism is probably related to high levels of bradykinin, prostaglandins, and substance P. The cough usually resolves within the first few days after discontinuing the ACE inhibitor.

Neutropenia. Neutropenia is a rare event that can occur during the first 3 months. Although it usually resolves with discontinuation of the drug, aplastic anemia has been reported. Therefore, blood tests should be performed during the first 2–3 months.

Other adverse effects. These include hyperkalemia due to inhibition of aldosterone; acute renal failure in patients with bilateral renal artery stenosis; angioneurotic edema with onset in first few hours to 1 week; and dermatitis, distortion of taste, and hypotension.

Indications *Congestive heart failure.* Multiple studies have shown that in patients with dilated cardiomyopathy and with an ejection fraction of 40% or less, regardless of etiology and New York Heart Association functional class, ACE inhibitors improve survival and functional class for symptomatic patients.[17]

After myocardial infarction. In patients following myocardial infarction, especially with left ventricular fractions of 40% or less, ACE inhibitors started as early as 24 hours after myocardial infarction have a beneficial effect on left ventricular remodeling, decrease reinfarction and angina, and improve mortality and heart failure symptoms. Patients receiving the most benefit are those with Killip class 2 or 3 symptoms, sinus tachycardia, and anterior myocardial infarction.[8,18]

Hypertension. ACE inhibitors are very effective antihypertensive agents, primarily in patients with a high renin state. ACE inhibitors also cause left ventricular hypertrophy regression. Left ventricular hypertrophy is a risk factor for both symptomatic coronary disease and sudden cardiac death.

Losartan Losartan is an angiotensin II receptor antagonist. Its efficacy in the treatment of hypertension has been established and it is considered second line therapy for heart failure if an ACE inhibitor cannot be tolerated. An important advantage over ACE inhibitors is that losartan may avoid side effects caused by elevated levels of bradykinin and prostaglandins, especially cough.

Answer to question 3

Digoxin

Cardiac glycosides or digitalis are obtained from the leaf of the foxglove plants *Digitalis purpurea* or *Digitalis lanata*. Several preparations are clinically available, including digoxin, digitoxin, ouabain, and deslanoside. Digoxin is the most frequently used glycoside.[19]

Mode of action The therapeutic effects are due to inhibition of the sarcolemmal membrane sodium/potassium adenosine triphosphate

(ATP)ase pump. This magnesium dependent pump actively transports potassium into the cell and sodium out of the cell via energy provided by hydrolysis of ATP. Digoxin binds to the α-subunit of the pump and inhibits it. This leads to an increase in intracellular sodium concentration, which subsequently produces an increase in intracellular calcium by inducing an alteration in the gradients for sodium/calcium exchange across the sarcolemma. Increasing intracellular calcium enhances excitation–contraction coupling and thus produces a positive inotropic effect.

An additional action of cardiac glycosides is due to a direct stimulating effect on the area postrema in the medulla, resulting in increased vagal efferent tone. This is the main mechanism by which digoxin slows atrioventricular conduction in atrial fibrillation.

Hemodynamics The hemodynamic effects of digoxin are dependent on the degree of left ventricular systolic dysfunction. In the normal heart, cardiac output is unchanged or slightly decreased. In heart failure, digoxin may increase cardiac contractility, increase cardiac output, decrease left ventricular end-diastolic pressure, decrease left ventricular volume, and decrease pulmonary artery and pulmonary capillary wedge pressures. These changes occur with minimal change in myocardial oxygen demand.

Absorption The therapeutic response is seen within 10 min after an intravenous dose and maximum response is within 1 hour. Orally administered, these responses are seen within 3 and 8 hours, respectively. Approximately 55–85% of the drug is absorbed in the gastrointestinal tract. Once a steady state is achieved the myocardial digoxin concentration may be 15–30 times that of plasma.

Elimination Digoxin is predominantly cleared by the kidney. In normal persons the half-life is about 36 hours. Thus, without a loading dose it may take up to 1 week to achieve a steady state.

Toxicity Digoxin has a narrow therapeutic to toxic ratio (a narrow therapeutic index). Determining serum digoxin concentration can be a useful guide to therapy. However, it is important to understand that, by itself, an elevated digoxin level is not diagnostic of toxicity without signs and symptoms, and a "normal" level does not exclude toxicity. Once in steady state serum levels should be checked 12 hours after an oral dose (before this, falsely high levels may be obtained) and, because physical activity will increase skeletal muscle binding and thus produce a substantially lowered plasma concentration, the patient should be at rest for at least 1 hour.

Extracardiac manifestations of toxicity. Symptoms primarily involve the gastrointestinal and neurologic systems, and include nausea, vomiting, anorexia, dizziness, fatigue, visual disturbances such as halos around bright objects, abdominal pain, diarrhea, headache, and delirium. Most of these manifestations are mediated via central nervous system mechanisms.

Cardiac manifestations of toxicity. Almost all arrhythmias have been reported in association with digoxin toxicity. Although there is no pathognomonic arrhythmia or electrocardiographic abnormality indicating digoxin toxicity, the combination of enhanced automaticity and impaired conduction is highly suggestive (for example, paroxysmal atrial tachycardia with block). Ventricular premature depolarizations and high degree atrioventricular block are common.

Factors associated with increased risk for digoxin toxicity. These include the following:

- renal insufficiency: by decreased excretion
- increased age
- electrolyte abnormalities, such as decreased potassium or magnesium, or increased calcium
- hypothyroidism: depresses sodium/potassium pump and decreases digoxin clearance
- type and severity of underlying heart disease: effects of digoxin are superimposed on a structurally abnormal heart and pre-existing rhythm abnormalities
- advanced pulmonary disease: these patients are at increased risk for supraventricular arrhythmias; hypoxia can increase sensitivity to digoxin
- other drug interactions: quinidine, amiodarone, verapamil, heparin, and certain antibiotics can lead to increased digoxin levels; diuretics may lead to electrolyte abnormalities.

Treatment of toxicity The following options are available for treatment of digoxin toxicity: discontinue further digoxin administration; correct electrolyte abnormalities; management of bradyarrhythmias by pacing or atropine; and suppression of other arrhythmias with phenytoin or lidocaine.

Digoxin specific F(ab) antibody fragments have been approved by the US Food and Drug Administration for "life-threatening arrhythmias" secondary to digoxin toxicity. This therapy is very expensive and should not be used for benign arrhythmias or asymptomatic elevation in serum digoxin concentration. The onset of action is very fast (19 min) and the antibody is quickly cleared by the kidney. The most common side effect is hypokalemia.

Indications *Chronic heart failure due to systolic dysfunction.* Patients with worse systolic function tend to respond the most. Digoxin chronically improves left ventricular function and exercise tolerance, and decreases plasma norepinephrine concentrations as compared with placebo. In combination with vasodilators, such as ACE inhibitors, the effects of digoxin are enhanced. Although digoxin has not been shown to improve survival in patients with heart failure, its withdrawal is associated with hemodynamic and clinical deterioration. Furthermore, in patients with chronic heart failure (and left ventricular ejection fraction <45%) digoxin therapy (when added to diuretics and ACE inhibitors) reduced the rate of hospitalization for heart failure.[20]

Atrial fibrillation. In acute atrial fibrillation, oral administration may take as long as 6 hours for rate control, which may be unacceptable if a patient is symptomatic. In this setting, intravenous administration may be more appropriate. In chronic atrial fibrillation, digoxin controls resting heart rate but is less effective in controlling heart rate during exertion. In this setting, β-blockers and calcium channel blockers are more effective for exertional heart rate control. Combination treatment may be particularly effective (digoxin plus a β-blocker or calcium channel blocker).

Acute myocardial infarction. In patients with heart failure following myocardial infarction, digoxin has a beneficial hemodynamic effect without increasing infarct size. However, these positive inotropic effects are small in comparison to those produced by intravenously administered catecholamines (dobutamine or dopamine).

Case 17.2 (continued)

For the first 7–10 days there is improvement on this medical regimen; however, despite entirely abstaining from alcohol consumption her heart failure progressively worsened. After about 1 month she developed a cough that was intractable and that persisted over the next 4 months. Ms Adair was evaluated as an outpatient; her left ventricular ejection fraction was found to be 22% by radionuclide angiography. Her physician considered alternative vasodilator therapy, including nitrates plus hydralazine. The captopril was stopped, and isosorbide dinitrate 40 mg orally three times daily and hydralazine 50 mg three times daily were started. Additionally, her physician started her on warfarin, in order to prolong the International Normalized Ratio of prothrombin time to 2·0–2·5. The cough immediately resolved and the heart failure symptoms stabilized.

Questions

4. Why might warfarin be of benefit in this setting? What is its mechanism of action?
5. Is there a relationship between her therapy and the chronic cough?
6. How do nitrates plus hydralazine benefit patients in congestive heart failure?

Answers

Answer to question 4

Warfarin

Patients with dilated and/or dyskinetic left ventricles are at increased risk for left ventricular thrombus, and thus cerebral and systemic embolization. Patients with heart failure also have an increased risk for venous thrombosis and pulmonary emboli. Warfarin therapy decreases the risk for these events.

Warfarin is the most commonly used oral anticoagulant. It inhibits vitamin K expoxide reductase in the liver (the enzyme required for recycling vitamin K to its active form). The active form of vitamin K is required for post-translational carboxylation of the vitamin K dependent proteins (factors II, VII, IX, and X, and proteins C and S). Without this carboxylation, these procoagulant proteins are biologically inactive. There is a lag period for therapeutic effect when warfarin is initiated because of the time required for the normal functioning procoagulant to be cleared from the blood and replaced by the inactive form. Factor VII and protein C have the shortest half-lives and are the first ones replaced. This early depletion of protein C may be responsible for an early paradoxic procoagulant effect. The antithrombotic effect is not maximal until plasma levels of factors IX and X are significantly depressed.

Administered orally, warfarin is rapidly absorbed. It binds to plasma proteins and accumulates in the liver. There is great variation among patients and dosage required. It is metabolized by the liver and excreted in the urine, and its half-life is 36 hours. The therapeutic effect traditionally was measured by the prothrombin time (PT). However, thromboplastin, the protein component of the reagent, varies markedly among preparations, leading to a great deal of variability between laboratories. A more standardized approach of measuring and reporting the anticoagulant effect of warfarin is the International

Normalized Ratio (INR). The INR is now the standard, preferred method of assessing the effect of warfarin.

Dosing If anticoagulation is required acutely, then the patient should be started on heparin as well as warfarin 10–15 mg for the first 1–2 days. In most circumstances, full anticoagulation from warfarin requires 72–96 hours and in the interim INR levels should be checked daily. Once a stable therapeutic dose of warfarin is obtained the frequency of INR monitoring may be decreased in a stepwise manner, but the patient should not receive warfarin for longer than 2 months without a known INR level. If the patient's INR levels are erratic, some of the common causes are medication non-compliance, interactions with other medications, or change in diet with either increase or decrease in vitamin K containing foods.

Drug interactions Many commonly used drugs interact with warfarin and can either potentiate or antagonize the therapeutic effect. Some of the most common cardiac drugs that interact with warfarin include amiodarone and aspirin. Both patient and physician should be aware of potential adverse drug interactions.

Side effects Bleeding is the most common complication. Risk for bleeding increases with higher levels of INR as well as with concomitant use of aspirin, which impairs platelet function and can produce gastric erosions. In cases in which reversal of anticoagulation is urgently required, fresh frozen plasma or prothrombin complex can be used. Administration of vitamin K restores normal INR levels within 24 hours, but patients may become resistant to warfarin for up to a week.

Warfarin skin necrosis is a rare complication. It usually occurs between days 3 and 8, and it is believed to be secondary to protein C deficiency leading to venule thrombosis.

Warfarin crosses the placenta and is teratogenic, and its use during the first trimester of pregnancy carries a significant risk to the fetus. Exposure in weeks 6–9 of gestation may produce the fetal warfarin syndrome, and spontaneous abortions, stillbirths, and neonatal deaths may occur. In a review of anticoagulant use in pregnant women with prosthetic heart valves, the use of oral anticoagulation throughout pregnancy was associated with warfarin embryopathy in 6·4% of live births, which was eliminated with substitution of heparin at or before 6 weeks of gestation.[21] When heparin was used between weeks 6 and 12, in place of continued warfarin therapy, the risk for valve thrombosis increased from 4% to 9%. The estimated risk for maternal hemorrhage in a woman taking anticoagulants is 2·5%, with the majority of episodes occurring at the time of delivery.

Indications

- Atrial fibrillation in patients with rheumatic mitral stenosis, and high risk patients in atrial fibrillation without rheumatic mitral stenosis (recommended INR 2–3).
- Mechanical prosthetic valves (recommended INR 2·5–3·5).
- After myocardial infarction: patients with large transmural anterior wall myocardial infarction are at increased risk for mural thrombi and subsequent thromboembolic events; in this group of patients, 3–6 months of anticoagulation is beneficial in preventing thromboemboli.
- Unstable angina: warfarin may be of benefit in some patients.

Answer to question 5

With regard to the mechanism of cough with ACE inhibitors, see page 549.

Answer to question 6

Nitrates plus hydralazine benefit patients in CHF by providing a balance of preload reduction (nitrates are powerful venous dilators and weak arteriolar dilators) and afterload reduction (hydralazine is a more powerful arteriolar dilator and may possibly attenuate the development of tolerance to nitrates).

Case 17.2 (continued)

Because of the progression in heart failure, Ms Adair was considered for cardiac transplantation. Her situation acutely worsened; she was admitted to the hospital in pulmonary edema. In addition to her previous regimen, she was started on an infusion of dobutamine, which produced symptomatic improvement and a diuresis. However, after 18 hours she had multiple episodes of ventricular tachycardia. The dobutamine was stopped, and intravenous amiodarone was initiated. Again, there was symptomatic improvement, with diuresis. She was stabilized and her usual oral medications for heart failure were restarted. On the night before planned discharge she developed ventricular fibrillation, from which she could not be resuscitated.

Question

7. What is the mechanism of action of dobutamine? How does it compare with other catecholamines?

Answer to question 7

Naturally occurring and synthetic catecholamines are commonly used in acutely ill patients with cardiovascular disease to increase cardiac contractility and to alter the tone of one or more vascular beds, which may have a subsequent effect on blood pressure. These drugs are almost always administered by controlled intravenous infusion; the therapeutic effect and adverse effects are critically dose related. Therefore, these drugs are often administered in the intensive care unit setting. Commonly used catecholamines include dopamine, dobutamine, phenylephrine, epinephrine, and norepinephrine.

All catecholamines bind to α- or β-adrenergic receptors, dopamine receptors, or a combination of receptors. α-Adrenergic agonists such as phenylephrine have little direct effect on the myocardium but produce vasoconstriction. β-Adrenergic agonists bind to β_1- and β_2-receptors, both of which are present in the myocardium, and produce an increase in intracellular cyclic adenosine monophosphate and a subsequent increase in the inotropic state of the heart, as well as an increase in heart rate. β-Receptors are also present in the vasculature; activation of these receptors can lead to vasodilatation and lower blood pressure. Dopaminergic receptors are present in the renal vasculature. When dopamine is administered in relatively low concentrations (2 micrograms/kg per min) there is a relatively selective effect on dopaminergic receptors, which leads to increased glomerular filtration and enhanced salt and water excretion (so-called renal dose dopamine). At higher concentrations (12 micrograms/ kg per min) dopamine activates cardiac β_1-receptors and α-receptors, leading to increased cardiac contractility, vasoconstriction, and an increase in blood pressure (Table 17.10).

Dosing (see Table 17.10) A drug whose mechanism of action is related to that of catecholamines is amrinone. This drug may be used for advanced heart failure. It produces a positive inotropic effect by inhibiting type III phosphodiesterase in tissues, including heart, resulting in increased cyclic adenosine monophosphate concentrations, and thus produces effects similar to those produced by β-adrenergic agonists. It also produces vasodilatation, resulting in an increase in cardiac output.

Table 17.10 Adrenergic agonist drugs

Drug	Typical dose	Receptor(s)	Effect
Dopamine	2 micrograms/ kg per min	Dopaminergic	Diuresis
Dopamine	12 micrograms/ kg per min	α, β_1	Vasoconstriction, positive inotropic effect
Dobutamine	2–15 micrograms/ kg per min	β_1	Positive inotropic effect
Phenylephrine	40–60 micrograms/min	α	Vasoconstriction
Epinephrine	1–2 micrograms/min	α, β_1, β_2	Depending on dose, vasodilatation or constriction; positive inotropic and chronotropic effect
Norepinephrine	2–4 micrograms/min	α, β_1, β_2	Positive inotropic and chronotropic effect, vasoconstriction

Table 17.11 Use of adrenergic agonist drugs

Drug	Indication	Adverse effects
Dopamine (low dose)	Heart failure	Tachycardia, arrhythmias
Dopamine (high dose)	Heart failure, hypotension	Hypertension, tachycardia, arrhythmias
Dobutamine	Heart failure	Hypotension, tachycardia, arrhythmias
Phenylephrine	Hypotension	Hypertension
Epinephrine	Heart failure, hypotension	Hypertension, tachycardia, arrhythmias
Norepinephrine	Heart failure, hypotension	Hypertension, tachycardia, arrhythmias

Indications and adverse effects (Table 17.11) Catecholamines are exceedingly potent and efficacious drugs that must be administered under extremely carefully controlled conditions. Potential for adverse effects is considerable.

Case 17.2 (continued)

Pharmacotherapy of advanced heart failure is difficult. Such patients typically have a predicted mortality of nearly 50% at 1 year;

about half of deaths are due to ventricular arrhythmias, as was the case for this patient. However, despite the limited ability to improve prognosis with pharmacotherapy, amelioration of symptoms is usually possible with skillful pharmacologic interventions.

References

1 Lauer MS. Aspirin for primary prevention of coronary events. *N Engl J Med* 2002;**346**:1468–74.
2 Manson JE, Tosteson H, Ridker PM, *et al.* The primary prevention of myocardial infarction. *N Engl J Med* 1992;**326**:1406–16.
3 Fuster V, Dyken ML, Vokonas PS, Hennekens C. Aspirin as a therapeutic agent in cardiovascular disease. AHA Medical/Scientific Statement. *Circulation* 1993;**87**: 659–75.
4 ISIS-2 (Second International Study of Infarct Survival) Collaborative Group. Randomised trial of intravenous streptokinase, oral aspirin, both, or neither among 17,187 cases of suspected acute myocardial infarction: ISIS-2. *Lancet* 1988;**2**:349–60.
5 Frishman WH. Carvedilol. *N Engl J Med* 1998;**339**:1759–65.
6 Califf RM, O'Connor CM. β-Blocker therapy for heart failure. The evidence is in, now the work begins. *JAMA* 2000;**283**:1335–7.
7 Parker JD, Parker JO. Nitrate therapy for stable angina pectoris. *N Engl J Med* 1998; **338**:520–31.
8 Hennekens CH, Albert CM, Godfried SL, Gaziano JM, Buring JE. Adjunctive drug therapy of acute myocardial infarction: evidence from clinical trials. *N Engl J Med* 1996;**335**:1660–7.
9 Fibrinolytic Therapy Trialists' (FTT) Collaborative Group. Indications for fibrinolytic therapy in suspected acute myocardial infarction: collaborative overview of mortality and major morbidity results from all randomised trials of more than 1000 patients. *Lancet* 1994;**343**:311–22.
10 Collins R, Peto R, Baigent C, Sleight P. Aspirin, heparin, and fibrinolytic therapy in suspected acute myocardial infarction [review]. *N Engl J Med* 1997;**336**:847–60.
11 Coplen SE, Antman EM, Berlin JA, Hewitt P, Chalmers TC. Efficacy and safety of quinidine therapy for maintenance of sinus rhythm after cardioversion. A meta-analysis of randomized control trials. *Circulation* 1990;**82**:1106–6.
12 Roden DM, Woosley RL. Flecainide. *N Engl J Med* 1986;**315**:36–41.
13 Hohnloser SH, Woosley RL. Sotalol. *N Engl J Med* 1994;**331**:31–8.
14 Mason JW. Amiodarone. *N Engl J Med* 1987;**316**:455–66.
15 Connolly SJ. Evidence-based analysis of amiodarone efficacy and safety. *Circulation* 1999;**100**:2025–34.
16 Campbell TJ. The place of amiodarone: an overview of the four recent large controlled trials. *Aust NZ J Med* 1997;**27**:582–90.
17 Brown NJ, Vaughan DE. Angiotensin-converting enzyme inhibitors. *Circulation* 1998;**97**:1411–20.
18 ACE Inhibitor Myocardial Infarction Collaborative Group. Indications for ACE inhibitors in the early treatment of acute myocardial infarction. *Circulation* 1998;**97**: 2202–12.
19 Hauptman PJ, Kelly RA. Digitalis. *Circulation* 1999;**99**:1265–70.
20 The Digitalis Investigation Group. The effect of digoxin on mortality and morbidity in patients with heart failure. *N Engl J Med* 1997;**336**:525–33.
21 Chan WS, Anand S, Ginsberg JS. Anticoagulation of pregnant women with mechanical heart valves: a systematic review of the literature. *Arch Intern Med* 2000; **160**:191–6.

18: Arterial vascular disease

KHETHER E RABY

Lower extremity arterial occlusive disease

Atherosclerosis is a common disease process that can affect arteries of any organ system. Among the most common sites to be affected are the coronary arteries, cerebral arteries, and lower extremity arteries; atherosclerosis in these three circulations accounts for virtually all of the mortality and much of the morbidity caused by this disease. The prevalence of lower extremity arterial occlusive disease is difficult to estimate but large epidemiologic studies have suggested it occurs in at least 1–15% of the population, depending on age. Men are more frequently affected than women and at a younger age; however, this gap narrows for postmenopausal women.[1]

Risk factors

The presence of diabetes and smoking appear to be particularly strong risk factors for the development of lower extremity atherosclerosis, and continued active smoking or uncontrolled diabetes adversely affect disease progression. The natural history of lower extremity arterial atherosclerosis is that of complete occlusion of vessels, ischemia of the distal extremities, and ultimately necrosis of tissue and gangrene. Although limb amputation is uncommon with appropriate medical management and surgical intervention, diabetic persons and active smokers still have a high amputation rate.[2]

Diagnosis

History

The diagnosis of claudication secondary to lower extremity atherosclerosis is most often made by history alone. In the presence of risk factors, a history of foot, calf, thigh, or buttock cramping brought on by exercise and relieved by rest is a classic presentation. The level of symptoms roughly correlate with the anatomic level of occlusive disease. For example, a patient with isolated right calf and foot pain is likely to have disease affecting the right superficial femoral artery at the knee; bilateral buttock and/or thigh pain is a likely presentation for occlusive disease at the distal abdominal aorta or both iliac arteries. As the severity of atherosclerosis progresses, symptoms worsen in intensity, frequency, and threshold of onset until they occur at rest. Many patients with advanced disease often complain of nocturnal pain that is only relieved by dangling the affected limb and using gravity to aid distal arterial circulation.

Examination

The major physical finding that confirms the presence of lower extremity atherosclerosis is the diminution or absence of pulses in the affected limb. Rarely, pulses at rest are intact but become absent with mild exercise. In a patient with right calf and foot pain and right superficial femoral artery disease at the knee, the popliteal pulse behind the knee, and the dorsalis pedis and posterior tibial pulses of the foot are likely to be diminished or absent, whereas the more proximal common femoral pulse may be intact (although bruits are often audible over the femoral artery, reflecting non-obstructive plaque). In the case of bilateral buttock/thigh pain and aortoiliac disease, bilateral common femoral pulses as well as distal pulses are likely to be diminished. Other physical signs of lower extremity atherosclerosis include distal hair loss, sclerosis, and yellowish discoloration of the nail beds. In severe cases there may be non-healing skin ulceration and dependent rubor, in which an affected foot appears pale white when elevated and bright red when dangling, reflecting maximal poststenotic distal capillary dilatation and the exaggerated effects of gravity.

Physical findings are important in distinguishing claudication from pseudoclaudication, a syndrome with similar symptoms that is caused by spinal canal stenosis and nerve compression, and is unrelated to atherosclerosis. The hallmark of this diagnosis is a history of claudication in the presence of normal pulses and no other physical signs of atherosclerosis. Patients with pseudoclaudication most often complain of bilateral leg fatigue with walking and experience no relief with standing, but need to sit down (and change the position of the spine) to get relief.

Investigations

The most helpful laboratory test to confirm the presence of lower extremity atherosclerosis is the measurement of systolic pressures of both arms, and comparison of the highest arm pressure with systolic pressures measured throughout the affected leg. Occlusive disease due to atherosclerosis will result in pressure drops, or gradients, in

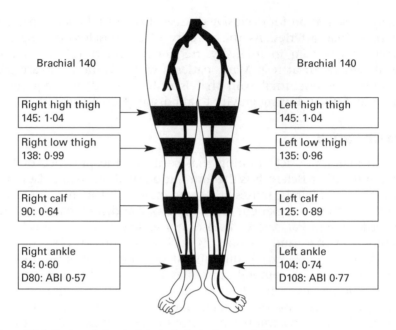

Figure 18.1 Segmental arterial study including systolic pressure measurements and brachial indices (systolic pressure index) of four standard sites of the lower extremities of a patient. Note that the greatest pressure gradient occurs between the lower thigh and upper calf on the right (138 mm to 90 mm), corresponding to a significant stenosis at the level of the right superficial femoral artery. Note also that the right and left ankle brachial indices (bottom two panels, systolic pressure at the ankle/highest systolic arm pressure) are diminished, which is consistent with bilateral lower extremity atherosclerosis

the distribution of the affected vessels. In the example of calf claudication and isolated superficial femoral artery disease, the systolic pressure at the low thigh is likely to be normal whereas that at the upper calf will be diminished (Figure 18.1). Similar information can be obtained by measuring pulse volume (by placing a Doppler probe over the arm and lower extremity vessels at various sites) and comparing volume amplitude in lieu of systolic pressures. The ratio of the pressure at the ankle to the highest arm pressure is called the ankle brachial index, and is a widely used indicator of lower extremity atherosclerosis severity. In general, severe ischemic symptoms (including non-healing ulcers) occur when the index drops to less than 0·5. Once lower extremity atherosclerosis is suspected and surgical intervention is contemplated, then angiography is used to ascertain the distribution and severity of disease (Figure 18.2).

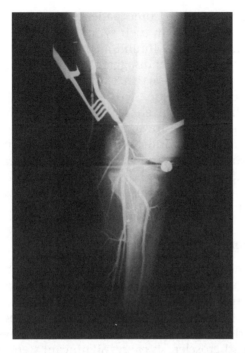

Figure 18.2 Intraoperative angiogram demonstrating successful anastomosis of a vein graft to the popliteal artery (see surgical clamp) bypassing a total occlusion of the right superficial femoral at the level of the knee, the most common site of occlusion and cause of right calf claudication

Treatment

Various treatment strategies are available for patients suffering from intermittent claudication and lower extremity atherosclerosis.

Non-surgical therapies

Non-surgical therapies aimed at relief of claudication include standardized exercise programs in which patients are encouraged to walk until they feel their symptoms, rest until their symptoms are resolved, and walk again. Exercise therapy improves the overall distance that patients can achieve before the onset of disabling symptoms, although it is unclear why exercise therapy works. Studies have failed to show that there is improvement in blood flow to affected limbs, and it is believed that exercise therapy alters skeletal muscle metabolism and makes aerobic respiration more efficient.

Pentoxifylline is a rheologic agent that is used for the treatment of intermittent claudication. Controlled studies on the use of the drug have been equivocal, with some patients experiencing benefit and others showing no change in their symptom complex. Cilostazol is a cellular phosphodiesterase inhibitor that is believed to improve claudication through platelet disaggregation, and recent studies again suggest modest improvements in exercise capacity among patients with mild to moderate disease.

Neither medicine nor exercise substantially alter the natural progression of the disease toward occlusion. Without question, the most important risk factor intervention to try and achieve in patients with lower extremity atherosclerosis is smoking cessation, which improves symptoms, slows disease progression, and reduces amputations. Similarly aggressive control of diabetes, hypertension, and cholesterol is very important.

Revascularization therapy

Revascularization therapy is aimed at restoring normal flow to the affected limb, and includes transluminal angioplasty with stenting and bypass surgery. Transluminal angioplasty and stenting is less invasive than surgery and does not require general anesthesia. However, experience with the technique thus far shows that it is most effective when atherosclerosis causes significant stenoses in the larger limb vessels (for example, iliac and proximal femoral arteries); in such cases surgery has excellent long-term benefits for both large and medium caliber vessels further downstream. Surgical therapy for intermittent claudication has been most successful at improving symptoms, but does not clearly alter the rate of amputations.

Association with coronary artery disease

Perhaps the most important issue to be addressed among patients with lower extremity atherosclerosis is that their disease is systemic and affects other circulations. In particular, patients with lower extremity atherosclerosis have a high prevalence of coronary artery disease, which is often asymptomatic because these patients are sedentary. The mortality of patients with peripheral lower extremity atherosclerosis remains extremely high as compared with that in a general population, and an overwhelming proportion of that mortality is accounted for by coronary artery disease. Therefore, when patients with intermittent claudication present for medical attention, an evaluation for the presence of coronary artery disease is at least as important as the evaluation and relief of their presenting symptoms.[3]

The relationship between lower extremity atherosclerosis and coronary artery disease is so strong that there is an inverse correlation between the ankle brachial index and the risk for death from coronary events (i.e. the lower the index, the higher the risk for cardiac death). In a landmark study conducted during the mid-1970s, coronary angiography was performed in all patients who presented with peripheral atherosclerosis. It was found that, by the time the patients presented with peripheral atherosclerosis, two-thirds had evidence of coronary atherosclerosis. Within this group, approximately half had clinically significant coronary artery disease. It is not surprising, therefore, that when patients with lower extremity atherosclerosis present for peripheral vascular surgery, their chances of surviving the surgery without significant cardiovascular morbidity are substantially poorer than in patients presenting for other types of surgery.

Cardiac risk stratification

In recent years the perioperative risk associated with vascular surgery has been decreasing. Although the approach to identifying coronary artery disease among patients with lower extremity atherosclerosis is still controversial, more clinicians are paying attention to this issue. It has become common for patients undergoing vascular surgery to undergo a preoperative clinical evaluation by an internist or a cardiologist. Patients are often stratified with respect to their risk for coronary artery disease by several clinical criteria, including age, the presence of diabetes, the presence of symptoms suggesting angina pectoris, past history of myocardial infarction, or the presence of cardiac arrhythmias. In combination, those factors may suggest a high prevalence of coronary artery disease.

Should all patients with peripheral atherosclerosis presenting for surgery receive non-invasive cardiac tests to establish the presence of coronary artery disease? This issue remains controversial because no cardiac non-invasive test is perfect. A reasonable approach is to identify those patients who are at highest risk for active coronary artery disease based on their age (for example, >70 years), and the presence of angina, myocardial infarction, cardiac arrhythmia, or diabetes. Patients who have any, or all, of these criteria are then tested with some non-invasive cardiac test to assess their risk further. Tests successfully used to identify cardiac risk among patients with lower extremity atherosclerosis include the following.

Exercise treadmill testing This is a procedure that requires patients to walk on a treadmill while serial electrocardiograms are obtained. Exercise capacity, presence of symptoms to suggest myocardial ischemia, and/or electrocardiographic changes that are diagnostic for ischemia confirm the presence of active coronary artery disease. The disadvantage of this test is that often patients are unable to walk because of claudication. The presence of a normal baseline electrocardiogram is also required for accurate interpretation.

Dipyridamole thallium/sestamibi imaging Dipyridamole is a coronary vasodilator that causes shunting of blood flow from coronary arteries with significant atherosclerotic stenoses to normal coronary arteries, resulting in a steal syndrome. Simultaneous radionuclide imaging can document hypoperfusion of areas of myocardium within the distribution of coronary atherosclerotic vessels. This is the most widely used cardiac test for assessing risk among patients with peripheral atherosclerosis. Although studies have suggested that this test is highly effective, it should not be used as a screening measure among all patients with peripheral atherosclerosis, but rather should be used for those at highest risk for coronary artery disease.

Holter monitoring for asymptomatic ischemia Patients wear a small tape recorder that monitors two leads of the electrocardiogram continuously over a 24-hour period. Patients with peripheral atherosclerosis have a high prevalence of coronary disease and may have frequent episodes of asymptomatic ST-segment depression due to spontaneous myocardial ischemia. The absence of ST-segment depressions predicts a very low risk for coronary artery disease or adverse cardiac events after vascular surgery, whereas the presence of ischemia predicts a higher risk.

Other studies These include the use of intravenous dipyridamole in conjunction with echocardiography, as well as the use of other stress agents such as dobutamine in conjunction with radionuclide imaging or echocardiography. Dobutamine stress echocardiography now has a well established track record for accurately predicting perioperative risk among vascular disease patients.

Management of peripheral atherosclerosis in the presence of high cardiac risk

Once a patient with peripheral atherosclerosis is identified as a high risk cardiac patient, what to do next is controversial. Conventional wisdom argues that those patients at high cardiac risk should undergo revascularization therapy (with coronary artery bypass graft surgery or coronary angioplasty/stenting). This aggressive approach should be used with caution. Patients with peripheral atherosclerosis are often poor candidates for coronary angiography and coronary bypass surgery because they tend to be older and have frequent comorbid diseases such as stroke, renal failure, or diffuse coronary atherosclerosis. This makes the techniques of revascularization risky or unsuitable. Hence, the overall risk of a strategy of myocardial revascularization may outweigh the risk associated with undergoing vascular surgery alone, and should only be undertaken if it will also substantially reduce long-term risk.[4] The combined morbidity and mortality of cardiac and peripheral arterial revascularization should not exceed the risk associated with vascular surgery alone in a patient with known, clinically relevant coronary artery disease. What has become very clear is that, in high risk patients, therapy with β-blockers reduces death from cardiac causes and non-fatal myocardial infarction, both perioperatively and on long-term follow up.[5]

Case studies

Case 18.1

A 67-year-old woman presented to a vascular surgery clinic with severe right calf pain at rest radiating to the foot. She was found to have adult onset diabetes mellitus 8 years previously. Over the prior 5 years she developed bilateral calf pain that occurred when she walked more than 50 feet on flat ground. The pains promptly resolved with rest and she was able to continue walking. For a 1 year period she was unsuccessfully treated with pentoxifylline, with no improvement in her exercise capacity or calf pain. She stopped the medication. Over the prior 4 months her calf pains had become more severe, particularly in the right leg, and she began to experience more frequent episodes of pain with less walking capacity. For 1 month she woke in the middle of the night with severe leg cramping that was not relieved unless she dangled her right leg outside of the bed. For the preceding 72 hours her right foot had become bright red and extremely painful to the touch.

She retired from her job as a school teacher at age 65 years. She was an active, 96 pack-year smoker. There was no history of prior myocardial infarction or angina.

Examination. Physical examination: the patient appeared chronically ill. She was afebrile. Pulse: 78 beats/min, regular, normal sinus rhythm. Blood pressure: 150/80 mmHg. Jugular venous pulse: normal. Cardiac impulse: normal. First heart sound: normal. Second heart sound: split normally on inspiration. No murmurs or added sounds. Chest examination: normal air entry, no rales or rhonchi. Abdominal examination: soft abdomen, no tenderness, and no masses. Normal liver span. No peripheral edema. Femoral arteries: loud bruits bilaterally. Left leg: faint popliteal pulse, and absent dorsalis pedis and posterior tibial pulses. Right leg: absent popliteal, dorsalis pedis, and posterior tibial pulses. The right foot was pale with the patient supine and red when the patient sat up and dangled the foot (dependent rubor). The nail beds of both feet were yellowed and sclerotic, and there was hair loss in a stocking distribution on both legs. Carotid pulses: normal, no bruits. Optic fundi: diabetic arterial changes.

Investigations. Laboratory studies: normal complete blood count and normal electrolytes, with the exception of a random serum glucose of 192 mg/dl (10·7 mmol/l). Electrocardiogram: normal sinus rhythm, normal axis, intervals, and no evidence of prior infarction or ST-T changes. A non-invasive arterial study comprising segmental pressure measurements was also obtained (see Figure 18.1): systolic pressure gradients throughout the right and left legs consistent with severe arterial occlusive disease that most affected the right leg in the distribution of the superficial femoral artery.

Progress

The consulting vascular surgeon recommended she undergo femoral angiography. Femoral angiography was carried out uneventfully via a left femoral arterial puncture approach and the right superficial femoral artery was found to be occluded. A cardiologist evaluated her. The interview with the cardiologist confirmed no history to suggest coronary artery disease or myocardial infarction, and physical examination failed to document any evidence of congestive heart failure. Accordingly, the cardiologist felt that her risks from general anesthesia, and femoral bypass surgery if this were required, were acceptable. The patient agreed to participate in a research study evaluating ST-segment changes on a Holter monitor 24 hours before surgery and up to 48 hours after surgery.

The patient underwent femoral/popliteal bypass surgery with an intraoperative angiogram documenting good run-off (see Figure 18.2). In the 8 hours following surgery the patient's vital signs were stable. She intermittently complained of pain in her leg throughout the night and received a total of four injections of narcotics. On the morning of her first postoperative day, the patient casually reported that she had a vague, heavy sensation in the center of her chest, which had occurred 2 hours previously and was gradually building in intensity.

She was sweating. Vital signs showed a blood pressure of 160/80 mmHg, heart rate of 100 beats/min, and a respiratory rate of 20/min. Her physical examination was not substantially changed from her preoperative state except her right foot was now pink in color, warm, and with a palpable dorsalis pedis pulse. An electrocardiogram was obtained and showed new, deep T-wave inversions in leads V_1-V_3. She was transferred to an intensive care unit and serial cardiac enzymes revealed an abnormal rise in creatine kinase to a peak of 475 mg/dl (7·9 µkat/l), and 16% of the rise was creatine kinase-MB fraction.

Intravenous heparin was administered. Her symptoms resolved with intravenous nitroglycerin, but returned abruptly on the second postoperative day. Electrocardiography failed to document new changes but because of unremitting chest symptoms the cardiology consultant recommended that she undergo coronary angiography. Angiography demonstrated severe three vessel coronary artery disease, and she was found to have mild anteroseptal hypokinesis with a left ventricular ejection fraction of 55%. She again complained of a dull ache returning to her chest approximately 2 hours after her coronary angiography. Intravenous metoprolol at a dose of 5 mg every four hours was instituted until her heart rate dropped to below 70 beats/min. Aspirin 325 mg was administered. A cardiac surgeon was consulted, and coronary bypass surgery was recommended as soon as possible.

The patient underwent uneventful three vessel coronary bypass grafting on the third day after her vascular surgery. She spent a total of 10 days in the hospital (7 days after cardiac surgery), slowly ambulating on her sore right leg. She had no further episodes of chest pressure, and was discharged taking aspirin, metoprolol, and glyburide. She saw her vascular surgeon 2 weeks after her discharge and his examination documented palpable pulses in her right foot. The patient remained well.

One year after her discharge from the hospital she received a telephone call from the cardiac research specialist who had enrolled her in the research study. Her Holter had demonstrated three, prolonged, asymptomatic ST-segment depression episodes during 24-hour monitoring before her femoral angiography. There were also extensive episodes of ST-segment depression detected during the 24 hours after surgery, preceding her complaints of chest pressure and documentation of myocardial infarction (Figure 18.3).

Comments

This case illustrates that asymptomatic myocardial ischemia and adverse cardiac events are most common in the 24–48 hour period after surgery (see Figure 18.3), a time period of heightened pain perception, increased adrenergic tone, higher average heart rates, and a hyperthrombotic state. Antiplatelet and β-adrenergic blocker therapies have established records for the control of myocardial ischemia via their effects on adrenergic tone and thrombosis, and could be easily concentrated during the high risk postoperative period. However, the use of antiplatelet and β-blocker therapy in patients with peripheral atherosclerosis, even when it is known that at least two-thirds of them have coronary artery disease, is remarkably low. β-Blocker therapy is often thought to be contraindicated in patients

Mary M. 67y female (femoral)

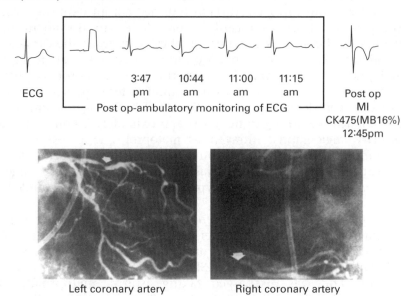

	3:47 pm	10:44 am	11:00 am	11:15 am	
ECG					Post op MI CK475(MB16%) 12:45pm

Post op-ambulatory monitoring of ECG

Left coronary artery   Right coronary artery

Figure 18.3 Relationship between postoperative myocardial ischemia and postoperative myocardial infarction in a patient undergoing femoral bypass surgery. The patient has a normal baseline electrocardiogram (ECG). On several occasions during the first 24 hours after surgery, the patient has episodes of asymptomatic ischemia manifest by ST-segment depression. All these episodes occur at a time when pain perception and average heart rates are at their highest, and precede the clinical event, a myocardial infarction (MI), by minutes to hours. Subsequent angiography demonstrates three vessel coronary artery disease. CK, creatine kinase; Post op, postoperative

with intermittent claudication because β-receptor antagonism in the peripheral circulation causes paradoxic vasoconstriction. Although this is theoretically plausible, a careful look at the medical literature reveals that the vast majority of patients with intermittent claudication can take β-blockers safely and with little change in their exercise capacity.

Thromboembolism

Arterial embolism from the heart is a complication of cardiovascular disease. There are three common clinical settings that make cardiac embolism a serious possibility in a differential diagnosis, namely recent myocardial infarction, atrial arrhythmia (more specifically, atrial fibrillation and/or flutter), and valvular heart

Table 18.1 Incidence of stroke, death, or myocardial infarction among patients on or off warfarin in the setting of prior myocardial infarction or atrial fibrillation

History	On warfarin	Placebo	Risk reduction with warfarin
History of atrial fibrillation ($n = 420$)[6]			
Incidence of stroke	1%	6%	86%
Incidence of death	5%	12%	62%
Prior myocardial infarction ($n = 1214$)[7]			
Incidence of stroke	3%	7%	55%
Incidence of death	15%	20%	24%
Incidence of reinfarction	14%	20%	34%

Presented is a summary of two studies[6,7]

disease. Arterial embolization from a cardiac source may affect any organ system, but common sites of embolization include the lower extremities, and the cerebral and visceral vessels. The potential for embolization should be considered particularly in the setting of a recent anterior myocardial infarction associated with a significant regional wall abnormality and/or left ventricular aneurysm. This can predispose to the formation of mural thrombus and arterial embolization. Similarly, atrial fibrillation causes abnormal asynchronous, atrial wall motion, creating areas of reduced blood flow that are highly susceptible to thrombus formation. This may be exacerbated by enlargement of the left atrial chamber. Finally, valvular disease in general, and mitral valvular disease in particular, predispose the heart to the formation of thrombus via left atrial enlargement and reduction in blood velocities.

In the setting of an anterior wall myocardial infarction or atrial fibrillation, the prevalence of thromboembolic disease is so high and the associated morbidity so troublesome that prophylactic anticoagulation is in order unless a specific contraindication exists. Numerous clinical trials have documented that the risk for stroke, death, or myocardial infarction due to thromboembolic disease is significantly reduced with anticoagulation in the setting of anterior infarction or atrial fibrillation (Table 18.1).[6,7]

Although thromboembolism originating from the left ventricle or atrium can involve any organ system or limb, one of the most common clinical syndromes caused by thromboembolism is cerebrovascular accidents with emboli to either the anterior circulation (carotid arteries) or the posterior circulation (vertebral arteries). The degree of deficit encountered with thromboembolic cerebrovascular disease largely depends on the abruptness of the event, the size of the embolus (and hence the size of the vessel being occluded), and the presence of adequate collateral circulation from other vessels. A large embolism that occludes a major cerebral vessel suddenly will usually cause a large stroke. By contrast, a small embolism affecting a branch vessel in the setting of excellent collateral flow from other cerebral vessels may cause minimal damage and be asymptomatic.

In the same manner, thromboembolism to the extremities can result in substantial ischemia versus no symptoms at all. In the more extreme spectrum, the junction of the distal aorta with the common iliac arteries is a frequent site of thromboembolism (the so-called "saddle embolism" of the aortoiliac junction). In the vast majority of such cases the presentation is dramatic, with severe pain, paresthesia, cyanosis from the waist down, and eventually paralysis of both extremities. More distal emboli are also common, frequently presenting with pain and paresthesia at a level roughly delineating the site of the occlusive embolus.

Intestinal ischemia can result from cardiac thromboembolism, which affects the superior mesenteric artery more commonly than the celiac axis or the inferior mesenteric artery. The onset of symptoms can be abrupt and dramatic but clinical examination of the abdomen may not be dramatic initially. The hallmark of acute intestinal ischemia is a paucity of physical signs in the setting of dramatic symptoms. Intestinal ischemia must be suspected, therefore, by the setting and clinical history. Specifically, risk factors for cardiac thromboembolic disease, such as a history of recent infarction, atrial fibrillation, or valvular disease, is most often present. Often, there is an associated low cardiac output state (as with anterior myocardial infarction) contributing to a slow flow state in the mesenteric vessels.

Laboratory findings are generally non-specific in the presence of thromboembolic disease. There is often a mild elevation in white blood cell count. In limb or visceral embolism, lactic acidosis may ensue from the anaerobic metabolism resulting from significant tissue ischemia or necrosis. This is manifest by a drop in the total carbon dioxide content in blood, a widened anion gap, and a drop in pH. In the case of cerebrovascular ischemia, radiographic findings are generally consistent with multiple infarctions, suggesting a shower of emboli, and this is often optimally demonstrated by computed tomography. In limb ischemia, angiography remains the gold standard for demonstrating the level of occlusion of the thromboembolism. Often the degree of ischemia is so dramatic (as, for example, with saddle embolus to the aortoiliac junction) and the site of the embolism so obvious based on the clinical findings that angiography is not needed before proceeding to definitive therapy. In the case of intestinal ischemia, standard or computed tomography angiography is almost always required and remains the gold standard for diagnosis. Identifying which of the three intestinal vessels is involved is of crucial importance to surgical intervention. In addition, angiography can often identify the presence or absence of collateral supply, which greatly affects the timing of surgery.

Surgical intervention is rarely, if ever, required in the case of cerebrovascular thromboembolism. Anticoagulation remains the mainstay of therapy both acutely and chronically. Surgery is often required in the case of limb ischemia, where anticoagulation is adjunctive or preparatory therapy. In only the most severely ill patients, in whom general anesthesia is felt to be too hazardous, is surgery deferred. Surgery often requires only thrombectomy at the site of thromboembolism and occasionally requires bypass surgery at the site. In the case of intestinal ischemia, surgery is almost always required. Even a minor delay in surgical intervention can result in intestinal necrosis and gangrene, a syndrome that carries with it an 80% mortality rate. Survivors of severe intestinal necrosis often have severe malabsorption syndromes because of major loss of their gastrointestinal absorptive area.

Acute intestinal thromboembolism is clinically distinct from intestinal vessel occlusion due to local atherosclerosis and/or thrombosis. An acute embolism to the mesenteric vessels is abrupt in onset and causes dramatic symptoms, making it relatively easy to diagnose. However, *in situ* occlusion/thrombosis of a mesenteric vessel, often in the setting of local atherosclerotic disease, can be a very subtle and difficult diagnosis. As with acute thromboembolism, presentation is often heralded by symptoms with no significant physical findings. Patients at risk for intestinal vessel occlusion from thrombosis are often the same as those at risk for thromboembolic disease; that is, patients with low cardiac output, recent myocardial infarction, atrial fibrillation, valvular disease, and those receiving digoxin therapy. The pain syndrome is different from acute thromboembolism in that it is quite insidious and vague in nature. There is sometimes a history of postprandial abdominal pain suggesting ischemia on a chronic basis due to fixed atherosclerotic narrowing of the mesenteric vessels. In contrast with embolic disease, in which the acute occlusion of one mesenteric vessel can cause ischemic bowel, a single vessel *in situ* occlusion/thrombosis occurs more slowly and rarely causes significant intestinal ischemia unless there is concomitant disease in the mesenteric vessels. Hence, the typical angiogram of patients with *in situ* occlusion/thrombosis and chronic ischemia is one of diffuse atherosclerotic disease of the celiac, superior mesenteric, and inferior mesenteric vessels together, with one or more vessels occluded.[8]

Case studies

Case 18.2

An 80-year-old man was transferred to a university hospital after having sustained his second myocardial infarction. His history began 5 years prior to this admission when he had his first onset of vague substernal chest pressure and diaphoresis while vacationing at a seaside resort. He was admitted to the local hospital 10 hours after the onset of his symptoms, where he was found to have sustained an inferior myocardial infarction. He received no thrombolysis due to his late presentation. He recovered from his inferior myocardial infarction uneventfully, and was discharged 6 days later on a regimen of isosorbide and aspirin.

He did well for 5 years, going for frequent quarter mile walks on the beach and remaining asymptomatic. One year before his admission he reported to his physician that he was having difficulty sleeping at night and would wake up because he felt somewhat uncomfortable with his breathing. He also reported some mild ankle swelling, particularly when he walked, and this prompted an evaluation, which revealed an enlarged heart on a chest x ray film. In addition to his isosorbide, his physician prescribed digoxin and furosemide. This resulted in resolution of his symptoms and return to his baseline until 4 days before this admission, when again he felt a recurrent episode of substernal chest pressure while vacationing at a seaside resort. After suffering angina for more than 24 hours he was admitted to hospital, where an anterior wall myocardial infarction was documented. He received no thrombolysis, but his pain resolved within 2–3 hours.

Examination. Physical examination: the patient appeared elderly and undistressed. No cyanosis or clubbing was noted, and he was afebrile. Respiratory rate: 20/min. Pulse: 88 beats/min, regular, normal sinus rhythm, normal character. Blood pressure: 148/80 mmHg. Jugular venous pulse: 6 cm above the sternal angle lying at 30°. Cardiac impulse: maximal impulse laterally displaced beyond the mid-clavicular line. First heart sound: normal. Second heart sound: not physiologically split. No murmurs. Third heart sound present. No fourth heart sound heard. Chest examination: decreased breath sounds at both lung bases, no rales or rhonchi. Abdominal examination: soft abdomen, no tenderness, and no masses. Liver span 14 cm, palpable 1 cm below the costal margin. Mild peripheral edema. Femoral, popliteal, posterior tibial, and dorsalis pedis pulses: all normal volume and equal. Carotid pulses: mildly diminished, no bruits. Optic fundi: normal.

Investigations. Blood counts: normal. Electrolytes: within normal limits with the exception of a blood urea nitrogen of 30 mg/dl (10·7 mmol/l) and a creatinine of 1·4 mg/dl (124 μmol/l). Maximum creatine kinase rise was at 1200 mg/dl (20·4 μkat/l). Electrocardiography: normal sinus rhythm, normal axis and intervals, evidence of an old inferior myocardial infarction, and a new anterior myocardial infarction with persistent ST-segment elevation in the anteroseptal leads. Echocardiography: moderately enlarged left ventricular chamber with inferior and anterior akinesis, and an overall ejection fraction of 30%. There was mild left atrial enlargement. There was no aneurysm or significant valvular abnormalities, and normal right sided chambers.

Progress

The patient was admitted to the cardiology step-down unit where he was maintained on digoxin, furosemide, isosorbide, and aspirin. The plan was to mobilize him slowly and begin afterload reduction therapy with angiotensin-converting enzyme inhibitors over the next 24–48 hours. The patient awoke at 2:00 am complaining of severe, sudden onset, diffuse upper abdominal pain. He had had a full supper at 6:00 pm and complained of no significant symptoms throughout the evening. He had a normal bowel movement earlier in the day but none since then. He described the pain as a severe cramp, initially felt in the epigastrium, but now spreading throughout the upper abdomen.

Examination. Physical examination: the patient appeared anxious and was writhing with pain. No cyanosis or clubbing noted. Temperature: 100°F (37·8°C). Pulse: 98 beats/min, irregularly irregular. Blood pressure: 160/90 mmHg. Cardiovascular examination: unchanged. Abdominal examination: mild guarding, no overt tenderness, no rebound tenderness, no masses. Liver span: 14 cm. Rectal examination: brown stool, negative for blood.

Subsequent progress

An attempt was made to treat the abdominal pain with antacids, but after half an hour of receiving 60 cm³ of Mylanta the patient continued to complain of severe upper abdominal pain. Intravenous nitroglycerin was instituted and an electrocardiogram showed new onset atrial fibrillation. Baseline laboratory examination including an arterial blood gas was obtained. A surgical consult was requested. The surgery resident who evaluated the patient documented similar examination findings. Laboratory examinations were notable for a mild elevation in white blood cell count to 10 000/mm³ without a

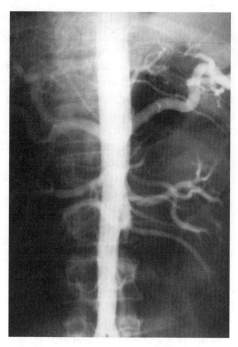

Figure 18.4 Angiography demonstrating occlusion of the superior mesenteric artery by a thrombus, causing acute intestinal ischemia

leftward shift, no change in the hemoglobin or hematocrit, and no change in electrolytes save for a drop in the total carbon dioxide content from a baseline of 26 to 18 mg/dl (from 26 to 18 mmol/l). There was an anion gap of 15 mEq/l (15 mmol/l). The arterial blood gas showed a pH of 7·35, partial carbon dioxide tension of 28 mmHg (3·7 kPa), partial oxygen tension of 91 mmHg (12 kPa), and a bicarbonate concentration of 17 mEq/l (17 mmol/l).

An abdominal radiograph was obtained and showed no free air in the abdomen, with non-specific bowel gas pattern and no evidence of mass. The patient underwent selective mesenteric and abdominal angiography (Figure 18.4). The angiogram documented complete occlusion of the superior mesenteric artery, without collateralization of the proximal intestinal vessels.

The patient was immediately begun on heparin and brought emergently to the operating room. He underwent an exploratory laparotomy where the proximal small bowel was found to be dusky. The superior mesenteric artery was opened. A thrombectomy was performed with immediate return of blood flow to the small bowel. The vessel was repaired. Over the course of the next 10 days the

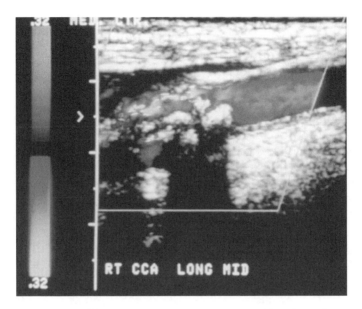

Figure 18.5 Duplex sonogram with color flow Doppler imaging of a moderate internal carotid artery stenosis at the carotid bulb. Note the shading change at the site of the stenosis, corresponding to high velocity flow

patient recovered slowly and uneventfully from his operation and his recent myocardial infarction. His regimen was changed to include enalapril, furosemide, isosorbide, atenolol, and warfarin (after a 4 day course of heparin). Two days after his surgical repair he was able to take oral medications, and his atrial fibrillation resolved 48 hours after the institution of this regimen. He left the hospital and had regular checks of his International Normalized Ratio.

Cerebrovascular disease

Atherosclerotic cerebrovascular disease remains the major cause of cerebrovascular accidents, accounting for significant mortality, and often devastating morbidity. The common carotid artery and its branches are a common site for atherosclerosis. In particular, the proximal internal carotid artery just after its take off at the carotid bulb is a very frequent site of atherosclerotic plaque (Figure 18.5). This is presumably because blood flow at the carotid bifurcation is at its most turbulent, contributing to increased shear force on the endothelial surface.

The proximity of the carotid artery to the skin surface makes it a particularly amenable vessel for study with ultrasound techniques, an invaluable tool in the diagnosis of this disease. Studies have shown that the initial change seen by sonography in carotid vessels with atherosclerosis is intimal thickening. As atherosclerosis progresses, thickening becomes more progressive, and eventually asymmetric, representing a plaque. In the more advanced state the plaque begins to calcify and become eccentric and irregular at its intimal surface, creating an excellent site for thrombus formation, which predisposes these vessels to occlusion. Eccentric plaques also act as sources of microemboli, which shower the distal branches of the internal carotid artery and cause transient ischemic episodes.

Transient ischemic episodes are extremely common among patients with cerebrovascular disease, and herald the development of more significant permanent damage associated with a stroke. In general, the identification of a transient ischemic episode warrants vigorous work up for its source, with particular attention to the internal carotid arteries. Common presentations of transient ischemic attacks related to the carotid circulation include sudden loss of vision in the ipsilateral eye or amaurosis fugax. The classic description of amaurosis is where the patient describes a shade of darkness that comes on suddenly and lasts minutes to hours. Other common symptoms of transient ischemic attacks include dizziness, difficulty with speech or articulating words (this is particularly the case in left hemispheric ischemia caused by left internal carotid artery atherosclerosis), as well as numbness, tingling, and weakness of the ipsilateral face or contralateral extremities.

Diagnosis

The ease with which the carotid arteries are examined by ultrasonography and Doppler interrogation makes these tests the cornerstone in the diagnosis and management of cerebrovascular disease. Distinct methods provide information on the morphology of the plaque (two-dimensional images) and the severity of the resultant stenosis (color flow and pulse wave Doppler interrogation). Pulse wave Doppler examination at the plaque site has been validated by angiography, and correlates strongly with the degree of stenosis. The more critical the stenosis, the higher the Doppler flow velocity detected at the plaque site (Table 18.2). Even increases in thickness of the intima, and media, of the carotid artery, as detected by ultrasound in older adults with no prior history of cardiovascular disease, are associated with an increased risk for stroke and myocardial infarction. Sonography has become so reliable that, in many cases of carotid disease, no further imaging is required before proceeding with surgery. More direct and detailed imaging can still be obtained with cerebral

Table 18.2 Pulse wave Doppler velocities and corresponding degree of carotid stenosis as validated by angiography

Peak systolic velocity (m/s)	Lumen stenosis (%)
<1·3	0–50
1·3–2·5	50–70
2·5–4·0	70–90
>4·0	>90

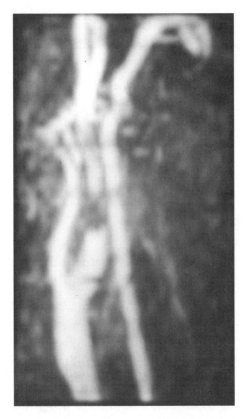

Figure 18.6 Magnetic resonance imaging (MRI) of the right carotid artery, demonstrating a subtotal occlusion at the origin of the internal carotid artery. MRI has the advantage of being non-invasive and not using intravenous contrast material

angiography and magnetic resonance angiography (Figure 18.6). The latter two techniques are often used if there is subtotal occlusion (i.e. 99% stenosis) that cannot be distinguished from total occlusion by sonography, and in which the plaque morphology is too complex to assess by sonography.[9]

Table 18.3 Incidence of stroke among patients randomized to carotid surgery (endarterectomy) or to medical therapy

Symptomatic versus asymptomatic carotid stenosis	Surgery	Medical therapy	Absolute risk reduction with surgery
Asymptomatic carotid stenosis Incidence of ipsilateral stroke and death at 5 years of follow up[10]	4·4%	10·4%	6%
Symptomatic carotid stenosis Incidence of ipsilateral stroke at 3 years[11]	2%	13·6%	11·6%
Incidence of ipsilateral stroke at 2 years[12]	9%	26%	17%

Presented is a summary of data from the Asymptomatic Carotid Atherosclerosis Study (≥70% [n = 374])[10], the European Carotid Surgery Trial (≥70% [n = 778])[11], and the North American Symptomatic Carotid Endarterectomy Trial (≥70% [n = 659])[12]

Treatment

Asymptomatic carotid disease

The management of patients who have asymptomatic carotid stenoses is still a difficult issue. It is clear that the presence of a carotid stenosis, in the absence of symptoms, increases the chances of a stroke among otherwise stable patients. The risk of a stroke, however, is significantly lower among asymptomatic patients than among patients with prior strokes or transient ischemic attacks in the distribution of the carotid stenosis. A large, randomized controlled trial showed that carotid endarterectomy of lesions with 60% or greater carotid artery stenosis in asymptomatic patients lowered the long-term risk for an ipsilateral stroke as compared with conventional therapy, including aspirin and significant atherosclerotic risk factor intervention.[10] This was provided that the procedure is performed with less than 3% operative morbidity and mortality, and modifiable risk factors (i.e. aspirin, low-density lipoprotein lowering) are aggressively managed (Table 18.3).[10]

Many now strongly advocate surgery for asymptomatic patients with significant carotid stenosis. If all asymptomatic patients who have significant carotid disease must be operated on, then should there now be worldwide sonographic screening of all adults at risk for developing atherosclerosis? Reduction in the incidence of strokes with such a strategy may be realized only at a very heavy price. In addition, although carotid endarterectomy may be superior to medical therapy in preventing strokes in asymptomatic patients, that advantage is only present if the surgical risk is very low (as is observed in the hands of the most expert surgeons). Furthermore, the overall risk among asymptomatic patients is already very low while on medical therapy, and the majority of asymptomatic patients will present with transient ischemic episodes before progressing to more disabling events, providing a window for surgical intervention even if medical therapy is chosen first.

The most prudent clinical practice at this point is to screen patients with obvious atherosclerosis, such as those with coronary artery disease and lower extremity disease, as well as persons who are in particularly high risk professions, such as airline pilots. If an asymptomatic stenosis is found, then the decision regarding whether to proceed with surgery is often made on an individual basis. It should be emphasized that medical therapy for carotid atherosclerotic disease is highly effective at lowering the risk for a stroke as well as other morbidities associated with atherosclerosis. In fact, all patients with carotid atherosclerosis, with or without symptoms, should be on antiplatelet therapy (with aspirin and/or new adenosine diphosphate blockers such as clopidogrel), regardless of whether they have surgery. In addition, it is clear that aggressive risk factor intervention also results in a reduction in long-term risk. Such strategies must include aggressive attempts at smoking cessation, meticulous control of diabetes and hypertension, and aggressive lowering of low-density lipoprotein cholesterol. Strategies to achieve the latter have been shown to decrease carotid atherosclerosis as measured by sonography, as well as to decrease the cardiac risk to which all these patients are subject.

Symptomatic carotid disease

Although the strategy to treat asymptomatic carotid disease may still be controversial, there is little controversy left regarding the role of carotid endarterectomy among patients with symptomatic carotid atherosclerosis. After a presentation with amaurosis fugax or other transient ischemic symptoms, medical treatment should be confined to minimizing the risk for acute thrombosis before carotid endarterectomy (including antiplatelet agents and intravenous heparin). Carotid endarterectomy in this patient subgroup is clearly superior to medical therapy in reducing the future risk for a stroke, as long as the surgical risk for a stroke is not prohibitive (see Table 18.3).[11,12] In patients with symptomatic, severe carotid stenosis (70–99% of luminal diameter) carotid endarterectomy is beneficial for up to 8 years after the procedure. In patients with symptomatic, moderate carotid stenosis (50–69% of luminal diameter) the benefits are decreased. (To prevent one ipisilateral stroke during 5 years of follow up, 15 patients would have to be treated with carotid endarterectomy.) Patients with less than 50% luminal diameter stenosis did not benefit from surgery.[11,12]

Association with coronary artery disease

Like patients with peripheral atherosclerosis of other end organs, the single biggest risk jeopardizing the long-term survival of patients with cerebrovascular disease is coronary artery disease. Hence, the greatest disservice that can be done to these patients is correction of their cerebrovascular problem without meticulous attention to the long-term cardiac risk. This is why all patients with manifestations of atherosclerosis should be on aspirin therapy at the very least, because this clearly minimizes the risk for myocardial ischemia. Other risk factor interventions including cholesterol lowering and smoking cessation have clearly been shown to pay a dividend in reducing the risk for atherosclerosis in all circulations. Finally, a low threshold could be observed in evaluating these patients more vigorously for coronary artery disease. A strategy involving frequent electrocardiography, exercise treadmill testing, and/or myocardial imaging for ischemia may yet prove prudent.

Case studies

Case 18.3

A 59-year-old commercial airline pilot presented for an annual screening evaluation mandated by his company. He had been in excellent health all his life and had never been hospitalized for any medical or surgical reason. He had been a pilot for 28 years, achieving senior status and flying transoceanic jets on a regular basis. There was no prior history of hypertension or diabetes. He had a 30 pack-year smoking history, quitting 18 years previously. There was no significant history of familial coronary artery disease or cerebrovascular disease. On his last routine evaluation, he was noted to have a total serum cholesterol of 248 mg/dl (6·4 mmol/l), with fractionation yielding a high-density lipoprotein (HDL) of 25 mg/dl (0·65 mmol/l) and low-density lipoprotein (LDL) of 177 mg/dl (4·6 mmol/l), with a cholesterol/HDL ratio of 9·9 (normal <5·0). In the interim he had been unable to lose weight or modify his diet. He was overweight, but he maintained vigorous activities in addition to his busy work schedule. He was an avid sailor and fond of racing yachts, which required enormous physical stamina.

Examination. Physical examination: the patient appeared overweight but fit, and was afebrile. Pulse: 66 beats/min, regular, normal sinus rhythm, normal character. Blood pressure: 130/70 mmHg. Jugular venous pulse: normal. Cardiac impulse: normal. First heart sound: normal. Second heart sound: split normally on inspiration. No murmurs or added sounds. Chest examination: normal air entry, no rales or rhonchi. Abdominal examination: soft abdomen, no tenderness, and no masses. Normal liver span. No peripheral edema. Femoral, popliteal, posterior tibial, and dorsalis pedis pulses: all normal volume and equal. No radial–femoral delay. Carotid pulses: normal, brisk upstroke, soft systolic bruit on right, near angle of jaw. Optic fundi: normal.

Investigations. Resting 12-lead electrocardiogram: normal. Chest *x* ray: normal. Routine blood tests: normal. Cholesterol profile: total cholesterol 266 mg/dl (6·9 mmol/l), HDL 25 mg/dl (0·6 mmol/l), LDL 189 mg/dl (4·9 mmol/l). He denied symptoms of syncope, near syncope, or transient visual loss.

As mandated by his employer, the patient underwent a full Bruce protocol treadmill exercise test, completing 12 min (13 METs workload) and achieving a heart rate of 170 beats/min, which was greater than his predicted maximum, in the absence of symptoms of angina or significant electrocardiographic changes suggestive of ischemia. The exercise treadmill study was interpreted as negative for myocardial ischemia at an excellent exercise workload.

Carotid non-invasive studies: duplex sonography showed no significant disease in the left common, internal, and external carotid arteries. The right internal carotid showed a calcified and eccentric plaque at its origin from the carotid bulb with abnormal color flow (see Figure 18.5). Pulse wave Doppler just beyond the plaque peaked at a maximum of 1·8 m/s, consistent with a 60–70% stenosis (see Table 18.2). The remainder of the study was within normal limits.

Progress

A discussion was held with the patient regarding the risks and benefits of having elective carotid endarterectomy, in the absence of symptoms, for carotid stenosis. He sought a second opinion and decided not to have surgery, but he started taking aspirin daily and 3-hydroxy3-methylglutary coenzyme A reductase inhibitor (statin), with the goal of reducing his LDL-cholesterol to below 100 mg/dl (<2·6 mmol/l). He retired from his job as an airline pilot.

Two years later, as a passenger on an international flight he experienced sudden onset, right sided, visual loss. He described the sensation as a shade being drawn from the top of the eye to the bottom. Rubbing his eyes and opening and closing them had no effect on this sensation. As he was doing this maneuver, he noticed that his left fingertips were somewhat numb. He experienced no other symptoms. In 15 min the visual loss gradually subsided and his hand once again felt normal. He remembered that he had not taken his aspirin that morning and immediately took it.

After evaluation in a hospital emergency room, where his neurologic and cardiovascular examinations were normal, he was admitted to the hospital and intravenous heparin was begun. Carotid sonography was once again performed. The left sided duplex imaging was again entirely within normal limits. On the right side, the internal carotid artery just distal to the carotid bulb showed a more eccentric plaque with pulse wave Doppler examination documenting velocities in excess of 4 m/s, consistent with a 95% stenosis. Magnetic resonance angiography performed on the second hospital day (see Figure 18.6) confirmed a subtotal occlusion at the origin of the right internal carotid artery. The remainder of the neck vessels and the circle of Willis were normal. On the third hospital day he underwent an uneventful right carotid endarterectomy. By the fourth hospital day he was up and about, and complaining only of mild swelling and itching at the carotid endarterectomy site. He was discharged on the fifth hospital day on coated aspirin once a day and his statin.

Comments

This case illustrates a classic history of the onset and progression of carotid arterial disease. In asymptomatic patients with carotid stenosis diameter narrowing of 60% or greater, the aggressive modification of risk factors (LDL lowering, treatment of diabetes and hypertension); aspirin therapy and carotid surgery (in a center that performs the procedure with less than 3% morbidity and mortality) will reduce the 5 year risk for an ipsilateral stroke. This patient elected to have aggressive medical therapy but decided not to undergo surgery. This was a debatable decision. After he became symptomatic it was clear that carotid surgery was indicated and the procedure was performed uneventfully.

Case 18.4

A 69-year-old man with a long history of essential hypertension has a 3 year history of stable angina pectoris. He leads an unrestricted recreational life in retirement. His medications include enteric coated aspirin, metoprolol, and sublingual nitroglycerin as needed.

During a routine 6 month evaluation by his primary care physician his physical examination was essentially normal, his blood pressure was controlled, and he was noted to have a more prominent pulsation of his aorta on palpation of his abdomen. Abdominal ultrasonography performed 4 days later revealed an aortic aneurysm measuring 6 cm in length and 5 cm in width, just inferior to the origin of the renal arteries, with an associated complex plaque proximal and distal to the border of the aneurysm. Routine blood tests revealed a normal complete blood count, normal electrolytes except for an elevated serum creatinine of 1·7 mg/dl (150 μmol/l), and elevated blood urea nitrogen of 28 mg/dl (10 mmol/l), which were unchanged from baseline. A routine electrocardiogram showed sinus rhythm, and evidence of left ventricular hypertrophy with a strain pattern. A routine chest radiograph showed mild cardiomegaly, but no evidence of heart failure.

A cardiologist evaluated him shortly before his scheduled abdominal angiogram, and it was decided that because of his angina pectoris a cardiac catheterization would also be performed. Coronary angiography (via the right femoral artery) revealed two vessel coronary artery disease with an occluded posterior descending branch of the right coronary artery and a 70% stenosis of a large obtuse marginal branch of the circumflex artery. Left ventricular function was normal, with mild ventricular hypertrophy. Abdominal angiography documented a non-obstructive complex plaque in the abdominal aorta at the area of the mesenteric vessels and a 5·5 cm wide infrarenal aneurysm. There was another ulcerated non-obstructive plaque at the aortoiliac junction. The left renal artery was found to be normal, and the right renal artery had a 60% stenosis at its ostium. The kidneys were found to be normal in size. The patient tolerated both procedures well. He remained in the hospital for approximately 9 hours after this procedure, receiving intravenous hydration at a rate of 150 cm³/hour of normal saline. He was discharged to go home and return in 7 days for elective abdominal aortic aneurysm repair. After a discussion regarding the risk for rupture of an aneurysm of this size, the patient decided to undergo elective aneurysm repair and was counseled that his risk for perioperative cardiac death or non-fatal myocardial infarction was approximately 4–6% (moderate to high).

One week later, on the day before the scheduled procedure, the patient developed severe pain and a purplish discoloration of his left great toe. Over the next few hours he developed severe pain in the left calf as well as the left foot, and noted numbness and tingling in both feet. He also had vague abdominal pain radiating to his back.

Examination. Physical examination: the patient was anxious and in pain. Mental status: normal. Temperature: 100·8°F (38·2°C). Pulse: 96 beats/min, regular, normal sinus rhythm, normal character. Blood pressure: 155/85 mmHg. Jugular venous pulse: normal. Cardiac

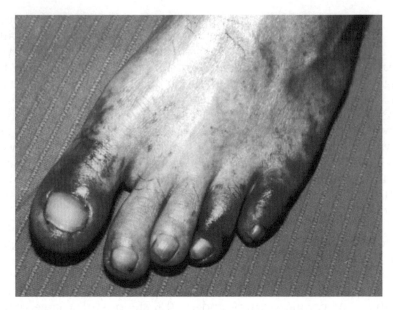

Figure 18.7 Left foot of a patient with atheroemboli demonstrating severe cyanosis and petechiae

impulse: normal. First heart sound: normal. Second heart sound: split normally on inspiration. No murmurs or added sounds. Chest examination: normal air entry, no rales or rhonchi. Abdominal examination: mild guarding and tenderness in the epigastrium. No rebound tenderness. Normal bowel sounds. Palpable, pulsating aorta as previously. Normal liver span. No peripheral edema. Femoral, popliteal, posterior tibial, and dorsalis pedis pulses: all normal volume and equal. There was a blotchy, purple rash over both anterior thighs consistent with livedo reticularis and the thigh muscles were tender to palpation anteriorly. The feet were warm with acrocyanosis of both sets of toes, with more profound cyanosis of the left great toe (Figure 18.7). Neurologic examination of the lower extremities showed hypersensitivity to touch and prick in a stocking distribution of both feet and ankles. Carotid pulses: normal, no bruits. Optic fundi: normal.

Investigations. Laboratory examination was now significant for a white blood cell count of 10 000/mm³ with 8% eosinophils; electrolytes were again within normal limits; but the creatinine was further elevated at 3·0 mg/dl (265 μmol/l) and the blood urea nitrogen was 44 mg/dl (15·7 mmol/l). Electrocardiogram: no changes from baseline. Serum amylase: 1000 mg/dl (16·7 μkat/l; normal 0·8–3·2). Erythrocyte sedimentation rate: 39 mm/hour (normal 0–20). Urine sediment was obtained and failed to show any eosinophils or casts.

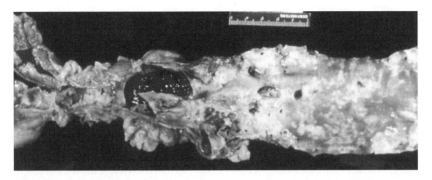

Figure 18.8 Pathologic specimen (not of the patient presented in Case 18.4) demonstrating extensive friable atherosclerotic changes and local thrombosis in a distal aorta and its branches, thus predisposing to atheroemboli

Progress

The patient was admitted to hospital and intravenous heparin and broad spectrum intravenous antibiotics were begun while blood cultures were sent for evaluation. The antibiotics were stopped when blood cultures returned 48 hours later as negative. Over the first 48 hours he had severe left calf and foot pain, which only resolved with narcotic injections. The distal leg pulses remained intact. Renal function deteriorated with serum creatinine rising to 5 mg/dl (442 µmol/l). A skin biopsy of the right thigh showed non-specific thrombosis in the arterioles of the skin vessels. On hospital day 3 hemodialysis access was achieved via a temporary left wrist shunt, and he was taken to the operating room for abdominal aortic repair with aorto-bifemoral bypass of the aneurysm and plaques (Figure 18.8).

An open kidney biopsy revealed multiple cholesterol clefts at the arteriolar level of both kidneys, with focal thrombosis in the same distribution. Postoperatively his serum creatinine climbed to 11 mg/dl (972 µkat/l) and hemodialysis was initiated. He made a slow recovery from his surgical wounds. Baseline blood tests showed a gradual decline of his eosinophilia back to the normal range, as well as a gradual decline in his amylase rise from a peak of 1200 mg/dl (20 µkat/l) back to normal over the course of 1 week. Renal function, however, never recovered and creatinine clearance measured by 24-hour urine collection was less than 1% of normal. He was discharged on hospital day 14 with resolution of his livedo reticularis and acrocyanosis, but on permanent hemodialysis scheduled for three times a week. His discharge medications included his baseline medicines, and no anticoagulation.

Comments

Multiple peripheral atheroemboli are a long recognized and feared complication of vascular procedures. This case illustrates an example of peripheral manifestations of atheroemboli in a very common setting – as an aftermath of cardiac catheterization and/or angiography. Although atheroemboli from complex plaques within the vascular system can occur spontaneously, a large proportion of reported cases follow instrumentation with endovascular catheters and wires such as after angiography or cardiac catheterization, or manipulation of the blood vessels during cardiovascular surgery. One presumed mechanism is that atherosclerotic plaque is dislodged mechanically and showers to any end organ in the body. The distribution of the embolization largely depends on the source of emboli. The example in this case is a manifestation of a common source, namely the abdominal aorta around the renal arteries.

End-organ damage is believed to be caused by the obstruction of small arteries and arterioles by cholesterol crystals with the triggering of local thrombosis. This syndrome is recognized by the clinical setting of the patient who recently underwent some endovascular manipulation or vascular procedure and who presents with multiorgan evidence of acute ischemia. Classically, symptoms can present as early as a few hours after a procedure, but have been reported as late as 1 month after a procedure. A frequent clinical presentation is pain, petechiae, and focal, patchy cyanosis of the distal lower extremities. An important feature of the diagnosis of atheroembolism as a cause of lower extremity ischemia is the presence of intact pedal pulses in the setting of obvious ischemia. Manifestations of ischemia can include the following: local cyanosis of one or more toes, the syndrome or acrocyanosis (a persistent bluish discoloration of the digits of the hands or the feet), and the presence of livedo reticularis (a mottled appearance with red/blue discoloration of the skin, usually of an extremity, with a pattern frequently resembling chicken wire). Another common end organ to be affected by atheroemboli is the kidney. Less common manifestations include ischemia to skeletal muscle, abdominal viscera (for example, pancreatitis), spinal cord, brain, and heart. Renal involvement greatly affects the prognosis of patients with this syndrome, because deterioration in renal function is often irreversible, with many patients sentenced to a lifetime of hemodialysis.[13]

Since the peripheral manifestations of atheroembolism are protean, the diagnosis is often made by history and physical examination alone. Atheroembolism to the kidney carries a particularly poor prognosis, however, and documentation of the syndrome is sometimes important to distinguish it from other causes of renal failure and peripheral lower extremity ischemia (for example, vasculitis, collagen vascular disease, or disseminated intravascular coagulation). Skin biopsies may be helpful among patients who have skin manifestations to suggest atheroembolism. However, dermal involvement generally affects arterioles that are relatively deep within the skin, and a superficial biopsy is often unrevealing, as was the case in this patient. Where there is evidence of myositis (for example, muscle tenderness over the thigh), biopsies can be useful but are often non-specific. Biopsy of the kidney, although risky, is definitive for establishing the presence of atheroemboli among patients with significant renal manifestations. Other manifestations of atheroembolism include pancreatitis, peripheral eosinophilia, and elevation in the erythrocyte sediment rate. Examination of urine sedimentation is not useful for making a diagnosis. In contrast to cardiac embolism, angiography is rarely useful diagnostically in this syndrome, reflecting the distal arteriolar embolization pattern.[14]

There is no definitive treatment for the aftermath of diffuse atheroembolism. Other causes of acute ischemia such as fixed atherosclerotic stenoses caused by plaque to an involved end organ should be addressed because this is frequently a reversible cause of end-organ damage. This patient's renal artery stenosis may have been a suitable target for revascularization after renal failure ensued, although improvement in blood flow with revascularization only infrequently results in improvement in renal function. If the abdominal aorta and/or the aortoiliac junction are the source of atheroemboli, then surgery is mandated to cut off the source emboli from the systemic circulation and prevent further embolization. Otherwise, surgical therapy is limited to amputation or salvage of affected limbs. There is no accepted medical therapy for atheroemboli. Anticoagulation and thrombolysis are controversial and do not appear to alter the course of the syndrome. Treatment with corticosteroids has been disappointing. Medical therapy has therefore been limited to supportive care such as control of hypertension associated with renal failure and initiation of hemodialysis where necessary.

Atheroembolism is not only an important cause of severe, irreversible renal failure, but it also carries a substantial mortality and severe morbidity, including stroke, myocardial infarction, and permanent paralysis due to spinal cord ischemia. Because treatment is basically palliative once the syndrome occurs, every effort should be made to prevent this syndrome from occurring in the first place. Hence, endovascular procedures such as angiography and cardiac catheterization, although extremely low risk in general, should be considered only if absolutely indicated. The cardiac risk of undergoing peripheral vascular surgery, even among patients with known coronary artery disease and symptoms of angina pectoris, is easy to identify and manage by non-invasive means, obviating the need for cardiac catheterization in the majority of cases. Increasingly, non-invasive imaging techniques such as sonography, computed tomography angiography, and magnetic resonance imaging are providing viable alternatives to angiography and should be considered where available. When angiography or cardiac catheterization is needed and abdominal aortic plaque is identified by non-invasive means, then one strategy for avoiding atheroemboli is to approach the heart or the proximal aorta via arm vessels rather than femoral vessels, because upper extremity vessels are less likely to be involved with the kind of severe atherosclerotic plaque that produce the syndrome.[14,15]

Case 18.5

A 26-year-old woman presented with left hand numbness. She had been well all her young life, maintaining a vigorous and active lifestyle with no significant past medical history save for wisdom teeth extractions. Six months before presentation she began to develop easy fatigue and she was unable to complete her day in graduate school without taking a nap. She also reported that on some evenings she would awaken with her clothes drenched with sweat. She developed poor appetite but did not lose any substantial weight, and occasionally reported feeling feverish, although she was unable to document this. She was seen by her family physician. Several blood tests were performed, and she was told that she had chronic fatigue syndrome. Over the prior month, she had experienced increasing fatigue, she was unable to carry out any of her daily activities, and she developed left hand numbness provoked by any activities using the left arm. She denied aching or pain in the arm, and described no other neurologic symptoms. Her right arm was entirely normal. Upon further questioning, she described a vague soreness over the area of her left shoulder and left collarbone.

Examination. Physical examination: the patient appeared anxious but was not in distress. Temperature: 100·2°F (37·9°C). Pulse: 60 beats/min, regular. Blood pressure: 145/70 mmHg in right arm, 90 mmHg by palpation in the left arm. Pulses: markedly diminished in the left radial and ulnar vessels. Loud, left subclavian bruit with some local tenderness to touch. Jugular venous pulse: normal. Cardiac impulse: normal. First heart sound: normal. Second heart sound: split normally on inspiration. No added sounds. Soft, diastolic decrescendo murmur heard at the base of the heart with the patient leaning forward in the expiratory phase of respiration. Chest examination:

normal air entry, no rales or rhonchi. Abdominal examination: soft abdomen, no tenderness, and no masses. Normal liver span. No peripheral edema. Femoral, popliteal, posterior tibial, and dorsalis pedis pulses: all normal volume and equal. The ankle pressures were equivalent to the right arm pressure. Carotid pulses: normal, no bruits. No lymphadenopathy detected in neck, axillae, or groin. Optic fundi: normal. Neurologic examination: normal mental status, cranial nerves, strength, and reflexes, and there was no sensory loss to pin prick or touch, especially in the left hand.

Investigations. White blood cell count: elevated to 11 000/mm³ with a mild leftward shift. Serum hemoglobin: 11·3 g/dl (113 g/l). Hematocrit: 34%. Coagulation tests, serum electrolytes, blood urea nitrogen, and creatinine: all normal. Liver function tests, serum albumin, calcium, and phosphate: all normal. Total protein: was 8 g/dl (80 g/l; normal 55–80), with an immunoglobulin fraction of 5 g/dl (50 g/l; normal 20–35). Erythrocyte sedimentation rate: elevated at 63 mm/hour (normal 0–20 mm/hour). Twelve-lead electrocardiogram and chest *x* ray: normal.

Elective outpatient angiography was recommended and performed within 48 hours. Arch angiography (Figure 18.9) revealed mild (1+) aortic insufficiency with opacification of the left ventricle. There was normal take off of the brachiocephalic trunk and the left common carotid artery. The proximal left subclavian artery and origin of the vertebral artery were normal. The mid-subclavian artery had a long 80% stenosis and mild poststenotic dilatation (Figure 18.10).

Progress

The case management was discussed extensively with the staff vascular surgeon and interventional radiologist. The option of left subclavian vessel angioplasty and stenting was considered and deemed feasible; however, given the patient's relatively mild left arm ischemic symptoms and more substantial constitutional symptoms, it was elected to start a trial of medical therapy with close follow up. She started prednisone 60 mg/day and enteric coated aspirin once a day, and was discharged home. Within 2 weeks her constitutional symptoms had improved substantially and the prednisone was tapered down to 15 mg. There was substantial improvement in her left hand numbness, and subsequent pressure measurements now revealed a right arm pressure of 140 mmHg systolic and a left arm pressure of 120 mmHg systolic. She complained of some bloating, weight gain, facial swelling, and mild dyspepsia, which was attributed to the prednisone and antacids were prescribed.

Four months after her angiogram, while working in her kitchen, she noted sudden onset light-headedness, blurring of the right eye, and

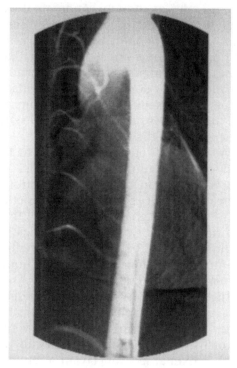

Figure 18.9 Ascending aortic angiogram demonstrating opacification of the left ventricle, which is mildly enlarged. These findings are consistent with the aortic valvular insufficiency that is seen with Takayasu's arteritis

recurrent numbness of the left hand. After approximately 2–3 min she had a syncopal episode, slumping to the ground, but sustaining no traumatic injury. She was found by her roommate and an ambulance was called. When the ambulance arrived the patient was conscious and feeling only mild, residual right eye blurring and left hand numbness.

She was transported to an emergency room where general and neurologic examinations were within normal limits, except for a new right neck bruit and the persistent 20 mmHg discrepancy of the right and left arm systolic blood pressures. Intravenous heparin was started, the prednisone dosage was increased to 60 mg, and on the second day she underwent repeat angiography. Arch angiography demonstrated the same mild aortic insufficiency, but the brachiocephalic trunk was now completely occluded with collaterals reconstituting the right carotid and vertebral arteries. The left carotid artery was still without disease, and there was persistent stenosis of the mid-left subclavian artery.

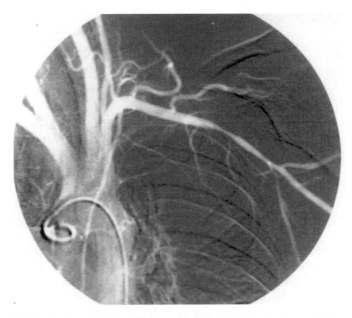

Figure 18.10 Arch angiogram demonstrating a long stenosis of the mid-left subclavian artery with poststenotic dilatation in a young woman with fever and malaise, consistent with Takayasu's arteritis

After a 4 day course of heparin, the patient was taken to the operating room where a Dacron graft was used to bypass her occluded brachiocephalic trunk to the right common carotid artery. The right vertebral artery was anastomosed to the limb of the graft, and a separate graft was used to connect the new brachiocephalic/right carotid graft to the distal left subclavian artery. Thus, with this reconstruction, complete revascularization of the right common carotid, right vertebral, and left subclavian arteries was achieved. Intraoperative angiography revealed patency of the three grafts.

On the first postoperative day, she complained of sudden onset palpitations and was documented to have a supraventricular tachycardia. She was uncomfortable from her palpitations but had a blood pressure of 140/70 mmHg and an overall pulse rate of 150 beat/min without chest pain or electrocardiographic changes to suggest ischemia. She was treated with intravenous adenosine, with prompt resolution of her tachycardia and return of sinus rhythm. After 4 days she was discharged from hospital taking prednisone 60 mg/day, Mylanta 30 cm³ twice daily, and enteric coated aspirin once daily. Pathologic examination of the native brachiocephalic artery specimen showed diffuse mononuclear cell infiltrates of the vessel intima and media with extensive fibrosis consistent with a diagnosis of Takayasu's arteritis.

Comments

Takayasu's arteritis is a rare inflammatory disease but an important cause of arterial ischemia in young patients. Its classic presentation, as illustrated in this case, is an excellent example of vasculitis, which is a cause of ischemia that must always be considered among patients too young to be at risk for atherosclerosis.

Takayasu's arteritis often affects large caliber vessels, particularly the aorta and its branches. Important features include its high predilection for affecting women, who account for more than 95% of cases. The average age of presentation is the mid-20s. As the disease was initially described in Japan, it was formerly thought to affect Asians more commonly. However, careful review of the literature shows that it is only slightly more common among Asians. There have been sporadic associations reported with some human leukocyte antigens, but no definite relationship has ever been established.

Most cases of Takayasu's arteritis involve the aortic arch and its branches. The subclavian, carotid, and vertebral arteries are the most affected vessels. Less commonly, the lower abdominal aorta and its branches (in particular the renal and iliofemoral vessels) are involved. The pulmonary artery is the most rarely involved vessel that has been reported. A classification is sometimes used to distinguish different presentations of Takayasu's arteritis. Pure aortic arch disease is often referred to as type I, pure lower abdominal aortic disease as type II, both arch and lower aortic disease as type III, and pulmonary involvement with or without any other vascular involvement as type IV.

Pathologically, the inflammatory response is a panarteritis, involving all layers of the vessel wall with mononuclear infiltrate and fibrosis. This process eventually results in long stenoses of affected vessels but can also cause aneurysmal dilatation.[16,17]

The initial symptoms of Takayasu's arteritis are often vague, resulting in a long lag between the onset of symptoms and definitive diagnosis. Patients at first complain of constitutional symptoms including weight loss, malaise, unexplained fever, night sweats, and arthralgia. During this phase vascular stenosis is rare, and more specific physical findings due to ischemia are not present. Eventually, pain occurs over the affected vessels, the stenotic phase begins, and ischemia ensues in the affected limb or end organ. In this later phase, presentations include syncope, stroke and transient ischemic attack, arm claudication, hand numbness, hypertension, and congestive heart failure secondary to aortic insufficiency. Angina and myocardial infarction are rare because coronary involvement in the disease is uncommon, but atrial and ventricular tachyarrhythmias are common.

Without medical or surgical intervention, Takayasu's arteritis is an aggressive, fulminant disease that leads to stroke and congestive heart failure (the number one cause of death). However, even without intervention, 20% of cases can remit spontaneously. With aggressive medical and surgical therapy, mortality has dropped significantly in recent times and is now estimated at about 10% on long-term follow up.[16,17]

Laboratory findings are non-specific and reflective of a general inflammatory response, including an elevation in erythrocyte sedimentation rate, elevation in white blood cell count, anemia, and a rise in immunoglobulin levels. In the late phase of Takayasu's arteritis, the physical examination is usually very impressive and crucial to the diagnosis. Bruits are frequently audible over affected subclavian, carotid, and vertebral vessels. Diminution of pulses is often noted in affected arm and neck vessels. Discrepant blood pressure between the two arms or between the arms and legs is also a frequent finding. Cardiac examination can be notable for the stigmata of congestive heart failure and aortic insufficiency. Hypertension is rare and when present always requires evaluation for renal artery stenosis. Although all such findings are relatively common in an elderly population at risk for atherosclerotic disease, they are exceedingly rare among women in their 20s. Hence, a patient presenting with constitutional symptoms, bruits, and discrepant blood pressures in the upper extremities has Takayasu's arteritis until proven otherwise.

Aortic or magnetic resonance angiography remains the mainstay of diagnosis and confirmation of Takayasu's arteritis. Studies classically demonstrate long stenoses of arch or lower aortic branch vessels, as well as occasional aneurysmal dilatations (see Figure 18.10). Pathologic confirmation is rarely required for diagnosis and is often not obtainable except after reconstructive surgery. In addition, in the age of immunosuppressive therapy, in the majority of patients with Takayasu's pathologic specimens obtained at surgery often do not show the characteristic inflammatory changes.

Although medical therapy clearly helps in reducing the symptoms of Takayasu's arteritis, no study has shown that medical therapy by itself improves survival. However, it is generally agreed that immunosuppressive therapy and surgery have acted in concert to prolong life. The most common immunosuppressive regimen is prednisone in high doses with rapid tapers over a 6 month period. Methotrexate and cyclophosphamide have also had reported successes. Surgical therapy generally involves bypass or reconstruction of diseased carotid, subclavian, or vertebral vessels, or less commonly reconstruction of renal or lower extremity branches. Percutaneous transluminal angioplasty and stenting, particularly of the subclavian and lower abdominal vessels, may be effective in restoring flow via a less invasive manner. Because congestive heart failure remains the most common cause of death among patients with Takayasu's arteritis, careful attention to systolic ventricular function and the degree of aortic insufficiency must always be maintained during follow up. Occasionally, patients do require aortic valve replacement for significant aortic regurgitation.[16,17]

References

1   Kannel WB, McGee DL. Update on some epidemiologic features of intermittent claudication: the Framingham Study. *J Am Geriatr Soc* 1985;**33**:13–18.
2   Jonason T, Bergstrom R. Cessation of smoking in patients with intermittent claudication. Effects on the risk of peripheral vascular complications, myocardial infarction and mortality. *Acta Med Scand* 1987;**221**:253–60.
3   Criqui MH, Langer RD, Fronek A, *et al*. Mortality over a period of 10 years in patients with peripheral arterial disease. *N Engl J Med* 1992;**326**:381–6.
4   Wong T, Detsky AS. Preoperative cardiac risk assessment for patients having peripheral vascular surgery. *Ann Intern Med* 1992;**116**:743–53.
5   Mangano DT, Layug EL, Wallace A, Tateo I. Effect of atenolol on mortality and cardiovascular morbidity after noncardiac surgery. Multicenter Study of Perioperative Ischemia Research Group. *N Engl J Med* 1996;**335**:1713–20.
6   The Boston Area Anticoagulation Trial for Atrial Fibrillation Investigators. The effect of low-dose warfarin on the risk of stroke in patients with nonrheumatic atrial fibrillation. *N Engl J Med* 1990;**323**:1505–151.
7   Smith P, Arnesen H, Holme I. The effect of warfarin on mortality and reinfarction after myocardial infarction. *N Engl J Med* 1990;**323**:147–52.
8   Bergan JJ, Yao JST. Acute intestinal ischemia. In: Rutherford RB, ed. *Vascular surgery*. Philadelphia: WB Saunders, 1984:138–48.
9   Polak JF. *Peripheral vascular sonography*. Baltimore: Williams and Wilkins, 1992.
10 Executive Committee for the Asymptomatic Carotid Atherosclerosis Study. Endarterectomy for asymptomatic carotid stenosis. *JAMA* 1995;**273**:1421–8.
11 North American Symptomatic Carotid Endarterectomy Trial Collaborators. Beneficial effects of carotid endarterectomy in symptomatic patients with high-grade carotid stenosis. *N Engl J Med* 1991;**325**:445–53.
12 Barnett HJM, Taylor DW, Eliasiw M, *et al*. Benefit of carotid endarterectomy in patients with symptomatic moderate or severe stenosis. *N Engl J Med* 1998;**339**: 1415–25.
13 Meyrier A, Buchet P, Simon P, Fernet M, Rainfray M, Callard P. Atheromatous renal disease. *Am J Med* 1985;**85**:139–46.
14 Halperin JL, Creager MA. Arterial obstructive disease of the extremities. In: Loscalzo J, Creager MA, Dzau VJ, eds. *Vascular medicine*. Boston: Little Brown and Co, 1992:835–65.
15 Colt HG, Begg RJ, Saporito JJ, Cooper WM, Shapiro AP. Cholesterol emboli after cardiac catheterization. *Medicine* 1988;**67**:389–400.
16 Gatenby PA. Vasculitis: diagnosis and treatment. *Aust NZ J Med* 1999;**29**:662–77.
17 Kerr GS, Hallahan CW, Giordano J, *et al*. Takayasu arteritis. *Ann Intern Med* 1994; **120**:919–29.

Index

Page references in **bold** text refer to figures in the text; those in *italic* refer to tables or boxed material